Neurology in
Pediatrics

Neurology in Pediatrics

by

PATRICK F. BRAY, M.D.
Professor of Pediatrics and Neurology
University of Utah Medical Center

35 EAST WACKER DRIVE • CHICAGO
YEAR BOOK *Medical Publishers, Inc.*

Copyright © 1969 by Year Book Medical Publishers, Inc. All rights reserved. No part of this publication may be reproduced, stored in a retrieval system, or transmitted, in any form or by any means, electronic, mechanical, photocopying, recording, or otherwise, without prior written permission from the publisher. Printed in the United States of America.

Reprinted, December 1970

Library of Congress Catalog Card Number: 75-83556

International Standard Book Number: 0-8151-1220-3

To MARILYN, PAUL, KATHERINE *and* MARGARET

Preface

DURING THE PAST GENERATION, diseases of the developing nervous system have increased in their relative importance primarily because of striking advances in other areas of child health. This change probably holds true the world over but it is especially true in the United States, where malnutrition, infectious diseases and fatalities resulting from secondary dehydration and electrolyte disorders have fortunately lost their epidemiologic preeminence.

We have attempted to make the book both practical and comprehensive. In an effort to approach the two goals, the book has been divided into two parts. Part I is organized according to symptoms, signs, syndromes and laboratory abnormalities—the way in which the patient commonly presents himself to the busy practitioner. Such common syndromes as mental retardation, behavior disorders, seizures, "cerebral palsy," abnormal head size and shape, and visual, hearing and language disorders are covered. Less common but equally important signs and syndromes such as strabismus, meningismus, increased intracranial pressure and brain herniation are also discussed. A chapter entitled Diagnostic Laboratory Tests is designed to clarify for the practitioner indications for ordering and interpreting the results of selected laboratory tests. Special attention is devoted to x-rays (plain films, air encephalograms, brain scans and spine films), electroencephalograms, cerebrospinal fluid study and muscle biopsy. In Part I emphasis is placed upon differential diagnosis, symptomatic treatment and, to a lesser extent, syndrome prognosis. Whenever possible the reader is cross-referred to Part II, which covers classic categories of disease.

In Part II diseases are discussed in a more conventional manner under Pathogenesis, Clinical and Laboratory Diagnosis, and Management and Prognosis. Greater detail has been provided in certain sections because of recent advances. In the chapter on congenital malformations of the nervous system the reader is presented with the important new concepts of chromosome anomalies as well as the difficulties encountered in the proper management of hydrocephalus. In another chapter, a modified working concept of idiopathic epilepsy is offered, based upon long-term clinical and electroencephalographic studies. A comprehensive description of drug intoxications and their management is provided, as well as a special section in the same chapter concerning adverse reactions to therapy. The rapidly growing list of inborn errors of metabolism is described in the chapter on hereditary metabolic and degenerative diseases, and special attention is devoted to those which can be diagnosed readily and those for which a specific treatment is available. A separate chapter is included to cover the neurologic complications of systemic diseases involving the blood and blood vessels, the kidneys and the lungs. Finally a short collection of appendixes includes such subjects as the treatment of prolonged convulsions and status epilepticus; the treatment of cerebral edema; water, electrolyte and transfusion therapy; treatment of shock; antimicrobial therapy; a deep-sedation mixture for diagnostic and therapeutic procedures in young children; normal values for head size and cerebrospinal fluid; and pneumoencephalographic estimation of ventricular size and position.

I am deeply indebted to a large group of people, both at the University of Utah and elsewhere, for the cooperation I received in preparing the text. Dr. Leonard W. Jarcho read the entire manuscript and offered critical and keen editorial advice. Dr. M. Eugene Lahey also provided helpful support and suggestions, and I owe a special debt to Dr. Alan K. Done for his constructive criticism of the chapter on intoxications. Cooperation and tolerance was given consistently from the Departments of Medical Illustration and Radiology. Case material and assistance were given by many, and my special thanks go to Drs. Jack A. Madsen, Theodore S. Roberts, Pasquale A. Cancilla, Anthony N. D'Agostino, Juan M. Taveras, Abner Wolf, Virgil R. Condon, and the Primary Children's Hospital. Finally I would like to say that the text would never have been finished without the patient, dedicated and consistent support of my secretary, Dorothy L. Holmgren.

PATRICK F. BRAY

Table of Contents

PART I

Neurologic Syndromes and Laboratory Abnormalities

1. **Mental, Behavior and Learning Disorders** **3**
    Mental Retardation 3
    Behavior Disorders 13
        Hyperactive Behavior 14
        Psychotic Behavior 18
        Withdrawn (Autistic) Behavior 20
        Psychogenic Disorders 20
        Hysteria 21
    Learning Disabilities 22

2. **Paroxysmal Disorders of the Nervous System** **24**
    Loss of Consciousness 25
        Cerebral Seizures 25
        Breathholding Spells 40
        Syncope 41
        Tetany 41
        Hypoglycemia 43
    Other Paroxysmal Disorders 47
        Headaches 47
        Nightmares (Night Terrors) 49
        Episodic Dizziness 49
        Excessive Sleepiness 50

3. **Chronic Motor Disorders ("Cerebral Palsy")** **52**
    Hypotonia 53
    Spasticity 54
    Ataxia 57
    Myoclonus 57
    Choreoathetosis 57
    Mirror Movements 58

TABLE OF CONTENTS

4. **Abnormal Head Size and Shape** **59**
   - Abnormal Head Size 59
   - Abnormal Head Shape 62

5. **Proptosis** **65**

6. **Language Disorders** **67**
   - Speech Disorders 68
   - Congenital Language Disorders 68
   - Acquired Language Disorders 72

7. **Visual and Hearing Deficits** **74**
   - Visual Deficit 74
   - Hearing Deficit 78

8. **Increased Intracranial Pressure, Papilledema and Brain Herniation Syndromes** . **82**
   - Increased Intracranial Pressure 82
   - Papilledema 84
   - Uncal and Cerebellar Herniation Syndromes 84

9. **Focal Deficit** **87**
   - Optic Atrophy 87
   - Retinal Hemorrhages 88
   - Nonparalytic Squint 88
   - Paralytic Squint and Diplopia 90
   - Spasmus Nutans 90
   - Oculomotor Apraxia 90
   - Bobble-head Doll Syndrome 91
   - Nystagmus 91
   - Ptosis 92
   - Pupillary Inequality (Anisocoria) 92
   - Papilledema 92
   - Facial Weakness or Asymmetry 92
   - Dizziness (Vertigo) 92
   - Hearing Loss 92
   - Dysarthria, Dysphonia and Dysphagia 93
   - Head Tilt 93
   - Acute Weakness 93
   - Acute Hypotonia 94
   - Ataxia 94
   - Other Movement Disorders 95
   - Acute Sensory Complaints 96

10. **Spinal Deformities and Meningismus** **97**
    - Spinal Deformities 97
    - Meningismus, Opisthotonus and Decerebrate Rigidity . . . 98

11. **Neuroendocrinologic (Diencephalic or Hypothalamic) Syndromes** . . **101**
    - Disturbance of Water and Electrolyte Metabolism 101

TABLE OF CONTENTS   XI

    Disturbances in Sexual Development 102
    Disturbances in Somatic Growth and Fat Deposition 103
    Disturbances of Carbohydrate Metabolism 104
    Disturbances in Body-Temperature Regulation, Sleep-Wake Cycle,
        Behavior and Appetite 104

12. Diagnostic Laboratory Tests **106**
    X-ray Studies 108
    Electrical Studies 114
    Clinical Chemistry 119
    Cerebrospinal Fluid Examination 119
    Muscle Biopsy 120

PART II

Conventional Categories of Disease

13. Congenital Malformations of the Nervous System **125**
    Structural Malformations of Obscure Etiology 127
        Incomplete Closure of the Neural Tube (Craniorhachischisis) 127
        Defects in the Development of the Ventricular System 136
        Occult Anomalies of the Brain 141
        Occult Anomalies of the Basal Ganglia, Cerebellum and Brain Stem . . 145
        Occult Anomalies of the Spinal Cord and Peripheral Nerves 147
        Occult Anomalies of the Autonomic Nervous System 150
        Vascular Malformations 151
        Skull and Spine Malformations 156
    Structural Malformations of Known Etiology 165
        Abnormalities in Chromosome Number 167
        Abnormalities in Chromosome Structure 170
        Malformations Due to Maternal Infections 173
        Malformations Due to Other Environmental Factors 175
    Low Birth Weight Infants 176
        Prematurity 176
        Intrauterine Growth Retardation 177

14. Idiopathic Epilepsy **183**
    Petit Mal 184
    Focal 186
    Grand Mal 189

15. Trauma **194**
    Postnatal Injury (Direct) 195
        Head 195
        Spine and Spinal Cord 217
        Peripheral Nerves 220
    Natal (Birth) Injury 221

TABLE OF CONTENTS

      Head 221
      Spinal Cord and Spine 224
      Peripheral Nerves 226
   Other Physical Injuries to the Nervous System 227
      Radiation Injury 227
      Electric Current 228

16. Hypoxia **230**
   Pathogenesis 231
      Prenatal Hypoxia 231
      Neonatal Hypoxia 231
      Postnatal Hypoxia 236
   Clinical and Laboratory Diagnosis 238
      Prenatal and Neonatal Hypoxia 238
      Postnatal Anoxia 239
   Management and Prognosis 239

17. Tumors of the Nervous System **241**
   Intracranial Tumors 242
      General Discussion 242
      Subtentorial or Posterior Fossa Tumors 245
      Supratentorial Tumors 252
      Metastatic Intracranial Tumors 263
   Intraspinal Tumors 266
      General Discussion 266
      Intramedullary Tumors 268
      Extramedullary Intradural Tumors 269
      Extradural Tumors 271
   Tumors of the Skull 276
      Congenital Tumors 276
      Primary Neoplasms (Osteomas and Sarcomas) 277

18. Infections **279**
   Meningoencephalitis 280
   Abscess Formation 296
   Infections with Neurotoxic Organisms 298
   Encephalomyelitis 300
   Disorders of Possible Infectious Etiology 303

19. Disorders of Muscle **314**
   Hereditary Myopathies 316
   Nonhereditary Myopathies 326
   Neurogenic Muscular Atrophies 326
   Myositis of Unknown Etiology 333
   Myositis of Known Etiology 336
   Nonhereditary Disorders of Neuromuscular Transmission 337
   Hereditary Disorders of Neuromuscular Transmission 341

TABLE OF CONTENTS　　XIII

　　　Congenital Defects 345
　　　Tumors of Muscle 348

20. **Intoxications and Adverse Reactions to Therapy** 352
　　　Poison Control Centers 354
　　　General Manifestations and Therapy 354
　　　Specific Manifestations and Therapy 359
　　　Poisonings 360
　　　　　Insecticides, Pesticides and Herbicides 360
　　　　　Fuels, Paints, Solvents and Antifreeze 362
　　　　　Food Poisoning 367
　　　　　Spider Bites and Snake Bites 368
　　　Adverse Reactions to Therapy 370
　　　　　Sedatives 371
　　　　　Stimulants 373
　　　　　Salicylates 374
　　　　　Antimicrobials 374
　　　　　Water and Electrolyte Therapy 376
　　　　　Hormones 377
　　　　　Anticancer Drugs 378
　　　　　Immunizations 378
　　　　　Diets and Supplements 378
　　　　　Miscellaneous 379

21. **Hereditary Metabolic and Degenerative Diseases** 385
　　　Dementia ± Seizures ± Spasticity ± Blindness 388
　　　　　Primary Aminoacidurias 388
　　　　　Carbohydrates 404
　　　　　Polysaccharidoses 407
　　　　　Cerebral Lipidoses 411
　　　　　Hormones 421
　　　　　Vitamins 426
　　　　　Hereditary Neoplastic Degenerative Disorders 427
　　　　　Dementias of Unknown Etiology 432
　　　Ataxia and Other Movement Disorders 433
　　　　　Hereditary Metabolic Defects (Amino Acids and Proteins) 433
　　　　　Hereditary Disease of Mineral Metabolism 436
　　　　　Degenerative Diseases of Unknown Etiology 438
　　　Weakness, Atrophy, Areflexia and Sensory Deficit 442
　　　　　Degenerative Diseases of Unknown Etiology 442
　　　Loss of Vision 443
　　　　　Hereditary Optic Atrophy (Leber) 443
　　　　　Pigmentary Degeneration of the Retina 445
　　　Familial Dysautonomia 445

22. **Demyelinating Disease** 452
　　　Primary Demyelinating Diseases 453

XIV TABLE OF CONTENTS

Encephalomyelitis 453
Multiple Sclerosis (Disseminated Sclerosis) 455

23. Neurologic Complications of Systemic Disease **458**
Diseases of the Blood and Blood Vessels 459
Hyperbilirubinemia with Kernicterus 474
Renal Disease 475
Chronic Respiratory Disease 475
Liver, Gastrointestinal and Other Systemic Diseases 476
Deficiency Diseases 476

APPENDIX 1. Treatment of Prolonged Acute Convulsions and Status Epilepticus 480
APPENDIX 2. Treatment of Cerebral Edema 481
APPENDIX 3. Water, Electrolyte and Transfusion Therapy (Parenteral) . . . 482
APPENDIX 4. Treatment of Shock 484
APPENDIX 5. Antimicrobial Therapy 485
APPENDIX 6. Deep-Sedation Mixture for Diagnostic and Therapeutic Procedures in Young Children 487
APPENDIX 7. Normal Head and Chest Circumferences 488
APPENDIX 8. Methods of Determining Ventricular Enlargement 489
APPENDIX 9. Normal Ventricular Measurements of the Lateral Pneumogram . 490
APPENDIX 10. Upper Limits of Normal Vertebral Interpediculate Distances . . 490
APPENDIX 11. Estimation of Enlargement of the Pituitary Fossa 491
APPENDIX 12. Normal Cerebrospinal Fluid Values 492
APPENDIX 13. Normal Blood Values 492
APPENDIX 14. Normal Urinary Values 493

Index **495**

PART I

Neurologic Syndromes and Laboratory Abnormalities

Mental, Behavior and Learning Disorders

Mental Retardation
    Mental Retardation
    Dementia
Behavior Disorders
    Hyperactive Behavior
    Psychotic Behavior
    Withdrawn (Autistic) Behavior
    Psychogenic Disorders
        Exaggerated habit disorders   Antisocial behavior
        Exaggerated neurotic reactions
    Hysteria
Learning Disabilities

Mental Retardation

NUMEROUS WRITERS have pointed out that two populations of mentally retarded are found in practice: (1) patients with "physiologic" mental retardation, i.e., those without other evidence of general or neurologic defects whose IQ scores range between 50 and 80 ("educable") and (2) patients with "pathologic" mental retardation, i.e., those who are moderately or severely retarded with other systemic or neurologic defects and whose IQ scores range from 50 to 0.

In the mildly retarded individuals ("physiologic" retardation), who fall at the lower end of the bell-shaped distribution curve (Fig. 1.1), the retardation is attributed by some workers to sociocultural deprivation and undereducation, whereas others feel that polygenic, organic factors account for the intellectual deficit in an unknown percentage of cases. It seems likely that both etiologies are important, but the age-old "nature versus nurture" controversy makes their relative importance uncertain. The group of patients with IQs between 50 and 0 ("pathologic" retar-

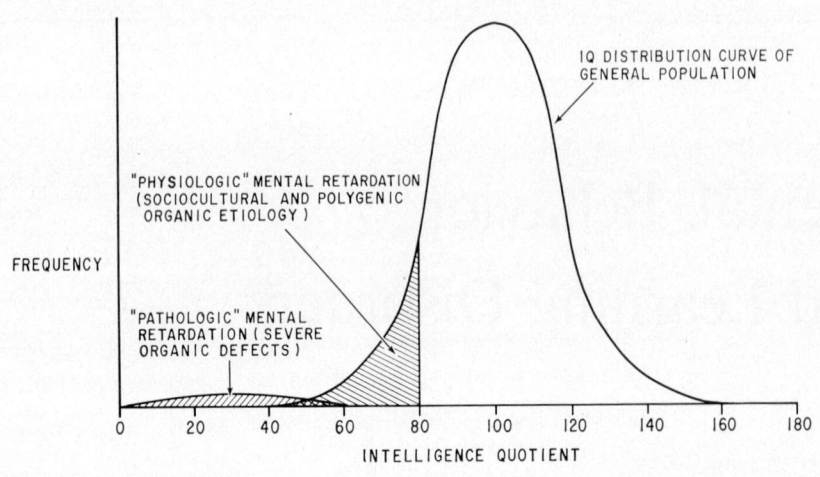

Fig. 1.1.—IQ distribution curve. Shaded areas indicate two populations of mentally retarded. See text for discussion.

dation) constitute a separate population (Fig. 1.1), and they commonly come to the physician's attention because they pose problems in medical diagnosis, therapy and counseling. This latter, smaller group of mentally retarded is subdivided for practical purposes into "trainable" (IQ 30–50) and "custodial" (IQ below 30). The mildly retarded, "physiologic" group (IQ 50–80) outnumbers the "pathologic" group by a ratio of about 10:1 and poses problems primarily for the educators, sociologists, economists and those concerned with social legislation. To a lesser extent psychologists and psychiatrists are involved in their management.

SYNDROME DIAGNOSIS.—The suspicion of retardation in infants often arises because of nonspecific symptoms, such as weak cry, poor suckle, swallowing difficulty, unexplained cyanosis, inactivity, slowness in reaching motor milestones (head support, gaze, sitting, standing, walking—Table 1.1) and delayed growth. In older children, slow or impaired speech development, behavior disorders and poor school performance (learning difficulty) commonly raise a question about defective intellect.

Great care must be used in the evaluation of infants and children with suspected mental retardation because of the shocking psychologic effect of the diagnosis upon some families. Thorough general and neurologic examinations are carried out with special attention to (1) head circumference (Appendix 7), (2) transillumination (e.g., Fig. 13.6, p. 134), (3) chronic motor deficit (Chapter 3), (4) abnormal infant reflex patterns (Table 1.1) and (5) a history of limited intrauterine fetal movement.

The precise quantitative measurement of infant development using formal tests requires expert experience (Gesell and Catell scales). Often, the physician experienced in the evaluation of young children can achieve reasonably accurate estimates by the combined use of Gesell's four areas of development (motor, social, language and adaptive).[6] However, studies have shown that the average pediatrician, despite experience, tends to *overestimate* IQ function in retarded children without other obvious physical defects.[10] Conversely, the pediatrician tends to

TABLE 1.1.—NORMAL AND ABNORMAL DEVELOPMENTAL SIGNS IN INFANCY*

	NORMAL MILESTONES	NORMAL REFLEXES AND MUSCLE TONE	PATHOLOGIC SIGNS AND MILESTONE FAILURES
Birth	Primitive reflex behavior and regular pattern to vital signs (see Gesell[6])	Suck, root, swallow, Moro and grasp present Extensor plantar reflex Flexion position of extremities	Stupor Abnormal Moro High-pitched or weak cry Abnormal temperature and respiratory pattern Opisthotonus Flaccidity or generalized hypertonia Abnormal eye signs Convulsive movements
2 mo.	Head support May smile Single vowel sounds		
3-4 mo.	Increased spontaneous movement Responds with coos and chuckles Inspects hands	Relative hypotonia generalized	No head support Chronic motor deficit usually demonstrable
5-6 mo.	Reaches and grasps Babbles Discriminates family and strangers	Moro and grasp disappear Gradual acquisition of muscle tone which leads to upright position (sitting)	
9 mo.	Creeps and pulls to stand Pincer and poking movements "Ma Ma," "Da Da" May "pat-a-cake" and drink from cup		Child does not sit alone
12 mo.	Stands alone, walks if led Tries to feed self	Flexor plantar (94%)	
15 mo.	Walks alone (9-14 mo.) Jargon 3-4 words Requests by pointing Interest in pictures and animal toys		Child does not walk by 16 mo.
18 mo.	Runs stiffly; hand dominance 6 words May obey commands Feeds self	Flexor plantar	
24 mo.	Runs well, climbs stairs, turns pages 2-3 word sentences Uses "you" and "me"		No words†

*Other primitive reflexes such as the stepping, crossed extensor, "parachutist" reflexes and the lateral curvature of the body in response to stimulation have value in expert hands. However, it is known that these reflexes may be normal in patients with anomalies such as microcephaly and anencephaly. Therefore they must be interpreted with caution.

†Rarely one sees otherwise normal children who do not develop speech until after age 2. Often this represents a pattern of language development on one side of the family.

underestimate IQ function in the child with chronic disabling systemic disease (e.g., rheumatoid arthritis, renal disease, cystic fibrosis). For children beyond infancy the Stanford-Binet test can be carried out to measure intelligence. Later the WPPSI (Wechsler Preschool and Primary Scale of Intelligence), the WISC (Wechsler Intelligence Scale for Children) and the WAIS (Weschler Adult Intelligence Scale) provide well-standardized psychometric yardsticks. Because these tests are time-consuming, expensive and require the services of a trained psychologist, many pediatricians prefer to employ a rapid screening test which they can administer without help. The Ammons' Quick Test provides such a tool and is quite accurate.[2,13] These and other tests which are designed to document (1) intellectual functioning and (2) "soft" signs of organic nervous system damage are outlined in Table 1.2.

The Bender-Gestalt and Memory for Design tests have special value because they document evidence of so-called perceptual-motor disabilities. Often these children with evidence of minimal cerebral dysfunction (e.g., the hyperactive child, p. 14) have no gross neurologic deficit but show inability to reproduce geometric designs, a reflection presumably of either impaired visual perception or mild motor deficit (clumsiness or awkwardness). So-called "projective" tests, such as the Rorschach and the Thematic Apperception Tests which are used to evaluate emotional disturbances, should not be interpreted by the general physician but should be reserved for the use of the psychiatric consultant.

DIFFERENTIAL DIAGNOSIS.—When the physician has concluded that a child is mentally retarded, he is then obligated to attempt an etiologic diagnosis in order to offer the most intelligent therapy, prognosis and counseling. Few definitive

TABLE 1.2.—PSYCHOMETRIC TESTS OF INTELLECTUAL FUNCTIONING

NAME OF TEST	USEFUL MENTAL AGE RANGE	WHAT THE TEST MEASURES
Common tests		
Stanford-Binet	2 yr. to adult	IQ and mental age
WPPSI (Wechsler Preschool and Primary Scale of Intelligence)	4-6½ yr.	Verbal, performance and full scale IQ
WISC (Wechsler Intelligence Scale for Children)	5-15 yr.	Verbal, performance and full scale IQ
WAIS (Wechsler Adult Intelligence Scale)	Over 15 yr.	Verbal, performance and full scale IQ
Visual-Motor Gestalt (Bender)		Perceptual-motor organization (minimal signs of organic brain damage)
Other tests		
Gesell Developmental Schedules	4 wk. to 6 yr.	Motor, social, language and adaptive development
Catell Infant Intelligence Scale	3-30 mo.	Similar to Stanford-Binet
Merrill-Palmer	18 mo. to 6 yr.	Performance test
Ammons Picture Vocabulary Test	2 yr. to adult	Nonverbal test
Draw-a-Man (Goodenough)	3-13 yr.	Nonverbal—requires normal motor status
Memory for Designs	5 yr. to adult	Same as Bender
Vineland Social Maturity Scale	From infancy	Social development

neuropathologic studies have been carried out on series of patients suffering from mental retardation. Those which have been done emphasize that *malformations* and *vascular deformities* cause the syndrome most frequently and that about 50% of the cases have a congenital origin.[5b] The diagnostic workup should be discussed fully with the parents after they have had a chance to recover from the impact of the presumptive diagnosis. Many cases will require a complete investigation, and one should generally try to carry out all of the studies at one time rather than do a piecemeal investigation over a prolonged period. If the parents insist upon limiting the diagnostic study to a search for medically treatable conditions, all of the various diagnostic procedures should at least be mentioned to them, so that in future conversations with well-meaning advisors the parents will not become anxious over the fact that certain studies were not considered. The sequence of diagnostic workup is outlined in Table 1.3.

1. Thorough *history-taking* and *physical examination* provide more important information than any single laboratory procedure. One should assess carefully the

TABLE 1.3.—DIAGNOSTIC WORKUP OF CHRONIC NEUROLOGIC SYNDROMES*

HISTORICAL COMPLAINTS	PHYSICAL FINDINGS	ROUTINE DIAGNOSTIC TESTS	SPECIAL DIAGNOSTIC TESTS
Delayed development	Microcephaly (App. 7) Increased head transillumination Congenital malformations Systemic findings (Table 1.4)	Skull x-rays Metabolic screening (Table 12.4)	Pneumoencephalography Chemical studies (Tables 12.4 and 21.1) Urine: chromatography Blood: calcium, phosphorus, sodium, potassium, chloride, PBI, uric acid, alkaline phosphatase, protein electrophoresis, ammonia, glucose CSF: protein
Seizures in infancy		Electroencephalography Vitamin B_6, 10 mg. I.M.	Cytologic Studies Buccal smear chromatin Chromosome study Biopsy Muscle
Floppy, "limp" baby	Hypotonia		Rectal mucosa (Chapter 21) Bone marrow (Chapter 21)
"Tense," "tight" baby	Spasticity		
Drooling, dysphagia, dysarthria	Pseudobulbar palsy		Viral and serologic studies
Poor coordination	Ataxia		
"Nervous" child	Choreoathetosis or other movement disorder		
Hyperactive child			
Speech problem			
Hearing defect			
Sight impairment			

*Mental retardation, seizures, cerebral palsy, behavior disorders and language, sight and hearing deficits.

history of the pregnancy, birth, neonatal course and behavior during infancy with the understanding that historical data must be interpreted cautiously. Pregnancies which are complicated by maternal infections, drug therapy, x-irradiation, blood group incompatibility, premature delivery and birth anoxia may lead to fetal brain damage. Similarly, a history of a transmissible neurologic disorder in an ancestor may account for retarded development in a child.

2. The presence of one or more *congenital malformations* in other organ systems raises the suspicion of a nervous system anomaly.

3. Occasionally a combination of *clinical abnormalities* will lead to the diagnosis of specific metabolic, degenerative or congenital disorders. Such systemic clinical signs are listed in Table 1.4 for aid in differential diagnosis. Especially important are skin and retinal lesions which may appear in patients with one of the neurocutaneous disorders or phacomatoses.

TABLE 1.4.—SYSTEMIC SIGNS IN PATIENTS WITH CHRONIC NEUROLOGIC DEFICIT

Skin	Eczema	Phenylketonuria
	Pellagra rash	Hartnup disease
	Areas of vitiligo	Tuberous sclerosis
	"Shagreen patches"	Tuberous sclerosis
	Café-au-lait spots	Neurofibromatosis
Hair	Blond	Phenylketonuria
	Fine and sparse	Cretinism, homocystinuria
	White and brittle	Argininosuccinicaciduria and sex-linked degenerative disease
Skeleton	Rickets	Vitamin-D–resistant rickets
		Lowe's syndrome
	Skull and skeletal deformities	Fanconi's syndrome
		Tyrosinosis
		Hypophosphatasia
Abnormal body size	Dwarfism	Turner's syndrome
		Fanconi's syndrome
		Tyrosinosis
		Lowe's syndrome
		Cystinosis
		Vitamin-D–resistant rickets
		Hypophosphatasia
	Tall stature	Homocystinuria
		Klinefelter's syndrome
Eyes	Cataracts	Lowe's syndrome
	Buphthalmos	Homocystinuria[15]
	Glaucoma	
	Ectopia lentis	Homocystinuria
	Chorioretinitis	Toxoplasmosis
		Cytomegalovirus infection
		Tuberous sclerosis
	Retinal exudates	Tuberous sclerosis
	Macula degeneration	Neural lipidoses
Hearing	Nerve deafness	Neonatal jaundice
Abnormal odor	Musty	Phenylketonuria
	Maple syrup	Branched-chain ketonuria
	Dried celery	Methionine malabsorption
	Sweaty feet	Isovaleric acidemia

TABLE 1.4 (CONTINUED) SYSTEMIC SIGNS IN PATIENTS WITH CHRONIC NEUROLOGIC DEFICIT

Organomegaly	Liver and spleen	Tyrosinosis Gaucher's disease; Niemann-Pick disease
Renal disease	Hematuria Albuminuria Aminoaciduria	Hydroxyprolinemia Hyperprolinemia Lowe's syndrome Fanconi's syndrome (cystinosis) Vitamin-D–resistant rickets
Stupor or coma	NH_3 intoxication Acidosis	Hyperammonemia Citrullinemia Argininosuccinicaciduria Congenital lysine intolerance Hyperglycinemia Fanconi's syndrome Lowe's syndrome Vitamin-D–resistant rickets Isovaleric acidemia Branched-chain ketonuria (maple syrup)
Seizures		Phenylketonuria Branched-chain ketonuria Hyperglycinemia Homocystinuria Argininosuccinicaciduria Vitamin-D–resistant rickets
Mental disorders (not retardation)		Hartnup disease Cystathioninuria
Thromboemboli		Homocystinuria

4. *Skull x-rays* yield useful diagnostic information very rarely, but they are performed almost as a matter of ritual largely because of tradition and mistaken concepts about their value. Occasionally bony abnormalities or intracranial calcifications are discovered.

5. *Metabolic screening tests* on urine and blood should be performed to uncover rare chemical disorders (see Table 12.4, p. 118). Even if no therapy is available, the information may have value in predicting recurrence risks to the family.

Table 12.4, page 118, and Table 21.1, p. 389, list some routine screening tests and special tests and indications for performing them.

6. *Electroencephalography* rarely provides useful information in retarded infants but, as in the case of skull x-rays, the anxious, worried layman may insist on a "brain-wave test" which he has been led to believe is very informative. Obviously, in infants with seizures or in older children with marked behavior disorders EEG studies may provide documentary proof of brain disease.

7. *Pneumoencephalography* (PEG) may also provide visible proof of a nervous system anomaly, hypoplasia or atrophy. Its value is primarily informative and it is useful in counseling, but it rarely leads to definitive therapy in retarded children. No positive relationship between IQ and the degree of ventricular dilatation has been demonstrated.[9] The physician should expect to find a considerable num-

ber of normal air studies in mildly retarded children, and the parents should be made aware of this fact in advance lest they conclude that a normal pneumoencephalogram lessens the clinical significance of the retardation. Furthermore, the regular occurrence of headache, nausea and vomiting as a result of a pneumogram must be balanced carefully against the values of the procedure. The author has rarely encountered a serious complication from an air study but stresses the need to use the greatest care in performing every study.

8. *Buccal smear chromatin study* can be performed easily and painlessly in children when the etiology of the retardation is obscure. It is known that an excessive number of chromatin-positive males and chromatin-negative females are mentally retarded.

MANAGEMENT OF SYNDROME.—A definitive disease diagnosis leads to specific therapy in an unfortunately small percentage of cases. Symptomatic medical therapy of mental retardation is limited largely to the occasional use of sedative and tranquilizing therapy for hyperactive, unmanageable older children (see p. 17). Needless to say, no drug has ever been developed which significantly alters intelligence, learning abilities or speech development.

COUNSELING.—The physician who sees retarded children must recognize the importance of his role as both diagnostician and counselor. All too often he has little to offer except an honest, sympathetic analysis to the family. To begin with, he must individualize his approach to each patient. In the course of a thorough workup, an analysis should be made of the family's ethnic background, education, emotional stability, socioeconomic status, parental agreement or disagreement about the significance of the problem, family size and feelings of guilt or blame (a common sentiment which may be well hidden). After the physician reaches a firm decision about the presence or absence of retardation, he should present his true convictions to the family calmly. If he is uncertain about the diagnosis of retardation, he should say so and advise observation and follow-up visits. If he is confident of his judgment in such matters, he should discourage "shopping" for medical opinions. If he is not so confident, he should seek consultation.

The parents should be told that the child has a "problem" or a "handicap." At the outset this kind of terminology may soften the blow incurred by terms such as "mental retardation," "brain damage" or "cerebral palsy," but eventually these terms may have to be brought into the open, if they are appropriate, so that the parents develop no illusions. The parents should be given time to discuss the matter so that they can pose all the questions which will arise. Sometimes a second visit will facilitate discussion and understanding of this emotionally charged diagnosis.

PROGNOSIS.—Because parents often tend to think of this diagnosis in "black and white" terms, they should be educated honestly to think of intelligence in terms of "shades of gray." The physician should also appreciate the fact, for example, that in a family of upper socioeconomic level in which both parents are college graduates, a child with an IQ of 90 is *relatively* retarded, especially if the siblings are bright, and the situation should therefore be managed accordingly. The need for follow-up observations and eventually for psychometric study at age 4 or 5 should be stressed. Usually after a short period of meditation parents raise

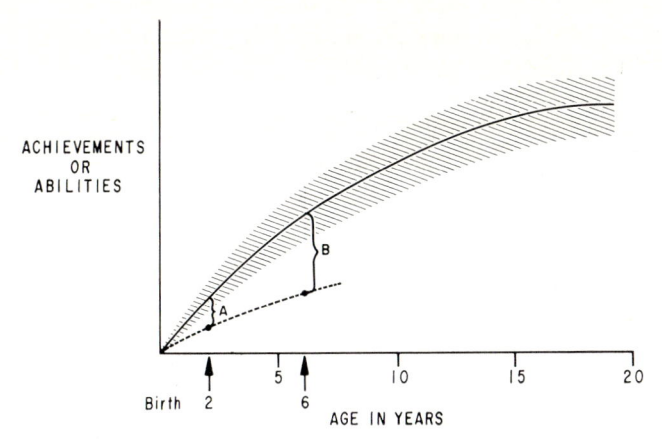

Fig. 1.2.—Diagram of a retarded child's developmental progress. Although new achievements can reasonably be expected with aging (interrupted curve from 2 to 6 years), the deviation from the normal child of the same age becomes more apparent (compare distances A at 2 years and B at 6 years). This diagram is useful in counseling.

questions about schooling, earning a livelihood and marriage. Despite the fact that these questions are of paramount importance, one should not try to guess at the answers. The need to "wait and watch" should be stressed, and the physician should not be pressured into predicting answers to such questions as whether the child will walk, talk, attend school, live an independent life, marry and have children of his own.

In our observations several types of mistakes are made, usually by going to extremes: (1) The physician jumps to conclusions about the presence or absence of retardation without firm evidence. (2) He is overly optimistic with parents and may reassure the parents not to worry, that "he'll grow out of it" or "he'll catch up." This leads to parental bitterness at a later date. (3) The physician is overly pessimistic and makes dire predictions that the child "will never walk" or "will never talk." This approach causes immediate bitterness in parents who are emotionally unable to accept this pronouncement, however accurate, and who later may return triumphantly to display what they consider errors in prediction.

It is helpful to draw the curves shown in Figure 1.2 to illustrate (1) the need for longitudinal observations, (2) the optimistic view that progress can be expected (and this is warranted in most cases) and (3) the realistic view that, despite progress, the discrepancy in achievements with the passage of time increases between the patient and other children of the same age. Often the handicap becomes most apparent when school starts or as the child meets academic failure in later school years.

Special Problems

Special education.—When the possibilities of medical therapy have been exhausted, parents of educable and trainable retarded children seek special educational help. A small number of tragic families with severely retarded children (IQ below 25–30) continue to seek special schooling because of their own inability to accept the problem. The physician must recognize and manage these persons sympathetically but he must avoid condoning unrealistic goals.

The facilities available for the mentally handicapped child vary greatly among communities, and advice will therefore depend upon a knowledge of the community resources. At first the most accurate psychometric evaluation possible should be obtained and this should be used by the educational administrators to place the child in the proper setting. Parents should be told that final decisions about school placement rest in the hands of the school authorities, since only they have an adequate overview of the total educational demands and resources in the community. Realistically one must understand that anxious parents who want their handicapped child to make maximal progress may pit the school authorities against the physician, hoping to keep the retarded child in regular classes for his age. This purposeless controversy can be avoided if the physician will take time at the outset to determine *the reason for seeking medical help* (a reason which is often well hidden by the parents).

The goals and techniques of special education and training schools lie beyond the scope of this text.

PLACEMENT OR INSTITUTIONALIZATION.—With the growing population, with an increasingly enlightened attitude toward the mentally retarded and with greater availability of special education in large communities, the population profile of institutions for the retarded has changed. An increasing percentage of the severely retarded populates these colonies, with the result that these institutions function more in a custodial capacity and less as training schools than they did a generation ago. The physician must not only bear this fact in mind when offering advice, but he should visit the institutions personally so that he will appreciate their strengths and weaknesses.

In general, we believe that the recommendation for institutionalization should rarely be made at the time of initial investigation. If institutionalization is recommended promptly and directly, many parents recoil bitterly from the suggestion and little will have been accomplished. Eventually, in the case of severely retarded children, one can expect that this suggestion will have been made to the parents by friends and relatives, and the matter can be approached indirectly by the physician if it seems appropriate. Sometimes it helps to inquire about long-term plans the parents have considered for their dependent child. This usually opens up the subject, and parents will respond by describing their attitudes toward placement "outside the home." The physician should sympathize with their point of view, but he should focus attention on the practical problems of (1) undue attention by the family to the severely retarded child with simultaneous neglect of normal children, (2) the possible permanent need for custodial care 10–20 years later and (3) the inevitable delay for admission to overcrowded state facilities if and when a decision is reached about placing the child outside the home.

RECURRENCE RISKS.—Young parents or those with small families usually inquire about the chances of subsequent children being similarly affected. In the rare instances in which a specific disease diagnosis is made (such as chromosome anomalies, viz., mongolism, hereditary metabolic defects and degenerative diseases), the doctor can counsel the parents with some precision *if* he has become informed about the genetic characteristics of different diseases. If he is not accurately informed, he should ask for appropriate consultation. In most instances the physician must offer advice without a specific diagnosis. We believe generally that the odds are against a recurrence of the same condition in most instances, but from observation the very fact that one child is affected with mental retardation increases the chances of its happening again.

PROMISCUITY.—Socially unacceptable sexual behavior and promiscuity naturally cause much concern in parents of mildly or moderately retarded older children and adolescents. In the younger child such acts may reflect simple curiosity or benign, uninhibited behavior. In retarded adolescent and young adult girls the threat of accidental pregnancy may compound a tragedy for the parents. This problem, which is basically not medical, must be avoided by means of intelligent, common-sense supervision and restrictions. Discussion of the question of sterilization, which has both personal and legal aspects, lies beyond the scope of this text.

ASSAULT.—Rarely, mentally retarded persons are implicated in cases of criminal assault such as rape and murder. One can only urge the responsible physician to look for these sociopathic tendencies in older children and adolescents. If such tendencies are noted or suspected, appropriate preventive steps should be taken with the help of social agencies, juvenile court authorities and the police. Admittedly, these episodes receive disproportionate notoriety when they occur, but the physician should take steps to protect other members of the community whenever he sees signs of assaultive, combative or sexually promiscuous behavior in a retarded youth.

The reader is referred to the excellent reviews by Wright[18,19] for a more detailed discussion of these specific problems in management.

Dementia

Among the many children who are seen because of slow development or faulty intelligence, the small segment of patients with signs of real deterioration must always be differentiated from those with simple mental retardation, those with true schizophrenia (rarely seen under age 5) and those with progressive impairment of vision, hearing or language. The recognition of progressive degenerative diseases depends heavily upon repeated observations. Examination of cerebrospinal fluid (CSF) protein and the electroencephalogram is also helpful. If psychotic behavior (thought disorder, delusions and hallucinations) or focal neurologic deficit develops under observation, a progressive process almost certainly exists.

The differential diagnosis should include (1) all of the hereditary degenerative metabolic diseases, especially the leukodystrophies and tuberous sclerosis, (2) subacute inclusion encephalitis and (3) slow-growing brain tumors. A small percentage of patients with heavy metal intoxication and severe, uncontrolled idiopathic epilepsy will become demented and psychotic.

Behavior Disorders

Medical help is now being sought with increasing frequency for children with disordered behavior largely because of greater public awareness of mental disorders as a disease and not a social stigma. Complaints may vary from mild difficulties with habit training (feeding, sleep and toileting problems) to common conduct disorders (lying, stealing and truancy) or to severe, pathologic problems that disrupt the home, school and neighborhood, unmanageable hyperactivity, psychosis and severe personality deviations. The physician must take a flexible, unprejudiced overview of these complex problems if he hopes to be effective. The rigid compartmentalized point of view which holds either that all behavior disorders in children result from environmental mismanagement or that they are all "organic" or constitutional (i.e., genetically determined) leads to diagnostic and therapeutic errors as well as to parental confusion and distress.

The physician must expect considerable overlap in the diagnostic importance of causative organic and environmental factors. If complaints persist and get worse, a careful medical diagnostic study should be carried out first; if this proves fruitless, neurologic consultation should be obtained, followed by psychiatric investigation when necessary. The presenting complaints discussed below are given in the approximate order of their practical neurologic importance.

Hyperactive Behavior

SYNDROME DIAGNOSIS.—All physicians who see children regularly are familiar with the syndrome of the hyperactive child. These patients (boys are affected much more frequently than girls) are seen because they "are continually on the go," they are impulsive and they are often unmanageable at home, at school and in the neighborhood. They exhibit a short attention span (some will become entranced only by television, especially commercials, but won't sit still for much else). This behavior pattern exhausts the parents, especially the mother, and disrupts the classroom to the point where the child cannot be tolerated for the sake of the rest of the class. These children learn very slowly from mistakes, exhibit sudden unpredictable mood swings and react to discipline by "going to pieces" in a catastrophic fit of fear and terror rather than the normal one of guilt.

These patients have been called "hyperactive," "brain damaged," or children with "minimal brain dysfunction."[12,14] It is true that one finds corollary clinical and laboratory signs of neurologic impairment in many of these children, but the physician should not jump to such conclusions without good confirmatory evidence (Tables 1.1–1.3). In a minority of these patients, follow-up observation and study may reveal that the behavioral abnormality largely disappears with maturation, or that it has an environmental or situational cause. The usual diagnostic workup for children with suspected chronic neurologic problems should be carried out, but one can expect normal results in some patients. Some of these children exhibit so-called "soft" neurologic signs, such as clumsiness, awkwardness, poor coordination or a nonparalytic eye muscle imbalance—no one of which has binding diagnostic significance since it may occur in a "normal" child. Obviously, if the patient exhibits clear evidence of mental retardation, cerebral palsy or a convulsive disorder, no major diagnostic problem exists. However, when the hyperactivity syndrome occurs by itself, one must bring to bear all his diagnostic skills before planning therapy or offering counsel.

Psychometric evaluation of perceptual-motor disability (Bender-Gestalt test,

BEHAVIOR DISORDERS 15

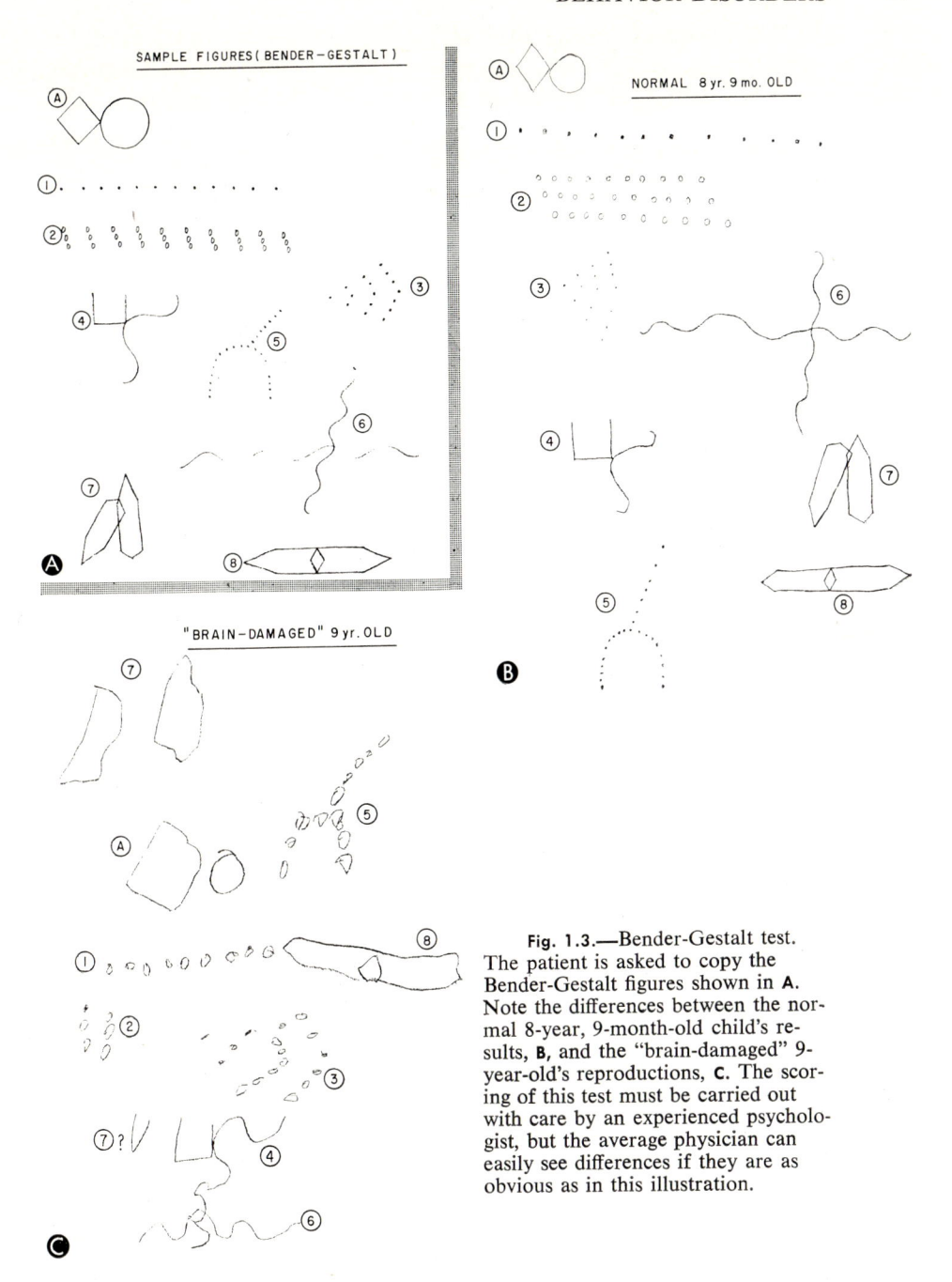

Fig. 1.3.—Bender-Gestalt test. The patient is asked to copy the Bender-Gestalt figures shown in **A**. Note the differences between the normal 8-year, 9-month-old child's results, **B**, and the "brain-damaged" 9-year-old's reproductions, **C**. The scoring of this test must be carried out with care by an experienced psychologist, but the average physician can easily see differences if they are as obvious as in this illustration.

Fig. 1.3) often provides the most valuable evidence of organic disability. This test may provide useful evidence of impaired ability to perceive whole images and reproduce them accurately, i.e., subtle evidence of abnormal brain function in children with normal intelligence. Obviously, many variables such as age, ability to cooperate, intelligence and emotional disturbances can influence the results of

3 years   **4 years**

○   +

Circle   Square Cross

5 years   **7 years**

□ △   ◇

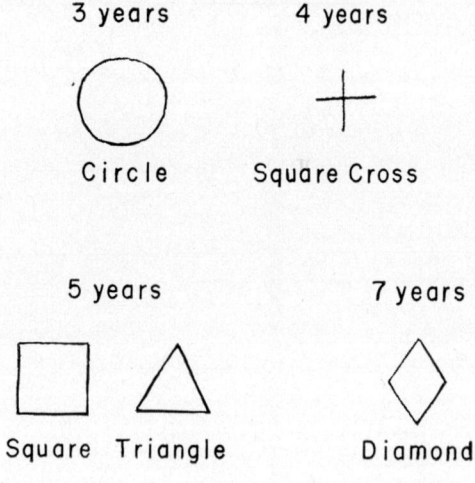

Square Triangle   Diamond

Fig. 1.4.—Gesell copying test for young children.

this test. A crude, simple guide to perceptual-motor function is shown in Figure 1.4. Normally the 3-year-old can copy a circle, the 4-year-old a square cross, the 5-year-old a square or a triangle and the 7-year-old a diamond.

Electroencephalography should be carried out in these patients. In as many as 50% of the patients with severe behavior disorders the electroencephalogram will exhibit definite abnormalities.[1]

The differential diagnosis in the child with "hyperactivity," "brain damage" or "minimal cerebral dysfunction" is identical to that in the child with mental retardation.

MANAGEMENT.—Management and counseling of these children prove difficult. After complete diagnostic study the problem should be discussed carefully and sympathetically with the parents. Often parents disagree about the severity of the problem because the father lives with it only a few hours each day whereas the mother is driven to distraction by the confusion, destruction and chaos that go on all day. She is often frustrated and agitated by her own inability to control the child and feels depressed and guilty because of her natural anger and hate. A sympathetic discussion of these parental reactions helps more than anything else.

If the child attends school, the teachers must be oriented to the problem. Many youngsters with perceptual-motor difficulties will benefit if placed in smaller classes in an environment with the fewest possible distractions. Strauss[16] has discussed this problem extensively and recommends special classrooms and special teachers for these children. Obviously, one should use such facilities when they are available or try to approximate them in the regular classroom when possible. Practically speaking, few facilities of this type are available regardless of the size of the community.

Parents can be given the honestly optimistic prognosis that hyperactivity tends to improve with maturation, almost regardless of the cause, and this attitude has considerable therapeutic value. If, after thorough study and observation, the physician is convinced that the syndrome is being caused or aggravated by environmental mismanagement, psychiatric help may be needed for distraught parents of the hyperactive child even if signs of organic deficit are found. However, we would urge the physician to avoid at all costs the practice of turning a brain-injured child over to a psychologically oriented person or group in which the parents and family are led to feel that the problem resulted from their own mismanagement of an otherwise normal child. This abhorrent practice occurs altogether too frequently and is usually seen when inadequately trained persons manage problems which they understand incompletely.

DRUG THERAPY

Occasionally drugs can be helpful in controlling the overactive and unmanageable child. When one looks critically at the literature on drug therapy for behavior disorders, he is struck with the few studies which have been carried out in a scientific manner, i.e., using a double-blind approach to treatment, using placebos and evaluating results with objective tests.[5] Nonetheless, it seems apparent from a number of empirical observations that drugs are useful in some patients. Drugs should be used only if such measures as education of parents and school teachers and manipulation of the environment fail. A list of drugs commonly used for this group of patients is given in Table 1.5 as a practical guide in management. The list is not intended to be encyclopedic, and most of these agents have no exclusive specificity.

Basically, two classes of drugs are used: stimulants and sedatives or tranquilizers. The *stimulants* were introduced over 30 years ago by Bradley.[3,4] Our experience suggests that the results are unpredictable and that these agents must be given on a trial-and-error basis. Their effectiveness probably depends either upon the euphoriant action they have in these irascible, perverse children or upon their ability to enhance work output by sustaining the attention or heightening motivation of patients who ordinarily have limited powers of concentration.[4a] One

TABLE 1.5.—DRUGS FOR TREATMENT OF BEHAVIOR DISORDERS

GENERIC NAME	TRADE NAME	PREPARATION	AVERAGE DOSE (MG./DAY)
Stimulants			
Methylphenidate	Ritalin	5, 10, 20 mg. tab.	5-30
Amphetamine	Benzedrine	5 mg. tab.	5-20
Dextroamphetamine	Dexedrine	5 mg. tab.	5-20
Dextroamphetamine	Dexamyl	5 mg. tab.	5-20
and amobarbital		10, 15 mg. caps.	10-15
Sedatives and tranquilizers			
Diphenhydramine	Benadryl	25, 30 mg. caps.	25-150
Thioridazine	Mellaril	10, 25, 50, 100 mg. tab.	10-150
Chlordiazepoxide	Librium	5, 10, 25 mg. tab. or caps.	5-30
Hydroxyzine	Vistaril	25, 50, 100 mg. caps.	25-150
Meprobamate	Miltown or Equanil	200, 400 mg. tab.	200-1200
Chlorpromazine	Thorazine	10, 25, 50, 100 mg. tab.	10-150
Phenobarbital	Phenobarbital	16, 32, 65, 100 mg. tab.	16-300

must be prepared for and warn parents about the common side effects of anorexia, weight loss, insomnia and the subjectively unpleasant "keyed-up" tenseness that often develops.

Sedatives and tranquilizers have definite value in managing children with moderate or severe behavior disorders. We think that the physician should become familiar with two or three agents and use them judiciously. He should not be overwhelmed by the huge assortment of drugs recommended by pharmaceutical houses for the treatment of this problem because it seems probable that the mode of action of all of these agents is primarily sedative and that their effect is related to the total dose. We do not ordinarily recommend the long-term use of these psychotropic drugs and most parents don't want to give them continually. Instead, the drugs can be used effectively to control the child in special outings (church, school, parties, etc.).

Psychotic Behavior

Mental confusion, delirium, mania (hyperactivity, irritability, flight of ideas and extreme talkativeness), disorientation, hallucinations and delusions occur quite often and usually result from acute organic disease. Uncommonly a true functional psychosis—schizophrenia in the conventional sense—occurs in childhood, but this disease is rarely seen under 5 years of age. *Infections* such as acute sepsis, dysentery, pneumonia, meningoencephalitis and pyelonephritis cause acute organic psychosis. Patients with severe rheumatic chorea may exhibit psychotic reactions and must be treated accordingly. *Intoxications* commonly cause psychotic behavior; less commonly head *trauma,* diffuse *collagen vascular* disease, *degenerative* diseases and *brain tumors* produce similar reactions. In fact, one should think seriously of brain tumors involving the limbic system in older children and adults with psychiatric symptoms.[11]

Convulsive disorders commonly cause confusion, disorientation and memory loss as part of the seizure or as a postictal neurologic phenomenon. Usually such signs are transient but occasionally they persist for several days and the behavior resembles that seen in a true psychosis. The syndrome has been described in detail by Goldensohn and Gold.[7] In addition, the author would stress the occasional occurrence of a prolonged "fugue" state, in which the patient appears confused and shows both motor slowing and mental dullness without a prior convulsion. This syndrome may be a reflection of a severe and at times continuous epileptiform brain-wave abnormality. One must investigate this puzzling clinical picture completely by searching for evidence of a neurodegenerative disease, a tumor, a subdural hematoma, an occult poison or infectious process or anything which produces increased intracranial pressure. An example of this confusional "fugue" state is shown in Figure 1.5.

All organic psychoses should be managed with specific therapy if an exact diagnosis can be made. Psychotropic drugs, such as chlorpromazine, which are of benefit in psychotic reactions, should be given in full dosage, and anticonvulsants should be used if the syndrome results from an epileptic process. Generally the response to anticonvulsant therapy is inconsistent and unpredictable. The reader is referred to psychiatric texts for information on the management of true childhood schizophrenia.

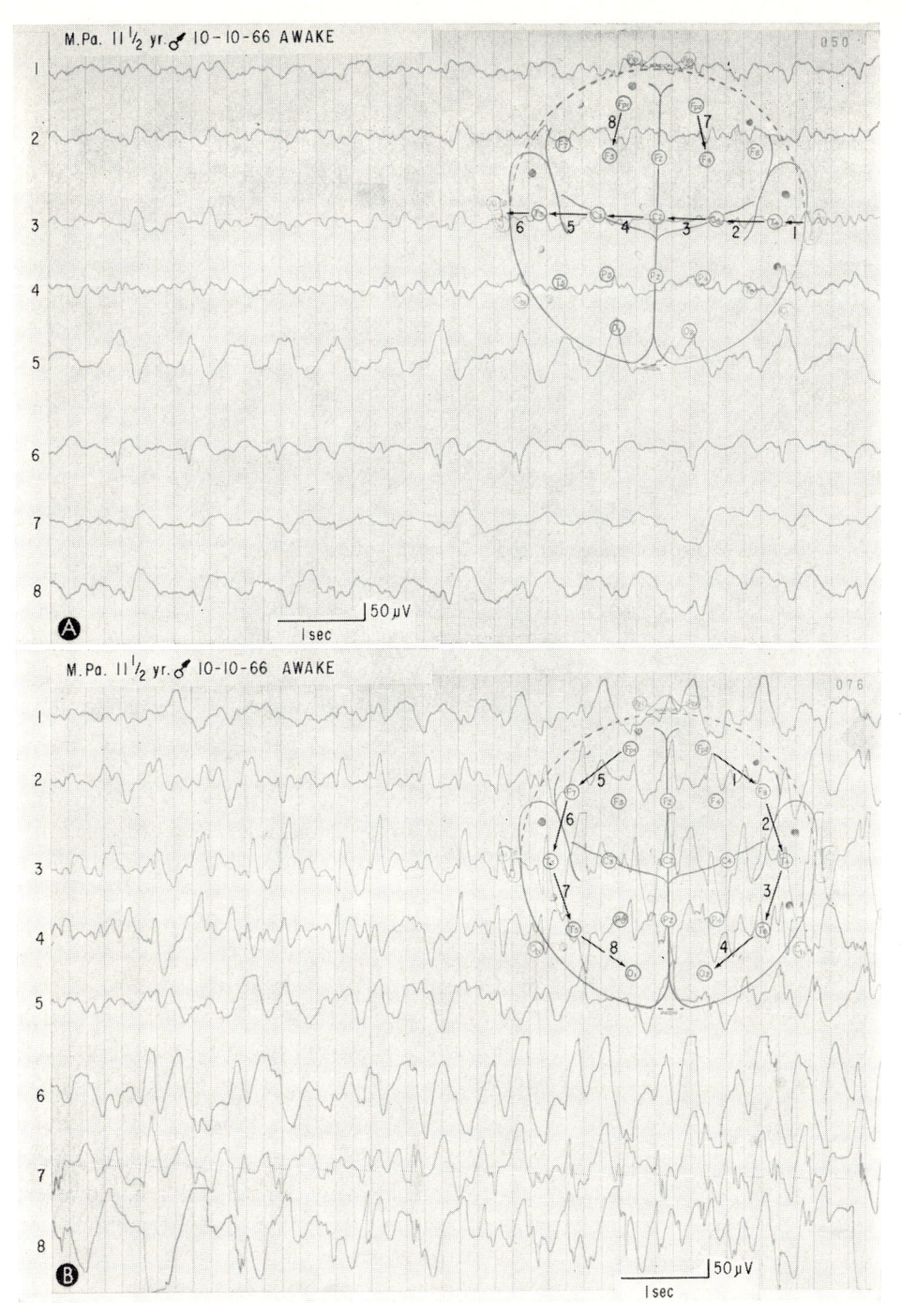

Fig. 1.5.—Acquired aphasia and confusional state (seizure). Boy, aged 11½, was well until early one morning when he had onset of right focal convulsions which became generalized. After a series of 30 seizures in 48 hours he regained consciousness but was very confused and unable to speak intelligibly. Thorough diagnostic study has not revealed the cause. Six weeks later he still had signs of a "fugue" state, with mental dullness and motor slowing, and aphasia—he was unable to name common objects (pencil, watch, tie) even though he was alert, cooperative and given ample time for recall. The aphasia and confusion cleared slowly during the next month. **A** and **B**, serial electroencephalograms show almost continuous epileptiform abnormalities. **A** shows long runs of rhythmic focal delta and sharp wave activity in the left temporal central area (compare bottom four channels with top four). This predominant activity gives way at times to diffuse, epileptiform abnormalities, **B**, which are most prominent over the left hemisphere (bottom four channels).

Withdrawn (Autistic) Behavior

SYNDROME DIAGNOSIS.—In 1943 Kanner[8] described children with distinctive and bizarre behavior characteristics which he called "early infantile autism." Since that time the syndrome has become well recognized. These children (1) have an impersonal, detached attitude in which they ignore other people, (2) develop a consuming interest in objects such as toys, (3) although they develop speech, do not use it to communicate with people and may appear mute, (4) exhibit good rote memory and (5) sometimes insist obsessively upon maintaining order and routine.

DIFFERENTIAL DIAGNOSIS.—Despite attempts by some to attribute all such cases to environmental situations and habits of parental management, we believe many of these children have demonstrable signs of organic disease of the nervous system or severe behavioral malfunction as measured by tests of intelligence, conditioning and learning. Thorough medical, neurologic and psychometric diagnostic study should be performed on all such patients. Of interest is the fact that White[17] found gross epileptiform EEG abnormalities in over 50% of a series of 149 children (58 with autism, 44 with schizophrenia and 47 with severe behavior disorders). Despite our strong plea to consider most of these patients organically damaged, we by no means exclude the fact that emotional trauma contributes to the cause in some patients. Our point of view is influenced by the experience of seeing autistic children with obvious organic deficit after the patient and the family have been in psychotherapy for several years.

Occasionally in children between the ages of 2 and 4 progressive dementia develops, and clinical features closely resemble those of autism or "schizophrenia." The disorder is sometimes called Heller's infantile dementia.[5a] Because this clinical syndrome is seen in known metabolic and degenerative diseases and because cortical neurons in some autopsied cases have shown lipid accumulations as well as other degenerative changes, we do not think that Heller's syndrome is a disease *sui generis*.

MANAGEMENT.—All would agree that special attention should be given to these withdrawn, "spellbound" children in special schools. However, until such efforts are evaluated scientifically we are not yet convinced that such efforts significantly influence the long-term outcome.

Psychogenic Disorders

All of these symptoms and signs are seen in many normal children. However, medical help is often sought when they become extreme because the antisocial or delinquent behavior has (1) caused increasing parental concern, (2) interfered with school performance or (3) caused serious conflict in the neighborhood or in the community as a whole. The symptoms and signs which create these parental and social conflicts are:

Exaggerated habit disorders: (1) feeding problems, (2) sleep problems (including nightmares and night terrors), (3) finger sucking, (4) body manipulations, especially masturbation, (5) rhythmic body movements such as prolonged head-banging or body-rocking and (6) temper tantrums.

Exaggerated neurotic reactions: (1) agitation and anxiety, (2) unwarranted fears or phobias, (3) obsessive-compulsive attitudes toward orderliness and routine.

Antisocial behavior: (1) disobedience, (2) stealing, (3) lying, (4) destructiveness or vandalism, (5) running away from home or school and (6) school conflict.

Because most of these problems have a functional, constitutional or psychogenic basis, no detailed discussion of their management will be presented here except to say that milder degrees of the problem can be handled by the family physician or pediatrician. More severe cases should be treated by a psychiatrist. The projective techniques, such as the Rorschach, may be useful in understanding the dynamics of emotional disturbances but such projective studies should be left to the psychiatrist who undertakes the long-term management. Moreover, we believe that the careful physician can usually obtain this important basic information by himself without such specialized techniques.

We would like to stress that severe habit disorders, neurotic reactions and antisocial behavior may represent the first symptoms in a child with mild mental retardation or, conversely, they may represent the frustrations and "acting out" behavior of the bright or "gifted" child whose talents and problems have not been recognized.

Hysteria

Very commonly, especially in adolescent girls, somatic complaints which have a hysterical basis are seen. Whether one wishes to describe the problem as "functional," "psychosomatic" or "hysterical" depends on the definition of terms. In effect these children are incapacitated by striking and often dramatic psychoneurotic symptoms of which they are not conscious. Hysteria must be distinguished clearly from *malingering,* which represents a conscious complaint designed to achieve some particular goal. Hysterical symptoms usually provide the patient some relief from his anxiety and lead to a bland, almost gay mood *(la belle indifférence)* which is in striking contrast to the severity of the apparent disability.

SYNDROME DIAGNOSIS.—The variety of ways in which hysteria can manifest itself is almost endless. Here we list some of the more common categories and characteristics of the patient's complaints. *Sensory symptoms* such as anesthesia, paresthesias and impairment of vision (usually of sudden onset) are seen frequently. The somatosensory deficit is often cut off exactly in the body's midline or in a glove-and-stocking distribution on an extremity and does not fit with other neurologic findings. Hysterical visual symptoms take the form of sudden onset of blindness or "tunnel" vision. However, the pupils react normally, and with close observation one sees that the patient usually avoids injurious collisions. *Headaches and abdominal pain* are common complaints. Because they are especially difficult to differentiate from organic disease, the patient almost inevitably is studied exhaustively by one or more physicians. In desperation, major diagnostic procedures and even exploratory laparotomy are sometimes carried out. *Motor deficit* such as weakness and paralysis of one or more limbs may be present. Examination discloses inconsistencies in tone, reflexes and posture which generally make it easy to distinguish from true neurologic deficit. Often such patients will complain of only generalized weakness, malaise and somnolence or stupor. Aphonia may occur, but patients with this sign usually disclose the functional basis to their problem by their normal ability to whisper and cough. Various movement disorders such as tics, dystonia, tremors or spasmodic twitching may require detailed study to determine their true nature. Complex *mental disturbances,* especially amnesia, are seen less commonly in children.

MANAGEMENT.—In general, if the hysterical complaint is persistent and incapacitating, the management should be taken over by a psychiatrist. However, the prevalence of this syndrome and the unavailability of psychiatrists in many areas may force the general physician to manage this problem by himself. Generally, he should avoid direct interpretation of the problem to the patient because such action is usually met with antagonism and protest. In some situations a direct approach to eliminate the symptom is warranted, but such efforts are best carried out by trained psychiatrists. Repeated interviews, when possible, may reveal the basis for the conversion reaction, and gradual interpretation of the underlying conflict to the patient will help not only to rid the patient of his symptoms but also to improve his over-all adjustment.

Learning Disabilities

In our experience the term "learning disability" too often is used euphemistically by educators and parents in a way which suggests that the child's problem is subtle, specific and highly specialized. Actually, the term is too vague to have much diagnostic medical value, although some physicians may want to use it to make the problem more palatable to parents and teachers.

In fact, most children who experience learning difficulty have below average intelligence. The level of intellectual functioning must be assessed accurately by a competent psychometrist. There is a small group of children who perform poorly in school because of behavior problems which result either from limited intellect, emotional disturbances or significant visual-motor perceptual difficulty. Factors which contribute significantly to poor school adjustment by mentally normal children (so-called "underachievers") include (1) poor socioeconomic background, (2) a disfiguring congenital defect, such as an ocular squint or a chronic motor disorder, and (3) seizures. In a small percentage of children one finds specific handicapping neurologic defects which impair learning and may be overlooked. These include (1) impaired vision, (2) impaired hearing, (3) specific language disorders, (4) oculomotor apraxia, (5) anomalies of the speech apparatus and (6) seizures. The bright, gifted children (who are easily detected by the alert physician and psychologist) may also do failing or mediocre school work because they are bored by an unchallenging system.

BIBLIOGRAPHY

1. Aird, R. B., and Yamamoto, T.: Behavior disorders of childhood, Electroencephalog. &. Clin. Neurophysiol. 21:148, 1966.
2. Ammons, R. B., and Ammons, C. H.: Quick Test (QT): Provisional Manual, Psychol. Rep. (monograph supp.) 1:111, 1962.

3. Bradley, C.: The behavior of children receiving Benzedrine, Am. J. Psychiat. 94:577, 1937.
4. Bradley, C.: Benzedrine and Dexedrine in the treatment of children's behavior disorders, Pediatrics 5:24, 1950.
4a. Conners, C. K., et al.: Effect of dextroamphetamine on children, Arch. Gen. Psychiat. 17:478, 1967.
5. Eisenberg, L., et al.: A psychopharmacologic experiment in a training school for delinquent boys: Methods, problems, findings, Am. J. Orthopsychiat. 33:431, 1963.
5a. Ford, F. R.: Heller's Infantile Dementia, in Ford, F. R. (ed.): *Diseases of the Nervous System in Infancy, Childhood and Adolescence* (5th ed.; Springfield, Ill.: Charles C Thomas, Publisher, 1966).
5b. Freytag, E., and Lindenberg, R.: Neuropathologic findings in patients of a hospital for the mentally deficient: Survey of 359 cases, Johns Hopkins M. J. 121:379, 1967.
6. Gesell, A.: *The First Five Years of Life* (New York City: Harper & Brothers, 1940).
7. Goldensohn, E. S., and Gold, A. P.: Prolonged behavioral disturbances as ictal phenomena, Neurology 10:1, 1960.
8. Kanner, L.: Early infantile autism, J. Pediat. 25:211, 1944.
9. Knobloch, H., et al.: The relationship between findings in pneumoencephalograms and clinical behavior, Pediatrics 22:13, 1958.
10. Korsch, B., et al.: Pediatricians' appraisals of patients' intelligence, Pediatrics 27:990, 1961.
11. Malamud, N.: Psychiatric disorder with intracranial tumors of limbic system, Arch. Neurol. 17:113, 1967.
12. Pincus, J. H., and Glaser, G. H.: The syndrome of "minimal brain damage" in childhood, New England J. Med. 275:27, 1966.
13. Pless, I. B., et al.: A rapid screening test for intelligence in children, Am. J. Dis. Child. 109:533, 1965.
14. Rapin, I.: Brain Damage in Children, in Brennemann-Kelley: *Practice of Pediatrics* (Hagerstown, Md.: W. F. Prior Company, Inc., 1964), Vol. IV, pt. 1, ch. 17.
15. Spaeth, G. L., and Barber, G. W.: Prevalence of homocystinuria among the mentally retarded: Evaluation of a specific screening test, Pediatrics 40:586, 1967.
16. Strauss, A. A., and Lehtinene, L. E.: *Psychopathology and Education of the Brain-Injured Child* (New York City: Grune & Stratton, Inc., 1947).
17. White, P. T., et al.: EEG abnormalities in early childhood schizophrenia, Am. J. Psychiat. 120:950, 1964.
18. Wright, S. W.: Mental Retardation: The Family and the Retarded Child, in Brennemann-Kelley: *Practice of Pediatrics* (Hagerstown, Md.: W. F. Prior Company, Inc., 1964), Vol. IV, pt. 1, ch. 13-N.
19. Wright, S. W., and Tarjan, G.: Mental retardation, Am. J. Dis. Child. 105:511, 1963.

2

Paroxysmal Disorders of the Nervous System

LOSS OF CONSCIOUSNESS

Cerebral Seizures
    Clinical Description
        Myoclonic seizures
        Head-bobbing episodes
        Salaam attacks
        Akinetic episodes
        "Absence" attacks or lapses
        Adversive attacks
        Focal motor seizures

        Psychomotor seizures
        Focal sensory seizures
        Visual seizures
        Visceral seizures
        Vertiginous seizures
        Major generalized seizures

    Syndrome Diagnosis, Drug Therapy and Prognosis
        Minor motor epilepsy
        Centrencephalic or "petit mal" seizures
        Generalized (grand mal) or focal seizures
        Febrile convulsions

        Status epilepticus
        Postseizure encephalopathy
        Neonatal seizures
        Reflex epilepsy

    Surgery for Seizures
    Prevention and Treatment of Severe Drug Reactions

Breathholding Spells
Syncope
Tetany
Hypoglycemia

        Hysterical Seizures
        Cardiac Seizures
        Coma from Other Causes

OTHER PAROXYSMAL DISORDERS

Headaches
Nightmares or Night Terrors

        Episodic Dizziness
        Excessive Sleepiness

Loss of Consciousness

MOST PAROXYSMAL DISORDERS of the brain cause loss of consciousness (e.g., convulsive seizures and fainting spells), although other periodic neurologic symptoms affect children occasionally. These various disorders will be discussed according to the usual presenting sign or symptom.

Cerebral Seizures

CLINICAL DESCRIPTION

In the past much attention has been devoted to a careful classification of the clinical seizure types, but we believe that, in contrast to the situation in adults, the nature of the clinical seizure in children, by itself, has limited diagnostic value. However, one must establish firmly (by history and electroencephalography) that actual cerebral seizures are occurring. The different clinical seizures are outlined and defined briefly here in order to insure proper understanding of clinical terms. The presumed origins of the different types of seizures are shown in Figure 2.1.[41]

Myoclonic seizures.—Momentary flexion movements of the arms and/or head and/or legs.

Head-bobbing episodes.—Momentary dropping forward of the head.

Salaam attacks.—Sudden flexion of the body at the waist.

Akinetic episodes.—Abrupt, often violent, falls from the erect position to the floor or ground, commonly causing secondary head injuries.

"Absence" attacks or lapses.—Staring, cessation of activity, often with rhythmic blinking, head nodding or mild flexion movements of the arms.

Adversive attacks.—Turning of the head and eyes to one side, often with focal motor activity of the limbs on that same side. In general, these seizures originate from an irritative process in the contralateral frontal cortex. (In contrast, destructive lesions in the same part of the frontal lobe, such as intracerebral hematomas and tumors, cause turning of the head and eyes toward the side of the lesion.)

Focal motor seizures.—Tonic-clonic movements of the limbs contralateral to the origin in the frontal motor cortex. "Jacksonian" seizures imply a gradual spread of the clinical convulsive activity, reflecting the gradual spread of the cortical epileptic process.

Psychomotor seizures.—Chewing, swallowing or mouthing movements associated with simple, stereotyped motor activity which is apparently purposeful but irrelevant, are often combined with peculiar subjective psychic experiences ("dreamy states") such as hallucinations of smell, taste, sight and sound. Also reported is a sense of undue familiarity *(dé jà vu)* or of impending danger as well as "impossible to describe" visceral symptoms (heat, cold, pressure, "rising fullness"). Most but not all psychomotor attacks originate in or involve secondarily the temporal lobe of the brain.

Focal sensory seizures.—Rarely focal numbness and tingling of one arm or leg appear as seizure symptoms, reflecting an irritative process in or near the parietal cortex. These symptoms must be interpreted with great caution in any patient because they often represent transient benign or functional complaints.

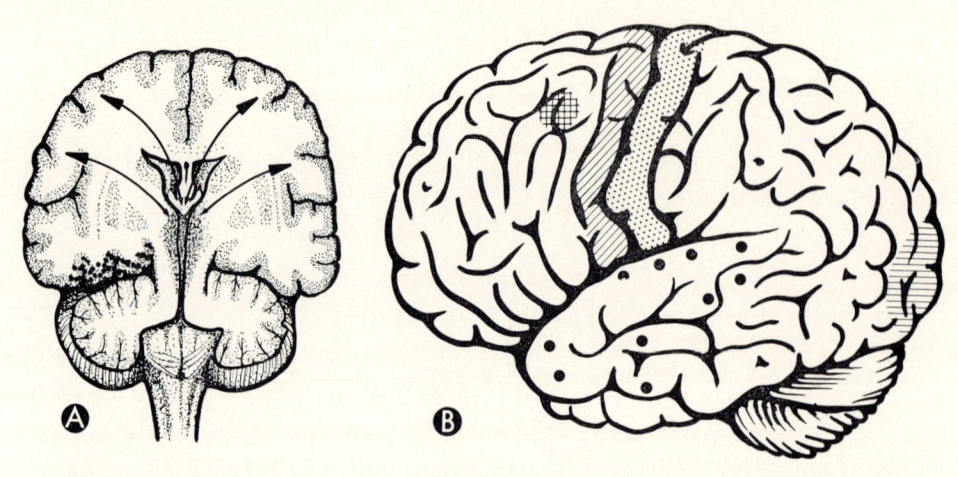

Fig. 2.1.—Diagrams of probable origin and spread of epileptic discharges. In **A**, arrows indicate the neural pathways (between reticular activating system and cortex) which subserve the epileptic process in patients with generalized seizures, both major and minor. Presumably the epileptic discharge traverses these pathways in patients with generalized seizures. In patients with "petit mal" or centrencephalic or *primary subcortical epilepsy* the discharge originates in the midline reticular formation of the brain stem. In patients with focal types of seizures which spread to become generalized, presumably the reticular activity system is excited secondarily by the focal cortical lesion. The latter type of seizure is sometimes referred to as *secondary subcortical epilepsy*. **B** points out the focal cortical origin of (1) adversive seizures (cross-hatch), (2) motor seizures (diagonal lines), (3) sensory seizures (dotted area), (4) visual seizures and (5) psychomotor seizures. The closed circles indicate the approximate widespread areas that have caused illusions, hallucinations and "dreamy states" in the experience of Penfield and Erickson.[41] (Visceral seizures also often arise from deep temporal lobe or upper brain stem structures.) Attention is called to the shaded area of the inferior, mesial temporal lobe in **A**. Sclerosis or scarring in this area of the uncus-hippocampus-amygdaloid is found in many patients with psychomotor attacks.

Visual seizures.—Rarely children experience scintillating scotomata, flashing lights which originate from or involve secondarily an epileptic process in the occipital cortex.

Visceral seizures.—Occasionally periodic bouts of head and abdominal pain, pupillary dilatation, sweating, flushing or pallor of the skin reflect epileptic discharges arising from deep structures such as hippocampus or diencephalic structures (Fig. 2.1,*A*). When these symptoms and signs occur in a consistent pattern and are associated with epileptiform EEG abnormalities, the syndrome has been called "abdominal migraine" or "abdominal epilepsy." The need to differentiate these subjective seizure phenomena from psychogenic or functional disorders is obvious.

Vertiginous seizures.—Occasionally parents report that children will periodically run to them, clutch them tightly and resist any movement of the body. Older children may report true vertigo with this behavior. Epileptiform EEG spike discharges have been recorded over the temporal lobe in some cases. Presumably the seizure involves the cortical center for balance in the temporal lobe. In our experience this type of complaint is usually difficult to explain, even after thorough diagnostic study. In most cases the complaint is not serious or prolonged, but posterior fossa brain tumors must be considered carefully.

Major generalized seizures.—Generalized convulsions can occur as the sole type of attack or they can complicate any of the minor or focal types that have been described. These seizures have no localizing diagnostic significance but they imply a diffuse spread of the epileptogenic process in the brain (Fig. 2.1,*A*). Generalized seizures may be characterized by an aura (warning) such as headache, nausea or "sense of impending doom," a high-pitched or guttural cry and falling to the floor. Generalized tonus followed by clonic movements of the arms and legs then ensues. The patient usually clenches the jaws (sometimes biting the tongue), salivates profusely, becomes cyanotic and may urinate or defecate. After 30 seconds to several minutes the clonic activity ceases, the patient gradually relaxes and enters a state of deep sleep. Common after-symptoms include headache, somnolence, nausea, vomiting and muscle soreness.

If the history is reliable or if an attack is seen, little diagnostic doubt about the true nature of the seizure remains. Careful electroencephalography usually provides graphic confirmatory evidence of a convulsive disorder, but electroencephalograms lack diagnostic specificity. The common occurrence of seizures and their commonly obscure etiology lead many physicians to treat them as disease entities without carrying out an adequate search for the basic cause. This practice delays the diagnosis of treatable disorders (such as subdural hematomas, tumors, meningitis, lead poisoning and some rare metabolic disturbances) and worsens the ultimate prognosis. Diagnostic studies should encompass all diseases for which specific medical or surgical therapy is available.

Syndrome Diagnosis, Drug Therapy and Prognosis

The common clinical seizure syndromes are discussed below according to age and EEG correlates, and these syndromes are discussed in terms of the sequence of diagnostic workup and management. When treatment is instituted with the drug of choice one must realize that the effective therapeutic dose in a given patient is reached only by a process of trial and error inasmuch as the serum level of the drug and dosages based upon body weight or surface area are *not* dependable guidelines.

Drugs are given initially in arbitrary, minimum doses and the amounts are increased until either the seizures are controlled or toxic side effects develop. If intoxication appears before seizure control, the drug dose is dropped below the toxic level and a second drug is added, the physician using the same principles of therapy. If the patient is receiving more than one anticonvulsant, we believe that changes in therapy should be limited to one drug at a time or the physician will be unable to interpret the clinical results and may become confused unnecessarily. In general, replacement of one drug with another should be carried out gradually.

Efforts should be made to avoid oversedation of children in school and to time the administration of sedative agents so that they coincide with the usual hours of sleep. Since the total dose of a drug is apparently more important to seizure control than the precise intervals between individual doses, it is usually possible for the patient to take all of the medication while he is at home, thereby eliminating the need for taking medication in public and lessening the chance of forgetting a dose.

Common mistakes in drug therapy made by physicians include (1) an insufficient trial period, (2) reluctance to raise the drug dose to toxic levels if necessary, (3) the sudden withdrawal of a previously used drug when a new medication is added and (4) the well-intentioned but unnecessary discontinuation of the drug prior to EEG study.

Minor Motor Epilepsy

Minor seizures as described above commonly occur in infants and young children and are usually correlated with diffuse epileptiform EEG abnormalities. The term "hypsarrhythmia" has been popularized by Gibbs to describe the gross and diffuse EEG abnormalities seen in some of these patients. The common correlation of "burst-suppression" EEG discharges as seen with minor motor attacks is shown in Figure 2.2. Unfortunately, these EEG findings have little diagnostic or prognostic specificity. This syndrome can result from congenital malformations, metabolic and degenerative diseases, anoxia, subdural hematoma, perinatal infections of the nervous system and intoxication and deficiency diseases. About 90% of these children are left with mental retardation, spasticity and continuing seizures of varying types; a small percentage of patients die.[29] Contrary to some reports we have found that the *etiology for this syndrome remains obscure in most cases despite extensive workup.*

A consistently good response to anticonvulsant therapy is rarely seen. What can be expected, however, is transient benefit from a variety of drugs with the gradual appearance of permanent neurologic deficit in most patients. In general, the standard anticonvulsants are tried, with unpredictable results. During the past 10 years adrenal corticosteroid therapy has been recommended, and experience has shown that striking transient clinical and electrographic changes can be expected in some cases. However, not only is the benefit usually temporary, but the effect upon the follow-up neurologic status has been dismal.[3,5,39] If one decides to use adrenal corticosteroid therapy, prednisone 1 mg./lb./day in divided doses may be given. Benefit will usually become apparent in seven to 10 days. If no improvement is noticed, the dose is tapered to nothing in three to four days. Treatment may be continued for weeks or months, but one should then expect signs of hyperadrenocorticism (excessive weight gain, moon facies, striae and hirsutism). If treatment is stopped after weeks or months, the daily dose should be tapered very gradually over several weeks. There is no reason to suppose that ACTH (which must be given intramuscularly) offers anything more than prednisone.

More recently the psychotropic and sedative agents, Valium and its analogues have shown some promise as clinically useful anticonvulsants for minor motor attacks. Valium may be given in 2, 5 or 10 mg. doses three times a day.

The value of the *ketogenic diet* is discussed under management of petit mal seizures.

Centrencephalic or Petit Mal Seizures

Centrencephalic or "petit mal" seizures consist of absence, akinetic or myoclonic episodes associated with the diffuse spike-wave dysrhythmia. The pathogenesis of centrencephalic epilepsy, which *nearly always* represents a genetic form

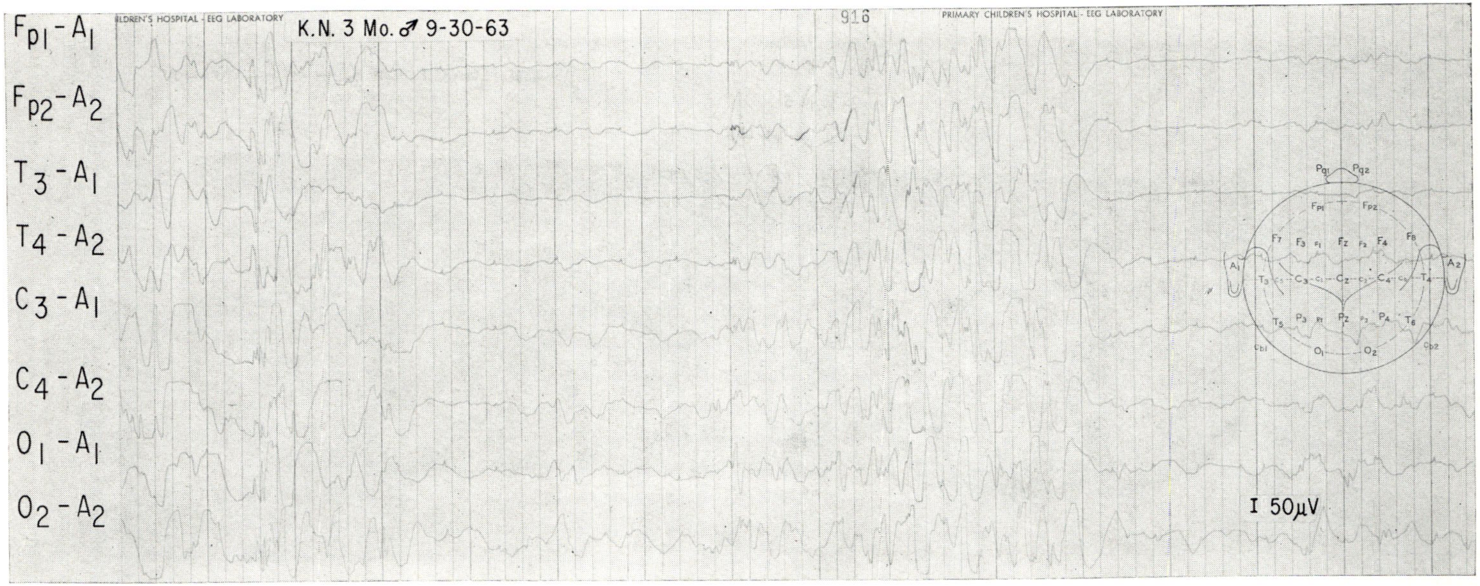

Fig. 2.2.—"Hypsarrhythmia" in 3-month-old infant with minor motor epilepsy. Myoclonic seizures began at age 1 week, were frequent and generalized and were not benefited by standard anticonvulsants. Physical examination revealed a retarded baby with mild spastic quadriparesis. Thorough laboratory workup revealed no abnormality except for EEG evidence of hypsarrhythmia. Seizures remained refractory to therapy, including adrenal corticosteroids, and the infant died at age 6 months.

of epilepsy, is discussed in Chapter 14. These episodes are usually treated with (1) barbiturates (phenobarbital and mephobarbital), (2) the succinimides (ethosuximide, phensuximide, methsuximide), (3) the oxazolidine drugs (trimethadione, paramethadione and dimethadione), or (4) a carbonic anhydrase inhibitor (acetazolamide). (See Table 2.1.)

Drugs are grouped below in the approximate order of clinical importance.

Phenobarbital is the drug of choice for the treatment of any seizure initially. Its low cost and safety make it an ideal agent for preschool children. It is usually given in divided daily doses. Infants and young children are usually started on 32 mg. per day and the dose raised to 50–65 mg. daily if necessary. Drowsiness, which is commonly observed, often disappears after the patient has been receiving the drug for a week or two. Some children will manifest irritable, hyperactive, obstreperous behavior on phenobarbital, requiring its replacement by another drug. Its sedative property can often be avoided completely when it is used in older children and adults by giving a larger single dose at bedtime. In this way an essentially equivalent anticonvulsant effect may be attained, with the sedative effect largely spent during the patient's usual hours of sleep.

Ethosuximide (Zarontin), the most recently developed succinimide, has become the drug of choice for the treatment of petit mal seizures if phenobarbital

TABLE 2.1.—DRUGS USED FOR TREATMENT OF PETIT MAL SEIZURES

Drug Generic Name (Trade Name)	Daily Dosage (Mg.) Infants	Children	Toxicity	Allergic Manifestation	Preparation
1. Ethosuximide (Zarontin)	250-500	500-1,500	Nausea, vomiting, drowsiness	Rash* Asplastic anemia* Leukopenia*	250 mg. caps.
2. Trimethadione (Tridione)	150-300	300-1,800	Photophobia, drowsiness	Nephrosis* Leukopenia† Rash*	300 mg. caps. 150 mg. tab. 150 mg./4 cc. elixir
3. Dimethadione‡ (Eupractone)	150-300	300-1,800	Drowsiness	Nephrosis*	300 mg. tab.
4. Acetazolamide (Diamox)	125-375	375-1,000	Anorexia	Leukopenia* Rash* Fever*	250 mg. tab.
5. Phensuximide (Milontin)	250-500	500-1,500	Drowsiness, nausea, vomiting, vertigo	Aplastic anemia*	500 mg. caps. 250 mg./4 cc. suspension
6. Methsuximide (Celontin)	150-300	300-900	Drowsiness, ataxia, vertigo	Aplastic anemia*	300 mg. caps.
7. Paramethadione (Paradione)	150-300	300-1,200	Drowsiness, photophobia	Aplastic anemia* Nephrosis* Neutropenia†	150, 300 mg. caps. 300 mg./1 cc. solution
8. Phenobarbital (Luminal)	32-50	50-200	Drowsiness, irritability, hyperactivity	Rash*	16 mg./4 cc. elixir 16, 32, 50, 65, 100 mg. tab.

*Indication for immediate discontinuation of the drug.   †See text for details.   ‡Not yet marketed.

alone is insufficient.[16,30] In young children 250–500 mg. per day can be used and in older children the daily dose is 500–1,500 mg. Not only has ethosuximide exhibited good clinical anticonvulsant action, but it has shown few serious side reactions. As often happens with prolonged, widespread usage of such agents, however, fatal cases of aplastic anemia have been reported.[37]

Trimethadione (Tridione) is also widely used for the treatment of petit mal. It is given to young children in a daily dose of 150–300 mg. and to older children in 300–1,800 mg. amounts. It commonly causes photophobia and drowsiness and not uncommonly causes bone marrow suppression and nephrosis. Whereas the photophobia is harmless and reversible, the other toxic or sensitivity reactions are serious. If leukopenia is discovered early, it is usually reversed by discontinuation of the drug. However, fatal bone marrow suppression has been attributed to trimethadione in 16 reported cases.[45] Trimethadione-induced nephrosis, as in the case of lipoid nephrosis of different etiology, generally has a good prognosis if treated properly, but fatalities have been reported.

Dimethadione (Eupractone), the more recently developed sister compound of trimethadione, holds promise as a useful drug, but it has not yet been marketed. It has the same indications for use as trimethadione, and the dosage range is quite similar (Table 2.1). Nephrosis can result from the use of this drug, as can rashes and leukopenia.[15] Since it has been used in only a limited number of patients, blood counts and urinalyses should be carried out at regular intervals.

Acetazolamide (Diamox), a carbonic anhydrase inhibitor, has properties in the experimental animal which suggest that it should have good clinical anticonvulsant properties. It has not become widely employed clinically because of its general ineffectiveness.[28] However, it may have a useful therapeutic role in some patients with petit mal. In view of its infrequent side effects, patients with refractory petit mal seizures should be given a clinical trial of acetazolamide. The daily dosage in infants ranges from 125 to 375 mg. and in older children from 375 to 1,000 mg.

Phensuximide (Milontin) and *methsuximide* (Celontin) have limited value in the treatment of petit mal. Both drugs commonly cause the reversible side effects of drowsiness, nausea and ataxia. Although methsuximide has been incriminated in one fatal case of bone marrow aplasia, phensuximide only rarely causes irreversible side effects.[45]

Paramethadione (Paradione) allegedly has fewer side effects than its sister compound, trimethadione. However, bone marrow suppression and nephrosis have been reported.[45] It is used in doses equivalent to trimethadione. The greater sedative property and greater expense of paramethadione tend to limit its use in the first place.

In general, one treats the patient's clinical seizures and not the electroencephalogram. However, one must remember that all patients who have had only minor seizures may experience grand mal attacks. In fact, the majority of patients with petit mal or centrencephalic epilepsy will have a major seizure at some time (Table 14.1, p. 191). In the experience of Livingston et al.,[30] the later the onset of petit mal the greater is the chance that the patient will have a convulsion. For this reason, in nearly all patients with petit mal we use phenobarbital either alone or in combination with ethosuximide or trimethadione.

The physician should familiarize himself completely with the toxic and allergic or sensitivity reactions to all of the drugs which he uses (Tables 2.1 and 2.2), and the patient should be alerted to the risks of therapy. Whereas the toxic phenomena are functions of dosage and are nearly always reversible, the allergic or sensitivity phenomena, although uncommon, are varied, often severe and may be fatal.

Ketogenic diet.—For many years the ketogenic diet has been recommended for the treatment of drug-refractory seizures, especially petit mal or minor motor attacks. However, we are not at all enthusiastic about this form of therapy, although we concede that occasionally a patient gets better with this approach. Whether the improvement results from a direct effect of the diet or by the elimination of toxic anticonvulsant drugs is in most cases an unanswered question.

In theory, the diet depends for its success upon keeping the patient in a state of ketosis. Such a long-term undertaking in young children is difficult because they often go into acidosis, which in itself is dangerous. In older children or adolescents a state of ketosis cannot be maintained without constant fluid restriction and a high fat diet, both of which are unpalatable and unpleasant. In our experience, most older children drink fluids when they are thirsty and steal tasty carbohydrates, especially if they have impaired intelligence. If the child cooperates and tolerates the diet with evidence of improved seizure control, the family must then be prepared to weigh and measure all meals for the patient and this requires careful instruction from a dietitian. The parents must also test urine specimens at least once a day for the presence of acetone in order to monitor the effectiveness of the diet.

The reader should consult the detailed recommendations of Keith[22] and of Low[35] if he decides to commit the patient, the family, a dietitian and himself to this demanding form of therapy. Institution of ketogenic diet therapy usually requires hospitalization for five to 10 days.

Generalized or Focal Seizures

These episodes are treated with (1) barbiturates (phenobarbital, primidone, mephobarbital and metharbital), (2) hydantoins (diphenylhydantoin, mephenytoin, N-3), (3) phenacemide and (4) bromides. (See Table 2.2.) The drugs are discussed in their approximate order of clinical choice. *These rules of medical therapy apply as well to "psychomotor" or "temporal lobe" epilepsy.*

Phenobarbital (see p. 30).

Diphenylhydantoin (Dilantin) is probably the most effective and widely used agent for the control of generalized and focal seizures of all types.[4] Infants and young children are started on a daily dose of 25–75 mg., whereas older children can tolerate from 75 to 300 mg. in a 24-hour period. In therapeutic doses it produces less sedation than any other standard anticonvulsant. For this reason the patient can often take his total daily requirement in one or two doses. The physician must strive carefully to attain the optimal dosage level, since the range between the amount producing seizure control and that causing toxicity may be very narrow.

The toxic effects of diphenylhydantoin therapy may be mild (gum hyper-

TABLE 2.2.—DRUGS USED FOR TREATMENT OF GRAND MAL AND FOCAL SEIZURES

	Drug Generic Name (Trade Name)	Daily Dosage (Mg.) Infants	Daily Dosage (Mg.) Children	Toxicity	Allergic Manifestation	Preparation
1.	Phenobarbital (Luminal)	32-50	50-200	Drowsiness	Rash (rare)*	16 mg./4 cc. elixir 16, 32, 50, 65, 100 mg. tab.
2.	Diphenylhydantoin (Dilantin)	25-75	100-300	Gum hyperplasia, ataxia, nystagmus and diplopia, hypertrichosis, nausea, vomiting and anorexia	Rash* Aplastic anemia* Hepatitis* Generalized hyperplasia of R-E system*	32, 100 mg. caps. 50 mg. tab. 100 mg./5 cc. suspension Parenteral solution in 250 mg. vial
3.	Primidone (Mysoline)	100-250	250-1,000	Nausea, vomiting and vertigo, drowsiness, ataxia	Rash* Megaloblastic anemia*	50, 250 mg. tab. 250 mg./5 cc. suspension
4.	Mephobarbital (Mebaral)	50-150	100-300	Drowsiness	Rash*	32, 50, 100 mg. tab.
5.	Metharbital (Gemonil)	50-100	100-300	Drowsiness	Rash*	100 mg. tab.
6.	Mephenytoin (Mesantoin)	50-100	100-300	Drowsiness, ataxia	Aplastic anemia* Rash and fever* Neutropenia*	100 mg. tab.
7.	Phenacemide (Phenurone)	250-500	500-1,500	Drowsiness, psychosis*	Jaundice (hepatitis)* Aplastic anemia* Neutropenia*	500 mg. tab.
8.	Bromides	—	500-1,500	Drowsiness	Rash Psychosis	

*Indication for immediate discontinuation of the drug.

plasia, hypertrichosis, gastric distress, nystagmus) or severe (ataxia, diplopia). In infants and young children vomiting often occurs as a toxic sign. Gum hyperplasia is common and represents both a cosmetic and a dental problem. It results from the high concentration of diphenylhydantoin secreted in the saliva and does not occur in edentulous areas of the gums. Good oral hygiene with massage may prevent the progress of this problem, but occasionally excision of the overgrown gum tissue by a dentist may be necessary. Hypertrichosis may become a psychologic problem in young girls, but discontinuation of the drug for this reason is rarely justified. Nausea, anorexia and weight loss, which often result from the irritative effect of this agent on the gastric mucosa, can be avoided by giving the medication after meals. Toxic reaction to this agent in infants and young children is usually manifested clinically by vomiting rather than ataxia. When ataxia of the trunk and limbs develops the drug dose must be lowered. Nystagmus alone is not a sufficient reason to change the dose.

An acute allergic reaction in the form of a morbilliform rash associated with fever and eosinophilia occurs during the second week of therapy in about 5-10% of patients. Less frequently an acute exfoliative dermatitis or a chronic acneiform eruption may develop in sensitive patients. The drug should be stopped when a rash of any type appears. Cautious retreatment with diphenylhydantoin after two or three weeks have elapsed is sometimes carried out, but the rash usually reappears, forcing the physician to use another anticonvulsant. Other unusual allergic reactions to the drug include hepatitis, lymphomas[21] and a syndrome resembling lupus erythematosus.[2,43] Slowly accumulating evidence, both clinical and experimental, suggests that in some patients who receive high doses of Dilantin over prolonged periods persistent ataxia[23] develops, possibly as a result of damage to the cerebellum. Similarly, signs of polyneuropathy in patients on long-term therapy have been observed by many and the findings have been documented.[34]

Kutt et al.[24,25] made some interesting observations on patients in whom signs of toxicity develop on small or average doses of Dilantin. By comparing the administered dose with circulating blood levels and the major urinary metabolite of Dilantin, a parahydroxylation product (HPPH), they showed that some of these patients have an inherently limited ability to metabolize the drug, possibly due to a hereditary enzyme defect. These same workers demonstrated the value of blood Dilantin levels in problem patients who show signs of intoxication or poor seizure control.[26]

Primidone (Mysoline), the drug of choice after phenobarbital and diphenylhydantoin have been tried, has good anticonvulsant properties against both focal and grand mal seizures. The physician should be warned about the method of instituting this particular therapy. *Nausea, vomiting and profound vertigo may affect patients who are placed abruptly on full therpeutic doses of this agent.* If, however, the patient is given small doses of the drug initially and the full therapeutic dose is approached gradually over four or five days, the unpleasant side effects can usually be avoided. The total daily dose is 100-250 mg. for infants and 250-1,000 mg. for older children.

Mephobarbital (Mebaral), a more expensive sister compound of phenobarbital, has less sedative effect in equivalent dosage. However, it is generally found that higher doses must be used to match the anticonvulsant effect in phenobarbital. One needs approximately twice the phenobarbital dose to achieve a similar therapeutic effect.

Metharbital (Gemonil), a weak, sister compound of phenobarbital, has limited clinical usefulness and is usually employed when other agents have failed. The dosage range is listed in Table 2.2.

Mephenytoin (Mesantoin) should be used only as a last resort to obtain seizure control and then only after the patient and the relatives are informed about the risks. It is employed in the same doses as diphenylhydantoin. *This drug has been implicated in the etiology of aplastic anemia more frequently than any other anticonvulsant,*[45] and it can also produce mild degrees of bone marrow suppression. Rashes similar to those seen with diphenylhydantoin therapy can also result. Drowsiness is seen as a common toxic side effect.

Phenacemide (Phenurone) is also used only as a last resort because of the serious toxic and allergic side effects. It may be used in patients with refractory focal or grand mal attacks. It can cause serious bone marrow suppression (including aplastic anemia), hepatitis, psychosis and skin eruptions. Less severe toxic side effects include nausea and drowsiness.

Bromides are now rarely used but they may be tried when all of the standard drugs fail. Drowsiness, psychosis and skin rashes complicate this form of therapy. Also, an adequate intake of salt must be maintained to prevent the development of bromism. Bromides may be used as the sodium or potassium salt in daily doses of 500–1,500 mg. in older children.

Summary.—In most patients with focal or generalized (grand mal) seizures (including "psychomotor" attacks), control will be obtained with diphenylhydantoin (Dilantin) and/or phenobarbital. If a combination of these two agents is not effective in doses raised to the point of toxicity, primidone (Mysoline) should be added to the regimen. If this combination does not control the attacks, the other agents that have been described should be tried *slowly* and *systematically,* with the understanding that complete control may not be possible and that the risk of reactions will be increased. The physician must become thoroughly familiar with the adverse reactions, both toxic and allergic, which are seen with anticonvulsant therapy.

When the physician encounters a patient with refractory seizures he should be reminded of several possible explanations: the patient is not receiving or taking his medication regularly, or the patient has a brain tumor (especially in patients with focal seizures), a degenerative disease, a metabolic disorder or a significant structural defect of the brain. An adequate diagnostic study should always be done before a diagnosis of idiopathic or genetic epilepsy is made in the refractory patient.

Febrile Convulsions

Seizures in infancy commonly result from fever secondary to infection. The eternal threat of unrecognized meningitis with its mortality and morbidity risks leads many experienced workers to recommend a diagnostic lumbar puncture in every infant with a febrile seizure. We support this point of view but concede that *experienced* physicians may want to risk exceptions to this inflexible rule. It has been well established that patients with recurrent febrile seizures have an increased incidence of idiopathic epilepsy in later life and that patients with *prolonged, focal* and *recurrent* febrile seizures may suffer permanent damage to the nervous system. The bulk of available evidence suggests that most permanent residua complicating febrile seizures (including the syndrome of "acute toxic encephalopathy") result from anoxic brain damage and cerebral edema. This subject is discussed under Postseizure Hemiplegia. If the child suffers from a febrile convulsion after age 3, one should consider a different basic etiology and that the fever has served only as a triggering mechanism in a patient with an abnormally low seizure threshold.

The electroencephalogram of patients with febrile convulsions is usually normal if (1) the record is taken a week or more after the seizure[11] and (2) the patient has not suffered anoxic or inflammatory brain damage during the seizure or (3) the patient does not have idiopathic epilepsy. Persistent occipital slow wave abnormalities and febrile seizures which occur after age 2½ increase the likelihood that patients will later exhibit epileptiform EEG abnormalities associated with idiopathic epilepsy.[11]

Most febrile convulsions appear to do no harm to most healthy children, and this makes it difficult for the neurologist (who sees many permanent complicacations) to practice what we consider good preventive medicine. Despite considerable controversy about the best way to manage febrile seizures,[20] we recommend that the child be placed on continuous maintenance anticonvulsant therapy after the first seizure, regardless of precipitating cause. Phenobarbital in a daily dose of 32–64 mg. or Dilantin in a dose of 50–150 mg. per day may be used. The drug is given until the patient has remained seizure free for two years or until he reaches 3 years of age, provided the electroencephalogram is normal. This recommendation is made because of the disturbingly high incidence of permanent residua, and it is made with the realization that about 5% of a pediatrician's or general practitioner's child clientele will have febrile convulsions. We shall hold this position until a statistically significant, controlled study shows that such a plan is not necessary or beneficial. We cannot support the alternative plan of using aspirin and anticonvulsants only at the time of fever because in many instances the convulsion occurs before the fever is recognized by the parents or the physician.

Status Epilepticus

Status epilepticus occurs when a patient has a series of successive major seizures without regaining consciousness. If this cycle continues without interruption, the patient may die of exhaustion or asphyxia. The situation therefore calls for prompt medical therapy. The management of status epilepticus is given in Appendix 1.[9,14,27,32,42]

Postseizure Encephalopathy

Figure 2.3 illustrates schematically the course of clinical events which may result from convulsions, anoxia and cerebral edema with uncal herniation. The commonest example of postnatal ischemic brain damage is the hemiparesis which follows a seizure. When this focal weakness is transient it is called *Todd's palsy* and when it persists it is called *acute infantile hemiplegia* (referred to in the past by some as Marie-Strümpell encephalitis or polioencephalitis). Although attention is usually directed first to this alarming physical sign, soon thereafter one or more of the other manifestations of chronic neurologic deficit develops (mental defect, a chronic convulsive disorder, hyperactive behavior disorder, retarded speech development or aphasia, hemianopia and astereognosis with impaired hand use). The sequence of events in such cases is detailed in Figure 2.3.

Often the syndrome of postseizure hemiplegia follows an episode of status epilepticus which is associated with high fever and severe stupor or coma. This syndrome, which has been called *acute toxic encephalopathy,* is characterized by evidence of increased intracranial pressure (papilledema and elevated cerebro-

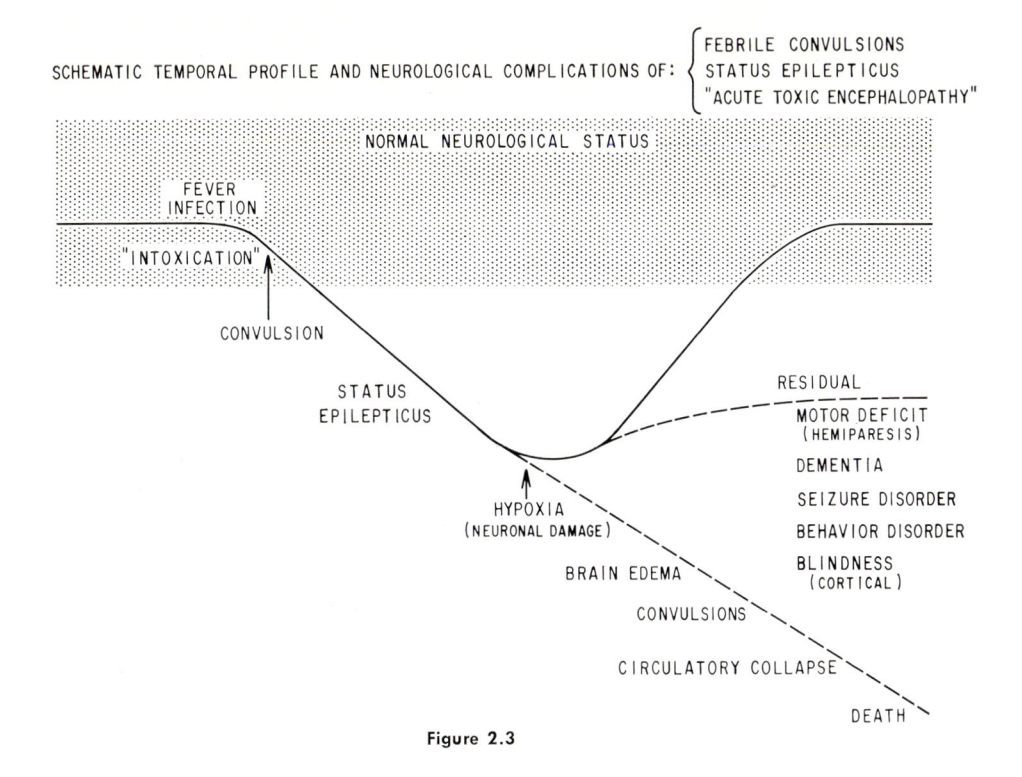

SCHEMATIC TEMPORAL PROFILE AND NEUROLOGICAL COMPLICATIONS OF: { FEBRILE CONVULSIONS / STATUS EPILEPTICUS / "ACUTE TOXIC ENCEPHALOPATHY" }

NORMAL NEUROLOGICAL STATUS

FEVER
INFECTION

"INTOXICATION"

CONVULSION

STATUS
EPILEPTICUS

RESIDUAL

MOTOR DEFICIT
(HEMIPARESIS)

DEMENTIA

HYPOXIA
(NEURONAL DAMAGE)

SEIZURE DISORDER

BEHAVIOR DISORDER

BRAIN EDEMA

BLINDNESS
(CORTICAL)

CONVULSIONS

CIRCULATORY COLLAPSE

DEATH

Figure 2.3

spinal fluid pressure in some cases) and signs of unilateral uncal herniation (third nerve palsy and contralateral hemiplegia) or bilateral uncal herniation (decerebrate rigidity). The cerebrospinal fluid usually contains no cells, has normal protein and sugar and is sterile. This clinical syndrome must always be differentiated from primary infections of the nervous system, such as acute encephalitis or meningitis, as well as from primary metabolic and vascular processes. In practice it may be difficult to make such a distinction with certainty. We believe that this syndrome in most cases represents a severe ischemic insult to the brain as a result of a seizure or a series of seizures. This point of view is based not only upon personal observations but upon the important clinicopathologic correlations made by Lyon and associates.[36] These authors found evidence of (1) anoxic neuronal damage and (2) cerebral edema in infants and children who present with the clinical syndrome of *acute toxic encephalopathy,* which in many cases is indistinguishable from status epilepticus. There is some reason to believe that occasionally acute infantile hemiplegia may result primarily from a cerebrovascular accident as it occurs in adults, i.e., an arterial occlusion, but this probably happens uncommonly. Proved thrombotic vascular accidents in young children are rare.

The same etiologic sequence need not cause a hemiparesis yet may lead to permanent and sometimes severe organic dementia or "mental retardation," serious personality change or a refractory convulsive disorder (Fig. 16.3, p. 234). Presumably many of the drug-refractory temporal lobe psychomotor seizure problems (with bizarre personality changes and often without marked mental defect) result from ischemic damage to the hippocampus of the temporal lobe.

Neonatal Seizures

Seizures in the neonate are worth considering separately because of their common occurrence, their atypical clinical and electrical signs and their high morbidity and mortality rates. The clinical signs of the seizure often differ greatly from the consistent generalized (grand mal) or focal attack in the older child and adult. Episodes may be fragmentary, migratory and inconsistent. They may vary in their focal features and are sometimes limited to altered breathing, such as bouts of apnea, with cyanosis, twitching or deviation of the eyes, posturing of a limb or mouthing movements. It is frequently necessary to differentiate the common "jitteriness" or diffuse myoclonus in the newborn from a true seizure. True "myoclonic jerks" (which closely resemble startle or Moro responses) carry an ominous prognosis, especially if they are associated with "hypsarrhythmia" on the electroencephalogram. Lombroso[31] emphasizes the value of early EEG study, preferably during the course of the attack. He concedes that later one may fail to demonstrate epileptiform brain wave abnormalities even while a seizure is taking place.

The etiology of the episodes is not uncovered in the majority of these infants. However, it is generally accepted that congenital malformations or metabolic disorders often are the cause. Hypoglycemia (associated with maternal diabetes or eclampsia) and transient hypocalcemia lead the list of metabolic disturbances which are incriminated. Of course, meningitis and intracranial bleeding must always be excluded. Actually, subdural hematomas at this age present with signs of a compressive mass more often than with seizures.

Reflex Epilepsy

Rarely, seizures are precipitated by specific sensory stimuli (sight, sound,[47] touch). The commonest form of reflex epilepsy is the clinical and electrographic seizure produced by flashing light (Fig. 14.2, p. 186). Much less often, patterned sound or language (music,[10] laughter, reading, speaking and writing) can provoke consistent types of seizures. Seizures evoked by reading ("reading epilepsy") are commonly associated with jaw-jerking, followed by loss of consciousness; convulsions may or may not occur. It seems likely that seizures provoked by reading and other language functions have the same anatomic foundations as those which are involved in centrencephalic epilepsy, inasmuch as the epileptiform EEG abnormalities are bilateral and not focal.[12]

SURGERY FOR SEIZURES

Surgical therapy for the removal of an epileptogenic focus is performed very rarely in children and then is done only after thorough diagnostic study by a team of experts. However, one should remain vigilant for the detection of small, slowly growing tumors, especially those arising in the temporal lobe.[1,7,19,44] Clinical suspicion of such lesions should arise in patients with (1) persistent "psychomotor," "temporal lobe" or focal seizures, (2) an EEG slow wave focus and (3) poor response to medical therapy (Fig. 17.4, p. 254).

TABLE 2.3.—STRUCTURE-ACTIVITY INTERRELATIONSHIPS OF COMMONLY USED ANTICONVULSANTS

NUCLEUS Generic Name	R$_1$	SUBSTITUENTS R$_2$	R$_3$	X	Trade Name
Barbiturates					
Phenobarbital	C$_6$H$_5$	C$_2$H$_5$	H	⎫	Luminal
Primidone*	C$_6$H$_5$	C$_2$H$_5$	H	⎬ —CO—NH—	Mysoline
Mephobarbital	C$_6$H$_5$	C$_2$H$_5$	CH$_3$	⎬	Mebaral
Metharbital	C$_2$H$_5$	C$_2$H$_5$	CH$_3$	⎭	Gemonil
Hydantoins					
Diphenylhydantoin	C$_6$H$_5$	C$_6$H$_5$	H	⎫ —NH—	Dilantin
Mephenytoin	C$_6$H$_5$	C$_2$H$_5$	CH$_3$	⎭	Mesantoin
Oxazolidinediones					
Trimethadione	CH$_3$	CH$_3$	CH$_3$	⎫	Tridione
Paramethadione	C$_2$H$_5$	CH$_3$	CH$_3$	⎬ —O—	Paradione
Dimethadione	CH$_3$	CH$_3$	H	⎭	Eupractone†
Succinimides					
Ethosuximide	C$_2$H$_5$	CH$_3$	H	⎫	Zarontin
Phensuximide	C$_6$H$_5$	H	CH$_3$	⎬ —CH$_2$—	Milontin
Methsuximide	C$_6$H$_5$	CH$_3$	CH$_3$	⎭	Celontin
Acetylureas‡					
Phenacemide	C$_6$H$_5$	H, H	H	NH$_2$—	Phenurone

*Carbonyl oxygen of urea moiety of phenobarbital is replaced by two hydrogen atoms.
†Not yet marketed.
‡Straight-chain compounds.

Prevention and Treatment of Severe Drug Reactions

The marked similarity in the chemical structures of the commonly used anticonvulsant drugs (Table 2.3) undoubtedly accounts for the high incidence of like reactions to these compounds. Bone marrow suppression represents the most serious threat from anticonvulsant therapy. Mesantoin or Tridione has been incriminated in most documented cases of aplastic anemia, according to Robins' review of the literature.[45] The occurrence of aplastic anemia is apparently not related to the age or sex of the patient, nor is it related to the drug dosage. However, in 80% of patients with aplastic anemia the symptoms develop within a year after institution of continuous therapy.

Since no clinical sign can be considered an accurate early indicator of bone marrow suppression, blood counts at regular intervals must be carried out. *Leukocyte and differential counts should be performed at monthly intervals for the first year and at least every two months thereafter.* If the *neutrophil* count falls below 2,500/cu. mm., the white cell counts and differentials should be done every two weeks. The drug or drugs should be stopped if the *total neutrophil* count falls below 1,600/cu. mm.

The mortality rate from anticonvulsant-induced aplastic anemia lies between 75 and 80%,[45] death occurring 30–60 days after the diagnosis is made. If the patients can be sustained during this early critical period, a gradual return to normal marrow function may occur. Treatment consists of (1) discontinuation of the offending drug, (2) repeated blood transfusions, (3) antibiotic therapy, (4) avoidance of intramuscular injections, (5) protective isolation and (6) steroid (testosterone and adrenocorticosteroid) therapy.

Nephrosis can result from trimethadione, paramethadione and dimethadione therapy. Consequently, routine urinalysis for albumin should be performed at the same time that blood counts are done. If albuminuria or the clinical picture of nephrosis develops, the offending drug should be stopped immediately. The prognosis for recovery is generally good, but at least five deaths have been reported.[48] In addition to discontinuation of the drug, these patients are usually treated in the same manner as those with idiopathic lipoid nephrosis. Adrenal cortical hormones, ACTH and antimetabolites, such as nitrogen mustard, are used.[50] It has been said that patients with trimethadione-induced nephrosis are more refractory to steroid therapy than patients with the idiopathic disorder, but this impression is not well documented.

Toxic hepatitis may complicate treatment with phenacemide (Phenurone). If the use of this agent seems indicated, the patient should have urinary urobilinogen tests carried out at the same time the blood counts are done. The drug should be stopped if an excessive output of urinary urobilinogen is noted.

Breathholding Spells

DIAGNOSIS.—Many children lose consciousness as a result of crying and breathholding. The attacks are usually precipitated by pain, anger, discipline or frustration. The nature of the episode varies clinically from apnea with cyanosis to an atonic ictal attack, a tonic seizure or a generalized convulsion. Critical to the diagnosis is a history that all attacks are precipitated by external factors such as those listed.[33] If an attack develops without provocation, one should not make the diagnosis of breathholding spells. The electroencephalogram in all patients with true breathholding episodes is normal.

MANAGEMENT AND PROGNOSIS.—Response to standard anticonvulsant drugs such as phenobarbital and Dilantin is somewhat unpredictable, but a therapeutic trial should be given. When a firm diagnosis has been established, parents should be given a good prognosis even though the response to therapy may be incomplete. True breathholding attacks rarely occur after age 3.

Syncope

Children, like adults, have fainting spells as a result of temporary circulatory insufficiency. Such episodes can be provoked by a sudden shift to the erect position (postural hypotension), prolonged standing in a fixed position, especially in hot weather, or severe psychologic or physical stress, including hunger. In some patients brief, clonic movements occur after consciousness is lost and the episode may be confused with a true convulsion. The diagnostic workup on these patients, including the electroencephalogram, gives normal findings and patients do not benefit from anticonvulsant therapy. Often one finds that a parent or other near relative has also had fainting spells.

Tetany

SYNDROME DIAGNOSIS.—In general, low blood calcium values (i.e., below 7.0 or 7.5 mg./100 ml.) are diagnostic of tetany. The clinical picture of tetany is quite constant, regardless of the cause or the age group affected, and reflects a state of increased neuromuscular excitability. In fully manifest tetany, tonic spasms of the muscles in the extremities *(carpopedal spasm)* may occur along with high-pitched, crowing respirations *(laryngospasm)* and/or seizures of varied type. In milder hypocalcemic states, only the more subtle signs may be elicited; these include Chvostek's sign—unilateral contraction of facial muscles on percussion of the facial nerve in front of the ear—and Trousseau's sign—carpal spasm resulting from constriction of the upper arm for two or three minutes (Fig. 2.4).

DIFFERENTIAL DIAGNOSIS.—In the differential diagnosis of tetany, tetany due to hypocalcemia must first be distinguished from tetany due to alkalosis (resulting from hyperventilation, excessive loss of chloride in vomitus or excessive intake of sodium bicarbonate). Table 2.4 outlines the differential diagnosis of hypocalcemic tetany. At present hypocalcemic tetany is seen most commonly in the newborn and results from a combination of transient functional hypoparathyroidism and the use of cow's milk with its high phosphorus content. Contributing factors in some cases of neonatal tetany are prematurity,[13] maternal diabetes mellitus[8] and unrecognized asymptomatic maternal hyperparathyroidism.[40] A generation ago tetany most often resulted from rickets due to a dietary deficiency of vitamin D. At present the rare disorder, familial hypophosphatemic vitamin-D–resistant rickets, is associated with tetany. If vitamin D, a critical factor in normal calcium-phosphorus metabolism, is deficient in the diet or if the patient has an inborn resistance to ordinary dietary amounts, the intestinal absorption of

TABLE 2.4.—DIFFERENTIAL DIAGNOSIS OF TETANY

Syndrome	Age of Occurrence	Familial	Serum Calcium	Serum Phosphorus	Serum Alkaline Phosphatase	Ectopic Calcium Subcutaneous	Ectopic Calcium Brain	Short Fingers, Stature	IQ	Moniliasis
Neonatal tetany (see text)	Birth to 3 wk. (cow's milk formula)	0	Low	High	Normal	0	0	0	Normal	0
Hypoparathyroidism*	Children and young adults	±	Low	High	Normal	0	+	0	± low	±
Pseudohypoparathyroidism*	Any age	+	Low	High	Normal	+	+	+	± low	0
Vitamin-D-deficient rickets	4 mo. to 3 yr.	0	Low	± high	High	0	0	0	Normal	0
Vitamin-D-resistant rickets	Any age	+ (sex-linked dominant)	± normal	Low	± high	0	0	+ (stature)	Normal	0
Celiac disease	6 mo. to 4 yr.	±	Low	Normal	Normal	0	0	0	Normal	0
Surgical or post-traumatic	Any age, adult	0	Low	Normal	Normal	0	0	0	Normal	0

*See Chapter 21.

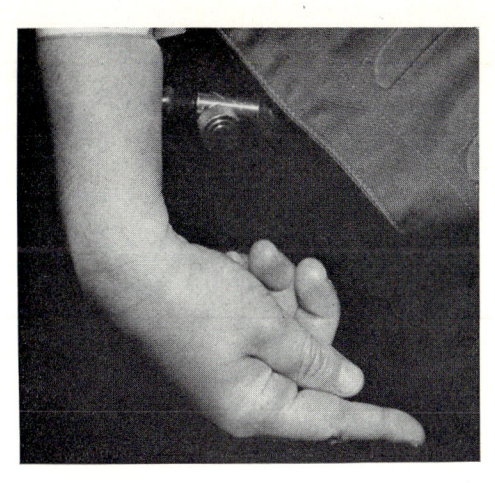

Fig. 2.4.—Typical Trousseau's sign (carpal spasm resulting from constriction of the upper arm) due to hypocalcemia. This patient had idiopathic hypoparathyroidism.

both calcium and phosphorus is reduced and the reabsorption of phosphorus by the renal tubules is decreased—a condition that may lead to hypocalcemia and tetany. In patients with malabsorption and steatorrhea secondary to celiac disease hypocalcemic tetany may occur due to poor intestinal absorption of calcium and phosphorus. Chronic renal insufficiency may cause hypocalcemic tetany as a result of phosphate retention and high serum levels of phosphorus.

MANAGEMENT.—The immediate correction of hypocalcemia is achieved with intravenous administration of 5–10 ml. of 10% calcium gluconate. Parathyroid extract, which is used only in the acute disease because it must be given parenterally and is expensive, may be given in doses of 25–50 units every six hours. These measures will readily control the seizures and diarrhea in the acute stage.

Hypoglycemia

The demonstration of hypoglycemia and its definitive differential diagnosis present some of the most difficult problems in the field of child health. A working classification of the types of hypoglycemia is shown in Table 2.5. The reader should understand clearly that most cases fall into the "idiopathic" category (in which multiple basic causes are probably involved) and the neonatal type. Only rarely are specific organic etiologies, such as endocrinopathies and enzymatic defects, demonstrated. Once the hypoglycemia is demonstrated, the physician must make every effort to rule out an insuloma because the treatment of such pancreatic tumors is operative and not medical.

SYNDROME DIAGNOSIS.—Symptoms of hypoglycemia are mainly neurologic since the brain, unlike other tissues, cannot utilize protein or fat but must depend upon a continuous supply of circulating glucose. Seizures, syncope, behavior disturbances, incoordination, focal weakness, headaches, tremulousness, speech and visual disturbances, and vegetative signs and symptoms such as sweating, pallor, hunger and tachycardia may reflect an abnormally low blood sugar. The clinical picture in the newborn may be more nonspecific. Neonates often exhibit cyanosis, subnormal temperature, poor feeding and respiratory irregularity; convulsions may not appear until later.

TABLE 2.5.—Classification of Hypoglycemia

I. Neonatal hypoglycemia*
   Low birth weight
   Maternal toxemia
   Maternal diabetes mellitus
   Twin pregnancy

II. "Idiopathic" spontaneous hypoglycemia (sometimes familial)
   Leucine sensitivity (hereditary)
   Leucine insensitivity†

III. "Functional," reactive or postprandial hyperinsulinism
   High carbohydrate meal
   Emotional stress
   "Ketogenic" hypoglycemia (see text)

IV. Organic hypoglycemia
   Insuloma
   Pituitary insufficiency
   Adrenal cortical insufficiency
   Hepatic insufficiency (cirrhosis, hepatitis, poisoning
     and tumor infiltrate)
   Malabsorption (celiac disease and chronic starvation)

V. Hereditary enzymatic defects
   Galactosemia
   Glycogen storage disease
   Fructose intolerance
   Maple syrup urine disease

*Neonatal hypoglycemia (20-30 mg./100 ml. blood glucose) may be asymptomatic or symptomatic.
†The majority of children with "idiopathic" hypoglycemia are *not* leucine-sensitive.

By general definition blood glucose levels below 40 mg./100 ml. in older children and adults are usually sufficient to explain the usual clinical symptoms, whereas newborn infants may be asymptomatic with levels of 20–40 mg./100 ml. Some patients with blood glucose levels of 25–30 mg./100 ml. will be completely free from symptoms, whereas others will show hypoglycemic signs and symptoms with levels of 60–70. The rapidity of the drop in blood sugar may be as important as the absolute level in explaining this paradox. Blood glucose levels which are low enough to cause clinical symptoms have many causes.

DIFFERENTIAL DIAGNOSIS.—Neonatal hypoglycemia, which occurs much more frequently in babies born of toxemic or diabetic mothers, tends to improve spontaneously with a few months' maturation, though residual damage to the nervous system is common (Fig. 21.7, p. 405).

Definitive diagnosis of hypoglycemia is difficult and is best broken down into (1) the demonstration of abnormally low blood glucose levels and (2) the definition of the exact etiology. In most cases of secondary hypoglycemia, which is less common, the definitive diagnosis depends on specific physical findings or laboratory tests. In this text attention will be directed to the tests of carbohydrate function which are critical for demonstrating both the hypoglycemic state and the etiologic mechanisms in the primary forms of hypoglycemia.

If the simple fasting blood sugar does not demonstrate hypoglycemia and the physician still suspects this disorder, the diagnostic sequence outlined in Table 2.6 is suggested and can be conducted in the following manner.

TABLE 2.6.—CLINICAL EVALUATION OF SUSPECTED HYPOGLYCEMIA

1. *Blood Sugar Determination*
   a) at time of an attack if possible, *or*
   b) after overnight fast

2. *I.V. Glucose Tolerance Test*

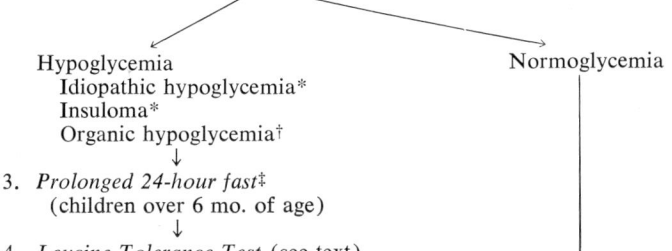

   Hypoglycemia
      Idiopathic hypoglycemia*
      Insuloma*
      Organic hypoglycemia†
   ↓

3. *Prolonged 24-hour fast*‡
   (children over 6 mo. of age)
   ↓

4. *Leucine Tolerance Test* (see text)

   Normoglycemia
   ↓
   5. *Oral Glucose Tolerance Test*
      Hypoglycemia   Flat curve
      Functional   Malabsorption
      Hyperinsulinism

*Wilkins[52] states that reliable tests have not yet been developed to differentiate all the causes of idiopathic hypoglycemia or to establish a reliable diagnosis of insuloma. Therefore, we believe all such cases should be referred to an endocrinologist for further study so that insulomas are not overlooked.

†Appropriate tests of pituitary, adrenal cortex and liver function should be done when organic hypoglycemia is suspected. (See Table 2.5, IV and V.)

‡The fast is carried out from the time the I.V. glucose tolerance test is started, and tests for acetonuria are carried out every four hours (see text).

1. Be certain that the child has had several days of full feeding to insure an adequate store of liver glycogen. If this is not done, interpretation of subsequent tests may be misleading. Blood sugars should then be obtained (*a*) at the time of an attack, (*b*) after an overnight fast or (*c*) after a prolonged 24-hour fast. The prolonged fast should not be carried out in infants under 6 months of age.

2. For the *intravenous glucose tolerance test,* give 0.7 Gm. of glucose/kg. (20 Gm./m²) as a 50% glucose solution over a period of four to five minutes. Obtain blood samples before and at 30 minutes, 1, 2, 3, 4 and 5 hours after the injection is completed. If the patient fails to restore the blood sugar level from hypoglycemic to normal between two and six hours, results are considered abnormal and suggest pancreatic adenoma or other organic cause.

Schotland *et al.*[46] have emphasized that the *tolbutamide tolerance test* fails to distinguish patients whose hypoglycemia results from insuloma, leucine sensitivity, ketosis or idiopathic causes.

Insulin tolerance tests are not recommended because of the potentially hazardous effect of inducing severe hypoglycemia and because the same information can usually be obtained from an intravenous glucose tolerance test.

3. *Fast the patient continuously for 24 hours* from the time the glucose tolerance test is started. Obtain serial urine specimens every four hours and test the sample for acetone. In a certain number of patients, especially those with "functional" hypoglycemia, marked ketonuria will develop after four to eight hours and will be associated with clinical symptoms of drowsiness and vomiting. Convulsions

are not usually seen. Ulstrom and Colle[49] have reported studies on a small series of these patients and suggest that the disorder may result from an unusual tendency to burn fat when glucose supplies are low. This type of disorder is called "ketogenic" hypoglycemia.

4. Perform a *leucine sensitivity test*. Give L-leucine, 150 mg./kg., by mouth or by nasogastric tube and obtain blood samples at 30, 60 and 90 minutes. If the patient is leucine-sensitive, abnormally low blood glucose levels will ensue.

It is commonly said that primary brain lesions can cause hypoglycemia, but it seems much more likely, in the absence of convincing evidence to the contrary, that the nervous system damage is the result and not the cause of low blood sugar.

Wilkins[52] states that mental retardation can be expected in 50% of babies in whom hypoglycemia develops before 6 months of age, whereas only 8% will be retarded if the disorder develops after 6 months of age.

MANAGEMENT.—If irreversible brain damage is to be avoided when the patient is acutely symptomatic, immediate administration of glucose, preferably intravenously, is mandatory. Hypoglycemia may also be reversed by giving epinephrine (0.03 ml. of 1:1,000 solution intramuscularly, with the total dose not to exceed 0.8 ml.) or low doses of adrenal cortical steroids (prednisone, 10–20 mg. daily). Whereas any or all of these treatment measures are indicated to prevent symptoms, one should be more careful and selective when giving dietary advice. Infants with neonatal hypoglycemia should be given high sugar formula feedings every two hours. If the patient is leucine-sensitive, he should be given supplemental carbohydrates (sweetened orange juice or glucose water in infants) 30 minutes after meals. In leucine-sensitive infants, a special low leucine milk formula should be used, such as Wyeth formula S-14. Cortisone or ACTH therapy is less effective in maintaining normoglycemia in leucine-sensitive patients than in those who are *not* leucine-sensitive. In the latter high carbohydrate meals should be avoided because they may aggravate the postprandial drop in blood sugar. Instead, high protein diets should be used to provide the slow formation of glucose from protein. When the above measures are ineffective, frequent feedings should be employed regardless of the type of hypoglycemia. Between-meal lunches and a lunch at bedtime are advocated to give at least six feedings a day.

A recent report suggests that sodium glutamate administration may relieve symptoms in hypoglycemic patients[17] during an attack (glutamate or Accent is a relatively cheap dietary supplement if its therapeutic value is confirmed). Also, recently a persistent hyperglycemic effect was obtained from diazoxide therapy (5–20 mg./kg./day) in infantile hypoglycemia.[38] Human growth hormone also has proved value in controlling blood glucose levels, but its limited availability has restricted its use.

If the hypoglycemic episodes are unresponsive to diet, corticosteroids and other drug therapy, the patient may require surgical exploration for pancreatic adenoma, assuming that diagnostic studies suggest this possibility. Wilkins[52] emphasizes this latter point, despite the rarity of insuloma. When a tumor is not found, some workers have recommended partial pancreatectomy, but the results of this procedure have not been impressive. One must be sure to treat patients with other, more specific measures if the hypoglycemia is shown to be secondary to other pathologic mechanisms (Table 2.5).

Hysterical Seizures

Convulsions occur rarely as a sign of a conversion reaction. The patients may pose a serious diagnostic problem but they do not have epileptiform EEG abnormalities unless both epilepsy and hysteria are present. Often the hysterical episodes have bizarre clinical features that cannot be explained on sound neurophysiologic grounds, and no confirmatory clinical or laboratory evidence is found. Careful observation of these patients and study of their personality traits with appropriate psychologic tests may provide evidence to support the diagnosis of hysteria.

Cardiac Seizures

In any child who loses consciousness partially, especially with pallor, sweating and cyanosis, and who does not have hypoglycemia or any definite epileptiform EEG abnormalities, the diagnosis of paroxysmal auricular tachycardia should be considered. The diagnosis is made by noting the tachycardia or by demonstrating an abnormal electrocardiogram during an attack. Sometimes attacks can be aborted by pressure on the eyeballs or the carotid sinus (vagal stimulation); if simple maneuvers fail, the patient may require digitalization.

Coma from Other Causes

If the patient is found unconscious and no seizure is witnessed, the many other causes for nonconvulsive loss of consciousness must be considered. *Poisonings* often cause stupor or coma in children and the diagnosis may be obscure unless the physician is alert to this common problem. Commonly, patients with *head injuries* are found unconscious with or without external signs of injury, and only careful history taking, observation and EEG study will differentiate a concussion from a true seizure. Very young infants may become stuporous or comatose because of *septicemia* or *meningitis* without exhibiting the usual signs of infection. In newborn infants a major *cerebral anomaly* such as anencephaly or hypoplasia must be considered, and head transillumination should be performed. *Rare metabolic disorders* such as hypoglycemia, hypocalcemia or ammonia intoxication (disorders of urea synthesis) can masquerade as convulsive disorders.

Management is discussed separately in Part II.

Other Paroxysmal Disorders

Headaches

Head pain is common in children and can be localized quite accurately after age 5. In younger children the symptom is not as well localized and sometimes cannot be reported at all. To simplify discussion, headache will be subdivided into organic headache and functional headache.

Organic Headache

Systemic infections (tonsillopharyngitis, viral respiratory tract infections and urinary tract infections) cause the majority of headaches in children and their management is obvious. Similarly, central nervous system infections (meningitis and encephalitis) cause head pain and generally present no great problem in diagnosis or therapy. In older children without evidence of infection, mass lesions such as brain tumor, brain abscess, subdural hematoma or subarachnoid hemorrhage from vascular malformations must be considered and managed appropriately. More uncommonly, children with hypertension secondary to renal disease and/or corticosteroid therapy will complain of headache as a result of the intracranial hypertension or associated hemorrhage. The author has been impressed that older children with the rare demyelinating disease, neuromyelitis optica, will report frontal headache which actually represents retro-orbital pain. The subtle distinction required in the latter case becomes important because brain tumor may be suspected erroneously on the basis of "headache and papilledema" and the patient may be subjected needlessly to diagnostic ventriculography and other procedures.

Functional Headache

DIFFERENTIAL DIAGNOSIS.—Intermittent headaches from nonorganic causes quite often lead children to the physician's office. Psychogenic factors, representing minor neurotic complaints from a disturbed home or school situation, account for most functional headaches in children. Occasionally more complicated conversion reactions or psychotic symptoms form the basis of the complaint. The fear of serious organic causes for headaches often leads to an extensive diagnostic study. One must use careful and delicate judgment in studying these problems and try on the one hand to avoid the mistake of overlooking a serious, treatable organic disease and on the other hand to avoid overstudying and thereby intensifying a psychogenic complaint. Occasionally children with seizures are seen with periodic head pain, which represents either "seizure fragments" in partially controlled epilepsy or visceral seizures.

Vascular or migraine headaches in children are sometimes seen but are much less common than are psychogenic functional headaches. The classic migraine headache is characterized by transient, scintillating scotomata, transient hemianopic visual field symptoms, transient third cranial nerve weakness, transient hemiparesis or hemisensory symptoms followed by severe headache, nausea and vomiting. Often a close relative has had migraine. In some cases the episodes tend to occur in "clusters" and these have been attributed to the oversecretion of histamine. Some workers believe there is a close etiologic relationship between true migraine and epilepsy,[51] but in our opinion good evidence for this theory is lacking. Admittedly, symptoms of "atypical migraine" and "epileptic equivalents" are very similar in that they are paroxysmal and EEG evidence has been presented to confirm their relationship. However, this evidence is not entirely convincing because the EEG abnormalities in patients with migraine are seen with the attack and the electroencephalogram is usually normal between attacks. We think that relatives and patients should be advised accordingly.

MANAGEMENT.—Most headaches should be managed by eliminating the basic cause, if possible. In those uncommon situations in which the head pain represents a seizure symptom, anticonvulsant drug therapy should be given (Table 2.2).

If true migraine is present and if the attacks are frequent and incapacitating, antimigraine drugs should be tried.

1. Cafergot tablets (1 mg. ergotamine tartrate and 100 mg. caffeine) may be given to children in a dosage of 1 tablet at the first sign of an attack and 1 additional tablet every half hour until relief occurs, for a maximum of 3 tablets; or ½ suppository may be given at the first sign of an attack, to be repeated once in one hour if no relief has occurred. The continued use of this medication will depend not only upon whether the severe headache is prevented but also upon whether the side effects of nausea and vomiting cause as much discomfort as the disease.

2. Methysergide maleate (Sansert), introduced about five years ago, must be used as a maintenance prophylactic drug in order to be effective. In the dose of about 1 tablet (2 mg.) three times a day it benefits a considerable number of patients. However, we cannot recommend the use of Sansert at this time because of the complications of retroperitoneal fibrosis[18] and vascular insufficiency syndromes[6] in a certain number of patients receiving the medication.

Patients with classic migraine, like those with tension and psychogenic headaches, often note that the headaches are precipitated by environmental stress. In addition to antimigraine drug therapy, every effort should be made to minimize the causes of stress. Psychiatric consultation should be sought, if necessary.

Nightmares (Night Terrors)

Frequently children are seen because they have severe night terrors or "bad dreams," in which they walk and talk, act terrified and may tremble and stiffen out. They are usually amnesic for the whole event. These periodic episodes bear a resemblance to seizures and therefore cause some parents and physicians to worry. Such episodes rarely represent seizures and are associated with no EEG abnormalities. Obviously, one's conclusions are based simply upon the differences between a typical nightmare and a typical seizure, as well as the EEG differences in doubtful cases. These night terrors usually are a phenomenon of childhood and are not a sign of serious psychopathology. If the attacks are frequent and sleepwalking is common, the child should be protected by the parents from potential accidental injury.

Episodic Dizziness

Periodic vertigo is seen fairly often in children but its cause remains obscure in a distressingly large percentage of cases. Older children can report the symptoms accurately but it often must be assumed that the young child is dizzy if he resists movement, prefers to remain motionless and shows nystagmus. The differential diagnosis must include head injury, acute labyrinthitis, acute cerebellitis or pontine encephalitis, intoxications, early symptom of brain tumor or increased intracranial pressure, demyelinating disease, tumors and vertiginous seizures, which presumably can originate from a focus in the temporal lobe. Childhood Ménière's syndrome is so rare it will be mentioned but not discussed. From experience we suggest that every effort be made to arrive at a specific diagnosis and so arrive at specific therapy. No useful symptomatic treatment can be recommended.

Excessive Sleepiness

In our experience the uncontrollable desire to sleep (narcolepsy) or the sudden transient loss of muscle tone (cataplexy) rarely affects children. However, occasional cases are reported.[53] These disorders of unknown etiology must be differentiated from true seizures, increased intracranial pressure, occult systemic disease and disease of the diencephalon or hypothalamus (Chapter 11). In general, the electroencephalograms in patients with narcolepsy show no abnormalities. Children with true narcolepsy are treated with Dexedrine, 2.5–5 mg. three times a day, or with methylphenidate (Ritalin), 10 mg. two to three times a day.

BIBLIOGRAPHY

1. Bailey, P.: Surgical treatment of psychomotor epilepsy: Five year follow-up, South. M. J. 54:299, 1961.
2. Benton, J. W.: Personal communication.
3. Bower, B. D., and Jeavons, P. M.: The effect of corticotrophin and prednisolone on infantile spasms with mental retardation, Arch. Dis. Childhood 36:23, 1961.
4. Bray, P. F.: Diphenylhydantoin (Dilantin) after 20 years, Pediatrics 23:151, 1959.
5. Bray, P. F.: The influence of adrenal steroids and corticotropin on massive myoclonic seizures of infancy, Pediatrics 32:169, 1963.
6. Buenger, R. E., and Hunter, J. A.: Reversible mesenteric artery stenoses due to methysergide maleate, J.A.M.A. 198:558, 1966.
7. Cavanagh, J. B.: On certain small tumours encountered in the temporal lobe, Brain 81:389, 1958.
8. Craig, W. S.: Clinical signs of neonatal tetany: With especial reference to their occurrence in newborn babies of diabetic mothers, Pediatrics 22:297, 1958.
9. Farmer, T. W.: *Pediatric Neurology* (New York City: Paul B. Hoeber, Inc., 1964).
10. Forster, F. M., et al.: Modification of musicogenic epilepsy by extinction technique, Tr. Am. Neurol. A. 90:179, 1965.
11. Frantzen, E., et al.: Longitudinal EEG and clinical study of children with febrile convulsions, Electroencephalog. & Clin. Neurophysiol. 24:197, 1968.
12. Geschwind, N., and Sherwin, I.: Language-induced epilepsy, Arch. Neurol. 16:25, 1967.
13. Gittleman, I. F., et al.: Hypocalcemia occurring on the first day of life in mature and premature infants, Pediatrics 18:721, 1956.
14. Gold, A. P., and Carter, S.: Pediatric Neurology in Shirkey, H. C. (ed.): *Pediatric Therapy* (2d ed.; St. Louis: C. V. Mosby Company, 1966).
15. Goldensohn, E. S.: Unpublished data.
16. Goldensohn, E. S., et al.: Ethosuximide in the treatment of epilepsy, J.A.M.A. 182:840, 1962.
17. Gomez, M. R., et al.: Effect of sodium glutamate on leucine-induced hypoglycemia, Pediatrics 28:935, 1961.
18. Graham, J. R., et al.: Fibrotic disorders associated with methysergide therapy for headache, New England J. Med. 274:359, 1966.
19. Green, J. R.: Temporal lobectomy, with special reference to selection of epileptic patients, J. Neurosurg. 26:584, 1967.
20. Hammill, J. F., and Carter, S.: Febrile convulsions, New England J. Med. 274:563, 1966.
21. Hyman, G. A., and Sommers, S. C.: The development of Hodgkin's disease and lymphoma during anticonvulsant therapy, Blood 28:416, 1966.
22. Keith, H. M.: *Convulsive Disorders in Children—with Reference to Treatment with Ketogenic Diet* (Boston: Little, Brown & Company, 1963).
23. Kokenge, R., et al.: Neurological sequelae following Dilantin overdose in a patient and in experimental animals, Neurology 15:823, 1965.
24. Kutt, H., et al.: Diphenylhydantoin metabolism, blood levels and toxicity, Arch. Neurol. 11:642, 1964.
25. Kutt, H., et al.: Insufficient parahydroxylation as a cause of diphenylhydantoin toxicity, Neurology 14:542, 1964.
26. Kutt, H., and McDowell, F.: Management of epilepsy with diphenylhydantoin sodium, J.A.M.A. 203:969, 1968.
27. Livingston, S.: Seizure Disorders, in Gellis, S. S., and Kagan, B. M. (eds.): *Current Pediatric Therapy* (Philadelphia: W. B. Saunders Company, 1966-67).

28. Livingston, S., *et al.*: Ineffectiveness of Diamox in the treatment of childhood epilepsy, Pediatrics 17:541, 1956.
29. Livingston, S., *et al.*: Minor motor epilepsy, Pediatrics 21:916, 1958.
30. Livingston, S., *et al.*: Petit mal epilepsy, J.A.M.A. 194:227, 1965.
31. Lombroso, C. T.: Neonatal Seizure States, in *Proceedings of the XI International Congress on Pediatrics* (Tokyo: University of Tokyo Press, 1965), pp. 38-49.
32. Lombroso, C. T.: Treatment of status epilepticus with diazepam, Neurology 16:629, 1966.
33. Lombroso, C. T., and Lerman, P.: Breathholding spells (cyanotic and pallid infantile syncope), Pediatrics 39:563, 1967.
34. Lovelace, R. E., and Horwitz, S. J.: Peripheral neuropathy in long-term diphenylhydantoin therapy, Arch. Neurol. 18:69, 1968.
35. Low, N. L.: Seizure Disorders in Children, in Brennemann-Kelley: *Practice of Pediatrics* (Hagerstown, Md.: W. F. Prior Company, Inc., 1964), Vol. IV, chap. 18.
36. Lyon, G., *et al.*: The acute encephalopathies of obscure origin in infants and children, Brain 84:680, 1961.
37. Mann, L. B., and Habenicht, H. A.: Fatal bone marrow aplasia associated with administration of ethosuximide (Zarontin) for petit mal epilepsy, Bull. Los Angeles Neurol. Soc. 27:1173, 1962.
38. Mereu, T. R., *et al.*: Diazoxide in the treatment of infantile hypoglycemia, New England J. Med. 275:1455, 1966.
39. Millichap, J. G., and Bickford, R. G.: Infantile spasms, hypsarhythmia, and mental retardation, J.A.M.A. 182:523, 1962.
40. Mizrahi, A., and Gold, A. P.: Neonatal tetany secondary to maternal hyperparathyroidism, J.A.M.A. 190:155, 1964.
41. Penfield, W., and Erickson, T. C.: *Epilepsy and Cerebral Localization* (Springfield, Ill.: Charles C Thomas, Publisher, 1941), chap. IV.
42. Prensky, A. L., *et al.*: Intravenous diazepam in the treatment of prolonged seizure activity, New England J. Med. 276:779, 1967.
43. Rallison, M. L., *et al.*: Lupus erythematosus and Stevens-Johnson syndrome: Occurrence as reactions to anticonvulsant medication, Am. J. Dis. Child. 101:725, 1961.
44. Rasmussen, T., and Branch, C.: Temporal lobe epilepsy: Indications for and results of surgical therapy, Postgrad. Med. 31:9, 1962.
45. Robins, M. M.: Aplastic anemia secondary to anticonvulsants, Am. J. Dis. Child. 104:614, 1962.
46. Schotland, M. G., *et al.*: The tolbutamide tolerance test in the evaluation of childhood hypoglycemia, Pediatrics 39:838, 1967.
47. Strobos, R. J.: Acousticomotor seizures, Electroencephalog. & Clin. Neurophysiol. 14:129, 1962.
48. Talamo, R. C., and Crawford, J. D.: Trimethadione nephrosis treated with cortisone and nitrogen mustard, New England J. Med. 269:15, 1963.
49. Ulstrom, R. A., and Colle, E.: Personal communication.
50. West, C. D.: Use of combined hormone and mechlorethamine (nitrogen mustard) therapy in lipoid nephrosis, Am. J. Dis. Child. 95:498, 1958.
51. Whitehouse, D., *et al.*: Electroencephalographic changes in children with migraine, New England J. Med. 276:23, 1967.
52. Wilkins, L.: *The Diagnosis and Treatment of Endocrine Disorders in Childhood and Adolescence* (3d ed.; Springfield, Ill.: Charles C Thomas, Publisher, 1965).
53. Yoss, R. E., and Daly, D. D.: Narcolepsy in children, Pediatrics 25:1025, 1960.

3

Chronic Motor Disorders ("Cerebral Palsy")*

Hypotonia (Amyotonia Congenita)
    Cerebral "Atonic Diplegia"
    Progressive Infantile Muscular Atrophy
    Benign Congenital Hypotonia
    Obstetric Cord Damage

    Hereditary Metabolic Disorders
    Congenital Myopathies
    Chronic Polyneuropathy

Spasticity
    Hemiplegia (or Hemiparesis)
    Diplegia
    Pseudobulbar Palsy

    Quadriplegia
    Paraplegia

Ataxia
    Congenital Cerebellar Ataxia
    Cerebral "Atonic Diplegia" (above)
    Congenital Internal Hydrocephalus

    Hereditary Spinocerebellar Ataxia
    Hereditary Metabolic Defects

Myoclonus
    Minor Motor Epilepsy
    Idiopathic Epilepsy

    Progressive Degenerative Diseases
    Paramyoclonus Multiplex

Choreoathetosis
    Kernicterus
    Anoxia
Mirror Movements

    Huntington's Chorea
    ? Congenital Malformation
        (Status Marmoratus)

*The specific disorders are considered in Part II. The differential diagnosis of acute motor disorders is discussed in Chapter 9.

Various other rare solitary and mixed movement disorders (tremor, chorea, rigidity, dystonia, and myoclonus) have been described, some of which are discussed in Chapter 21.

INFANTS AND YOUNG CHILDREN with chronic disorders of movement and tone come to medical attention because of (1) delayed motor development, (2) "floppy" or "limp" muscle tone, (3) "tense" or "tight" muscle tone, (4) swallowing or speech difficulty, (5) poor coordination and (6) "nervousness."

The motor syndrome diagnosis is based upon the neurologic physical findings (Table 1.3, p. 7).

Hypotonia

SYNDROME DIAGNOSIS.—Hypotonia is characterized by flaccid muscle tone, variable muscle mass (best evaluated by soft-tissue x-rays of the extremities), hyperextensibility of the joints, deep tendon reflexes which vary from normal to absent and in some cases a mild "ataxic" tremor.

Many different descriptive diagnostic terms have been used in these patients and this has created unnecessary confusion. We use the term "amyotonia congenita" (as does Brandt[2]) as a descriptive term for any hypotonic infant, not to indicate a specific disease. Most floppy babies have motor retardation because of disorders in the central nervous system, usually congenital malformations of the brain (Table 3.1). The latter children have cerebral hypotonia or "atonic diplegia,"[6] they have *normal* deep tendon reflexes (Fig. 3.1), and they have mental retardation of varying severity.[16] Infants with progressive spinal muscular atrophy exhibit hypotonia, atrophy and areflexia. Muscle biopsy is diagnostic in these patients (Chapter 19).[9] A few floppy babies without evidence of neurogenic atrophy, myopathy or systemic disease have hypotonia and hyporeflexia (or normal reflexes) and reach their motor milestones later than the average. The term "benign congenital hypotonia" has been applied to them by Walton.[15] Muscle biopsy and electrical studies in this group of patients give normal findings, except for small fiber size in some cases.[5,9] However, extreme care must be taken to differentiate the latter group from babies with cerebral atonic diplegia. Much more rarely one will find that hypotonia results from hereditary metabolic diseases, polyneuritis (including mercury poisoning in acrodynia), congenital myopathies and pseudoparalysis from conditions such as scurvy. Obstetric stretching injury to the cervical cord at breech delivery will also cause diffuse hypotonia.

MANAGEMENT.—The management of children with hypotonia depends upon the specific diagnosis. In general, such patients do not require and do not benefit significantly from physiotherapy unless signs of joint contracture are found. Par-

TABLE 3.1.—DIFFERENTIAL DIAGNOSIS OF HYPOTONIA*

CLINICAL SYNDROME	BASIC ETIOLOGY	ASSOCIATED SYMPTOMS AND SIGNS
Cerebral hypotonia ("atonic diplegia")	Congenital malformations Hereditary metabolic disorders	Small head size Malformations in other organs Signs of mental retardation Normal tendon reflexes
Spinal hypotonia	Infantile spinal muscle atrophy Polyneuritis Intraspinal tumor Cord trauma Intoxications and adverse reactions	Muscle atrophy Hyporeflexia Muscle biopsy evidence
Muscular hypotonia	Primary myopathy	Muscle atrophy and hyporeflexia Muscle biopsy evidence

*The specific etiologies are listed in their approximate order of frequency.

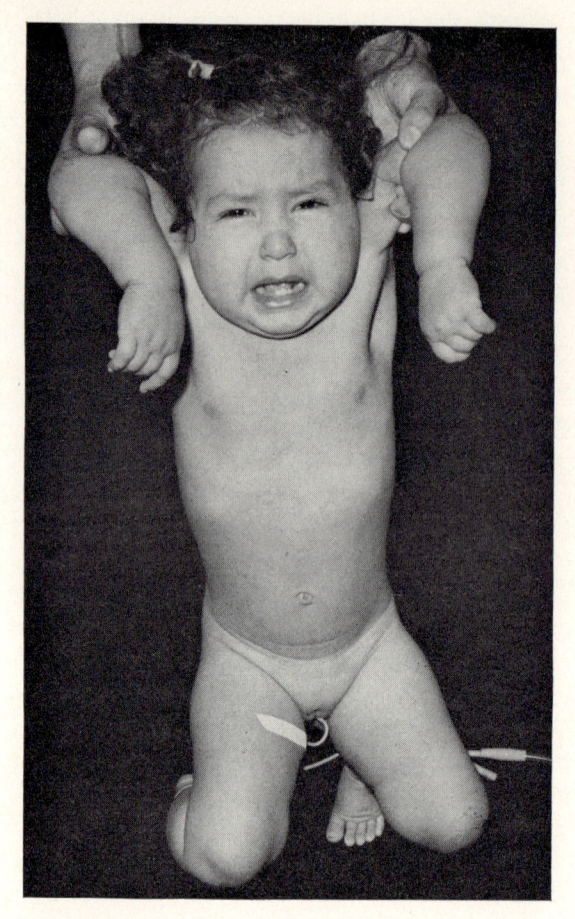

Fig. 3.1.—Cerebral hypotonia (atonic diplegia). This little girl and three siblings had moderate mental retardation and were very hypotonic. No specific diagnosis could be made. Three other siblings were normal.

ents should be reassured that the usual "tender loving care" and stimulation given to infants and young children will suffice to promote progress within the limits of physical development.

Spasticity

SYNDROME DIAGNOSIS.—The syndrome of spasticity accounts for the large majority of patients with "cerebral palsy." Spastic infants usually exhibit delayed motor development and parents often report "tenseness" and "tightness." Paradoxically, however, parents often wrongly attribute motor retardation to diminished muscle tone, whereas the problem in fact results from increased muscle tone. Patients with spasticity show increased tone, hyperreflexia and pathologic reflexes in the affected limbs. Those with bilateral involvement may exhibit *pseudobulbar palsy* (dysphagia, excessive drooling and dysarthria) as a result of bilateral corticospinal tract lesions. On examination, the latter patients exhibit a relatively immobile face at rest, hyperactive gag and jaw jerk, slowed succession movements of the lips and tongue, excessive pooling of saliva and "emotional incontinence" (mild emotional stimuli cause an exaggerated grin or giggle, a so-called cortical "release phenomenon," which relatives often wrongly interpret as a sign of normal intelligence). *Hemiplegia* implies involvement of the arm, leg and face on one side; *diplegia* implies involvement of all four extremities but with greater involvement of the legs than the arms; *quadriplegia* (or *tetraplegia*) implies equal involvement of all four extremities; *paraplegia* signifies involvement of the legs only.

Hemiplegia

One of the commonest types of cerebral palsy, spastic hemiplegia often has either a congenital basis or complicates a series of severe convulsions (see Chapter 16, acute infantile hemiplegia or acute toxic encephalopathy). Despite this generalization the possibility of other causes must always be carefully considered, particularly treatable conditions such as subdural hematoma, slow-growing tumors (especially in the brain stem and spinal canal), multiple sclerosis and degenerative or metabolic disorders. In the neonate the subtle signs of hemiparesis are often overlooked or the findings are attributed to a brachial plexus injury, since the arm is usually more affected than the leg. Later the unilateral spastic weakness and hyperreflexia become obvious. The patient postures the arm in about 90-degree flexion at the elbow, he does not swing it normally and he circumducts or drags the affected leg. In mild cases the leg involvement may be reflected only by greater wear on the toe rather than the heel of the shoe.

Perlstein and Hood[12,13] documented the frequency of seizures and mental retardation in these patients. Among 173 patients, 76 had seizures and the mean IQ score was about 80 (average of general population = 100). Hemiplegic children with seizures had an average IQ of 70 compared to an average of 82 among patients without seizures.

If the patient does not have normal cortical sensation (stereognosis) in the affected hand, the hand cannot be expected to become a useful one. Patients with long-standing hemiparesis, both congenital and acquired, often show a typical constellation of skull x-ray changes—the so-called Davidoff-Dyke-Masson syndrome—and a dilated ventricular system on the side of the lesion. Both of these x-ray abnormalities give evidence of a chronically shrunken hemisphere but tell nothing about the basic cause of the lesion.

MANAGEMENT.—Patients who have spastic hemiplegia should be given the benefit of careful evaluation, anticonvulsant therapy if necessary, special education according to their intellectual potential and continuous physical therapy.[4] Although nobody has yet devised a drug, an operation or a manipulative program to abolish or reduce spasticity satisfactorily, good rehabilitative therapy is essential. Physical therapy is intended (1) to prevent deformities with range-of-motion and stretching exercises as well as braces and night splints; (2) to treat the deformities, i.e., if intensive stretching and adequate bracing does not correct a deformity, wedging casts, tenotomies, muscle transplants and neurectomies may be necessary; (3) to train the affected extremities with the aid of specialists in physical therapy, and (4) to concentrate upon teaching the activities of daily living (eating, brushing the teeth, combing the hair). Activities which require two hands, such as dressing, tying bows and cutting food, may be very difficult, especially if there is astereognosis in the paretic hand.

In a certain number of patients an increasingly troublesome organic behavior disorder develops with age. This may be modified with tranquilizing or sedative drug therapy (Chapter 1). A highly selected, small percentage of them may be considered candidates for hemispherectomy[14] if they have (1) a severe spastic hemiplegia, (2) drug-refractory seizures and (3) an unmanageable behavior disorder. In carefully selected patients the results are surprisingly good in terms of behavioral improvement,[11] better seizure control, no worsening of the motor deficit and no loss of speech (in patients with a congenital defect) even if the left hemisphere is removed.

Diplegia

This syndrome can result from a variety of causes, but a high percentage of cases are due to congenital malformations or to prematurity with or without neonatal asphyxia. Bilateral spasticity and pseudobulbar phenomena predominate. In older children kyphosis or kyphoscoliosis often develops from spastic muscles in the trunk. Mental retardation is present in most of these patients, usually to a degree greater than that seen in spastic hemiplegia. Exceptional patients with spastic diplegia have only motor deficit with no demonstrable intellectual deficit. Convulsive disorders are also common.

Pseudobulbar Palsy

The pseudobulbar signs account for the common feeding difficulties in infancy, the persistent drooling later and the apparently "happy" attitude of these patients.

MANAGEMENT.—Treatment closely resembles that described for patients with hemiplegia. Therapy must be tailored, however, to the patient's intellectual potential, and the physician must use careful judgment before recommending extensive physiotherapy, bracing and reparative surgery in patients who are severely retarded mentally.

Quadriplegia

The distinction between diplegia and quadriplegia is often a fine one and depends upon the greater degree of upper extremity spasticity. The differential diagnosis, workup and management are identical for the two syndromes.

Paraplegia

This term is applied when corticospinal tract signs involve the legs only and are caused by a lesion in the spinal cord. If ancillary clinical signs of cerebral disease are found, the term "diplegia" is generally used. In the differential diagnosis intraspinal tumors must be considered carefully—even in newborn infants (Fig. 17.14, p. 274)—along with demyelinating disease. Therapy depends upon the specific diagnosis. Chronic spasticity in the legs is managed in the same manner as other clinical forms of spasticity (see Hemiplegia).

Ataxia

This chronic motor disorder is not as common as spasticity. It causes incoordination of the extremities and/or trunk, a coarse tremor of the arms and hands with intentional movements, titubation (tremulous, rocking movements of the head and trunk when erect) and an unsteady, wide-based, staggering gate. In many cases hypotonia and hyporeflexia occur with ataxia. Rapid, alternating hand movements are slow and irregular, and increased excursion of the movement is noted. Most cases occur with congenital cerebellar defects or as a result of hypotonia in patients with cerebral atonic diplegia. In patients with advanced hydrocephalus ataxia follows compression of the midline vermis. The differential diagnosis is considered in Chapter 9.

Symptomatic therapy of ataxia is limited largely to gait training by a physical therapist.

Myoclonus

Rhythmic, repetitive, involuntary jerking of a group of muscles is called *myoclonus*. It occurs most commonly in patients with epilepsy, but it can be a symptom of a wide range of nervous system diseases.[1]

DIFFERENTIAL DIAGNOSIS.—Myoclonic seizures of infants and children under about 5 years of age constitute a common form of minor motor epilepsy. Older children and adults may have myoclonic jerking as a manifestation of idiopathic epilepsy. In both cases one finds epileptiform EEG abnormalities and the patients exhibit loss or lapses of consciousness.

In rare situations, when myoclonus is associated with dementia and neurologic deficit, the constellation of clinical signs is caused by diffuse neuronal disease. Examples of such diseases include the cerebral lipidoses, subacute leukoencephalitis and progressive familial disorders (Unverricht's disease, Lafora's disease and the Ramsay-Hunt syndrome). Occasionally diffuse myoclonus is seen in patients without seizures, dementia or other neurologic deficit. This nonprogressive disorder has been called *paramyoclonus multiplex*.[7] Its etiology and neuropathologic basis are poorly understood. In these cases diagnosis depends upon tissue examination, either from biopsy or autopsy specimens.[8]

MANAGEMENT AND PROGNOSIS.—Treatment of myoclonus as a manifestation of epilepsy is covered in Chapter 2. No other specific therapy is helpful.

When myoclonus appears in infancy, about 90% of the patients are mentally retarded. In the case of idiopathic epilepsy the prognosis is much better (Chapter 14).

Choreoathetosis

Choreoathetosis is not as common as spasticity and is characterized by fine, jerking movements of small and large skeletal muscles *(chorea),* often associated with slow, twisting, "wormy" movements *(athetosis).*[3] Neonatal hyperbilirubinemia causes most cases of choreoathetosis or kernicterus, but some are caused by severe perinatal anoxia. The syndrome also appears in patients with Huntington's chorea and, according to some, is a sign of congenital malformation of the basal ganglia.

MANAGEMENT.—Patients with this type of movement disorder often are benefited by tranquilizing drug therapy (chlorpromazine, Serpasil). In exceptional cases of nonprogressive choreoathetosis, pallidotomy is considered but operation is contraindicated in the presence of diffuse neurologic deficit.

The differential diagnosis of choreoathetosis and the extremely rare chronic movement disorders such as *rigidity, tremor* and *dystonia* are covered in Chapter 9.

Mirror Movements

With the natural movements of a hand or extremity one occasionally sees the mirrored replica of the movements (with a smaller excursion) in the opposite hand or extremity. Such movements may follow a dominant pattern of inheritance and may occur with or without other signs of congenital neurologic defects. Incomplete medullary decussation of the corticospinal tracts has been suggested as the explanation for this curious phenomenon.[10] In children with mirror movements, look especially for malformations of the spine and spinal cord, as are seen in the Klippel-Feil deformity and syringomyelia.[6]

BIBLIOGRAPHY

1. Aigner, B. R., and Mulder, D. W.: Myoclonus, Arch. Neurol. 2:600, 1960.
2. Brandt, S.: Amyotonia congenita—a symptom and not a separate disorder, J. Child. Psychiat. 1:266, 1948.
3. Byers, R. K., *et al.*: Extrapyramidal cerebral palsy with hearing loss following erythroblastosis, Pediatrics 15:248, 1955.
4. Deaver, G.: Treatment of the spastic hemiplegic, Am. J. Phys. Med. 35:32, 1956.
5. Engel, W. K., and Hogenhuis, L. A. H.: Genetically determined myopathies (Symposium Review of Current Concepts of Myopathies), Clin. Orthop. 39:34, 1965.
6. Ford, F. R.: *Diseases of the Nervous System in Infancy, Childhood and Adolescence* (5th ed.; Springfield, Ill.: Charles C Thomas, Publisher, 1966).
7. Friedreich, N.: Paramyoklonus multiplex, Arch. path. Anat. 86:421, 1881.
8. Greenfield, J. G.: *Neuropathology* (2d ed.; Baltimore: Williams & Wilkins Company, 1963).
9. Greenfield, J. G., *et al.*: The prognostic value of the muscle biopsy in the "floppy infant," Brain 81:461, 1958.
10. Haerer, A. F., and Currier, R. D.: Mirror movements, Neurology 16:757, 1966.
11. Munz, A., and Tolor, A.: Psychological effects of major cerebral excision: Intellectual and emotional changes following hemispherectomy, J. Nerv. & Ment. Dis. 121:438, 1955.
12. Perlstein, M. A., and Hood, P. N.: Infantile spastic hemiplegia: I. Incidence, Pediatrics 14:436, 1954.
13. Perlstein, M. A., and Hood, P. N.: Infantile spastic hemiplegia: III. Intelligence, Pediatrics 15:676, 1955.
14. Ransohoff, J., and Carter, S.: Hemispherectomy in the treatment of convulsive seizures associated with infantile hemiplegia, Neurol. & Psychiat. Childhood 34:176, 1956.
15. Walton, J. N.: Amyotonia congenita: Follow-up study, Lancet 1:1023, 1956.
16. Yannet, H., and Horton, F.: Hypotonic cerebral palsy in mental defectives, Pediatrics 9:204, 1952.

4

Abnormal Head Size and Shape

Size
    Small Head Size   Closure of the Anterior Fontanel
    Large Head Size
Shape
    General Asymmetry   Prominent Temporal Area
    Specific Deformities   Localized Bulging
    Frontal Bossing   Facial Deformities (Orbital Hypo- and Hypertelorism)
    Prominent Occiput

Abnormal Head Size

DESPITE THE COMMON OCCURRENCE of *small head size* (microcrania), parents rarely seek medical help for this reason alone unless the patient has the severe form of so-called "true" microcephaly which behaves as an autosomal recessive trait. In this case the head appears grotesquely small and even parents notice the problem. Usually the physician makes this observation first and investigates it. In contrast, *large head size* (macrocrania) is often noted by parents or relatives and they seek diagnostic help. In other cases, associated symptoms lead the patient to the physician's office.

SYNDROME DIAGNOSIS.—The diagnosis of abnormal head size is made either by comparing single measurements of the OFC (occipital frontal circumference) with the normal average head size for age and sex (Appendix 7) or by noting excessive head growth after serial measurements (Fig. 4.1). All physicians who see children routinely in their practice should measure and record head size since it reflects brain growth accurately.[7] Deciding whether head size is normal or abnormal on the basis of one measurement is important but at times difficult. In general, disease is suspected if the head circumference deviates *more than 2 standard deviations* below (bottom 2% of the population) or above (top 98% of the population) the mean measurement for that age and sex.[10]

Two extenuating circumstances complicate interpretation in borderline cases: (1) the comparison of head size to general body size (as measured by chest circumference or body length) and (2) the factor of prematurity. Unfortunately, as yet no dependable statistical rules can be laid down to compensate for these

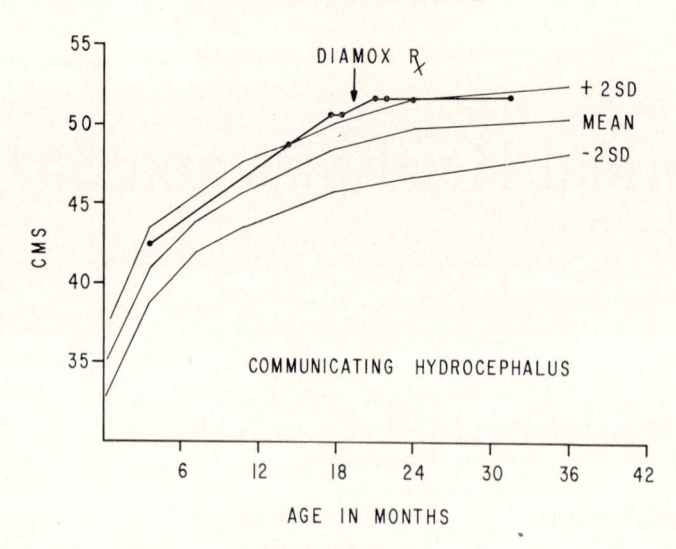

Fig. 4.1.—Serial measures of head size. This patient exhibited head enlargement, delayed motor development and mild ventricular dilatation. Diagnosis was low-grade communicating hydrocephalus. Therapy with acetazolamide (Diamox) arrested head growth (see Chapter 13).

two variables in clinical diagnosis. However, we believe that a discrepancy between head growth and somatic growth (either chest circumference or body length) has more diagnostic significance than absolute head size measurements alone. In other words, an OFC falling 2 standard deviations below the mean and the chest circumference near the mean suggest the diagnosis of microcrania. Conversely, an OFC of 1–2 standard deviations above the mean in a patient with neurologic symptoms and signs and with a chest circumference that is average or below may signify excessive head growth. If the general body size is 1–2 standard deviations below the mean for sex and age and the head is also 1–2 standard deviations below average, it is more difficult to conclude that one is dealing with microcephaly. However, some workers have suggested that brain growth (or head size) continues, independent of poor somatic growth,[8] and we would agree with this proposition on the basis of our experience. Dependable clinical rules of thumb for evaluating head size in prematures have not been collected, so that we use the same general principles as outlined here but make interpretations cautiously.

DIFFERENTIAL DIAGNOSIS.—*Small head size (microcrania).*—Basically only two conditions cause true microcrania: (1) *microcephaly,* the failure of normal brain growth, and (2) severe *craniostenosis,* which prevents the head from expanding normally. Because microcephaly causes microcrania much more commonly than does craniostenosis, the term is generally used loosely by the clinician to indicate small head size. Microcephaly is characterized by clinical signs of retardation (Table 1.3, p. 7) and essentially normal head shape. It should be understood that skull x-rays in patients with microcephaly may show early suture closure but, to repeat, the head is not misshapen (see discussion under Abnormal Head Shape). In our experience the coexistence of true craniostenosis and normal or small head size without head deformity occurs rarely and should suggest the diagnosis of hypophosphatasia (Chapter 21).

Microcephaly has several different causes: a variety of congenital malformations, a variety of metabolic and degenerative diseases, hypoxia, and infections of the nervous system, either prenatal or postnatal, which have caused irreparable damage to the brain. A recent study[6] suggests that cytomegalovirus infection should be considered in any infant with microcephaly if another good explanation is not available, even though systemic evidence of the disease is lacking. It has been established that excessive irradiation to the fetus can cause microcephaly,[9,11] but the effect of radiation upon the infant and child after birth is not yet known. The management and counseling of parents of children with retarded development is covered under Mental Retardation in Chapter 1.

Large head size (macrocrania).—The many causes of head enlargement and a working approach to the differential diagnosis are presented in Table 4.1. We wish to stress that subdural hematoma should be considered before all other diagnoses because the most experienced physicians often tend to think first of hydrocephalus. They proceed with workup accordingly and sometimes overlook a subdural collection. The other considerations are obvious (Table 4.1) and depend upon appropriate clinical and laboratory findings, nearly all of which cause head enlargement by producing some type of obstructive hydrocephalus. A rare group of bony deformities of the skull and spine—Klippel-Feil deformity, chondrodystrophy, gargoylism, platybasia and osteopetrosis—causes communicating hydrocephalus, presumably by crowding the structures in the posterior fossa. When all other diagnoses have been excluded, one should remember that occasionally enlarged heads are caused by excessive brain size—megalencephaly. In most of

TABLE 4.1.—DIFFERENTIAL DIAGNOSTIC WORKUP IN PATIENTS WITH HEAD ENLARGEMENT

	ROUTINE STUDIES	SPECIAL STUDIES
Subdural hematoma Brain tumor Hydrocephalus	Skull x-rays Electroencephalography Subdural taps	Lumbar puncture, funduscopy and pneumoencephalography (under sedation)
Lead poisoning	Urine sugar and coproporphyrin determination Blood smear for basophilic stippling	
Chronic meningitis	Complete CSF examination (cell count, chemistries, routine and special culture)—acid fast and India ink stains	
Bony anomalies of skull and cervical spine		Cervical spine x-rays
Gargoylism		Urine test for mucopolysaccharides
Cerebral lipidoses		Bone marrow examination Biopsy of rectal mucosa, spleen or liver
"Megalencephaly"		

the latter cases diagnosis can be established only at autopsy. We do not advocate brain biopsy in such patients unless it can be done at the time of ventriculography. Even then one can expect a low diagnostic yield except in cases of suspected Tay-Sachs disease. Most of the time brain biopsies prove fruitless because the neurosurgeon is understandably reluctant to remove enough tissue to satisfy the pathologist.

Macrocrania is managed according to the specific diagnosis which is made. Many of these patients suffer permanent neurologic deficit, and appropriate counseling should be given.

Closure of the anterior fontanel.—In any large series of normal infants the time at which the anterior fontanel closes varies greatly, and the examiner should therefore be cautious in making clinical interpretations based upon the size of this fontanel. In a series of 1,677 babies, the age of closing varied from 7 to 19 months with the mean being about 1 year of age.[1] Excessively early closure should suggest underlying microcephaly, craniosynostosis or hypophosphatasia. Delayed fontanel closure may result from increased intracranial pressure (Chapter 8) and the various causes of retarded somatic growth, including hypothyroidism.

Abnormal Head Shape

SYNDROME DIAGNOSIS.—Many patients are seen because of a misshapen head and, in contrast to observations about head size, many overinterpretations are made. One should cautiously review all of the clinical, x-ray and laboratory findings before attaching significance to a misshapen head. Obviously, in severe cases no great caution is needed and a thorough workup is undertaken. The various head deformities can be divided arbitrarily into the following categories: (1) generalized asymmetry, (2) gross head deformity suggesting premature suture closure, (3) frontal bossing, (4) prominent occiput, (5) prominent temporal areas and (6) localized, circumscribed bulging.

Generalized asymmetry of the head, usually with parietal-occipital flattening on one side and bulging of the diagonal frontal area, results from positioning of the head in an infant who does not sit. It is seen commonly in the premature whose skull is soft and who reaches his motor milestones slowly. It also is seen for the same basic reason in the infant who is retarded because of mental defect or parental neglect. As indicated in Chapter 19 (p. 347), skull and facial asymmetry may result from congenital torticollis.

The head circumference should be checked carefully in patients with misshapen heads, and in unusual cases skull x-rays may be necessary. In general, no therapy is needed and parents should be reassured that if the head size is normal, the deformity will clear as the child ages or will become less noticeable as the hair grows longer. If the physician suspects parental neglect, appropriate psychosocial investigation is indicated. Obviously, when the deformity is associated with microcephaly or other signs of neurologic deficit, the prognosis must be guarded.

Gross head deformities which suggest premature suture closure are listed, along with associated physical defects, in Table 13.1 (p. 157). The physician should never forget that proved craniostenosis may occur as one of a constellation of anomalies or as a solitary defect. A complete discussion of this subject is covered in Chapter 13. Many normal premature infants exhibit prominent anteroposterior head growth which gives a scaphocephalic appearance, a finding which should be interpreted conservatively.

Frontal bossing may represent a normal familial variant and should be interpreted only in conjunction with other physical and laboratory evidence. Subdural hematoma, hydrocephalus and, rarely, rickets should be considered in babies with this sign.

A prominent occiput is quite often the reason one is asked to examine an infant. In many cases no disease is uncovered, but when rapid head growth or delayed development is noted, the Dandy-Walker form of obstructive hydrocephalus should be considered. The latter anomaly allegedly causes preferential enlargement of the posterior fossa by virtue of the atresia of the fourth ventricular foramina. We have been impressed with the fact that many normal infants have a prominent occiput yet in some patients with the Dandy-Walker anomaly it fails to develop. Hence the finding by itself has only equivocal significance.

Prominent temporal areas may not indicate intracranial disease, especially if this prominence is found bilaterally in husky children. Occasionally, however, bulging signifies a localized intracranial mass, often unilateral, which has gradually "ironed out" the calvarium and caused prominence of the temple or temples. A long-standing subdural hematoma in the middle cranial fossa or a slow-growing temporal lobe tumor may cause the deformity (Fig. 15.5, p. 207).

Localized or circumscribed bulging of the skull suggests (1) a primary tumor of the skull, (2) a slow-growing meningioma—a rare brain tumor in children, (3) a benign exostosis, (4) an encephalocele, (5) a cephalhematoma or caput succedaneum, if it occurs in the newborn, or (6) dura bulging through a surgical or traumatic defect. Appropriate x-ray studies are diagnostic of these specific diseases, which are managed according to the descriptions in Part II.

FACIAL DEFORMITIES.—It is well known that severe deformities of the eyes, the nose, the lip and the palate are often associated with defects in the development of the skull and the brain. Excessively large and small heads call one's attention to intracranial disease and represent an important factor in prognosis. In addition, eyes which are situated too close together (hypotelorism) or too far apart (hypertelorism) may be associated with significant anomalies of the nervous system. The clinician can usually make a dependable diagnosis of orbital hypotelorism or hypertelorism by simple inspection, but sometimes he is misled by a flat nasal bridge, epicanthal folds, convergent or divergent squints and anomalies of the eyebrows, the lids or the inner canthi. In such cases it is useful to refer to objective normal standards of interorbital distance, as defined by Gerald and Silverman.[5] These measurements vary with age.

Orbital hypotelorism.—Eyes which lie too close together are associated in a high percentage of cases with arhinencephaly (holoprosencephaly) or trigonocephaly.[2] Several workers have suggested different categories of arhinencephaly based on the severity of associated anomalies involving the eyes, the nose, the lip and the palate.[4] Trigonocephaly may be seen without an associated anomaly of the nervous system or in association with arhinencephaly.

Orbital hypertelorism.—The eyes may show abnormal separation by objective measurement and this may be associated with other facial anomalies (V-shaped hairline, occult cranium bifidum and cleft nose, lip or palate) and with extrafacial defects. Such findings may be associated with neurologic defect, but this is not seen as frequently as it is in cases of orbital hypotelorism.[3]

BIBLIOGRAPHY

1. Aisenson, M. R.: Closing of the anterior fontanelle, Pediatrics 6:223, 1950.
2. Currarino, G., and Silverman, F. N.: Orbital hypotelorism, arhinencephaly and trigonocephaly, Radiology 74:206, 1960.
3. DeMyer, W.: The median cleft face syndrome, Neurology 17:961, 1967.
4. DeMyer, W., *et al.*: The face predicts the brain: Diagnostic significance of median facial anomalies for holoprosencephaly (arhinencephaly), Pediatrics 34:256, 1964.
5. Gerald, B. E., and Silverman, F. N.: Normal and abnormal interorbital distances, with special reference to mongolism, Am. J. Roentgenol. 95:154, 1965.
6. Hanshaw, J. B.: Cytomegalovirus complement-fixing antibody in microcephaly, New England J. Med. 275:476, 1966.
7. Nellhaus, G.: Head circumference from birth to eighteen years, Pediatrics 41:106, 1968.
8. O'Connell, E. J., *et al.*: Head circumference, mental retardation, and growth failure, Pediatrics 36:62, 1965.
9. Plummer, G.: Anomalies occurring in children exposed in utero to the atomic bomb in Hiroshima, Pediatrics 10:687, 1952.
10. Vickers, V. S., and Stuart, H. C.: Anthropometry in the pediatrician's office—norms for selected body measurements based on studies of children of north European stock, J. Pediat. 22:155, 1943.
11. Yamazaki, J. N., *et al.*: Outcome of pregnancy in women exposed to atomic bomb in Nagasaki, Am. J. Dis. Child. 87:448, 1954.

5

Proptosis

Congenital Malformations
    Orbital Encephalocele   Polyostotic Fibrous Dysplasia
    Vascular Malformation (Hemangioma)
Tumors
    Dermoid Cyst   Neurofibroma (von Recklinghausen's Disease)
    Teratoma   Metastatic Neuroblastoma
    Optic Nerve Glioma   Rhabdomyosarcoma
Infections
    Chronic Orbital Cellulitis with Myositis
    Granuloma (Congenital Syphilis)

EXOPHTHALMOS, which occurs uncommonly in children, calls for a differential diagnosis of "tumors" of the orbit. In most reported series the etiology of the exophthalmos corresponds closely to the order of the conditions listed in the outline above.[1,2]

    Occasionally parents will seek medical help for a young child because of a prominent or bulging eye. More often the complaints will be those of facial asymmetry, ptosis, ocular squint or diplopia, eye pain or headache, or signs of inflammation of the lid and conjunctiva. With any of these complaints one should consider orbital tumor and, as part of a complete examination, one should ask an ophthalmologist to carry out exophthalmometry. When the proptosis becomes advanced, the globe is displaced forward, downward and either out or in. Limited range of motion of one or more extraocular muscles can often be demonstrated, and it may be difficult by examination alone to distinguish true neurologic from muscular deficit. Associated abnormalities of the pupil and optic nerve head are common. The examiner should listen for a bruit over the eyeball and look for evidence of systemic disease. In particular, examination should include abdominal palpation for tumor and a search for café-au-lait spots and subcutaneous nodules. X-rays of the skull, orbits (including optic foramen views), chest, abdomen and long bones should be obtained. When a metastatic lesion is suspected, intravenous urography is carried out.

MANAGEMENT.—Treatment of this clinical problem requires expert consultation because few physicians have accumulated enough experience to avoid diagnostic pitfalls. Obviously, operation is necessary for many of these lesions, but one must guard against surgical intervention in cases of infectious processes in the orbit, such as inflammatory pseudotumor. When operation is indicated, most experienced neurosurgeons prefer to do a transfrontal craniotomy rather than an anterior exploration because they are better able to manage a tumor which has an intracranial extension with this technique.

BIBLIOGRAPHY

1. Ingraham, F. D., and Matson, D. D.: *Neurosurgery of Infancy and Childhood* (Springfield, Ill.: Charles C Thomas, Publisher, 1961).
2. MacCarty, C. S., and Brown, D. N.: Orbital Tumors in Children, in *Clinical Neurosurgery,* Proceedings of Congress of Neurological Surgeons, Vol. 11 (Baltimore: Williams & Wilkins Company, 1964).

6

Language Disorders

Congenital Language Disorders
    Mental Retardation
    Deafness
        Rubella   Nephritis
        Kernicterus   Osteogenesis imperfecta
        Turner's syndrome
    Visual Deficit or Oculomotor Apraxia
    Chronic Motor Disorders (Cerebral Palsy)
    Anomalies of Peripheral Speech Organs
        Palate   Teeth
        Lips   Tongue
    Developmental Language Disorders
        Developmental dyslexia (congenital word blindness)
        Developmental agraphia
        Stuttering
        Developmental dysarthria
        Developmental word deafness (congenital auditory imperception)
        Developmental motor aphasia
Acquired Language Disorders
    Aphasia
        Convulsive disorder   Tumor
        Post-traumatic   Cerebrovascular accident
        Postencephalitis   Degenerative disease
    Dysarthria
        Bell's palsy   Tumor of the brain stem
        Poliomyelitis   Muscle disease—myasthenia gravis
        Degenerative disease—Friedreich's ataxia
    Psychogenic Language Disorders
    Sociocultural Deprivation

Speech Disorders

SYNDROME DIAGNOSIS.—Medical help is often sought for children who exhibit (1) slow speech development, (2) poor pronunciation, (3) poor reading ability and (4) poor writing ability. In general, if a child is not saying understandable words by age 2, one should search for an explanation. A few children who are otherwise quite normal have close relatives with a history of equally slow speech development, and they are simply "slow talkers." The average child says his first single words between 10 and 12 months of age, has a vocabulary of about 18 words and is beginning to say phrases at 18 months, and uses sentences at 30 months. A diagnostic study should be carried out in those children whose speech articulation, reading ability and writing ability are clearly substandard for their age.

The following studies should be carried out in every child in whom the language problem is severe enough to worry the family, the physician or the teacher: (1) complete general and neurologic examination, (2) tests of intelligence, (3) hearing tests and (4) vision tests.

DIFFERENTIAL DIAGNOSIS.—The various causes of language disorders are given in the outline at the beginning of the chapter.

MANAGEMENT.—Speech therapy is recommended and given to numerous slow talkers and those with speech impediments. However, we have no objective evidence to determine how much benefit is derived from this effort. If speech therapists are conveniently available, if the family is anxious to obtain help and if the investment of time and effort does not seriously drain a family's financial resources, it certainly seems worth the effort. However, when the effort is undertaken, it is incumbent upon the physician to keep an objective, sympathetic attitude and to have the family maintain reasonable expectations for improvement.

Congenital Language Disorders
MENTAL RETARDATION, DEAFNESS, BLINDNESS AND CEREBRAL PALSY

Most children whose speech and language development is significantly delayed or impaired have defective intellect. This can be detected by careful observation, examination and intelligence testing. One must rule out defective hearing and vision in all such patients because, obviously, partially deaf patients will have impaired speech development and partially blind patients will have trouble learning to read and write. Many patients with chronic motor deficit, including those with spasticity, athetosis, ataxia and chorea, have speech problems. The centrally caused speech difficulties in the latter group result from either dysarthria or associated mental retardation. On rare occasions examples of so-called congenital aphasia may occur,[5] but we believe this is a poorly conceived term which is misused in most cases.

ANOMALIES OF SPEECH ORGANS

Patients with structural anomalies of the peripheral speech apparatus (i.e., the palate, lips, teeth and tongue) also have speech defects, especially those with cleft palate, cleft lip and severe jaw deformities.

Developmental Language Disorders

Among the vast number of slow learners, poor readers and poor speakers in the world, a small, hard core exhibit selective language disability whose basic nature is poorly understood but which is presumably present at birth. In 1937 Orton[7] classified these different but related conditions into the categories listed in the outline on page 67. Despite a proliferation of terms to describe these clinical syndromes over the past generation, relatively little additional factual information on etiology and pathogenesis has been introduced. Better clinical descriptions and more accurate data about incidence, prognosis and therapy have clarified our working concepts and management to some extent.

These disorders represent categories of clinical convenience and not disease conditions per se.

ETIOLOGY AND PATHOGENESIS.—In developmental word blindness (dyslexia), stuttering (or stammering), word deafness and some cases of agraphia a definite familial incidence has been noted.[4] Poorly established cerebral dominance with a high incidence of left-handedness and ambidexterity has been noted among affected patients and their relatives. To the best of our knowledge no neuropathologic studies have ever been reported on a series of these patients and so the structural basis for the disorders is unknown. Convincing studies about the etiologic role of prenatal and natal disease have not been done. Sir Russell Brain[1] has said that the failure to establish a dominant hemisphere is probably the result and not the cause of congenital disabilities in speech, reading and writing.

Developmental Dyslexia (Congenital Word Blindness)

SYNDROME DIAGNOSIS.—The physician must be keenly aware of the variation in language skills exhibited by the normal population and realize that, whereas one person can become fluent in several languages simultaneously, another may never develop facility of expression in his native tongue despite average or superior general intelligence. However, among the world's many thousands of backward readers there is a small percentage with a selective disability that does not result from mental retardation, poor motivation, inattention, poor vision, inadequate teaching or neurotic behavior. The practical handicap consists of reading retardation, often associated with poor spelling and poor writing. Usually the reading age lags 20% or two school years behind the mental age despite two or more years of regular school attendance.

These children have a fundamental disability in (1) breaking up the written word into sounds and letters—this leads to mispronunciation—and in (2) separating the spoken word into phonic units—this causes much misspelling; or (3) they have the tendency to read words from right to left wholly or in part—this leads to many mistakes in spelling, with partial letter reversals of long words and complete letter reversal of short words. This combination of disabilities accounts for the common correlation between reading, spelling and writing difficulty. In addition to reversals the dyslexic child often exhibits mirror writing (see Differential Diagnosis). Mirror writing in the dyslexic is considered secondary to mirror reading because the patient, when asked to copy words, reverses the order of letters and reverses single letters.

Critchley,[2] who has studied the problem extensively, has found a familial incidence of dyslexia in most cases studied and a 4:1 ratio of affected boys to girls. He has also found a high incidence of left-handedness and ambidexterity among dyslexic children and their near relatives as well as nonspecific clumsiness or awkwardness.

DIFFERENTIAL DIAGNOSIS.—Before making a diagnosis of this specific and uncommon language disorder, the physician should carry out a careful evaluation of intelligence, vision, neurologic status and emotional state of the child. Mental retardation, impaired vision, emotional disturbances and poor motivation are most often the causes of poor reading. If psychologic problems are recognized in children with marked reading disability, one should realize that they may be the result and not the cause of the language disorder. Children with dyslexia may be rejected by their parents, considered lazy or stupid by the teacher and be outdone by their younger siblings.

Another uncommon cause of reading disability, congenital oculomotor apraxia, should be considered in the differential diagnosis. This disorder is discussed on page 90.

It is generally well known that normal children exhibit mirror writing for a short time while they are learning to write and that many adults can perform mirror writing, especially when they are using both hands simultaneously. Mirror writing is also seen more frequently in mentally retarded patients and in some patients who acquire a right hemiparesis.

MANAGEMENT AND PROGNOSIS.—Prompt diagnosis, which is the most important factor in treatment, may require expert consultation whenever the diagnosis of dyslexia is being considered. The children must have special, intensive instruction which emphasizes the "phonic" system of learning to read rather than the "flash" system of "look–say." At times, curriculum time usually devoted to other subjects must be sacrificed in order to save the child from ending up as an illiterate adult. As Critchley has pointed out, the problem should be treated with optimism, not hopelessness, realizing that dyslexics may never read for simple enjoyment but may develop the ability to read road signs, bus signs, the telephone book and newspapers—critical and basic abilities in urban societies of the 20th century.

Developmental Agraphia

This syndrome often occurs in left-handed children or in those who have been forced to write with their right hand. The disability is frequently associated with dyslexia but occasionally occurs as a solitary disability. Diagnosis and treatment are approached in the same way as in patients with dyslexia.

Stuttering (or Stammering)

SYNDROME DIAGNOSIS.—This easily recognized disorder of articulation is characterized by (1) repetition of syllables and (2) prolonged articulation of words. The additional features of facial contractions, tics, hissing and grunting usually reflect the stutterer's attempt to correct the defect or result from emotional stress. Many stutterers add additional, pointless phrases to their speech in order to lubricate the flow of words. Of interest is the fact that they can often sing or recite without difficulty. One must realize that the young child learning to talk normally repeats sounds, words and phrases; this should not be confused with real stuttering which is a severe, persistent speech defect.

As in developmental dyslexia, there is a high incidence of left-handedness or ambidexterity in stutterers and their close relatives. Boys are affected 4 times as often as girls. In some patients the defect appears to result when handedness has been shifted from left to right. In individual cases psychiatrists have attributed the problem to emotional conflicts in early childhood, but the common association with signs of impaired cerebral dominance suggests a physiologic disability.

MANAGEMENT AND PROGNOSIS.—Mild stuttering often disappears spontaneously, as evidenced by the much higher incidence in children than in adults. Patients with severe disability can benefit from therapy, but some residual deficit often lasts a lifetime.

Patients should be managed with patience, understanding and reassurance. If the stutterer has not established dominance, he should be aided gently in a choice of handedness. If he has been forced to use his right hand after he has demonstrated natural left-handedness, this change should be reversed. Therapy should be sought from a speech pathologist or an expert teacher. These specialists teach breathing exercises and methods of relaxation, often aided by the use of diagrams of the vocal apparatus. We advise against routine psychiatric management of the problem.

Developmental Dysarthria

SYNDROME DIAGNOSIS.—This common but less serious disorder of language development is characterized by the faulty pronunciation of consonants. Affected children have trouble with the following consonants in this approximate order: r, sh, th (that), s, l, k, ch (church), dg (dodge), g, f, v, p, and b.

DIFFERENTIAL DIAGNOSIS.—As in the other language disorders one must certify that these patients have normal intelligence, normal hearing and no other neurologic deficits. Severe forms of developmental dysarthria are difficult if not impossible to distinguish from developmental motor aphasia, which in turn is difficult to differentiate from mental retardation.

MANAGEMENT.—Patients with uncomplicated developmental dysarthria usually respond well to conventional speech therapy of the type used in stutterers. The prognosis is quite good.

Developmental Word Deafness (Congenital Auditory Imperception)

For all practical purposes we have not been able to diagnose developmental word deafness or developmental motor aphasia. The distinction between these selective disabilities and the global syndrome of mental retardation is, in our experience, difficult or impossible.

SYNDROME DIAGNOSIS.—At an age when children usually start to talk (15 months) it is said that these children do not respond when spoken to and they do not learn to mimic words. At this time their hearing impairment must be differentiated from true deafness, which also hinders normal speech development.

Children with developmental word deafness are said to have normal hearing and normal intelligence. Eventually they develop a language of their own which resembles "baby talk" and has been called "idioglossia." Their comprehension of speech is greatly impaired when they cannot watch the speaker's lips, which indicates that they learn to read lips spontaneously.

As in developmental word blindness and stuttering, this disorder affects males more than females in a ratio of 5:1.

DIFFERENTIAL DIAGNOSIS.—As just indicated, these patients must be distinguished primarily from patients with true deafness. Because of the poor speech development, they appear mentally retarded, and because of their apparent mutism or failure to pay attention to speech, they can be confused with autistic children (Chapter 1). Especially important to differentiate from congenital auditory imperception is selective, high-tone deafness. The inaudible high tones lead to a defective type of speech development which resembles idioglossia. Therefore, the medical workup should include careful observation by the physician, psychometric tests and an audiometric examination which covers the complete range of tones.

MANAGEMENT AND PROGNOSIS.—These children, if taught to read lips, generally show improvement although there will be much variation in their progress.

Developmental Motor Aphasia

Children who are said to suffer this disability in its frank form are brought to the physician because they have no speech. Since they can often only grunt or make unintelligible sounds, they are frequently considered mentally defective. If they show good comprehension by following commands and making intelligent gestures, there is reason to consider the basic intelligence normal. If the disorder exists in the pure state, it must be extremely rare. In our experience the vast majority of such children are retarded for practical purposes.

Acquired Language Disorders

Most acquired disorders of language result from organic structural disease of the nervous system. However, many children from socially and culturally deprived homes come to one's attention in the early school years because of reading retardation. Eisenberg[3] has emphasized the need to be aware of this great problem and to attack it both prophylactically and therapeutically.

Hysterical dysphonia also occurs rarely in children.

APHASIA

Severe damage to the motor speech area as the result of a head injury, encephalitis, cerebrovascular accident, tumor or degenerative disease (e.g., Schilder's disease) can cause aphasia in children as well as in adults. Children who have a left hemispherectomy for a congenitally atrophic hemisphere do not become aphasic, indicating that speech centers can develop in the minor hemisphere if the pathologic lesion is acquired early enough in life. One cannot expect such a transfer of speech in older children who have already acquired speech.

Acquired aphasia also occurs as a manifestation of epilepsy. This phenomenon, which is illustrated in Figure 1.5 (p. 19), and well described by Landau and Kleffner,[6] often causes considerable clinical confusion. A diagnosis of deafness or psychosis is also often made in these patients. Although the electroclinical syndrome may reflect only a static seizure disorder, one must rule out such progressive processes as brain tumor, degenerative diseases, brain abscess, subdural hematoma, intoxications, rare metabolic disorders and diffuse collagen vascular disease.

Dysarthria

Defective articulation of words (dysarthria) results from weakness caused by disease of the muscle or lower motor neuron. Bell's palsy (inflammation or injury of the facial nerve), poliomyelitis, tumors of the brain stem, myasthenia gravis and some degenerative diseases (e.g., Friedreich's ataxia) commonly cause dysarthria.

Psychogenic Language Disorders

Serious psychologic disorders in the home or in the child's past experience can delay speech development and perpetuate "baby talk." Relatives often attribute a child's slow speech development to parental or sibling overindulgence ("he gets everything he wants without talking"). However, this explanation is rarely valid and one should search for more convincing explanations. The mutism which is seen in patients with infantile autism is discussed in Chapter 1 (p. 20).

Occasionally, dysarthria in which the child speaks in a faint whisper or very softly but with good articulation appears as an hysterical conversion reaction in middle childhood and should be handled with psychiatric help.

Sociocultural Deprivation

Among the many slow readers in the early school years one finds a certain number in whom the etiology seems to be a severely deprived background. These children must not be considered mentally retarded or labeled as dyslexic. Efforts should be made to better their home environment and enroll them in classes that will enrich their social experiences and stimulate language development in general. They may benefit from remedial reading classes and active social casework.

BIBLIOGRAPHY

1. Brain, W. R.: *Speech Disorders* (Washington, D. C.: Butterworth & Co., Ltd., 1961).
2. Critchley, M.: *Developmental Dyslexia* (London: William Heinemann, Ltd., 1964).
3. Eisenberg, L.: Reading retardation: I. Psychiatric and sociologic aspects, Pediatrics 37:352, 1966.
4. Ingram, T. T. S.: Specific developmental disorders of speech in childhood, Brain 82:450, 1959.
5. Landau, W. M., et al.: Congenital aphasia: A clinicopathological study, Neurology 10:915, 1957.
6. Landau, W. M., and Kleffner, F. R.: Syndrome of acquired aphasia with convulsive disorder in children, Neurology 7:523, 1957.
7. Orton, S. T.: *Reading, Writing and Speech Problems in Children* (New York City: W. W. Norton & Company, Inc., 1961).

7

Visual and Hearing Deficits

Visual Deficit
    Neurologic Causes
    Ocular Causes—Amblyopia
        Ocular squint (amblyopia ex anopsia)   Unknown cause
        Refractive error
Hearing Deficit
    True Deafness
        Nerve deafness
        Conduction deafness
    Apparent Deafness

Visual Deficit

SYNDROME DIAGNOSIS.—Impaired sight may be noted (1) on routine medical or school examination or is suspected or discovered because of: (2) clumsiness, frequent falls or bumping into objects, (3) the child's habit of holding objects unusually close to his eyes, (4) slow or poor reading, (5) abnormal eye movements, (6) strabismus, (7) proptosis, (8) a family history of high-grade refractive error, squint, nystagmus or poor vision, and (9) other eye or neurologic abnormalities.

Evaluation of vision in newborn infants is limited to a blinking response to bright lights and hand threat and the pupillary reaction to light. At 1 month or 6 weeks of age the child can fixate on bright objects and follow them jerkily for a short distance. The principle of opticokinetic ("railroad") nystagmus can be used to obtain a rough idea about the adequacy of visual acuity, visual fields and ocular movements. Conscious infants and children with normal mentality will develop opticokinetic nystagmus when a piece of cloth with alternating colored stripes or designs is drawn horizontally across the field of vision, from right to left and then left to right. This technique will sometimes demonstrate a hemianopic visual field defect.

The visual acuity gradually increases from the normal myopic state in infancy to adult acuity at age 7 years. Keeney[7] reports the following changes in acuity with aging:

```
4 months = 20/400      3 years   = 20/30
1 year   = 20/200      6-7 years = 20/20
2 years  = 20/40
```

However, up to 3 years of age accurate assessment of acuity is difficult or impossible. After age 3 some cooperative preschool children with normal intellect can be tested either with the Snellen picture chart or with the illiterate E test, after proper instruction. School-age children who have learned the names of letters can be tested easily with the standard Snellen chart since they usually like to demonstrate their knowledge.

The remainder of the evaluation should include: (1) the pupillary responses to light, examination of (2) the media, including the cornea and lens, (3) the optic nerve head and (4) the retina, (5) search for squint and (6) detection of nystagmus. The pupils of young children (except prematures) usually show brisk reactions to light and may show some size inequality which is often insignificant. Opacities of the media are visualized best with a +8 or +10 ophthalmoscope lens. One should also estimate refractive errors as follows: After the disc or macula is seen in clear focus, the ophthalmoscope lenses are rotated until the image just blurs; the preceding lens reading represents the approximate refractive error in diopters. If the final lens is plus, the patient is hyperopic; if minus, the patient is myopic. A completely accurate estimate is obtained only with a mydriatic.

Cogan[5] states that if *pendular* nystagmus is noted, i.e., if eye oscillations are approximately equal in the two horizontal directions when the eyes are looking straight ahead, *and* the patient has impaired central vision, one can assume that loss of vision in both eyes took place under 2 years of age. Between ages 2 and 6 loss of central vision results in irregular, roving eye movements, and after age 6 loss of central vision causes no abnormal eye movements. A discussion of ocular squint and more details about nystagmus are given in Chapter 9.

If there is evidence of an organic eye lesion, such as abnormal pupillary responses, medial opacities, abnormalities of the optic discs or retina, or nystagmus, a complete general neurologic investigation is in order. This should include (1) visual field examination, if possible, (2) skull x-rays for signs of increased pressure, calcifications and anomalies, (3) lumbar puncture, (4) optic foramen films and if necessary (5) a pneumoencephalogram.

REGIONAL AND DIFFERENTIAL DIAGNOSIS.—The various causes of defective vision are listed in Table 7.1. Only the more important conditions are discussed below, and others are covered in Part II.

Neurologic Causes

Lesions of optic nerve and chiasm.—Patients with lesions in the nerve usually have impaired central vision (Snellen chart), a sluggish, direct pupillary reaction to light and a brisk consensual light reaction. They may have papillitis in the acute stage and optic atrophy late, and scotomata may be demonstrated if a visual field study can be done. If the optic chiasm is affected by a compressive lesion, impairment of both temporal fields of vision is typically found. In addition, hypothalamic signs (Chapter 11) and obstructive hydrocephalus at the level of the third ventricle may occur. Increased intracranial pressure, regardless of etiology, repre-

TABLE 7.1.—DIFFERENTIAL DIAGNOSIS OF VISUAL DEFICIT

NEUROLOGIC CAUSES

Optic Nerve
  Increased intracranial pressure
    Acute (papilledema)
    Chronic (optic atrophy)
  Anomalies of optic apparatus

  Avulsion of optic nerve

  Tumors
    Optic nerve glioma
    Craniopharyngioma
    Frontal lobe tumor

  Infections
    Purulent and chronic meningitis

Optic Tract
  Intracerebral mass

Occipital Cortex (cortical blindness)
  Anoxia
    Cardiac arrest
    Status epilepticus
    CO poisoning

  Venous thrombosis
    Meningitis
    Metastatic tumor
      (neuroblastoma)

Intoxications
  Methyl alcohol
  Thallium

Degenerative and metabolic disease
  Hereditary optic atrophy
  Neurofibromatosis
  Spinocerebellar degeneration
  Cerebral lipidoses
  Pigmentary degeneration of retina

Demyelinating disease
  Optic neuritis
  Neuromyelitis optica

Malnutrition

Uncal herniation
  Subdural hematoma
  Supratentorial neoplasm

Disease in both occipital lobes
  Schilder's disease
  Brain abscesses

OCULAR CAUSES

Medial opacities
  Congenital rubella
  Excessive oxygen to prematures

Amblyopia
  Ocular squint (amblyopia ex anopsia)
  Refractive error
  Unknown cause

---

sents the commonest neurologic threat to vision. Congenital hydrocephalus and slow-growing tumors cause optic atrophy in a high percentage of the patients who survive the basic disease. In the obscure clinical syndrome, pseudotumor cerebri (Chapter 8), the physician must maintain adequate intracranial decompression over a period of weeks and months or expect to find some degree of optic atrophy at a later date.

Lesions of optic tract.—Any intracerebral lesion which affects the optic pathways behind the chiasm will cause a homonymous hemianopia, i.e., a left-sided cerebral lesion will produce a defect in the right field of vision but will spare the macular area, the dead center of the visual field. Most of these lesions are located in the optic radiations as they fan out in the temporal, parietal and occipital lobes behind the lateral geniculate body. Tumors, intracerebral blood clots, areas of encephalomalacia and brain abscesses commonly produce a hemianopia.

Cortical (central or cerebral) blindness.—This term refers to loss of vision resulting from damage to the calcarine or visual cortex via the basilar-vertebral system. The specific etiologies in children include anoxic damage from (1) cardiac arrest, often secondary to arrhythmias with congenital heart disease, (2) status epilepticus (Fig. 16.9, p. 238), (3) carbon monoxide poisoning, (4) venous thrombosis secondary to meningitis or metastatic tumor, (5) uncal herniation with compromise of the posterior cerebral circulation (secondary to subdural or epidural hematoma or other mass lesions) and (6) embolization. Much less commonly the syndrome results from a progressive degenerative disease involving the white matter of the occipital lobe, such as Schilder's disease (Fig. 21.15, p. 421), and bilateral occipital lobe abscesses.

Transient central blindness after seemingly trivial head injury has been reported in children by Griffith and Dodge.[6] The exact pathogenesis is unclear, but the absence of abnormal eye signs, the eventual return of vision to normal and the posterior slowing of brain waves suggest a temporary cerebral dysfunction.

Ocular Causes

If the patient has visual deficit without any evidence of an organic lesion of the eye (i.e., amblyopia), one should seek ophthalmologic consultation. *Amblyopia* is important because it represents the single most common cause of visual loss in children. Amblyopia can result from (1) an ocular squint (amblyopia ex anopsia—Chapter 9), (2) a refractive error, especially if the other eye has a smaller error or none at all or (3) no obvious cause.[9] Amblyopia ex anopsia or the "lazy eye" syndrome results from disuse of a squinting eye through an unconscious attempt by children under 6 to suppress diplopia. This type of visual impairment should not be considered irreversible. The reader is referred to ophthalmology texts for a discussion of amblyopia resulting from refractive errors and obscure causes.

MANAGEMENT AND PROGNOSIS.—The neurologic causes of visual deficit are discussed in Part II. Only amblyopia ex anopsia will be covered here.

Normal binocular, i.e., three dimensional or stereoscopic, vision in young children depends upon the development of *fixation* and *conjugate deviation* reflexes along with development of the *maculae*. If the patient has a squint, he either uses both eyes alternately, thereby maintaining normal acuity but failing to develop binocular vision, or he uses only one eye to avoid diplopia. The eye which is not used loses visual acuity, i.e., becomes amblyopic. It is important to realize that macular vision develops rapidly during the first 2 years of life and is completed by age 5. Therefore, if the squint develops in the first year of life and treatment is delayed until the third or fourth year, the resulting amblyopia may be irreversible to some extent (although improvement in acuity with occlusion or patching can be expected). If such a patient should lose the good eye for any reason, vision could be reduced to semi-blindness. When such children have, in addition, a severe refractive error which is not corrected with glasses until age 5, the visual acuity may not approach normal. Unless the vision in the squinting eye improves with treatment to within one line (on the Snellen chart) of the straight eye, stereoscopic vision cannot be expected. It is recommended that an ophthalmologic examination be carried out before the age of 9 months on all children of families with a history of gross refractive error or strabismus.[8]

Early detection and ophthalmologic therapy of an ocular squint is essential if one expects to obtain (1) good visual acuity, (2) stereoscopic vision and (3) a good cosmetic appearance. The "cross-eyed" or "cock-eyed" appearance causes embarrassment and anxiety to children and may interfere in some cases with occupational success in adult life.

Treatment by the ophthalmologist beginning at 6–9 months of age consists of (1) occlusion or patching of the turning eye, (2) operation on eye muscles, (3) corrective lenses (glasses) and (4) eye coordination exercises (orthoptics). Laws[8] states that orthoptics has value preoperatively to make the brain "fusion conscious" and postoperatively to promote fusion. Orthoptics has no therapeutic value in curing a crossed eye and its use by anyone other than an ophthalmologist is to be condemned.

CONSERVATION-OF-SIGHT PROGRAMS.—Routine eye examination by a physician as outlined previously is considered optimal. If this is impractical among economically deprived groups or if an inadequate number of physicians is available, some other responsible unit, such as the school, or the preschool nursery, should carry out accurate screening tests. Both medical and school examinations should include measurements of acuity with the illiterate E or Snellen letter chart and some test for ocular squint. The physician can use the cover test and the school screening program can use the Atlantic City Eye Test.* The latter test serves only as a gross screening measure.

Hearing Deficit

SYNDROME DIAGNOSIS.—The question of hearing loss usually arises because of a lack of speech, poor speech, or inattention or unresponsiveness. In early infancy, hearing loss may be overlooked because affected babies have a normal primitive coo and are not expected to respond regularly. Later in the first and second years of life, partially or totally deaf babies fail to develop speech normally and remain inattentive. Also, parents and the physician may note the typically monotonous cry and the absence of variation in the pitch of the voice. Patients with a composite hearing loss of more than 30 decibels are socially handicapped because they cannot perceive ordinary speech. Those with about 80 decibels loss have almost complete loss of hearing usable for speech.

When the possibility of hearing defect is raised by the parent, the teacher or another physician, one must decide whether the defect represents *true deafness* (the inability to detect sound—either noise or speech) or the inability to understand or respond to speech (Table 7.2). True deafness can be differentiated from apparent deafness fairly easily in most cases. An accurate history should be obtained from the parents, who have usually conducted their own simple hearing tests at home, and from an examination in which the physician (without letting the child see him) whispers the patient's name, offers an attractive reward, makes a loud noise, rattles coins or presents a stimulus such as a bell or a tuning fork. A careful examination of the eardrum should be done. If the patient has had recurrent ear infections, mastoid x-rays may be necessary. Accurate and thorough psychometric and neurologic examinations should be conducted to rule out mental retardation, developmental word deafness, an unusual manifestation of epi-

---

*From William Freund, 1415 Pacific Avenue, Atlantic City, New Jersey.

TABLE 7.2.—DIFFERENTIAL DIAGNOSIS OF TRUE AND APPARENT DEAFNESS

TRUE DEAFNESS	APPARENT DEAFNESS
Nerve Deafness (see text for diagnosis)	

1. Congenital—structural anomalies of the inner ear, the middle ear and the cochlear nuclei
    Rubella
    Cretinism
	1. Mental retardation
	2. "Differential deafness" (see text)

2. Infections
    Purulent meningitis
    Mumps
    Acute labyrinthitis
    Tuberculosis
    Other acute infections (scarlatina, measles, influenza)
	3. Aphasia
	    Acquired—epilepsy
	    Developmental word deafness
	4. Autism
	5. Dementia

3. Intoxications
    Hyperbilirubinemia
    Drugs (streptomycin, kanamycin)	

4. Tumors
    Neurofibroma (including von Recklinghausen's disease)
    Brain stem glioma	

5. Heredodegenerative diseases
    Hereditary nerve deafness
    Osteogenesis imperfecta
    Gargoylism
    Retinitis pigmentosa
    Hereditary nephritis[4]	

Conduction Deafness	
1. Recurrent otitis media and mastoiditis	
2. Hereditary otosclerosis	

lepsy, degenerative diseases and behavior disorders such as autistic mutism. At the outset one should also consider the "differential deafness" of the child who is preoccupied or is "turning a deaf ear" to an overdemanding parent.

If the question of true hearing loss is not settled by these simple techniques, more definitive, objective methods should be used. Obviously an audiometric examination through the whole range of frequency tones is most desirable, but it is often impossible in the preschool child because the test requires cooperation and concentration. In normal persons a loud noise during a light-sleep electroencephalogram causes a so-called K-complex or arousal response. This response is easily demonstrated and its absence can be used as a crude indication of hearing loss in infants and young children. Recently computer averaging of EEG-evoked responses to repetitive clicks and tones has been reported to be useful in the diagnosis of deafness, but this technique has not yet been developed to the point of being clinically practical.[1,10,11] Theoretically, the psychogalvanometric skin-resistance (PGSR) test has value in the young child who cannot cooperate in a formal audiometric test. The child is conditioned to sweat, thereby lowering the measured skin resistance by pairing an audiometric tone with a slight electric shock. Eventually the tone alone will cause sweating and lowered skin resistance. Actually, this test is not very practical either, because it frightens the young child by causing pain and so loses its value.

Audiograms are interpreted in terms of the range of frequency impairment (high tones vs. low tones) and air conduction deficit versus bone conduction deficit.

DIFFERENTIAL DIAGNOSIS.—Most instances of true deafness in children result from so-called *nerve deafness* which includes disease of the inner ear (bony labyrinth and cochlea, including the end-organ of Corti) and of the eighth nerve itself.[3] It is extremely rare to find deafness resulting from disease of the neural pathways from the brain stem to the auditory cortex because of the extensive decussations of the afferent pathways in the brain stem and the bilateral representation of hearing in the cerebral cortex. Nerve deafness causes high-tone hearing loss and impaired bone conduction. This is measured by audiometry and in some cases by the Weber and Rinne tests. All these tests require cooperative patients, and results may be difficult to interpret with bilateral hearing loss. A severe hearing deficit almost always indicates nerve deafness.

Conduction deafness results most often in children from fibrosis in the middle ear following recurrent serous or purulent otitis or mastoiditis. Rarely hereditary otosclerosis causes conduction deafness beginning in late childhood. Patients with conductive hearing loss exhibit defective air conduction (Rinne's test or audiometry), normal bone conduction and a deficit over all frequency ranges which does not exceed 60 decibels.

The reader is referred to other sections of the text for a discussion of most of the causes of true and apparent deafness listed in Table 7.2. The exact mechanism responsible for congenital deafness often remains obscure unless such deafness results from congenital rubella or cretinism. Infections, intoxications and tumors cause most additional cases of nerve deafness. Assorted rare degenerative diseases are also associated with hearing loss.

MANAGEMENT.—Most deaf children receive only limited benefit from mechanical hearing aids because the intelligibility of speech in patients with inner ear disease or nerve deafness does not increase proportionately with the intensity of the sound. In contrast, patients with conduction deficit from middle ear disease approximate normal hearing of speech with a hearing aid.

Patients with a "composite" or "better ear" hearing deficit of 25 decibels or more should be referred for speech training and lip reading after medical therapy is exhausted. If the child has a 30-decibel loss, the use of a hearing aid should be considered. If, despite medical therapy, mechanical hearing aids and instruction in lip reading, the patient with normal intellect fails in regular school, he should be referred to a special school for the hearing handicapped.

CONSERVATION-OF-HEARING PROGRAMS.—School children should have hearing tested every 3 years because the success of therapy depends upon early detection. The complexity of the problem often requires the combined talents of the family physician, the neurologist, the otologist, the psychometrist, the speech and hearing pathologist and the special educator.

Hearing loss can be prevented to some extent by (1) the intensive and adequate treatment of otitis media, (2) the avoidance of swimming when acute ear infections or middle ear effusions develop and (3) adequate immunization.

BIBLIOGRAPHY

1. Barnet, A. B., and Lodge, A.: Diagnosis of deafness in infants with the use of computer-averaged electroencephalographic responses to sound, J. Pediat. 69:753, 1966.
2. Bergman, P. S.: Cerebral blindness, A.M.A. Arch. Neurol. & Psychiat. 78:568, 1957.
3. Byers, R. K., *et al.*: Extrapyramidal cerebral palsy with hearing loss following erythroblastosis, Pediatrics 15:248, 1955.
4. Cassady, G., *et al.*: Hereditary renal function and deafness, Pediatrics 35:967, 1965.
5. Cogan, D. G.: *Neurology of the Ocular Muscles* (2d ed.; Springfield, Ill.: Charles C Thomas, Publisher, 1956).
6. Griffith, J. F., and Dodge, P. R.: Transient blindness following head injury in children, New England J. Med. 278:648, 1968.
7. Keeney, A. H.: *Chronology of Ophthalmic Development* (Springfield, Ill.: Charles C Thomas, Publisher, 1951).
8. Laws, H. W.: Strabismus in general practice, Canad. M. A. J. 90:76, 1964.
9. Parks, M. M.: Strabismus, A.M.A. Arch. Ophth. 56:138, 1956.
10. Rapin, I., and Graziani, L. J.: Auditory-evoked responses in normal, brain-damaged and deaf infants, Neurology 17:881, 1967.
11. Ritvo, E. R., *et al.*: Clinical application of the auditory averaged evoked response at sleep onset in the diagnosis of deafness, Pediatrics 40:1003, 1967.

8

Increased Intracranial Pressure, Papilledema and Brain Herniation Syndromes

Increased Intracranial Pressure
    Pseudotumor cerebri
Papilledema
Uncal Herniation
Cerebellar Herniation

Increased Intracranial Pressure

USUAL SYMPTOMS.—Headache, vomiting and drowsiness should always raise the question of increased intracranial pressure. Obviously, the common occurrence of these complaints with a variety of acute and chronic illnesses means that they will often turn out to be nonspecific. The symptom of double vision is a more specific complaint and should receive careful attention. "Blurring" of vision is also reported by some patients. With acutely increased pressure, enlargement of the blind spot will be found (in testable children) as well as slight constriction of the peripheral fields and no impairment of central acuity (Snellen chart). Patients with long-standing increase of pressure will have varying degrees of central visual loss and greatly constricted peripheral vision.

SYNDROME DIAGNOSIS.—If these complaints reflect increased pressure, one can expect to find papilledema and sometimes unilateral or bilateral sixth nerve palsy (a "false localizing sign"). Babies will often exhibit a tense or bulging fontanel and palpably separated sutures. These findings must be interpreted cautiously since their interpretation is rather subjective and is dependent on the examiner's experience and on whether the baby is relaxed or crying. In all patients suspected of having increased pressure, skull films should be obtained to look for (1) suture separation, (2) increased convolutional markings ("hammered silver") and (3) erosion or demineralization of the dorsum sellae. Caution is needed for the accurate interpretation of abnormalities of sutures, markings and changes of the sella in infants. With older children who are able to cooperate with accurate visual field testing, it is often possible to map an enlarged blind spot, a safe and useful sign of elevated pressure. If a conclusive diagnosis of increased pressure is reached on the basis of the above findings, a neurosurgical consultation should be sought promptly and the differential diagnostic workup continued cautiously. If the diagnosis of increased pressure remains in doubt after careful and repeated examinations, the physician should, after alerting the neurosurgeon, perform a spinal puncture with the child quiet (sedated if necessary) and obtain an accurate pressure reading. Unfortunately, upper normal limits of CSF pressure have never been established for children of different ages and sizes, but any reading over 180 mm. of water should be considered suspicious and any reading over 200 mm. should be considered abnormal. We would like to stress the need to carry out this procedure carefully and with good technique in every patient. If the pressure is obviously elevated, only enough fluid should be removed to do the routine CSF studies (not more than 2-3 ml.). The patient is kept flat after the procedure.

DIFFERENTIAL DIAGNOSIS.—This will depend largely upon a consideration of all the other clinical and laboratory findings in the case. In their approximate order of clinical frequency, the following conditions cause increased intracranial pressure: (1) *intracranial hemorrhage* (subdural, epidural or intracerebral), (2) *congenital obstructive hydrocephalus,* (3) *status epilepticus* with *cerebral edema* (acute toxic encephalopathy), (4) *brain tumor,* (5) *central nervous system infections* (chronic granulomatous meningitis, such as tuberculosis and cryptococcosis, and brain abscess), (6) *intoxications that cause cerebral edema* (lead, adrenal corticosteroid therapy,[2] vitamin A overdosage[7] and water overloading with hyponatremia) and (7) *craniostenosis* (coronal suture). Much less commonly in children one finds (8) a *vascular* etiology for the increased pressure (hypertensive encephalopathy with renal disease or sinus thrombosis with or without hypernatremia) and (9) *Schilder's disease*.

The reader is referred to Part II for a full discussion of the diagnosis and management of disease conditions.

Pseudotumor cerebri.—This syndrome is also known as meningeal hydrops, benign intracranial hypertension, otitic hydrocephalus and chronic adhesive arachnoiditis. It is defined as unlocalized increased intracranial pressure of unknown cause. Most experienced workers agree that a more definitive diagnosis may frequently be made if these patients are followed. Brain tumors are often found, or the syndrome may result from long-term, high-dose glucocorticoid therapy or its rapid discontinuation.[3,10] It also occurs with conditions that cause cerebral edema, such as infections, intoxications and trauma, and may be associated with venous thrombosis.[9] Therefore, we urge thorough study of every patient with this syndrome to the point where all other causes are excluded. Then and only then should the diagnosis of pseudotumor be made.

When air encephalography is done on patients with this syndrome, the ventricles may appear unusually small, presumably because of diffuse compression.[4] In fact, the surgeon may have great difficulty in finding the ventricle with the cannula when he attempts ventriculography. Patients with pseudotumor of obscure cause usually appear disproportionately well despite signs of pressure.

MANAGEMENT.—It is most important to provide definitive treatment when a diagnosis is established. In patients with true pseudotumor cerebri an attempt should be made to keep the pressures in the normal range by frequent lumbar punctures (1–2 times weekly) and by suppressing CSF production with acetazolamide (5–25 mg./kg./24 hours) in order to prevent loss of vision. The medical management of cerebral swelling[6] or edema using mannitol[1] and cortisone[8] is outlined in Appendix 2. These agents should be used with caution because subdural hematoma may complicate the excessively rapid administration of hypertonic urea.[5] In exceptional cases surgical shunt procedures may be necessary.

Papilledema

SYNDROME DIAGNOSIS.—The term "papilledema" is used here to refer to the physical abnormality of the optic nerve head and is not intended to carry any connotation about etiology.

Papilledema is characterized by *a group of signs:* (1) blurring or obliteration of disc margins, (2) increased vascularity, (3) venous engorgement and tortuosity, (4) retinal hemorrhages and (5) a brush-streaked appearance to the retina around the disc. Most physicians are not able to distinguish papilledema of increased intracranial pressure ("choked discs") from papillitis due to other causes. One must differentiate true papilledema from (1) papillitis seen in optic neuritis, (2) the small pink disc seen in patients with hyperopia (farsightedness), a common cause of "pseudopapilledema," and (3) rare congenital anomalies of the optic nerve head. So-called drüsen (round, hyaline masses in the optic papilla) may simulate papilledema; they represent myelinated nerve fibers which run radially from the optic disc.

DIFFERENTIAL DIAGNOSIS.—A careful search should be made first for other signs of increased intracranial pressure and, if these are not found, consideration is then given to (1) demyelinating disease (optic neuritis and neuromyelitis optica), (2) postinfectious optic neuritis (including polyneuritis), (3) hereditary optic neuritis and atrophy (Leber), (4) metabolic causes, such as chronic pulmonary disease with hypercapnia (as in cystic fibrosis, Chapter 23), hypoparathyroidism, hypophosphatasia and (5) intoxications with adrenal steroids, lead, tetracycline or vitamin A.

MANAGEMENT.—The problem is managed according to the specific disease (Part II).

Uncal and Cerebellar Herniation Syndromes

PATHOGENESIS.—*Uncal herniation.*—Almost all of the causes of increased intracranial pressure (p. 83) can lead to herniation downward of the inferior, mesial aspect of the temporal lobe (the uncus or hippocampal gyrus) through the opening in the tentorium, the incisural notch. The reader should make a special effort to understand this pathologic mechanism fully so that he can make the diagnosis early and prevent the important and disastrous consequences which result from inaction due to ignorance of the syndrome.

The displacement and deformity of the important brain structures are illustrated in Figure 8.1, *A*. Increased supratentorial pressure squeezes one or both

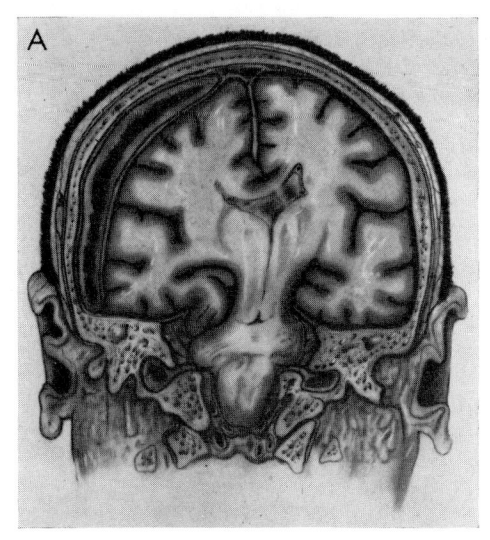

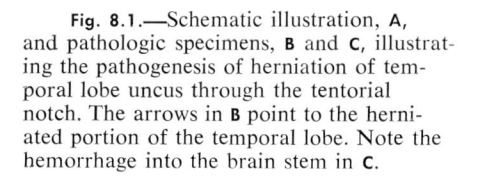

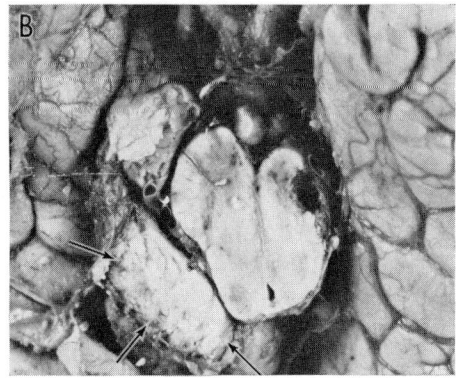

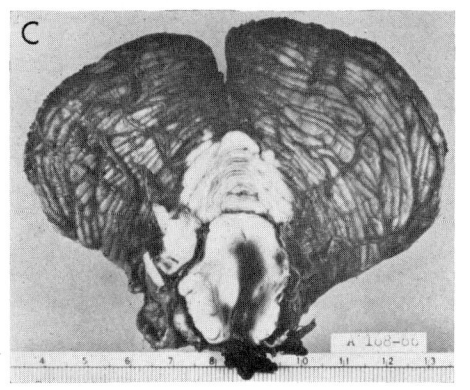

Fig. 8.1.—Schematic illustration, **A**, and pathologic specimens, **B** and **C**, illustrating the pathogenesis of herniation of temporal lobe uncus through the tentorial notch. The arrows in **B** point to the herniated portion of the temporal lobe. Note the hemorrhage into the brain stem in **C**.

temporal lobe unci through the tentorial opening (Fig. 8.1,*B*) and causes the following serious events: (1) compression of either the ipsilateral or contralateral third cranial nerve, (2) compression of either the opposite or ipsilateral cerebral peduncle against the free edge of the tentorium, (3) hemorrhage into the brain stem (Fig. 8.1,*C*), and (4) necrosis and ischemic infarction of the hippocampus, the calcarine cortex and the cerebral peduncle (or pyramidal tract). Without entering into all of the speculation about the pathogenesis of the resultant brain damage, one can say that the problems of mortality and morbidity are caused by (1) direct ischemic compression of structures such as the third nerve, temporal lobe and peduncle, (2) compromise of posterior cerebral arteries, (3) venous hemorrhages into the brain stem from pressure and (4) cerebral edema.

Cerebellar herniation.—Herniation of the cerebellar tonsils results from increased intracranial pressure, especially when it is caused by a mass in the posterior fossa. The tonsils are displaced inferiorly into the cisterna magna.

SYNDROME AND DIFFERENTIAL DIAGNOSIS.—*Uncal herniation.*—Patients have the usual symptoms and signs of increased intracranial pressure. In addition, unilateral herniation is followed by (1) ipsilateral or contralateral third nerve palsy, ushered in by a poorly reactive or fixed, dilated pupil, (2) ipsilateral or contralateral hemiparesis (so-called "false localizing sign" from compression of the opposite cerebral peduncle against the free edge of the tentorium), and (3) increasing stupor or coma (from both increased intracranial pressure and brain stem hemorrhage).

Many patients die in this state, or, if they survive, are often left with permanent residual deficit, including mental retardation or dementia with unilateral or bilateral ventricular dilatation (Fig. 16.8, p. 237), hemiparesis with a shrunken cerebral hemisphere (Fig. 16.8), seizure disorders, especially psychomotor attacks (Figs. 16.3, p. 234, and 16.8), and cortical blindness (Fig. 16.9, p. 238). Other chronic disabilities are noted, such as behavior disorders, speech and language disorders and astereognosis in the hemiparetic limb. Some workers have attributed chronic pituitary-hypothalamic disturbances such as diabetes insipidus to pituitary vascular insufficiency at the time of the acute insult.

Cerebellar herniation.—Patients exhibit symptoms and signs of increased intracranial pressure along with head tilt, neck stiffness and suboccipital tenderness.

MANAGEMENT.—Treatment is directed toward (1) adequate oxygenation and support of blood pressure, (2) immediate surgical decompression if indicated by the basic diagnosis, (3) treatment of cerebral edema (Appendix 2) and (4) specific therapy of the underlying disease.

BIBLIOGRAPHY

1. Cirksena, W. J., et al.: Use of mannitol in exogenous and endogenous intoxications, New England J. Med. 270:161, 1964.
2. Dees, S. C., and McKay, H. W.: Occurrence of pseudotumor cerebri (benign intracranial hypertension) during treatment of children with asthma by adrenal steroids, Pediatrics 23:1143, 1959.
3. Greer, M.: Benign intracranial hypertension: II. Following corticosteroid therapy, Neurology 13:439, 1963.
4. Jacobson, H. G., and Shapiro, J. H.: Pseudotumor cerebri, Radiology 82:202, 1964.
5. Marshall, S., and Hinman, F.: Subdural hematoma following the administration of urea for diagnosis of hypertension, J.A.M.A. 182:813, 1962.
6. Matson, D. D.: Treatment of cerebral swelling, New England J. Med. 272:626, 1965.
7. Morrice, G., et al.: Vitamin A intoxication as a cause of pseudotumor cerebri, J.A.M.A. 173:1802, 1960.
8. Rasmussen, T., and Gulati, D. R.: Cortisone in the treatment of postoperative cerebral edema, J. Neurosurg. 19:535, 1962.
9. Rose, A., and Matson, D. D.: Benign intracranial hypertension in children, Pediatrics 39:227, 1967.
10. Walker, A. E., and Adamkiewicz, J. J.: Pseudotumor cerebri associated with prolonged corticosteroid therapy, J.A.M.A. 188:779, 1964.

9

Focal Deficit

Optic Atrophy
Retinal Hemorrhages
Nonparalytic Squint
Paralytic Squint and Diplopia
Spasmus Nutans
Oculomotor Apraxia
Bobble-head Doll Syndrome
Nystagmus
Ptosis
Pupillary Inequality
Papilledema
Facial Weakness or Asymmetry
Dizziness (Vertigo) (Chapter 2)

Hearing Loss (Chapter 7)
Dysarthria, Dysphonia and Dysphagia
Head Tilt
Acute Weakness
Acute Hypotonia
Ataxia
Other Movement Disorders
   Chorea
   Tremor-rigidity
   Akathisia
   Dystonia
Acute Sensory Complaints

THE COMMONEST FOCAL NEUROLOGICAL SYMPTOMS and signs are discussed here in their approximate order of importance. We have not attempted to describe the detailed techniques of physical diagnosis, but we expect the material to help in the regional localization of lesions.

Optic Atrophy

Two criteria must be satisfied before the diagnosis of optic atrophy can be made: (1) pallor of the optic nerve head and (2) impairment of visual acuity or visual fields. Deciding that optic nerves are abnormally pale is often difficult since in young infants, especially prematures, the papillae normally have a grayish cast instead of the usual orange-pink color seen in the older child and adult. In marginal or equivocal cases the examiner may not be able to interpret his findings with certainty, especially if he has any degree of red-green color blindness. Atrophic optic nerves are often smaller than normal, but one also finds smaller-than-average discs in patients with hyperopia (farsightedness), a common refractive error in children. Hence, it becomes important to decide whether the patient has noncorrectable reduction in visual acuity (as seen in optic atrophy). In other words, the acuity and fields can only be tested accurately after the patient is fitted with glasses to correct any refractive error (hyperopia, myopia or astigmatism).

Symptomatic treatment of optic atrophy, if it is severe enough, consists of special education in a facility for the blind. Corrective lenses have no value unless an associated refractive error is discovered. Specific therapy for the underlying condition should be provided.

Retinal Hemorrhages

Recognition of retinal hemorrhages usually provides no difficulty except for the mistakes of overinterpretation. Occasionally the examiner reports small "splinter hemorrhages" which on careful and repeated observation prove to be normal blood vessels.

Nonparalytic Squint

SYNDROME DIAGNOSIS.—The recognition of a squint (or strabismus) in a young child is not always easy. It is generally noted on routine examination, is brought to one's attention by a parent or a teacher noticing a "cross-eyed" appearance or is found in association with loss of vision in one eye (amblyopia ex anopsia or "lazy eye"). Parents may for many years overlook a squint which is obvious to the examining physician. Occasionally a nonparalytic squint will appear abruptly, suggesting paralysis of an extraocular muscle. Often when this happens there will be a definitive refractive error. It is well known that young infants may have a "cross-eyed" appearance until binocular fixation is established at 6–8 weeks of age.

The full range of extraocular movements should be tested by having the child fixate on the examiner's finger or a light. In addition, the *cover test* should be carried out in questionable cases. For the cover test the child fixates on the examiner's nose or on a light while one eye is simultaneously covered by a 3×5 card. When fixation is established, the covered eye is uncovered quickly and in the same motion the uncovered eye is covered. If this procedure is repeated several times, the lag of the deviating or paretic muscle (heterophoria) can be easily seen.

Once the squint is detected, it is important to decide whether the extraocular muscle imbalance has a nonparalytic (concomitant) or a paralytic (comitant) basis. It is important to realize that a patient with long-standing squint may exhibit apparent muscle paralysis. For example, a child with severe, chronic esotropia (internal strabismus) may be unable to abduct the squinting eye fully as a result either of muscle contracture or of operative shortening of a muscle. Generally speaking, patients with paralytic squint have diplopia and patients with nonparalytic squint do not have diplopia. However, one must be very careful about this assumption because children do not report diplopia regularly and accurately. Further, children with nonparalytic squint may report diplopia transiently, so that care must be taken to exclude a true paralytic basis for any squint in childhood. We have seen corrective eye muscle operations performed on children with sixth nerve palsy from a brain stem tumor.

The absence of diplopia in patients with nonparalytic squint is attributed to "suppression" (in the visual cortex) of the image from the squinting eye. In a minority of patients only one eye is used for fixation and the other eye is constantly deviated. The macular area in the visual cortex is constantly suppressed and this results in *amblyopia ex anopsia*. In most cases the patient alternately fixates and suppresses with both eyes and thus prevents loss of vision.

The suffix *-phoria* is used to describe a transient tendency to eye deviation (a situation in which the eyes appear straight when the child is fixating but eye deviation is noted when the cover test is performed), and the suffix *-tropia* is applied to an obvious, persistent deviation which does not require the cover test for its recognition. Prefixes are used to specify the direction of the deviation: *eso* for inward deviation or convergence, *exo* for outward deviation or divergence, *hyper* for upward deviation and *hypo* for downward deviation.

Convergent squint (internal strabismus).—This type of squint is the commonest and is usually associated with hyperopia or farsightedness. Farsighted children are forced to accommodate to see near objects clearly and, since the mechanisms of accommodation and convergence are closely allied and usually function simultaneously, the nonfixating eye turns inward. As indicated, most patients with convergent squints alternate the fixating eye and thus do not develop amblyopia ex anopsia. However, it should be understood that the severity of the squint has no dependable relationship to the severity of the amblyopia. In other words, children with mild squint or those who appear to "outgrow" the squint may have the most severe degree of visual loss because they have stopped trying to fuse with both eyes and are simultaneously developing loss of vision (amblyopia).

Divergent squint (external strabismus).—This less common type of squint is often associated with myopia or nearsightedness. The child does not need to accommodate or converge with near vision because of his myopic refractive error. The lack of stimulus for accommodation and convergence leads to an external strabismus.

Whereas lateral squints are usually associated with refractive errors, vertical squints are usually paralytic.

DIFFERENTIAL DIAGNOSIS.—As indicated previously cross-eyedness usually results from a refractive error or the failure to develop reflexes which insure stereoscopic or three-dimensional vision. However, any organic ocular lesion which obstructs vision in one eye will cause inward deviation of that eye under the age of 2 years. Intraocular disorders which cause squints include congenital cataracts, retrolental fibroplasia, congenital glaucoma, congenital microphthalmus and a tumor such as retinoblastoma.

MANAGEMENT AND PROGNOSIS.—Extraocular muscle imbalances are treated with (1) *patching,* (2) *lenses* (glasses) to correct the associated refractive error, (3) eye muscle *operation* and (4) orthoptic *exercises.* These problems should be managed by an ophthalmologist unless they are associated with other neurologic or neuromuscular deficits. In the latter case the patient should be cared for jointly by a physician who is fully aware of the general problems and an eye specialist. Infants with a manifest squint should be referred to an ophthalmologist not later than 6–9 months of age in order to avoid irreversible loss of vision.

Paralytic Squint and Diplopia

Chronic nonparalytic squints which represent extraocular muscle imbalance affect children much more commonly than acute paralytic squints. Occasionally nonparalytic squints appear abruptly in young children and, if associated with diplopia, should alert the physician to the possibility of an underlying refractive error. A thorough neurologic examination should be carried out, including a range-of-motion test of *all eye muscles in both eyes* as well as a lens refraction, if necessary. When paralytic squints occur, there is usually evidence of a sixth or third nerve palsy. The child may or may not report double vision. Sixth nerve palsies occur more frequently because this cranial nerve is especially sensitive to increased intracranial pressure, and malfunction of this nerve is the most commonly encountered "false localizing neurologic sign." In addition, brain tumor, myasthenia gravis, trauma and disease in the tissues of the orbit must be considered. Occasionally benign, transient, sixth nerve palsies are seen in children. These presumably result from otitis media or complicate a viral illness.[6] Third nerve palsies are seen infrequently, either as a reflection of uncal herniation (Chapter 8), multiple sclerosis, myasthenia gravis or, rarely, ophthalmoplegic migraine. One should avoid at all costs the mistake of calling a squint nonparalytic when it is in fact paralytic. Such errors lead to mismanagement, such as placing a child in glasses or doing an unnecessary eye muscle operation when symptoms are due to increased pressure, a tumor or myasthenia gravis.

Spasmus Nutans

This peculiar constellation of neuromotor signs includes (1) slow, inconstant head-nodding, (2) unilateral or bilateral pendular nystagmus (rotary, horizontal or vertical) and (3) torticollis. This clinical syndrome of unknown cause usually appears between 4 and 12 months of age and disappears in every case within a year or two, usually sooner.

This benign syndrome seems to be occurring with decreasing frequency. If the diagnosis is correct, no treatment is necessary.

Oculomotor Apraxia

Patients with this rare and subtle disorder of eye movement usually complain of reading disability. Cogan[4] has described these children in some detail. Although they have normal random, involuntary eye movements, they are unable to carry out voluntary horizontal eye movements and, as a result, cannot read a line of print normally. They compensate for the disability by acquiring quick, jerking head movements which are often overlooked. Other static motor disorders, such as ataxia and delayed walking, are described, suggesting that the eye disorder represents only one of a number of nervous system anomalies. Altrocchi and Menkes[1] point out that all reported cases have been in males.

Predictions about development and intellectual abilities should be guarded because of the circumstantial clinical evidence of multiple nervous system anomalies in many patients. The number of documented cases which have been followed long enough for conclusions to be drawn is limited, but it is said that these patients have permanently slow reading habits despite therapy.

Bobble-head Doll Syndrome

A rare and unusual 2–3 per second bobbing tremor of the head and trunk has been described in two patients.[2] In both patients a large cyst near the third ventricle caused marked obstructive dilatation of both lateral ventricles. Another patient with the same unusual sign had hydrocephalus secondary to aqueductal stenosis.[7]

Nystagmus

An important neurologic sign, nystagmus by itself rarely has specific localizing value in regional diagnosis of nervous system disease. It must be considered with all the other positive findings in the history, physical examination and laboratory studies. However, one can generalize with caution about the approximate meaning of the different types of nystagmus—horizontal, vertical and rotary. In our experience intoxication with drugs such as phenobarbital, Dilantin and many other sedatives and tranquilizers, which has become increasingly common in children, can cause all three types of nystagmus and so must always be considered.

Horizontal nystagmus results from lesions in the cerebellar pathways all the way from the cerebellum itself to the cerebrum (such as frontal lobe mass lesions involving the corticopontocerebellar fibers) to the upper cervical spinal cord (such as syringomyelia and syringobulbia involving the medial longitudinal fasciculus). Coarse horizontal nystagmus is often seen ipsilateral to tumors in the cerebellar hemisphere, and fine horizontal nystagmus is characteristic of lesions in the brain stem.

Vertical nystagmus is considered the hallmark of intramedullary lesions of the brain stem (such as tumors and demyelinating disease) but is also seen commonly with drug intoxications.

Rotary nystagmus suggests disease in the inner ear or anywhere in the vestibular pathways to the cerebellum. In children it occurs with acute drug intoxication, head trauma, posterior fossa tumors, spinocerebellar degenerations, syringomyelia and labyrinthitis.

Nystagmus can be induced normally by douching the ear with 5 cc. of ice water (Barany's caloric test), being sure that the water makes contact with the drum. The test is used to see whether the labyrinth and eighth nerve are intact. This should be done in the morning before breakfast because it can cause severe nausea in sensitive patients. As the water is instilled the patient is told to look to the opposite side, and for a few seconds one normally sees coarse nystagmus with the fast component in the direction of gaze. If nystagmus does not develop with repeated testing, a "dead" labyrinth is suggested. This is seen with eighth nerve tumors (especially acoustic neurinoma), streptomycin toxicity and purulent labyrinthitis, the last being a rare disease at present.

A peculiar type of "nystagmus" or *opsoclonus* characterized by periodic eye oscillations is seen in acute ataxia of unknown etiology (cerebellitis or pontine encephalitis, Chapter 18). The fundamental mechanism of this eye movement disorder is poorly understood, and the condition is seen in very few neurologic disorders of children other than this syndrome of acute ataxia.

Ptosis

Rarely ptosis comes on acutely and represents (1) one sign of a third nerve palsy, along with paralysis of eye adduction and a dilated pupil which fails to react to light, (2) myasthenia gravis, in which case the ptosis is often bilateral, or (3) one fragment of a Horner syndrome (together with miosis, enophthalmos and absent sweating on the same side of the face) as a result of a lesion in the cervical sympathetic chain. In addition to myasthenia gravis the differential diagnosis should include myotonic dystrophy, congenital ptosis, progressive bulbar ophthalmoplegia and conditions which cause proptosis and ophthalmoplegia.

Oculomotor paralysis may occur in *cycles* and the differential diagnosis must include multiple sclerosis, myasthenia gravis, tumors in the brain stem or those compressing the third, fourth or sixth cranial nerves behind the orbit, migraine and obscure causes.[11]

Pupillary Inequality (Anisocoria)

Patients with this complaint and who are otherwise well usually have no neurologic disease. Occasionally anisocoria may be a manifestation of Adie's syndrome—a benign, static condition in which the larger pupil reacts normally in accommodation but sluggishly to light. Adie's syndrome is commonest in young women and is associated with diffuse hyporeflexia. As mentioned in the description of uncal herniation, this sign may be one reflection of a third nerve palsy.

Papilledema

This "focal" finding is considered separately in Chapter 8.

Facial Weakness or Asymmetry

The acute or gradual onset of facial weakness or asymmetry has many different causes. Some are obvious, as in the case of head injury, but some may be obscure, e.g., Bell's palsy, brain tumor and postconvulsive paralysis. If the patient has no obvious asymmetry and moves both sides equally well, the possibility of bilateral facial weakness (as seen in actue infectious polyneuritis) must always be considered.

Management depends upon the specific diagnosis.

Dizziness (Vertigo)

See Chapter 2.

Hearing Loss

See Chapter 7.

Dysarthria, Dysphonia and Dysphagia

When there is a change in the quality of a child's speech or voice or a swallowing difficulty develops, the general differential diagnosis includes (1) nasopharyngeal obstruction due to inflammatory disease or hypertrophied adenoid tissue, (2) a neuromuscular cause (posterior fossa brain tumor, poliomyelitis, polyneuritis, myasthenia gravis, progressive bulbar palsy) and (3) a psychogenic etiology. Dysphonia is seen occasionally as a clinical manifestation of hysteria or severe psychoneurosis in children (Chapter 1).

Head Tilt

The observation that a child is beginning to cock his head abruptly to one side usually indicates an attempt to splint the neck muscles because of pain or meningismus. However, it may represent his way of avoiding diplopia. Consequently, in addition to benign, localized trauma, one must consider increased intracranial pressure as the cause of sixth nerve palsy and all other causes of diplopia and third nerve weakness. An especially important diagnostic consideration is a mass in the posterior fossa which is causing herniation of the cerebellar tonsils into the cisterna magna. Head tilt will also be seen as a sign of cervical spine subluxation (Fig. 15.8, p. 219). Chronic head tilt often results from congenital torticollis.

Acute Weakness

Many patients and parents use the term "weakness" in a general, nonspecific way to describe the inactivity and lassitude of the sick child. The term is used here only to describe true paresis or paralysis. An attempt should be made first to decide whether acute weakness is of neural or muscular origin. In neurogenic weakness the lesion involves either the upper motor neuron (pyramidal tract) or the lower motor neuron (anterior horn cell, root or peripheral nerve). *Upper motor neuron* lesions are usually eventually associated with increased muscle tone (spasticity), hyperreflexia, pathologic reflexes (clonus or Babinski signs) and normal sensation. Mild muscle atrophy of disuse appears late. With *lower motor neuron weakness* the opposite signs are found, i.e., flaccid muscle tone, depressed or absent reflexes, no pathologic reflexes, muscle atrophy and some sensory deficit within a week or 10 days after the onset of the disease. When the type of weakness cannot be distinguished with certainty, electromyography and conduction velocity studies may have diagnostic value (Chapter 12). Fibrillation potentials on electromyography and delayed conduction velocity suggest lower motor neuron disease, whereas normal studies would favor corticospinal tract weakness.

Acute upper motor neuron lesions result most commonly from postconclusive hemiparesis (Todd's palsy or acute infantile hemiplegia—Chapter 2). Less commonly they complicate acute infectious encephalomyelitis or are caused by brain tumors, spinal cord tumors or acute demyelinating disease. Only occasionally do true cerebrovascular accidents occur in children. Lower motor neuron weakness has in the past been most often due to enterovirus infections (poliomyelitis), but the incidence has plummeted since the introduction of polio vaccine. Now it is appearing relatively more often as a result of polyneuritis, postinjection (sciatic and radial) neuropathy or direct trauma to peripheral nerves and as a complication of drug therapy or horse-serum sensitivity. Chronic multiple polyneuropathy can result from many different causes: intoxication, nutritional deficiencies, polyarteritis nodosa and the Guillain-Barré syndrome. Other more uncommon causes have been reviewed by Byers and Taft.[3]

In older patients localized shoulder-girdle weakness and atrophy are infrequently seen and the cause is usually obscure.[10] Prior injections and trauma should be considered carefully in a search for the etiology.

Certain rare insect and snake bites can cause diffuse flaccid weakness. Mixed upper and lower motor neuron lesions are seen with such uncommon lesions as avulsion injury to the spinal cord at birth and tumors in the spinal canal and rarely with transverse myelitis.

Weakness can result acutely from unusual disorders of muscle. Periodic muscle weakness is seen with myasthenia gravis, with rare hereditary forms of periodic paralysis and with electrolyte disorders. Both hypokalemia and hyperkalemia can cause clinical signs of muscle weakness, as can hypernatremia.[8] Hypokalemia is most common in patients with metabolic alkalosis, which often is due to prolonged dehydration associated with intestinal obstruction.

In the disorders of neuromuscular transmission there is transient flaccid weakness without reflex changes or atrophy in the acute stages.

Management depends upon the specific diagnosis which is established.

Acute Hypotonia

Acute forms of flaccidity, seen most commonly at birth, have many causes: (1) CNS depression from obstetric analgesia and anesthesia, (2) CNS hemorrhage and hypoxia, (3) neonatal or prenatal meningitis or sepsis, (4) CNS anomalies, including prematurity and intrauterine growth retardation, (5) birth trauma, that is, stretching injury to the cervical cord—usually from a breech delivery—and brachial plexus injuries, (6) neonatal myasthenia gravis and (7) rare inborn errors of metabolism.

In older children the acute development is seen most often in the early "shock" stage of an upper motor neuron lesion and with any of the conditions previously described which cause lower motor neuron or myoneural junction disease. Therapy consists of supportive care and depends upon a specific diagnosis.

Ataxia

Table 9.1 lists the many diseases which cause ataxia.[9] These are discussed separately in Part II.

Acute ataxia is common and results from a variety of poisonings and from acute head injury. Care must be taken to differentiate acute weakness (as seen in polyneuritis) and hysteria from true ataxia. Ataxia is associated with a broad-based, unsteady gait, terminal intention tremor on finger-to-nose movements, impaired ability to perform rapid alternating hand movements and nystagmus. Naturally, brain tumors must always be considered in the differential diagnosis, and the read-

TABLE 9.1.—DIFFERENTIAL DIAGNOSIS OF ATAXIA*

Chronic
    Congenital malformations (cerebellum)
    Metabolic and degenerative diseases
        Friedreich's ataxia
        Hereditary ataxia with muscle atrophy (Lévy-Roussy)
        Progressive neural atrophy (Charcot-Marie-Tooth)
        Hereditary ataxia with myoclonic epilepsy (Ramsay-Hunt)
        Ataxia-telangiectasia
        Hartnup disease
        Cerebral lipidoses (Niemann-Pick and metachromatic leukodystrophy)
    Obstructive hydrocephalus
    Slow-growing gliomas (brain stem)

Acute
    Intoxications (accidental or iatrogenic)
    Head injury
    Brain tumor (posterior fossa)
    Cerebellitis or pontine encephalitis
    Metabolic diseases
    Polyneuritis
    Spinal cord tumor
    Hysteria
    Multiple sclerosis

*Each disease is discussed separately in Part II.

er's attention is called especially to the syndrome of "acute cerebellar ataxia of unknown etiology" (acute cerebellitis or pontine encephalitis). Rare metabolic disorders can also cause acute intermittent ataxia.

Other Movement Disorders

Most involuntary movement disorders have a chronic course, but a few develop acutely. *Chorea,* which can vary greatly in severity, should always be considered a sign of rheumatic fever or rheumatic heart disease unless another good explanation is apparent. Differentiation of true chorea from the normal "herky-jerky" behavior of the young child who cannot sit still presents a difficult and delicate clinical decision. Often the answer comes only from repeated observations and the accumulation of definitive laboratory data.

Intoxications with stimulant drugs can cause marked *hyperactivity*. This continuous, purposeless movement subsides fairly quickly under observation and therapy. A variety of unusual movements (*restlessness* or *akathisia, dystonia* and *tremor*) complicates chlorpromazine therapy. In children the clinical picture is often caused by overdosage with suppository forms of the drugs. The differential diagnosis and management of movement disorders caused by phenothiazines are discussed in Chapter 20. Of special interest is the recent observation of a transient "extrapyramidal" disturbance in an infant born of a psychotic mother who had received phenothiazines during pregnancy.[5]

Rarely brain tumors and inborn errors of metabolism produce acute or subacute extrapyramidal signs such as tremor and choreoathetosis. Hysteria must always be considered when obscure movement disorders appear in older children and adults.

Acute Sensory Complaints

Numbness and tingling occur commonly and may have little clinical significance. These symptoms are caused by an irritative lesion of the afferent pathway anywhere from the distal peripheral nerve to the ascending pathways in the spinal cord up to the sensory cortex in the brain. The commonest organic bases for these complaints in children include polyneuritis, intoxications which affect peripheral nerves, mononeuropathies (postinjection or direct trauma), spinal cord tumors and rarely brain tumors or seizures. Functional factors, such as mild transient ischemia from compression of the extremities during sleep and true conversion hysteria, frequently cause these complaints.

Pain of neural origin results most often from compression of nerve roots, plexuses or peripheral nerves. Primary intraspinal tumors (especially extramedullary and extradural masses), metastatic tumors or paraspinal masses which extend into the spinal canal should be considered first. Pain can also result from direct injury or postinjection trauma to peripheral nerves or as a result of drugs which have a direct neurotoxic effect, e.g., nitrofurantoin and mercury and the chemotherapeutic agents used for the treatment of cancer.

BIBLIOGRAPHY

1. Altrocchi, P. H., and Menkes, J. H.: Congenital ocular motor apraxia, Brain 83:579, 1960.
2. Benton, J. W., *et al.*: The bobble-head doll syndrome, Neurology 16:725, 1966.
3. Byers, R. K., and Taft, L. T.: Chronic multiple peripheral neuropathy in childhood, Pediatrics 20:517, 1957.
4. Cogan, D. G.: A type of congenital ocular motor apraxia presenting jerking head movements, Tr. Am. Acad. Ophth. 56:853, 1952.
5. Hill, R. M., *et al.*: Extrapyramidal dysfunction in an infant of a schizophrenic mother, J. Pediat. 69:589, 1966.
6. Knox, D. L., *et al.*: Benign VI nerve palsies in children, Pediatrics 40:560, 1967.
7. Nellhaus, G.: The bobble-head doll syndrome: A "tic" with a neuropathologic basis, Pediatrics 40:250, 1967.
8. Pleasure, D., and Goldberg, M.: Neurogenic hypernatremia, Arch. Neurol. 15:78, 1966.
9. Siekert, R. G.: Introduction to symposium on ataxia in childhood, Proc. Staff Meet. Mayo Clin. 34:569, 1959.
10. Spillane, J. D.: Localized neuritis of the shoulder girdle, Lancet 2:532, 1943.
11. Stevens, H.: Cyclic oculomotor paralysis, Neurology 15:556, 1965.

10

Spinal Deformities and Meningismus

Scoliosis and Kyphoscoliosis
Meningismus
Opisthotonus
Aseptic Meningitis
Decerebrate Rigidity

Spinal Deformities

Scoliosis or *kyphoscoliosis* occurs commonly and in most cases from non-neurologic causes. In fact, the etiology of spinal curvature is unknown in the majority of cases. The condition can be recognized clinically if it is well advanced, but in many cases it can only be demonstrated on x-rays. The commoner known causes for this chronic spine deformity are listed in Table 10.1 and are divided into neural and non-neural types. In most instances the spinal deformity is secondary

TABLE 10.1.—Etiologies of Scoliosis and Kyphoscoliosis

	Neural	Non-neural
Congenital malformations	Syringomyelia Spina bifida with meningomyelocele	Spinal anomalies (hemivertebrae) Klippel-Feil syndrome
Metabolic and degenerative disorders	Spinocerebellar degeneration (e.g., Friedreich's) Neurofibromatosis Dystonia musculorum deformans	Marfan's syndrome Chondrodystrophy
Tumors	Intraspinal	
Infections	Poliomyelitis	Tuberculous spondylitis (Pott's disease)
Muscle disease	Muscular dystrophy Progressive muscle atrophy Arthrogryposis	Congenital torticollis Congenital elevation of scapula
Syndromes	Cerebral spastic diplegia (Chapter 3) Other movement disorders (Chapter 3)	Idiopathic

to some other disease which requires orthopedic therapy and so the scoliosis per se usually has no major neurologic importance. Occasionally, however, the curvature becomes so severe that the cord is stretched to a thin ribbon, causing a spastic paraplegia, as in patients with achondroplastic dwarfism.[2]

The gradual evolution of a scoliosis whose cause is obscure suggests the following neurologic disorders: (1) intraspinal tumor, (2) syringomyelia, (3) neurofibromatosis, (4) poliomyelitis in the remote past and (5) spinocerebellar degeneration, e.g., Friedreich's ataxia. Patients should have, in addition to a detailed neurologic examination, complete spine x-rays, skull x-rays, CSF examination, and myelography in selected cases. Electromyography, conduction velocity studies and muscle biopsy may also provide useful information if other studies are normal. All children with scoliosis secondary to an intraspinal tumor should have intravenous urography because of the relatively high incidence of neuroblastomas which "dumbbell" into the spinal canal from the paravertebral tissues. The diagnosis of hypophosphatasia depends upon the finding of a low serum alkaline phosphatase. If a patient with scoliosis has signs of Marfan's syndrome, urinary amino acid chromatography should be carried out to consider the diagnosis of homocystinuria, since some workers now believe that some patients with Marfan's syndrome may in fact have this hereditary aminoacidopathy.

Treatment of scoliosis is directed (1) at the primary etiologic disease and (2) to orthopedic appliances, braces and corrective surgery.

Meningismus, Opisthotonus and Decerebrate Rigidity

Meningismus.—Patients resist movement of the neck, back and hamstring muscles when they have meningeal irritation (i.e., *meningismus*), and they assume a position of hyperextension or opisthotonus if they have serious diffuse brain disease either acute or chronic. Meningismus is a sign of acute meningeal irritation. Opisthotonus and decerebrate rigidity are ominous signs of acute or chronic central nervous system decompensation.

Most patients in whom meningismus develops acutely have some degree of increased intracranial pressure. In addition to acute bacterial meningitis, signs of meningeal irritation may be due to a variety of acute, fulminating systemic infections such as pneumonia, otitis media, pyelonephritis, tonsillitis, bacillary dysentery, the prodromal phase of acute exanthematous diseases, acute rheumatic fever and rheumatoid arthritis. The patient may exhibit meningismus while he is recovering from a convulsive seizure or after an episode of anoxia. Mass lesions which threaten uncal herniation, such as an intracranial hematoma, cerebral edema or an abscess, may produce the syndrome. Obviously, one must take a quick but judicious diagnostic approach to this problem in order to treat infections and relieve elevated pressure as promptly as possible.

Opisthotonus.—Normally, muscle tone in the neonate is characterized by increased extensor tone in the paraspinous muscles and increased flexor tone in the extremities, a pattern which normally approaches a state of mild generalized hypotonia at 3 months of age. Exaggeration of this normal spinal extensor tone with arching of neck and back *(opisthotonus)* is considered an ominous though nonspecific prognostic sign, especially if it is associated with an abnormal cry, irritability, poor suck, an abnormal Moro reflex and abnormal vital signs. If the newborn assumes the position of opisthotonus intermittently and has no signs of acute disease of the central nervous system, congenital malformations and anoxic encephalopathy[1] must be considered strongly. When these signs develop in older infants and children after a period of well-being, other etiologies must be considered (Table 10.2).

Aseptic meningitis.—We define the syndrome of *aseptic meningitis* as one in which the patient has acute clinical signs of meningitis and the cerebrospinal fluid shows an elevated cell count and sometimes a slightly elevated protein level. Differential diagnosis should include viral meningoencephalitis, brain abscess, "acute toxic encephalopathy" (Chapter 2), subdural effusion complicating unrecognized meningitis, brain tumor, chronic forms of meningitis, the prediarrheal stage of dysentery and intoxications with agents such as lead or aminophylline. We would like to emphasize that, as more experience is gathered with the uncommon hereditary metabolic disorders, it is clear that those with an early onset such as maple syrup disease, pyridoxine dependency, hyperglycinemia and even phenylketonuria may simulate aseptic meningitis in the neonate.

Even in hospitals with elaborate virus laboratories one can expect to identify the agent in only about two thirds of the cases, compared to a proved etiology in 50% of patients with clinical encephalitis.[3]

Decerebrate rigidity.—When opisthotonus is associated with unconsciousness and sustained extension of the extremities, the patient is in the state of *decerebrate rigidity*. Acute decerebrate states often reflect hypoxia or increased intracranial pressure with impending herniation of supratentorial structures through the tentorial notch (Chapter 8). Chronic decerebrate states often signify diffuse irreversible nervous system damage and/or chronic increased intracranial pressure. Table 10.2 lists the usual causes of meningismus, opisthotonus and decerebrate rigidity in the newborn infant and the older child. A distinction is made between acute and chronic forms because etiologies differ. Chronic states of decerebrate rigidity result from (1) irreversible damage to the central nervous sys-

TABLE 10.2.—Etiologies of Meningismus, Opisthotonus and Decerebrate Rigidity

	Acute or Subacute	Chronic
Newborn	Perinatal meningitis Neonatal meningitis Intracranial hemorrhage Asphyxia	Congenital malformations

Infant and Older Child	Meningitis
	  Bacterial
	  Viral
	  Chronic granulomatous
	Meningismus with systemic infection
	Hypoxia
	Seizure state
	Trauma with intracranial hemorrhage
	Cerebral edema
	Abscess
		Progressive cerebral disease
		Leukodystrophies
		  (Krabbe, Schilder, metachromatic)
		Subacute sclerosing leukoencephalopathy
		Terminal brain tumor

tem as a result of acute disease and (2) slowly progressive metabolic, degenerative and infectious diseases.

Management.—This depends upon accurate diagnosis and in nearly all cases the etiology can be identified without difficulty. In patients with increased intracranial pressure aggravation of impending uncal herniation must be avoided. Lumbar punctures and pneumoencephalography should be undertaken with caution and only after weighing all other diagnostic evidence. The controversy and concern about doing lumbar punctures in such serious and life-threatening situations are discussed in Chapter 12 (p. 110). Definitive therapy is directed at the specific disease condition.

BIBLIOGRAPHY

1. Banker, B. Q., and Larroche, J.: Periventricular leukomalacia of infancy, Arch. Neurol. 7:386, 1962.
2. Duvoisin, R. C., and Yahr, M. D.: Compressive spinal cord and root syndrome in achondroplastic dwarfs, Neurology 12:202, 1962.
3. Lennette, E. H., *et al.*: Viral central nervous system disease, J.A.M.A. 179:687, 1962.

11

Neuroendocrinologic (Diencephalic or Hypothalamic) Syndromes

Hyponatremia with
    Inappropriate ADH Secretion
Isosexual Precocity
Hyperglycemia-Glycosuria
Gigantism, Froehlich's Syndrome
Hyperthermia

Diabetes Insipidus
Sexual Infantilism
(CNS Hypoglycemia)
Emaciation Syndrome (Russell)
Hypothermia

    Pathologic Somnolence
    "Sham Rage"
    Excessive Hunger (Bulimia)

SYNDROME DIAGNOSIS.—Many different neuroendocrinologic syndromes can result from primary brain disease (Table 11.1). However, one must speculate for the most part about the pathologic physiology which causes the metabolic disturbance. Presumably, the neural or vascular connections between the brain or telencephalon and the pituitary-hypothalamus are affected by irritative or destructive mechanisms. As a result, overactivity or underactivity of the pituitary gland gives rise to one of the syndromes described here.

Disturbance of Water and Electrolyte Metabolism

Central diabetes insipidus.—Patients with diabetes insipidus exhibit polydipsia and polyuria and may become very dehydrated if deprived of water. The pathologic thirst may lead to self-intoxication with water and convulsions may ensue. The urine specific gravity is very low and does not exceed 1.007 with a standard urine concentration test. Presumably, diabetes insipidus of the central type is caused by inadequate secretion of the antidiuretic hormone (ADH, pitressin).

TABLE 11.1.—ENDOCRINOLOGIC COMPLICATIONS OF NEUROLOGIC DISEASE

Endocrine Function	Clinical-Laboratory Syndromes	
	Excessive Secretion	Inadequate Secretion
Water and electrolyte metabolism (antidiuretic hormone secretion)	Inappropriate ADH secretion Seizures Hyponatremia Hypertonic urine (spec. grav. > 1.029) Neurogenic hypernatremia	Diabetes insipidus (too little ADH) Polyuria, polydipsia Hyperelectrolyteuria Hypotonic urine (spec. grav. <1.007)
Sexual development (gonadotropin secretion)	Isosexual precocity Elevated 17-ketosteroids (urine) Elevated gonadotropins (urine)	Sexual infantilism (Froehlich)
Somatic growth and fat deposition (growth hormone secretion)	Gigantism ± mental retardation Extreme obesity (Froehlich's syndrome) Advanced bone age	Emaciation, lipodystrophy Hyperactivity, euphoria ± elevated CSF protein
Carbohydrate metabolism		Hyperglycemia Glycosuria Polyuria, polydipsia
Body temperature regulation	Hyperthermia	Hypothermia
Sleep-wake cycle	Pathologic somnolence	
Behavior	"Sham rage"	
Appetite	Excessive hunger (bulimia)—Kleine-Levin syndrome	

Specifically, tumors, trauma, meningitis, encephalitis and the reticuloendothelioses cause this syndrome. Lesions which cause diabetes insipidus are usually located in the anterior hypothalamus and are often associated with ocular signs such as papilledema, optic atrophy, nystagmus and visual field cuts.

Occasionally one sees chronic, persistent elevation of serum electrolytes (sodium, potassium and chloride) without evidence of diabetes insipidus following head injury or other intracranial lesions.[14] Although the mechanism of this so-called "neurogenic hypernatremia" is not well understood, it is probably mediated by way of the suprasegmental autonomic apparatus including the hypothalamus.

Inappropriate secretion of ADH.—At other times an opposite type of water and electrolyte disturbance is seen. It is that of inappropriate ADH secretion and leads to hyponatremia, mental confusion and seizures in some patients. The urine is hypertonic, usually with a specific gravity exceeding 1.030 even after a water load. This chronic condition results from a variety of lesions of the central nervous system, including trauma,[3] meningitis,[9,11] subarachnoid hemorrhage,[6] pituitary tumor,[5] cerebral thrombosis,[5] diffuse, nonprogressive brain damage,[10] and infectious polyneuritis (Landry-Guillain-Barré).[12]

Disturbances in Sexual Development

Central sexual precocity.—Precocious sexual development resulting from lesions in the central nervous system is always isosexual, i.e., boys show abnormally early masculinization and girls manifest premature feminization. Children with sexual precocity must be studied very carefully in a search for neoplasms arising not only in the central nervous system[8] but in the adrenal cortex, the gonads and even the liver. The reader is referred to standard references on endocrinology such as Wilkins[18] for appropriate laboratory methods of differentiation. In contrast to the situation in diabetes insipidus, lesions which cause sexual precocity are located in the *posterior hypothalamus* and associated ocular signs are seldom seen. Pinealoma is associated with sexual precocity in some cases.

Sexual infantilism.—Hypothalamic damage that is due to head injury causes sexual infantilism more frequently than it causes precocity. The syndrome of delayed sexual development and obesity (and sometimes diabetes insipidus) has been called "adiposogenital dystrophy" or "Froehlich's syndrome." The latter term should be restricted to those cases of extreme obesity in which a known hypothalamic lesion exists (Fig. 17.6, p. 257). Lesions which cause hypogonadism are more often located in the anterior hypothalamus and frequently are associated with diabetes insipidus and obesity. Before a diagnosis of post-traumatic hypothalamic damage is made, the patient must be studied fully to rule out tumors in the region of the sella turcica and third ventricle as well as third ventricular dilatation in patients with hydrocephalus. Gonadal agenesis can be distinguished readily by abnormalities in smears for sex chromatin and chromosome studies. Patients with the Laurence-Moon-Biedl syndrome resemble closely those with adiposogenital syndrome, but in the former condition (a clinical constellation of anomalies sometimes behaving as a recessive trait) one expects to see mental defect, polydactyly and sometimes retinitis pigmentosa.

The remaining hypothalamic syndromes are seen with great rarity. As in the case of the above two clinical situations, special care must be taken to exclude treatable conditions such as infections, tumors, intoxications and specific metabolic disorders before resorting to the diagnosis of fixed irritative or atrophic post-traumatic hypothalamic conditions.

Disturbances in Somatic Growth and Fat Deposition

Emaciation syndrome of Russell.[15]—Whenever one sees a markedly emaciated child who otherwise seems active, well and happy, the diagnosis of a diencephalic tumor should be considered seriously, especially if abnormal ocular signs are found. This paradoxical syndrome is seen in infants who appear terminally ill despite good food intake and a happy disposition.[1] Disproportionately large hands and feet have been noted with this syndrome.[4] In most cases a "silent," low-grade glioma is found in the parasellar region.[2] If a tumor is demonstrated, it is handled according to its location. An example of this syndrome is shown in Figure 17.7 on page 259.

Gigantism.—Recently several examples of cerebral gigantism with excessive growth of the hands and feet have been reported.[7,17] The cerebral etiology of the syndrome has been based upon the common occurrence of mental retardation and ventricular dilatation. The patients also exhibit acromegalic facies, excessively rapid growth, large skulls and advanced bone age.[13] The syndrome has also been seen in patients with pituitary tumors.[16]

Froehlich's syndrome.—This syndrome is discussed in the preceding section on sexual infantilism.

Disturbances of Carbohydrate Metabolism

Rarely hyperglycemia and glycosuria occur without other laboratory and clinical evidence of diabetes mellitus. The disorder of sugar metabolism can be controlled with insulin, but this measure is not usually warranted since the patient remains asymptomatic and does not become hyperlipemic, ketotic or acidotic. Although some authors state that hypoglycemia can arise secondary to lesions of the central nervous system, until more convincing evidence is presented one should presume that the neurologic symptoms and signs result from rather than cause the hypoglycemia.

Disturbances in Body-Temperature Regulation, Sleep-Wake Cycle, Behavior and Appetite

Because these conditions are extremely rare, the diagnostic evidence should be examined with great care. Hypothermia and hyperthermia can follow damage to or irritation of areas in the hypothalamus. However, the diagnosis of central hyperthermia should be made only as a last resort after a thorough and exhaustive search for a site of infection.

Hypothalamic disease can cause pathologic states of somnolence aside from conditions of true coma or stupor. It can also cause ravenous increases in appetite (bulimia). States of "sham rage," like the other vegetative symptoms and signs, can be produced by properly placed experimental lesions in the hypothalamus of animals. Rarely, similar states of inappropriate, violent behavior have been reported in patients with hypothalamic disease.

DIFFERENTIAL DIAGNOSIS.—Many different neuroendocrinologic syndromes can result from primary disease of the brain. The most common basic etiologies of hypothalamic or diencephalic syndromes are (1) head trauma, (2) brain tumor, (3) ischemia, (4) complications of infections of the nervous system, (5) congenital malformations and (6) neoplastic degenerative diseases such as neurofibromatosis and tuberous sclerosis.

MANAGEMENT.—*Diabetes insipidus.*—Pitressin can be given in either the powder or snuff form (posterior pituitary powder), the intramuscular form (pitressin tannate in oil) or as a solution to be used nasally. Previously, cotton pledgets soaked in pitressin solution were employed, but recently a new synthetic product, lysyl-8-vasopressin has been used as a nasal spray. Rallison and Tyler[14] report that the latter solution has caused no serious allergic reactions, but nasal irritation is not uncommon.

Other symptomatic therapy is well outlined in Wilkins' textbook,[18] and the specific neurologic treatment is covered in other chapters.

BIBLIOGRAPHY

1. Bain, H. W., *et al.*: The diencephalic syndrome of early infancy due to silent brain tumor: With special reference to treatment, Pediatrics 38:473, 1966.

2. Braun, F. C., and Forney, W. R.: Diencephalic syndrome of early infancy associated with brain tumor, Pediatrics 24:609, 1959.
3. Carter, N. W., et al.: Hyponatremia in cerebral disease resulting from the inappropriate secretion of antidiuretic hormone, New England J. Med. 264:67, 1961.
4. Gamstorp, I., et al.: Diencephalic syndromes of infancy, J. Pediat. 70:383, 1967.
5. Goldberg, M., and Handler, J. S.: Hyponatremia and renal wasting of sodium in patients with malfunction of the central nervous system, New England J. Med. 263:1037, 1960.
6. Joynt, R. J., et al.: Hyponatremia in subarachnoid hemorrhage, Arch. Neurol. 13:633, 1965.
7. Kjellman, B.: Cerebral gigantism, Acta paediat. scandinav. 54:603, 1965.
8. Loop, J. W.: Precocious puberty: Pneumoencephalography demonstrating a hamartoma in the absence of cerebral symptoms, New England J. Med. 271:409, 1964.
9. Mangos, J. A., and Lobeck, C. C.: Studies of sustained hyponatremia due to central nervous system infection, Pediatrics 34:503, 1964.
10. McCrory, W. W., and Macauley, D.: Idiopathic hyponatremia in an infant with diffuse cerebral damage, Pediatrics 20:23, 1957.
11. Nyhan, W. L., and Cooke, R. E.: Symptomatic hyponatremia in acute infections of the central nervous system, Pediatrics 18:604, 1956.
12. Posner, J. B., et al.: Hyponatremia in acute polyneuropathy, Arch. Neurol. 17:530, 1967.
13. Poznanski, A. K., and Stephenson, J. M.: Radiographic findings in hypothalamic acceleration of growth associated with cerebral atrophy and mental retardation (cerebral gigantism), Radiology 88:446, 1967.
14. Rallison, M. L., and Tyler, F. H.: Treatment of diabetes insipidus in children with lysyl-8-vasopressin, J. Pediat. 70:122, 1967.
15. Russell, A.: A diencephalic syndrome of emaciation in infancy and childhood (abstract), Arch. Dis. Childhood 26:274, 1951.
16. Saxena, K. M., and Crawford, J. D.: Acromegalic gigantism in an adolescent girl, J. Pediat. 62:660, 1963.
17. Sotos, J. F., et al.: Cerebral gigantism in childhood, New England J. Med. 271:109, 1964.
18. Wilkins, L.: *The Diagnosis and Treatment of Endocrine Disorders in Childhood and Adolescence* (3d ed.; Springfield, Ill.: Charles C Thomas, Publisher, 1965).

12

Diagnostic Laboratory Tests

X-ray Studies
    Plain Skull X-rays
        Sutures, head size and thickness of calvarium
        Suspected brain tumors
        Intracranial calcification
    Pneumography
        Hypotensive hydrocephalus
        Hypertensive hydrocephalus
        Choice between pneumoencephalography and ventriculography
        Analgesia and anesthesia
        Complications
    Angiography
    Radioisotopic Brain Scans
    Echoencephalography
    Spine X-rays
    Myelography
    Visual Field Study
Electrical Studies
    Electroencephalography
        Principles of recording
        Interpretation
        Diagnostic value
    Electromyography and Conduction Velocity Studies
Clinical Chemistry
    Urine Chromatography
Cerebrospinal Fluid Examination
Muscle Biopsy

MATERIAL IN THIS CHAPTER covers interpretation of test results and offers selected comments about the strengths and limitations of the more important laboratory procedures. The busy clinician quickly learns which diagnostic studies help him most, but he usually must depend upon laboratory experts for accurate interpretation. However, he should develop as much personal interpretive skill as possible

TABLE 12.1.—Diagnostic Laboratory Tests

Suspected Disease	Tests	Cross References to Figures
Congenital malformations	Skull x-rays	13.3, 13.18,B, 13.22, 13.23, 13.25,B, 13.28
	Pneumography	13.6,B, 13.8,A & B, 13.13, 13.14,B, 13.19,C, 13.28
	Cervical spine films	13.27
	Angiography	13.19,C, 13.20,A & B, 13.21
Epilepsy	Electroencephalography	14.1,B–D, 14.2, 14.3,B–D, 14.4,B & C
Trauma	Skull x-rays	15.5,B, 15.6,A–C, 15.9
	Pneumography	15.4,A, 15.7
	Angiography	15.4,B, 15.5,C
	Spine x-rays	15.8,A & C
	Myelography	15.10,D
Hypoxia	Lumbar puncture and CSF study	16.4
	Electroencephalography	16.1,A, 16.8,B
	Pneumography	16.1,B, 16.8,C
Tumors	Skull x-rays	17.6,B & D, 17.8,B & C, 17.10
	Electroencephalography	17.4,A & B, 17.5,A
	Pneumography and Pantopaque ventriculography	17.1,A–C, 17.2, 17.3,C, 17.7,A, 17.8,D, 17.9
	Angiography	17.5,B
	Radioisotope scan	17.1,D & E, 17.7,B & C
	Spine x-rays	17.11,A
	Myelography	17.11,B, 17.12,A, 17.13,A–C, 17.14,A & B
Infections	Skull x-rays	18.6
	Electroencephalography	18.3
Muscle diseases	Biopsy (muscle and liver)	19.1,C, 19.3,C
	Electromyography	19.2,B, 19.7,B & C
Intoxications	Skull & bone x-rays	20.2,A
Metabolic and degenerative diseases	Chemical tests	
	Urine	21.6,B
	Blood	21.2
	CSF	21.13
	Biopsy (bone marrow, muscle, liver, rectum)	21.10,A & B, 21.11,B
	Skull x-rays	21.17, 21.18,A
	Electroencephalography	21.15,B
	Pneumography	21.7,B, 21.12,B
Demyelinating disease		
Neurologic complications of systemic disease	Electroencephalography	23.1, 23.3,D, 23.4

and maintain a critical attitude about the laboratory expert's opinion. Also, he should avoid the mistake of leaning too heavily upon any single diagnostic study. Instead he should consider *all* of the historical data, the physical findings and the laboratory results in order to insure diagnostic success.

Table 12.1 summarizes the many tests which have diagnostic value in different categories of disease. Diseases are listed in their chapter order, the tests are listed in their approximate order of importance and the reader is referred to exemplary illustrations in Part II.

X-ray Studies[19]

Plain Skull X-rays

This type of examination is commonly used, but one must guard against certain pitfalls in the process of interpretation.

SUTURES.—In normal infants the sutures may appear abnormally separated and the erroneous diagnoses of increased intracranial pressure or defective bone formation are made in these cases. At other times the differentiation of normal sutures from linear skull fractures may be extremely different and expert interpretation is often required before a decision can be reached.[8] This question has special importance when litigation arises involving infants and young children who have suffered head injuries.

EVALUATION OF HEAD SIZE.—The diagnosis of microcrania or macrocrania can be suspected on an x-ray of the skull, but the clinician can come to such a decision with greater accuracy than the radiologist by using simple measurements of occipital-frontal head circumference (Appendix 7) or serial head measurements.[23a] Efforts have been made to estimate brain size by measurements of intracranial volume. However, such techniques have not yet reached the stage of practical clinical use.

THICKNESS OF THE CALVARIUM.—Although thickening of the skull often has no clinical significance, it can signify an adjacent slow-growing tumor, such as a meningioma, or an area of fibrous dysplasia. Thinning of the calvarium can result from uncommon lesions such as subdural hematomas of the middle fossa (Fig. 15.5, p. 207), slow-growing gliomas and porencephalic cysts.[11]

SUSPECTED BRAIN TUMORS.—A plain skull series should be obtained on all patients in whom tumor is suspected. Special attention is paid to signs of increased intracranial pressure, such as separated sutures, erosion or demineralization of the dorsum sellae and the posterior clinoids, and to abnormally prominent convolutional markings. Guard especially against overinterpretation of the latter finding since the markings normally become prominent between 5 and 7 years of age. Approximately 10–15% of older patients with supratentorial tumors exhibit a shifted, calcified pineal gland on plain skull x-ray examination, but in children this helps very little unless a pineal gland tumor is suspected. Occasionally a slowly growing mass (not necessarily neoplasm) will thin the calvarium by eroding the inner table (Fig. 15.6, p. 209). In addition to changes from generalized pressure, the sella turcica may show enlargement or ballooning, as in craniopharyngioma or pituitary adenoma, undermining of the anterior clinoids with a resulting J-shaped (optic chiasm glioma) abnormality or suprasellar calcification (75% of craniopharyngiomas).

Special views are necessary to see the optic foramina, which are enlarged in gliomas and other infiltrating tumors of the optic nerve. An optic foramen is considered to be enlarged if it exceeds 6.5 mm. in its greatest diameter and, even though some size asymmetry between the two sides is common, an abnormality should be suspected if the difference is 2 mm. or more.[35] Occasionally views of the internal auditory meatus and the acoustic canal (Stenvers' projection) are needed to aid in the diagnosis of an acoustic neurinoma, an uncommon tumor in childhood. Calcification in tumors other than craniopharyngiomas is seen only rarely in children but may appear in any slow-growing glioma, especially oligodendroglioma, or in congenital tumors such as teratomas.

INTRACRANIAL CALCIFICATIONS.—A variety of uncommon diseases cause intracranial calcifications. Among the more common lesions which calcify are brain tumors (especially craniopharyngiomas and slow-growing gliomas), perinatal forms of meningitis (toxoplasmosis and cytomegalovirus infections), metabolic and degenerative diseases (pseudohypoparathyroidism, hypoparathyroidism and tuberous sclerosis) and congenital vascular malformations. Chronic subdural hematomas calcify rarely.

PNEUMOGRAPHY

Instillation of air into the lumbar subarachnoid space or into the ventricles is performed to demonstrate the size, the shape and the position of the ventricles. In addition, pneumoencephalography outlines the surface subarachnoid pathways and the basal cisterns of the brain. The techniques have wide usefulness in diagnostic neurology, as indicated in Table 12.1.

HYPOTENSIVE AND HYPERTENSIVE HYDROCEPHALUS.—It is helpful to divide all cases of hydrocephalus (i.e., ventricular enlargement) into *hypotensive* and *hypertensive* types. In patients with hypotensive hydrocephalus (sometimes called *hydrocephalus ex vacuo*) the ventricles enlarge because of underdevelopment (hypoplasia), atrophy or shrinkage of the brain. In hypertensive hydrocephalus the ventricles enlarge because of an obstruction to the normal flow or absorption of cerebrospinal fluid.

Differentiation of hypotensive from hypertensive hydrocephalus is usually not difficult. It depends upon a consideration of all the clinical data. The important factors are compared in Table 12.2. Patients with hypotensive hydrocephalus often have abnormally small heads, whereas those with the hypertensive type have enlarged heads. The hypotensive type is more often associated with evidence of chronic neurologic deficit such as mental retardation, seizures and spasticity. However, spasticity can be seen in the obstructive hypertensive type because the slowly enlarging ventricles can stretch the corticospinal tracts and cause pyramidal tract signs. No good correlation exists, however, between the pneumographic findings and the severity of clinical deficits such as mental retardation and convulsive disorders.[10, 16a]

TABLE 12.2.—CLINICAL DIFFERENTIATION OF VENTRICULAR ENLARGEMENT

	HYPOTENSIVE HYDROCEPHALUS	HYPERTENSIVE HYDROCEPHALUS
Small head	+	0
Enlarged head	0	+
Symptoms, signs and laboratory evidence of increased intracranial pressure (Chapter 8)	0	+
Mental retardation	Common	Uncommon
Seizures	Common	Uncommon
Spasticity	May be present in either type	

CHOICE BETWEEN PNEUMOENCEPHALOGRAPHY AND VENTRICULOGRAPHY.—The decision about when to do pneumography and the choice between pneumoencephalography and ventriculography should be made only by experienced neurologists and neurosurgeons. In general, a pneumoencephalogram is preferable to a ventriculogram if the procedure can be carried out without undue risk to the patient and at the same time obtain diagnostic information. In the course of ventriculography needles are passed through the brain and this is not an innocuous procedure. Often in situations in which increased intracranial pressure exists, one encounters normal or small-sized ventricles in such conditions as pseudotumor cerebri. Even in cases of increased intracranial pressure with obstructive hydrocephalus and moderate ventricular dilatation the operator may have to make several passes with the cannula before he hits the ventricle. We have seen several patients who later had focal seizures on the side opposite the brain needling. Obviously it is not certain that the seizures resulted from the procedure rather than from brain damage secondary to obstructive hydrocephalus, but the association is suggestive.

Choice of ventriculography.—In general, one recommends ventriculography when increased intracranial pressure is of an acute nature or when one suspects a mass lesion. Once air has been instilled into the ventricles through a burr hole, the operator and the x-ray technician must spend sufficient time manipulating the patient's head to fill the critical pathways (both lateral ventricles, the third ventricle, the aqueduct of Sylvius and the fourth ventricle) if diagnostic evidence is to be gained. Such maneuvers may or may not be successful, their success usually depending upon the degree of obstruction and the operator's technique. Also the experience and the interpretive skill of the physician reading the x-rays influence greatly the amount of information obtained from air-contrast study.

Choice of pneumoencephalography.—In general, air is instilled through a lumbar spinal puncture needle if one suspects an atrophic lesion of the brain, if long-standing increased intracranial pressure is present (subdural hematomas and congenital hydrocephalus) or if ventriculography has not been diagnostic. The combined ventriculogram-pneumoencephalogram is often necessary if a tumor is suspected.

Instillation of air from below is generally considered dangerous because of the risk of (1) cerebellar tonsillar herniation in the case of a posterior fossa mass lesion or (2) herniation of the temporal lobe uncus in the case of a supratentorial neoplasm. However, this issue remains a matter of controversy among neurologists and neurosurgeons. Prince and Wiener[27] performed lumbar pneumoencephalograms on 133 patients with brain tumors and concluded that this procedure remains the procedure of choice for visualizing the ventricular system, even in patients with increased intracranial pressure. Most workers would disagree with this point of view.

In our opinion, pneumoencephalography may be undertaken when the patient's condition is well compensated, when the signs and symptoms of pressure are not severe, when the clinical indications warrant it and when the neurosurgeon and anesthesiologist are available. A careful, small (10–15 cc. of air) positive-pressure procedure (i.e., without removal of any cerebrospinal fluid) can be carried out using a No. 22 gauge lumbar puncture needle. It is done under deep sedation (Appendix 6), using local anesthesia for the spinal tap. Properly timed and positioned x-ray films are then obtained. If air fails to enter the ventricular system (as often happens with cerebellar or brain stem tumors) at the time of an otherwise technically satisfactory study, this fact in itself enhances the likelihood of finding a mass lesion, as pointed out by Scheinberg and Yahr.[30]

PANTOPAQUE VENTRICULOGRAPHY.—This technique is indicated in carefully selected cases, usually in patients suspected of having an obstructive lesion of the aqueduct or the fourth ventricle in whom air-contrast studies from above and below are not diagnostic. Pantopaque, 2–3 cc., is instilled into the lateral ventricle by way of a burr hole and a ventricular tap without removing any fluid. When carefully performed this procedure can be very helpful, but proper manipulation of the patient's head is essential in order to maintain the oily Pantopaque in a bolus, direct it to the critical portion of the ventricular system and avoid spreading it in droplet form to all parts of the ventricular system and subarachnoid space.

ANALGESIA AND ANESTHESIA.—The type and dose of sedation used for painful diagnostic procedures such as pneumoencephalography are outlined in Appendix 6. In general, we prefer deep sedation to general anesthesia for these procedures because of its relative safety.[24]

COMPLICATIONS.—Different types of vascular accidents occasionally complicate pneumography, although the risks are generally lower in children than in adults. It has been known for many years that bloody fluid may accumulate in the subdural space. This occurs most often in children under age 2, especially when a large amount of air is instilled accidentally into the subdural space.[32] We think this complication is an uncommon problem in the hands of experienced operators. If the spinal tap is done carefully, if good flow is obtained before proceeding and if scout films are obtained after 10 or 20 cc. of air is injected, this complication is obviated. When an inadequate flow of fluid is encountered or when the scout films reveal a subdural injection of air, the procedure should either be terminated or the needle should be withdrawn and reinserted at the next higher interspace. It is well known, also, that the incidence of unsatisfactory pneumoencephalograms is much higher in patients who have had a lumbar puncture a week or two prior to the attempted air study.

Ischemic vascular accidents (both coronary occlusions and cerebral "strokes") complicate a certain number of diagnostic air studies in adults, probably as a result of associated hypotension.[33] Such complications have also been seen in children but their incidence is fortunately low. We usually wrap the legs with elastic bandages in children over 4 years of age to avoid postural hypotension.

ANGIOGRAPHY

Injection of positive-contrast radiopaque media (50% Hypaque or 60% Renografin) into the blood vessels, usually the arteries, is helpful in the diagnosis of supratentorial mass lesions such as neoplasms, subdural hematomas and brain abscesses as well as vascular malformations. Since these lesions are rather uncommon and since the procedure requires greater technical skill and usually a general anesthetic in children, its use is restricted in most centers. Whereas percutaneous carotid injection can usually be performed without difficulty in adults, other techniques such as retrograde brachial, femoral or subclavian injection are often used and often require surgical exposure of the vessel. When the procedure is indicated, it should be carried out with care by an experienced person who is doing angiograms regularly. If this approach is used, few complications will be encountered.

Angiography is generally indicated whenever a patient has localizing or lateralizing, supratentorial neurologic signs or when a vascular lesion is suspected on the basis of subarachnoid bleeding or the clinical picture of "stroke."

Radioisotopic Brain Scans

The technique of scintillation scanning of the brain following the intravenous injection of radioactive isotopes (mercury, iodine or technetium) has now become a useful, dependable, well-established procedure in most large hospitals.[7,22,39,41,43] This test has entered widespread use because it can be carried out easily and without hazard. Indications for its use are similar to those for angiography. Since the radioactive material is trapped in areas of increased vascularity, the procedure is used primarily to localize supratentorial neoplasms and to some extent hemorrhages, abscesses and posterior fossa tumors.[41]

False-positive studies have been encountered[42] for a variety of reasons, so it is essential not only to realize that they do occur but why they occur and what should be done to avoid them. Some false positives result from trapping of the radioisotope in vascular structures such as the choroid plexus; this can be avoided to some extent by giving the patient 200–400 mg. of potassium perchlorate by mouth 15–30 minutes before the scan is done.[44] In other instances extracranial contamination of the skin and hair from saliva or gastric juice has led to false-positive studies. We have had the even more disconcerting experience of encountering false-negative scans in several patients with malignant tumors of the cerebral hemisphere. Expert interpretation is essential.

Echoencephalography

Instruments utilizing ultrasonic impulses can localize intracranial structures having a normally midline position.[2,6] This simple and safe procedure has already become an established method for detecting shift of midline structures secondary to neoplasm or hematoma. More recently it has been extended to recognize the presence and thickness of hematomas and the existence of dilated ventricles.

Spine X-rays

The physician should seek expert advice for the interpretation of all spine films, especially when there is suspected trauma to the cervical spine, because of normal variations and because of the differences from adult spine films.[9,37] A complete set of spine films should be obtained first whenever the diagnosis of an intraspinal mass is considered. Anteroposterior and lateral views should be obtained routinely and oblique spot films can be ordered to investigate suspicious areas. Widening of the spinal canal can be documented with careful measurements of the interpediculate distance (Appendix 10) on the anteroposterior views. In the lateral projection a mass is suspected if one sees increased concavity of the posterior aspects of the vertebral bodies. Erosion of the pedicles, thinning of the laminae and enlargement of the intervertebral foramina can be seen well in the oblique views. Vertebral anomalies should be looked for carefully since they may coexist with "congenital" tumors. Lumbar puncture and CSF examination often provide valuable diagnostic information, but caution should be taken before this procedure is done. Patients with established neurologic deficit can worsen precipitously when a spinal tap is done and fluid removed. In patients in whom tumor is strongly suspected, one should be ready to proceed directly to a myelogram, and the neurosurgeon should be prepared to do a laminectomy immediately if necessary. Difficulty in entering the subarachnoid space should point to a large intraspinal mass. Similarly, xanthochromic fluid may indicate a complete block. In such situations manometric study of the CSF dynamics or myelography should be performed with caution for reasons already mentioned. A myelogram from below attempted at a later time may be impossible because the small reservoir of fluid in the lumbar sac below the block has been drained. In such situations, or if the subarachnoid space was never entered, a cisternal myelogram under general anesthesia may be necessary to localize the mass. If the neurosurgeon wants to know the upper and lower limits of the lesion, a combined lumbar and cisternal Pantopaque study must be carried out.

Calcified intervertebral disk.—Occasionally calcified intervertebral disks are seen in children, but for all practical purposes these findings have no clinical significance.[23]

Myelography

Although a detailed description of the technique and interpretation of myelograms goes beyond the scope of this text, some summary information is presented. Data obtained from myelography permit individual tumors to be classified according to three categories: (1) extradural, (2) intradural extramedullary and (3) intramedullary. This classification, the value of which depends upon accurate interpretation, has great usefulness not only because it narrows the range of diagnostic possibilities when combined with other clinical information, but because it helps the neurosurgeon greatly. The accurate differentiation of extradural from intradural lesions often prevents unnecessarily extensive surgical exploration and needling of the cord and obviates the need to open the dura—all of which increase the operative morbidity.

Myelograms in patients with *intramedullary* tumors (most often astrocytomas or ependymomas) usually show fusiform widening of the spinal cord with tapering of the Pantopaque away from the midline at the site of the block. *Extramedullary intradural* neoplasms (neurofibroma, meningioma or a medulloblastoma which has seeded) are typified by a tumor mass which is sharply outlined by contrast medium and which displaces the cord shadow in the frontal or lateral prone projections. *Extradural* masses (leukemic infiltrate, extended paraspinal lesions such as neuroblastomas and sarcoma) are characterized either by sweeping indentations of the dye column over several segments of the spinal column or by a gradual attenuation or constriction of the Pantopaque shadow to a point of complete obstruction (malignant metastatic lesions such as leukemia). An intravenous urogram should be taken routinely whenever it is suspected that the intraspinal mass has extended from the common neuroblastoma or neurofibroma in the paraspinal area.

Visual Field Study

Patients must be old enough to cooperate before these techniques can be used. Visual acuity determinations should be carried out in every patient prior to field testing. In patients with signs of papilledema one expects essentially normal acuity with enlarged blind spots but without any significant field cut except for mild constriction of the peripheral fields with long-standing pressure. Tumors in the parasellar region may compress the optic chiasm and produce a bitemporal hemianopia, and large scotomata may be demonstrated in patients with gliomas of the optic nerve. We have been struck with the frequent observation of apparently severe visual field constriction in children without other evidence of neurologic or ocular disease. In some patients this "tunnel vision" represents a hysterical conversion reaction but in many children it simply reflects their misunderstanding of the test instructions.

Electrical Studies

Electroencephalography

Electroencephalographic diagnosis is discussed in more detail than other laboratory procedures because of its frequent use in neurologic disorders of children. Also, in some instances neurologists either supervise laboratories or need some guidelines in evaluating interpretation by others. We think that electroencephalography is a very helpful procedure when used properly and we believe that most mistakes result from overzealous interpretation. A glossary of EEG terminology has been set forth by the International Federation of Societies for Electroencephalography and Clinical Neurophysiology.[38]

Principles of recording.—About 20 electrodes are applied to the scalp with a conductant paste, and electric potentials produced by the brain are run into the machine where they are amplified about 1,000 times. This electrical energy is then converted into the mechanical energy of 8–16 ink-writing pens on moving paper. A permanent record is produced.

The electrodes are positioned symmetrically on the scalp in a precise fashion according to distances measured from bony landmarks. The so-called "10-20 International System" of electrode placement has entered widespread use and is recommended.[29] The recording is made in a quiet or soundproof room so that the patient will relax and a record of optimal quality will be obtained. When dealing with restless, active children it is often advisable to secure the electrodes to the scalp with an elastic bandage.

Both monopolar (scalp to interconnected ears) and bipolar (scalp to scalp) recordings are obtained in most laboratories. Standard recording patterns (montages) can be selected by the turn of a switch, but the technician should be encouraged to record independent patterns, especially if he sees what looks like a focus of abnormal activity. The technician should also note eye opening and closure, and he should be familiar with all kinds of artifacts. Adjustment or changes in the electrodes may be necessary during recording in order to eliminate artifacts.

In every case recordings should be made with the patient (1) awake and (2) asleep, and using the activation or provocative techniques of (3) hyperventilation and (4) photic stimulation.[5] Instructions should be given the patient or the parents to limit the patient's sleep to four or five hours the night before the test so that he will go to sleep readily. It helps to have patients avoid stimulating drinks such as coffee or "coke" before coming to the laboratory. Contrary to common belief it is not necessary to discontinue drug therapy before the study. In fact, this practice should be avoided so that patients do not run the risk of status epilepticus.

Special electrode placements can be used. Nasopharyngeal electrodes can be inserted with only minor discomfort to the patient and have great value in cases of psychomotor epilepsy. They aid in the localization of foci on the inferior mesial aspect of the temporal lobe, i.e., in the region of the uncus and hippocampus. In carefully selected, older children and adults sphenoidal electrode recording and electrocorticography can be used if the total workup suggests that the patient may be a suitable candidate for surgical therapy. In general, the latter techniques should be used only in large centers where a team has developed a major interest in and commitment to the operative treatment of epilepsy.

INTERPRETATION.—The most useful EEG interpretation is obtained from the subjective impression of an experienced electroencephalographer. Not only does he recognize all types of artifacts, but he considers normal variation with age, level of consciousness, drug effects and the range of normal responses to activation techniques. So far, machine analyses of clinical records have not made important contributions to EEG diagnosis.

Hyperventilation, consisting of two three-minute periods of continuous deep breathing, is carried out in all patients who are able to cooperate. This measure effectively precipitates petit mal discharges in many patients (Chapter 14). However, many normal children show diffuse high-voltage slow activity which by itself should not be considered pathologic. We think that *sleep recordings should be obtained in every patient with seizures* because a certain percentage of patients will exhibit epileptiform discharges only during light sleep.

Photic stimulation, using commercially available electronic stroboscopes, should also be employed routinely.[16] The details of this activation technique have been fully described.[5] So-called photic driving or photic recruitment has no particular clinical significance. Photic stimulation has its greatest diagnostic value in patients with petit mal epilepsy (Chapter 14) and in some with myoclonic seizures. In patients who are known to be light-sensitive, this activation method should be used cautiously in the EEG laboratory so that clinical convulsions are not precipitated.

When other provocative techniques fail to elicit epileptiform EEG abnormalities in a patient with seizures, it helps to get an EEG recording after *sleep deprivation*. The patient is kept awake for 24 hours before the recording and this can be done most dependably, in our experience, by hospitalization. A report by Pratt et al.[26] shows that this technique activates epileptiform discharges in 41% of patients who previously had normal or borderline recordings. In contrast, Bennett and Ziter[3] have shown that in a normal young adult control group EEG abnormalities did not develop with sleep deprivation.

DIAGNOSTIC VALUE.—Electroencephalography has its main value in the diagnosis of convulsive disorders and, to a lesser extent, in the localization of mass lesions.[5] Electroencephalograms from patients with hemisphere tumors often exhibit a slow wave focus or a sharp wave epileptiform focus combined with a consistently well-localized slow wave discharge in the theta (4–7 cycles/sec) or delta (1–3 cycles/sec) frequency range. Generalized slowing has no diagnostic specificity since it occurs commonly in a variety of other neurologic disorders and is a common reflection of increased intracranial pressure. Even the generalized, paroxysmal, spike wave abnormality which typifies the brain wave disorder of centrencephalic epilepsy has been noted in patients with tumors often enough to suggest that the tumor itself and not a coincidental idiopathic seizure disorder has caused the epileptiform discharge (Table 12.3). We have been impressed also with the value of the electroencephalogram in patients with behavior and personality disorders in whom the clinical evidence may otherwise fail to distinguish between a functional and an organic etiology. It is especially helpful in patients with acute delirium, organic psychosis and psychomotor seizures which may suggest hysteria. However, one finds little correlation between the type of abnormality and the exact nature and severity of the mental disturbance.

Prognostic value has been attached to the electroencephalogram in patients with head injuries or infections of the cerebrum, either bacterial or viral. Serial recordings, particularly in young children in whom the added variable of a developing nervous system complicates the prognosis, may aid the physician in predicting the long-range outcome. It is said that EEG recordings may help in the evaluation of the therapy of meningitis and head injuries, but most clinicians rightfully base their evaluation regarding duration of therapy on other laboratory evidence or on clinical grounds.

Since children with febrile convulsions and breath-holding spells usually have normal electroencephalograms, definite EEG abnormalities in such patients may mean that fever or anoxia simply evoked the seizure in a child who may later exhibit true epilepsy. Some value has been attached to the electroencephalogram in the diagnosis of suspected deafness in young children, evidence being provided by the absence of an arousal response to loud sounds (Chapter 7). Encephalopathies which result not from infections of the nervous system but from anoxia and drug, water or metabolic end-product intoxication often produce significant EEG changes, but these are usually highly nonspecific. Similarly, certain endocrinopathies, such as hypothyroidism, hypoadrenocorticism (Addison's disease) and hypoglycemia secondary to hyperinsulinism, may produce real but nonspecific slow wave EEG changes.

A summary of the most important types of EEG abnormalities is given in

TABLE 12.3.—EEG ABNORMALITIES USEFUL IN DIAGNOSIS

	CROSS REFERENCES TO FIGURES
Seizure disorders	
"Petit mal" (diffuse spike and wave)	
Primary bilateral synchrony*	14.1, 14.2
Secondary bilateral synchrony*	17.4,*B*
Focal	
Midtemporal	14.3
Anterior temporal	14.3, 16.3
Hypsarrhythmia	2.2
"Petit mal variant"	—
Mass lesions	
Slow wave focus	17.5,*A*, 18.4,*A*, 23.1, 23.3,*D*
Spike focus	17.4,*A*
Voltage asymmetry	15.8,*B*, 23.3,*D*
Behavior disorders	
Spike focus	—
Spike and slow wave focus	1.5,*A*
Generalized slowing	21.15,*B*
"14 and 6 c/s positive spikes"†	—
6-per-second spike and wave‡	—
Aphasia (acquired speech and hearing defects)	1.5,*A* & *B*
Meningoencephalitis	
Slowing	18.3
Periodic sharp waves with slow background frequencies ("burst-suppression")§	—

*Diffuse spike and wave EEG discharges are seen most commonly in petit mal or centrencephalic epilepsy. The term "primary bilateral synchrony" has been used to describe the origin and spread of these epileptiform discharges. Occasionally, however, similar spike and wave discharges are seen in patients with focal lesions in one hemisphere which presumably spread to activate the brain stem reticular-activating system. The resulting diffuse EEG abnormality is called "secondary bilateral synchrony." The latter phenomenon is well documented in the literature,[1,20,21,34] and an example is shown in Figure 17.4,*B*, page 254.

†Gibbs and Gibbs[14] called attention to this type of EEG discharge and suggested that the finding correlates with a variety of clinical syndromes, including autonomic symptoms and behavioral abnormalities, especially rage reactions. They consider this EEG finding a manifestation of thalamic or hypothalamic epilepsy. Other reports have confirmed and denied[18] their impression. Recently another group has correlated this brain wave finding with migraine in childhood.[40] We believe the clinical significance of this occasional EEG wave form has not yet been clearly established.

‡Six-per-second spike and wave ("wave and spike phantom") discharges resemble petit mal morphologically and resemble "14 and 6 c/s positive spikes" in their diffuse, nonspecific clinical correlates. Some workers consider this electrical phenomenon a normal variant.[36]

§Diagnostic specificity has been attached to the periodic sharp wave discharges ("burst-suppression") seen in patients with subacute sclerosing leukoencephalitis[28] (Chapter 18), but other workers have seen similar abnormalities in a variety of other conditions.[12,17]

Table 12.3 and cross references to illustrations are listed. In general, the search for diagnostic or pathognomonic wave forms and patterns has so far not proved very helpful. Most clinicians agree that the clinical electroencephalogram has a limited diagnostic repertoire. Undue significance should not be given to minor or equivocal abnormalities. Rather, the findings should be considered in the context of all other clinical and laboratory observations.

Schwab and others[31] have suggested that the electroencephalogram be used to define "life or death" in patients who have suffered severe cerebral anoxia and who appear to be living only with the help of artificial respirators and heart stimulators. If the patient has no spontaneous respirations and is areflexic, a "flat EEG" which persists for at least 24 hours may be a good guide to irreversible brain damage and may indicate that efforts at resuscitation will prove fruitless.[15]

Diagnostic Laboratory Tests

Electromyography and Conduction Velocity Studies

Electromyography has not entered widespread clinical usefulness because of its relative lack of diagnostic specificity. The experienced clinician usually finds that he obtains as much or more accurate diagnostic information from a careful neurologic examination (including muscle check) and muscle biopsy. However, the electromyogram may show fibrillation potentials in equivocal cases (evidence

---

TABLE 12.4.—Diagnostic Tests for Metabolic and Degenerative Disorders Affecting the Nervous System

Screening Tests	Disorders*
Urine	
1. FeCl₃	
2. DNPH	Aminoacidopathies
3. NaCN-nitroprusside[33a]	
4. Reducing substance	Carbohydrate diseases
5. Toluidine blue "spot test"	Polysaccharidoses
Blood	
Calcium and phosphorus	Tetany
Glucose	Hypoglycemia
PBI	Cretinism
CSF	
Protein	Leukodystrophies
Therapeutic Trial (seizures in early infancy)	
Vitamin B₆, 10 mg. I.M.	Pyridoxine dependency
Special Tests†	
Urine	
1. Amino acid chromatography	Aminoacidopathies
2. Phenolic acid chromatography	Phenylketonuria
3. Indolic acid chromatography	Hartnup disease
4. Keto acid	Maple syrup disease
5. Quantitative estimation of polysaccharide excretion	Gargoylism, other polysaccharidoses
6. Metachromatic stain of sediment	Metachromatic leukodystrophy
7. Copper excretion	Wilson's disease
Blood	
1. Serum chromatography	Aminoacidopathies
2. Protein electrophoresis	Ataxia-telangiectasia / Acanthocytosis / Wilson's disease
3. Blood ammonia	Disorders of urea synthesis
4. Serum uric acid	Primary hyperuricemia
5. Serum alkaline phosphatase	Hypophosphatasia
6. Sodium, potassium, chloride	Diencephalic syndrome (Chapter 11)
Biopsy (bone marrow, sural nerve or rectal mucosa)	Neural lipidoses

*See Chapter 21 for details.
†Indications for complete metabolic studies:
 1. History of neurologic disease in sibling or close relative
 2. History of neurologic disease with cousin marriages
 3. Any child with a progressive or unmanageable neurologic disorder
 4. Any retarded child who fails to thrive when the following conditions have been ruled out:
   a) Improper feeding
   b) Disease in other organ system (gastrointestinal or genitourinary tract, heart, lung, etc.)

of denervation in patients with lower motor neuron disease) and serves as an interesting tool for clinical teaching and research.

Conduction velocity studies, on the other hand, have value in documenting evidence of lower motor neuron disease by showing slowed nerve conduction times (e.g., polyneuritis). Together electromyography and conduction velocity studies help to differentiate upper motor neuron from lower motor neuron weakness in equivocal cases.

Clinical Chemistry

Urine chromatography, especially amino acid analysis, is now being performed by many clinical laboratories, but the reports are often too vague to satisfy the clinician. In our opinion the interpretation of two-dimensional paper chromatography or quantitative measurements of amino acids depends upon the experience and conservative judgment of a person with a research interest in the field of the rare metabolic disorders. The man in practice must familiarize himself with the accurate methods available for the diagnosis of phenylketonuria. If he suspects any of the other hereditary metabolic defects on the basis of the clinical findings (Table 12.4), he should seek consultation at a facility with a dependable clinical chemistry laboratory.[13]

Cerebrospinal Fluid Examination

Many physicians make the mistake of getting insufficient information at the time of a diagnostic lumbar puncture. This is due to the failure routinely to obtain (1) pressure measurements, with the patient relaxed (presedated if necessary), (2) immediate total cell count and differential cell count using freshly cleaned equipment, (3) protein and sugar determination, (4) Gram stain and India ink stain of sediment in *any* patient with the possible diagnosis of meningitis and (5) culture for bacteria, acid-fast organisms and fungi, if necessary.

CELL COUNT.—A CSF white cell count of more than 5 cells/cu. mm. occurs in meningoencephalitis (Table 18.2, p. 287), brain abscess, tumors (especially if they are malignant or near the ventricle), and some cases of demyelinating disease. Bloody taps are encountered in patients of any age but are especially common in children. If a bloody tap occurs, the fluid can be cultured and a smear made, with dependable results, but interpretation of the cell count is difficult. The fluid should be centrifuged and the supernatant inspected for xanthochromia. Gross xanthochromia should suggest subarachnoid hemorrhage, but faint degrees of xanthochromia may result from the yellowness of contaminating blood serum. One must always suspect intracranial hemorrhage, in which the fluid remains bloody in all three tubes. It is often suggested that the CSF erythrocyte-leukocyte ratio be compared to that in the peripheral blood to detect a real pleocytosis, but in practice one is often left in doubt. Theoretically one can allow 1,000 red blood cells for each milligram of protein to estimate the CSF protein, but such results are often equivocal.

A pleocytosis is seen with many malignant tumors which lie next to the subarachnoid space.

CSF PROTEIN.—All hospital laboratories can handle CSF protein determinations, but few can provide accurate, reproducible measurements because of the dilute concentrations of protein in the cerebrospinal fluid. Unless many determinations are being done regularly by one or two technicians in the laboratory, results may be inconsistent and the clinician will not be able to depend upon them.

In patients with definite and repeated CSF protein elevations (especially if the level exceeds 100 mg./100 ml.), one should suspect a tumor, a degenerative disease (Fig. 21.13, p. 418) or a chronic form of meningitis. It is obvious that acute diseases such as head trauma, severe anoxia and acute bacterial meningitis also cause marked elevation in CSF protein content.

Active efforts to obtain additional diagnostic information by fractionating the CSF proteins have been carried out in the past 20 years. In our opinion, useful information can be expected at present in only a few conditions. These findings are discussed under *multiple sclerosis* (p. 455) and *subacute sclerosing leukoencephalitis* (p. 309). Abnormalities are also seen in neurosyphilis and sarcoidosis which can affect the nervous system, but these problems are extremely rare in children.

CSF SUGAR.—Normally the CSF sugar level approximates two-thirds that found in the blood. In patients with purulent meningitis or a diffuse infiltration of the meninges[4,25] or spinal cord with tumor, the glucose concentration falls to abnormally low levels (hypoglycorrhachia—Fig. 17.12, p. 270).

Muscle Biopsy

This valuable diagnostic procedure is used (1) to decide whether muscle weakness has a *myopathic* or *neurogenic* basis, (2) to differentiate the *different types* of myopathies and (3) to provide definitive evidence for the diagnosis of *systemic disease,* such as collagen, vascular and metabolic disorders which involve skeletal muscle. Other diagnostic steps such as electromyography and serum enzyme levels should be undertaken before biopsy is carried out. The following factors should be considered carefully before performing the procedure.

1. *Selection of the biopsy site.*—Ideally, one should pick a large muscle which is actively involved by the disease. Muscles which are severely involved and muscle from an area which has been probed by EMG needles should be avoided.

2. *Operative technique.*—Biopsies in young children should be done under general anesthesia. In older children and adults local anesthetic can be used, with care taken to avoid infiltrating the specimen with the anesthetic. The surgeon should take a specimen about 1.5 cm. long, 1 cm. wide and 1 cm. thick.

3. *Handling the specimen.*—The surgeon should fasten the specimen to a piece of cardboard with pins so that it is extended in its horizontal plane and place it in a Petri dish containing normal saline to prevent shrinkage, drying out and distortion, all of which can create confusing microscopic artifacts. In 15–30 minutes the specimen can be placed in the fixative. Ideally, one should consult the pathologist before fixing the tissue. Altogether too many specimens wind up in the wrong fixative solution, sometimes rendering useless an expensive, time-consuming operative procedure.

For routine histologic examination fixation with 10% neutral Formalin or Zenker's solution is satisfactory. If both routine and electron-microscopic studies are planned, glutaraldehyde is considered a good fixative. Decisions about staining techniques should be made by the pathologist after he is told what you are looking for. It may be necessary to carry out special stains at a later date.

Typical examples of the most common biopsy findings in children with neuromuscular diseases are illustrated in Chapter 19.

BIBLIOGRAPHY

1. Andermann, F.: Absence attacks and diffuse neuronal disease, Neurology 17:205, 1967.
2. Barrows, H. S., et al.: The diagnostic applications of ultrasound in neurological disease, Neurology 15:361, 1965.
3. Bennett, D. R., and Ziter, F. A.: Electroencephalographic study of sleep deprivation in flying personnel (abstract), American Academy of Neurologists Meeting, San Francisco, April 27, 1967.
4. Berg, L.: Hypoglycorrhachia of non-infectious origin: Diffuse meningeal neoplasia, Neurology 3:811, 1953.
5. Bray, P. F.: Electroencephalography, in Brennemann-Kelley: *Practice of Pediatrics* (Hagerstown, Md.: W. F. Prior Company, Inc., 1964), Vol. IV, ch. 2.
6. Brinker, R. A., et al.: Echoencephalography, Am. J. Roentgenol. 93:781, 1965.
7. Bucy, P. C., and Ciric, I. S.: Brain scans in diagnosis of brain tumors, J.A.M.A. 191:437, 1965.
8. Caffey, J.: *Pediatric X-ray Diagnosis* (4th ed.; Chicago: Year Book Medical Publishers, Inc., 1961).
9. Cattell, H. S., and Filtzer, D. L.: Pseudosubluxation and other normal variations in the cervical spine in children, J. Bone & Joint Surg. 47:1295, 1965.
10. Charash, L. I., and Dunning, H. S: An appraisal of pneumoencephalography in mental retardation and epilepsy, Pediatrics 18:716, 1956.
11. Childe, A. E.: Localized thinning and enlargement of the cranium with special reference to the middle fossa, Am. J. Roentgenol. 70:1, 1953.
12. Cobb, W., et al.: Cerebral lipidosis: An electroencephalographic study, Brain 75:343, 1952.
13. Ghadimi, H.: Diagnosis of inborn errors of metabolism, Am. J. Dis. Child. 114:433, 1967.
14. Gibbs, F. A., and Gibbs, E. L.: *Atlas of Electroencephalography* (Reading, Mass.: Addison-Wesley Publishing Co., Inc., 1952), Vol. II, ch. 13.
15. Hamlin, H.: Life or death by EEG, J.A.M.A. 190:112, 1964.
16. Hughes, J. R.: Usefulness of photic stimulation in routine clinical electroencephalography, Neurology 10:777, 1960.
16a. Knobloch, H., et al.: The relationship between findings in pneumoencephalograms and clinical behavior, Pediatrics 22:13, 1958.
17. Lesse, S., et al.: The electroencephalogram in diffuse encephalopathies; significance of periodic synchronous discharges, A.M.A. Arch. Neurol. & Psychiat. 79:359, 1958.
18. Lombroso, C. T., et al.: Ctenoids in healthy youths; controlled study of 14- and 6-per-second positive spiking, Neurology 16:1152, 1966.
19. Low, N. L.: Diagnostic radiologic procedures, in Brennemann-Kelley: *Practice of Pediatrics* (Hagerstown, Md.: W. F. Prior Company, Inc., 1964), Vol. IV, ch. 2.
20. Madsen, J. A., and Bray, P. F.: The coincidence of diffuse electroencephalographic spike-wave paroxysms and brain tumors, Neurology 16:546, 1966.
21. Marsan, C. A., and Lewis, W. R.: Pathologic findings in patients with "centrencephalic" electroencephalographic patterns, Neurology 10:922, 1960.
22. McAfee, J. G., et al.: Tc-99m pertechnetate for brain scanning, J. Nucl. Med. 5:811, 1964.
23. Melnick, J. C., and Silverman, F. N.: Intervertebral disk calcification in childhood, Radiology 80:399, 1963.
23a. Nellhaus, G.: Head circumference from birth to eighteen years, Pediatrics 41:106, 1968.
24. Nellhaus, G., and Chutorian, A.: Narcosis for neuroradiologic procedures in children, Arch. Neurol. 10:485, 1964.
25. Oliver, D. G., et al: Diffuse glioma of the spinal cord with hypoglycorrhachia, Neurology 16:911, 1966.

26. Pratt, K. L., *et al.*: EEG activation of epileptics following sleep deprivation, Electroencephalog. & Clin. Neurophysiol. 24:11, 1968.
27. Prince, D., and Wiener, L. M.: Pneumoencephalography in patients with brain tumor, Neurology 14:677, 1964.
28. Radermecker, J., and Poser, C. M.: The significance of repetitive paroxysmal electroencephalographic patterns: Their specificity in subacute sclerosing leukoencephalitis, World Neurol. 1:422, 1960.
29. Report of the Committee on Methods of Clinical Examination in Electroencephalography, Electroencephalog. & Clin. Neurophysiol. 10:370, 1958.
30. Scheinberg, L., and Yahr, M. D.: The unsatisfactory pneumoencephalogram, Tr. Am. Neurol. A. 80:221, 1955.
31. Schwab, R. S., *et al.*: EEG as an aid in determining death in the presence of cardiac activity (abstract), Electroencephalog. & Clin. Neurophysiol. 15:147, 1963.
32. Smith, H. V., and Crothers, B.: Subdural fluid as a consequence of pneumoencephalography, Pediatrics 5:375, 1950.
33. Solomon, S., and Barron, K. D.: Complications of pneumoencephalography associated with internal carotid thrombosis, Neurology 7:373, 1957.
33a. Spaeth, G. L., and Barber, G. W.: Prevalence of homocystinuria among the mentally retarded: Evaluation of a specific screening test, Pediatrics 40:586, 1967.
34. Stewart, L. F., and Dreifuss, F. E.: "Centrencephalic" seizure discharges in focal hemispheral lesions, Arch. Neurol. 17:60, 1967.
35. Taveras, J. M., and Wood, E. H.: *Diagnostic Neuroradiology* (Baltimore: Williams & Wilkins Company, 1964).
36. Tharp, B. R.: The 6-per-second spike and wave complex, Arch. Neurol. 15:533, 1966.
37. Townsend, E. H., and Rowe, M. L.: Mobility of the upper cervical spine in health and disease, Pediatrics 10:567, 1952.
38. van Leeuwen, W. S., *et al.*: Proposal for an EEG terminology, Electroencephalog. & Clin. Neurophysiol. 13:646, 1961; 20:303, 1966.
39. Webber, M. M.: Technetium^{99m} normal brain scans and their anatomic features, Am. J. Roentgenol. 94:815, 1965.
40. Whitehouse, D., *et al.*: Electroencephalographic changes in children with migraine, New England J. Med. 276:23, 1967.
41. Witcofski, R. L., and Roper, T. J.: A technique for scanning the posterior fossa, J. Nucl. Med. 6:754, 1965.
42. Witcofski, R. L., *et al.*: False positive brain scans from extracranial contamination with ^{99m}technetium, J. Nucl. Med. 6:524, 1965.
43. Witcofski, R. L., *et al.*: The utilization of ^{99m}technetium in brain scanning, J. Nucl. Med. 6:121, 1965.
44. Witcofski, R. L., *et al.*: Visualization of the choroid plexus on the technetium^{99m} brain scan, Arch. Neurol. 16:286, 1967.

PART II

Conventional Categories of Disease

13

Congenital Malformations of the Nervous System

STRUCTURAL MALFORMATIONS OF OBSCURE ETIOLOGY

Incomplete Closure of the Neural Tube (Craniorachischisis)
- Spina Bifida with Meningomyelocele
- Cranium Bifidum with Meningoencephalocele
- Anencephaly and Hydranencephaly
- Anomalies of Optic and Olfactory Apparatus

Defects in the Development of the Ventricular System
- Congenital Hydrocephalus

Occult Anomalies of the Brain
- Agenesis of Corpus Callosum
- Porencephalic Cysts
- Cerebral Hypoplasia
- Micropolygyria
- Pachygyria
- Heterotopia
- Micrencephaly
- Megalencephaly
- Incontinentia Pigmenti
- Infantile Hypercalcemia Syndrome

Occult Anomalies of the Basal Ganglia, Cerebellum and Brain Stem

Occult Anomalies of the Spinal Cord and Peripheral Nerves
- Syringomyelia and Syringobulbia
- Congenital Insensitivity to Pain (also Hereditary Sensory Radicular Neuropathy)

Occult Anomalies of the Autonomic Nervous System
- Aganglionic Megacolon (Hirschsprung)
- Megaloureters, Achalasia, Pyloric Stenosis
- Familial Dysautonomia (Chapter 21)

Vascular and Skin Malformations
- Angiomas
- Arterial Aneurysms

Skull and Spine Malformations
- Craniosynostosis (Craniostenosis)
- Diastematomyelia
- Klippel-Feil Deformity
- Platybasia
- Chondrodystrophy (Achondroplasia)
- Osteopetrosis
- Fibrous Dysplasia

126 CONGENITAL MALFORMATIONS OF THE NERVOUS SYSTEM

STRUCTURAL MALFORMATIONS OF KNOWN ETIOLOGY

Abnormalities in Chromosome Number
    Autosomes
        21 Trisomy   "D" Trisomy
        18 Trisomy
    Sex Chromosomes
        Turner's syndrome
        Klinefelter's syndrome
    (Mosaicism)
Abnormalities in Chromosome Structure
    Translocation   "Ring" Chromosomes
    Deletions
Malformations Due to Maternal Infections
    German Measles (Rubella)   Other Maternal Virus Infections
    Toxoplasmosis, Cytomegalic Inclusion Disease and Syphilis
Malformations Due to Other Environmental Factors
    Drugs   Maternal Diabetes, Malnutrition and Anoxia
    Irradiation

LOW BIRTH WEIGHT INFANTS

Prematures
Intrauterine Growth Retardation (Undergrown Neonates)

CONGENITAL MALFORMATIONS of the nervous system are defined here as gross structural abnormalities which are present at birth. Hereditary disorders which may be associated with malformations at the cellular or molecular level, such as epilepsy, metabolic defects and degenerative diseases, are discussed separately in other chapters.

Baumgartner[1d] has shown that congenital malformations, in general, represent the second leading cause of death in infants under age 1, being exceeded only by prematurity. Among the few large and meaningful studies on this subject is that of McIntosh et al.,[51] who found nervous system malformation was the second most frequent type of organ-system anomaly, occurring in 1.3% of total births. Neel[59a] made similar observations in a large Japanese study. Other studies by Malpas[48b] and by Stevenson and Warnock[84] have indicated that nervous system anomalies occur more frequently than those of any other organ system. Thus, it can be seen that the worker's definition and the geographic variation influence the conclusions of different studies. Minor anomalies which do not become manifest until later in infancy would add to this incidence. Although many clinicians suspect that the morbidity from nervous system anomalies, i.e., chronic neurologic disability, is higher than generally assumed, objective studies on this question have not yet been reported.

PATHOGENESIS.—No specific etiology has been found for the majority of congenital malformations, but it is thought by Warkany and Kalter[96] and by Fraser[23] that most anomalies result from the complicated interaction of a genetic predisposition and subtle factors in the intrauterine environment. Despite an intensive search, the number of environmental factors which are known to be teratogenic for the human nervous system is limited. These factors include maternal infections during pregnancy (rubella,[29,85] toxoplasmosis[16,17] salivary gland virus disease[101]), irradiation[56,64] and drug-induced folic acid deficiency.[90] Mongolism, discussed later in this chapter, represents the only malformation which has a genetic etiology in nearly all cases.[63] The familial occurrence of certain neurologic anomalies such as anencephaly[62] and spina bifida is well recognized. Although the latter anomalies do not occur in a consistent mendelian pattern of inheritance, it is thought that they probably result from a genetic predisposition coupled with familial environmental factors.

In the isolated clinical syndrome, e.g., anencephaly, the problem is complicated by the fact that the phenotype (the clinical form of a genetically determined trait) cannot be distinguished readily from the radiation-induced phenocopy (a clinical form which mimics the phenotype but is caused by an environmental factor). Classifying anomalies according to time of insult to the embryo or fetus has a logical appeal, especially to embryologists and pathologists. However, this stage-specific etiologic concept of certain anomalies has failed to achieve practical clinical value. Furthermore, symptoms of an occult congenital defect often do not become manifest until after three or four months of postnatal life because the brain of the newborn is largely unmyelinated and has a limited capacity to reflect structural defect. This set of circumstances may lead the physician to attribute the cerebral damage erroneously to some postnatal event, a treacherous line of reasoning in patients whose response to any illness is often extreme.

The classification outlined at the beginning of the chapter is based primarily upon etiology and secondarily upon morphologic defect. Scientific progress in this important area should gradually increase the number of conditions in which the etiology is known.

Structural Malformations of Obscure Etiology

Epidemiologic data indicate that the most common and the most severe anomalies are caused by obscure factors which result in incomplete closure of the neural tube. The neural tube defects apparent at or shortly after birth include spina bifida with meningomyelocele, cranium bifidum with meningoencephalocele and anencephaly. All of these conditions show a familial tendency of occurrence but do not usually behave as simple dominant or recessive traits.

Incomplete Closure of the Neural Tube (Craniorhachischisis)

Malformations which result from incomplete closure of the neural tube probably have their origin during the fourth week of embryonic life. Spina bifida and

128   CONGENITAL MALFORMATIONS OF THE NERVOUS SYSTEM

anencephaly may occur together in the same individual or in different members of a sibship. Some workers have suggested that spina bifida occulta occasionally results from the expression of the heterozygous state, but this proposition is conjectural. Stern[83] suggests that anencephaly and spina bifida, like some other abnormalities, can probably be produced by more than one genotype as well as by environmental agents.

Spina Bifida with Meningomyelocele

PATHOGENESIS.—This anomaly results from incomplete closure of the lower end of the bony spinal canal and occurs about once in every thousand births. Clinical types vary in the following order of decreasing severity.

Complete rhachischisis.—The bony vertebral arches are missing in the lumbar region, the cord is underdeveloped or aplastic and the nerve elements have no covering.

Meningomyelocele.—An obvious soft-tissue sac projects over the lumbosacral spine and a transparent membrane overlies the cord and cauda equina (Fig. 13.1). The neural elements may be attached to this membrane and the cerebrospinal fluid may leak to the outside as a result of minor trauma, introducing the threat of secondary meningitis.

Meningocele.—A soft-tissue sac, covered by atrophic skin, covers a bony defect in the spine. The spinal cord is usually intact, and the lumbosacral roots may be functioning with little apparent deficit.

Spina bifida occulta.—A defect in the bony canal, often discovered incidentally on x-ray examination, does not involve the neural elements in the vast majority of cases. The overlying skin may be the site of a pilonidal dimple, a tuft of hair or a birthmark. Sometimes such minor skin anomalies may be associated with a *dermal sinus* which is continuous with the subarachnoid space.[49b] Such der-

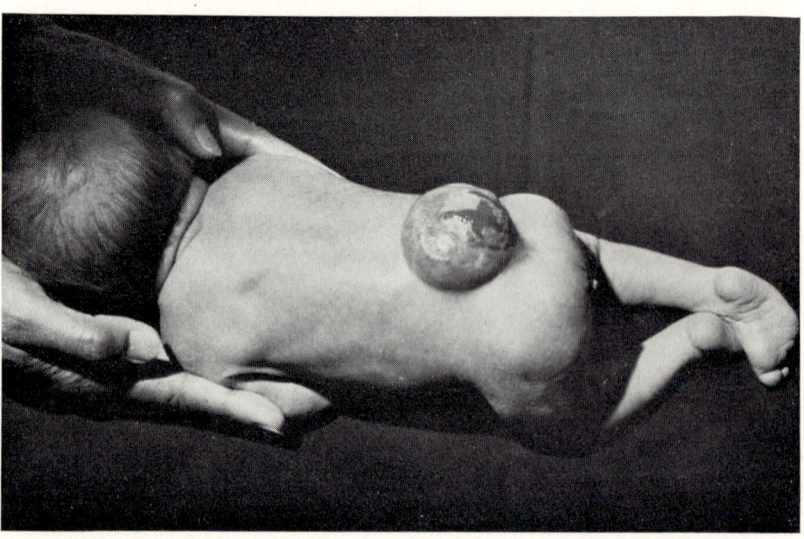

Fig. 13.1.—Lumbar meningomyelocele. Soft-tissue sac covered by a thin, transparent membrane through which cerebrospinal fluid oozes.

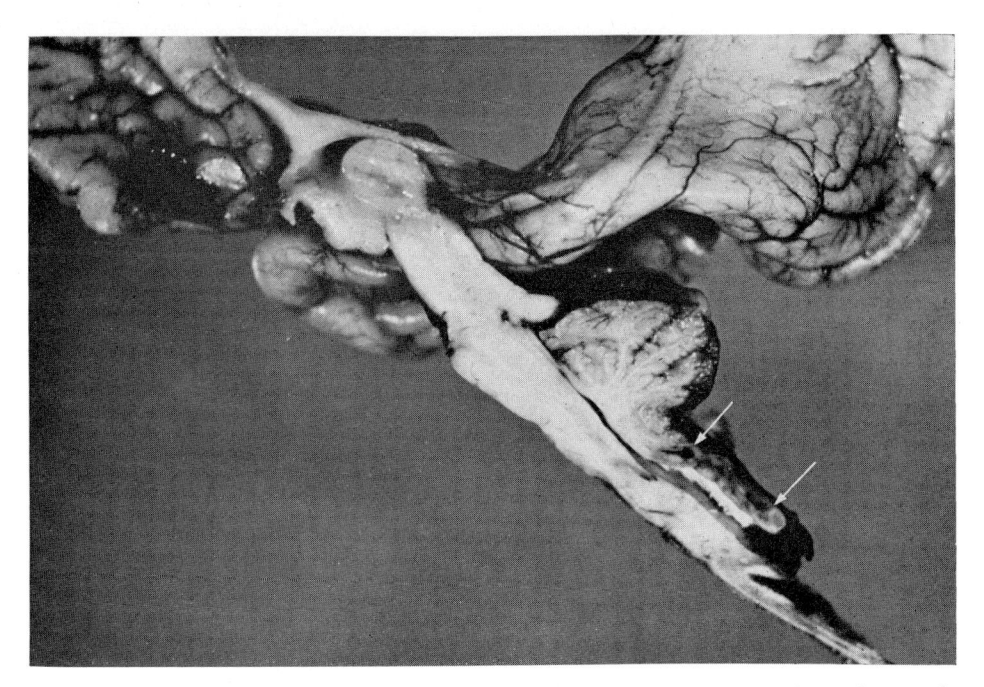

Fig. 13.2.—Arnold-Chiari malformation with hydrocephalus. Brain specimen from a 3-week-old baby who was born with large dorsolumbar meningomyelocele. Examination showed a complete flaccid paraplegia with anesthesia below the waist and incontinence of both urine and feces. In addition to head enlargement, x-rays showed a lacunar skull (Fig. 13.3) and multiple anomalies of vertebrae and ribs; a ventriculogram showed markedly dilated ventricles. Pathologic study of the brain revealed a typical Arnold-Chiari malformation (arrows) and an associated hydrocephalus. Additional vascular and renal anomalies were found.

mal sinuses can cause recurrent bouts of meningitis. The diagnosis of occult dermal sinuses and the treatment of recurrent meningitis are covered in Chapter 18.

Several other anomalies are commonly associated with spina bifida and myelodysplasia. The *Arnold-Chiari malformation,* characterized by inferior displacement of cerebellar or medullary tissue through the foramen magnum into the spinal canal (Fig. 13.2), is often seen concurrently, and it, in turn, is often associated with progressive hydrocephalus. It is also well known that Arnold-Chiari deformity can appear by itself, usually in adults, without associated bony anomalies of the cranium, the spine or the spinal cord.[89a] *Syringomyelia* and *syringobulbia* often are seen concurrently, but they may become manifest only in later childhood. A variety of anomalies in other organ systems may be seen but not with any real consistency.

CLINICAL AND LABORATORY DIAGNOSIS.—The neurologic deficit varies with the severity of the defect, the sacral roots showing involvement in all but the mildest form of defect and the lumbar roots being involved in only the severest anomalies. Motor deficit, with weakness and atrophy, usually affects the muscles below the knee and sometimes below the waist. Sensory loss is commonly seen in the "saddle area" and over variable areas of the feet and legs. The ankle jerks and the superficial anal reflex are usually lost, whereas the knee jerks are preserved except with the most severe defects. The anus is patulous and the sphincter tone is poor.

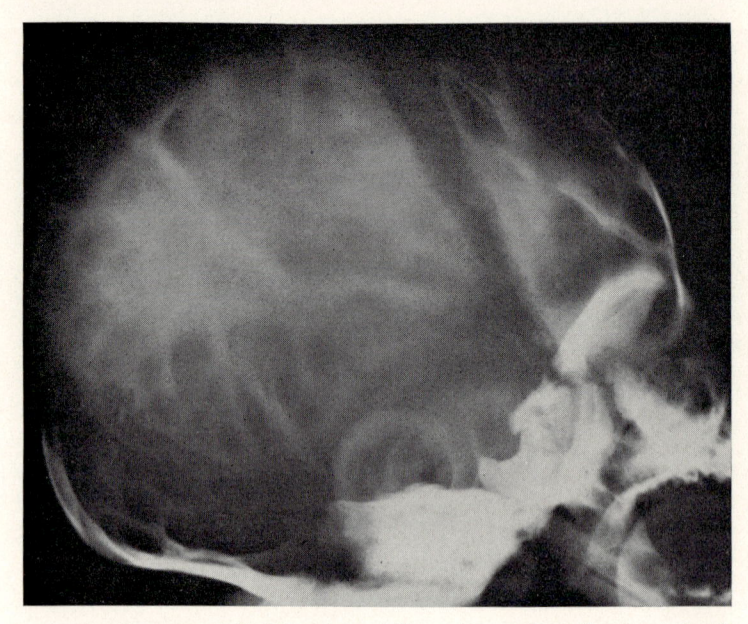

Fig. 13.3.—Lacunar skull. Note the weblike pattern of varying bone density.

Bladder-bowel dysfunction results when the sacral roots are involved and this is manifested by frequent urinary dribbling, chronic constipation and fecal soiling. In severe cases, there are trophic skin changes in the feet and legs, with coldness, cyanosis and ulcerations at pressure points. Secondary musculoskeletal deformities in the form of pes cavus, equinovarus and dorsiflexion of the great toes are common. The clinical signs and symptoms which accompany the associated anomalies of hydrocephalus and syringomyelia are discussed under the specific headings.

A fluctuant, soft-tissue mass which can be transilluminated and which can be palpated or seen on x-ray presents no diagnostic difficulty. Other tumors in this area, such as lipomas, dermoids and teratomas, may be differentiated by their differences in consistency, the absence of defects in the bony spine or their association with soft-tissue calcification, or may require myelography and operative exploration. If no soft-tissue mass is present but the syndrome of flaccid paralysis or hypotonia is evident in the newborn, one should exclude obstetric injury to the spinal cord, progressive infantile muscular atrophy and arthrogryposis, neonatal myasthenia gravis, amyoplasia congenita and congenital intraspinal tumors.

"Lacunar skull" (craniolacunia or *Lückenschädel*) is a term applied to the weblike areas of translucency which are demarcated by strips of increased density on the skull x-rays of some newborn infants[78e] (Fig. 13.3). It is seen in nearly all babies who are born with a meningocele or an encephalocele and it usually disappears by the age of 3 months. The etiology has been ascribed by some to prenatal increased intracranial pressure and by others to a developmental defect of membranous bone ossification.

MANAGEMENT AND PROGNOSIS.—Much controversy surrounds the management of meningomyelocele, some of which is philosophical rather than directly medical in nature. If the child is free from other major defects, most physicians have recommended and parents have requested closure of the defect in order to avoid meningitis secondary to rupture of the sac and to facilitate home management. In following such a course, one cannot expect to produce any improvement in the neurologic deficit. In fact, further damage to the sacral roots may take place unknowingly during the surgical closure, and the development of hydrocephalus may be accelerated, probably because of removal of the available absorptive surface in the meningocele sac. The parents may wish to defer closure of the sac, especially if the neurologic deficit is severe, if hydrocephalus is already apparent and if other anomalies are present. If a vigorous, all-out effort is used at the outset and equally dedicated follow-up and habilitative therapy is provided, one can expect a longer survival and greater self-sufficiency in these patients.[1f] When slowly progressive hydrocephalus develops after a meningocele is repaired, decompression of the basal cisterns by suboccipital craniectomy and high cervical laminectomy may arrest the process. Constant ventricular drainage is recommended

Fig. 13.4.—Chronic urinary tract damage in patient with myelomeningocele. Intravenous urogram shows chronic hydronephrosis, hydroureters, pyelonephritis and poor renal function (upper left arrow). Note severe scoliosis which was associated with clinical signs of syringomyelia.

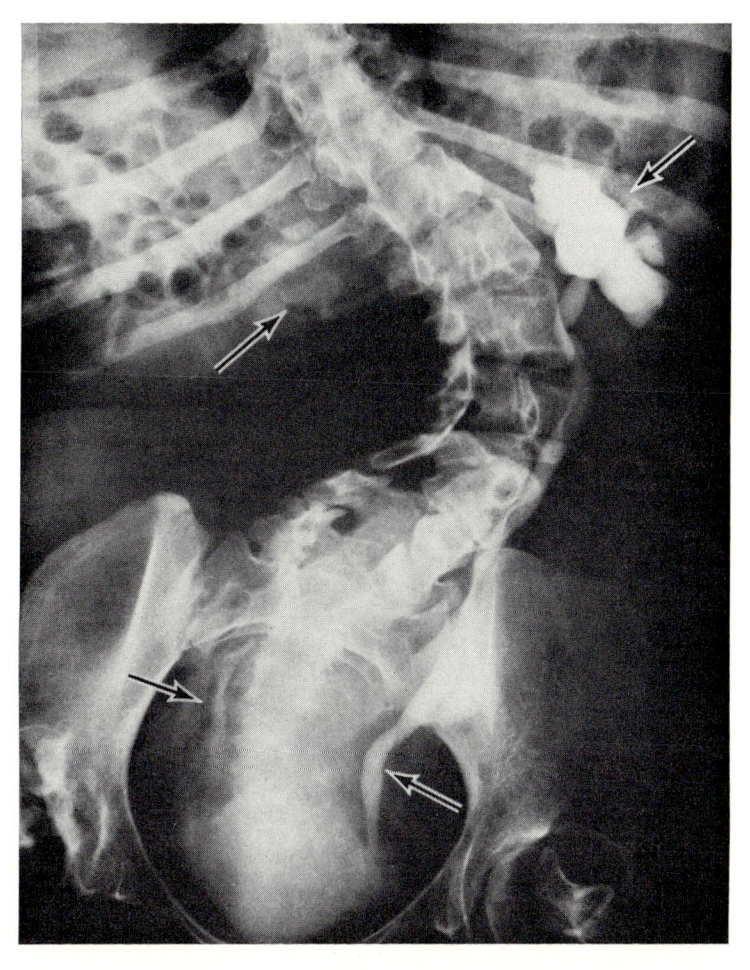

in some cases by Ingraham and Matson[35] for a period after meningocele repair or after a "universal shunt." The more detailed management of hydrocephalus is discussed on page 139. When the lumbar sac is not removed, it has shown a tendency in some instances to collapse and scar down. As yet too few series have been reported for evaluation of the results of this approach, but it may prove more effective if it does nothing more than to reduce the severity of subsequent lumbosacral root deficit.[41a] The latter deficit has been seen almost uniformly following the traditional surgical treatment. The long-term clinical picture in the patients surviving to late childhood and adult life varies from bladder-bowel dysfunction alone to moderate weakness and sensory loss below the knee to flaccid paraplegia and anesthesia below the waist. Also seen are moderate to severe degrees of intellectual deficit as well as seizures and behavior disorders that may be proportional to the severity of the hydrocephalus.

In the surviving child, the bladder-bowel dysfunction often leads to ascending urinary tract infection, chronic pyelonephritis and eventual renal failure[54a] (Fig. 13.4). Careful observation for these complications should be made and appropriate chemotherapy should be instituted when they occur. The constant odor of urine in the incontinent serves to ostracize these children socially and completes the pathetic picture. Recent surgical attempts have been carried out by Bradley and co-workers[2] to evacuate the bladder periodically by radio stimulation of an implanted bladder electrode. If this technique can be refined, it may help to prevent the chronic urinary tract disease.

Most patients with an occult spina bifida are neurologically intact, and the bony lesion is discovered only incidentally on x-ray examination performed for other reasons. If the patient exhibits neurologic deficit, bladder-bowel dysfunction or skeletal deformity, operation should be carried out after myelography in a search for congenital intraspinal tumors.

Cranium Bifidum with Meningoencephalocele

PATHOGENESIS.—Much less frequently, the neural tube fails to close at its cranial end and soft-tissue masses containing meninges, brain tissue and a portion of the ventricular system project through bony defects in the skull or cervical spine. The commonest meningoencephalocele is occipital, often arising from midline structures in the posterior fossa, particularly the roof of the fourth ventricle and occasionally the roof of the third ventricle. Various occult anomalies of the nervous system are associated with the obvious encephalocele and they are discussed separately. At times the meningocele or encephalocele protrudes through a bony defect in the cribriform plate into the nasal cavity or through the roof of the orbit into the orbital cavity.

CLINICAL AND LABORATORY DIAGNOSIS.—Encephaloceles vary in size and position. Although the lesion is commonest by far in the occipital area, the bony defect can occur at any point on the skull and it is usually, though not necessarily, in the midline. Rarely the soft-tissue mass projects into the nasal cavity, causing cerebrospinal fluid rhinorrhea, and simulates a nasal polyp; it may project into the orbit, causing exophthalmos (Fig. 13.5). In some cases the glial tissue is simply ectopically placed, as pointed out by Low et al.,[47] and in other situations

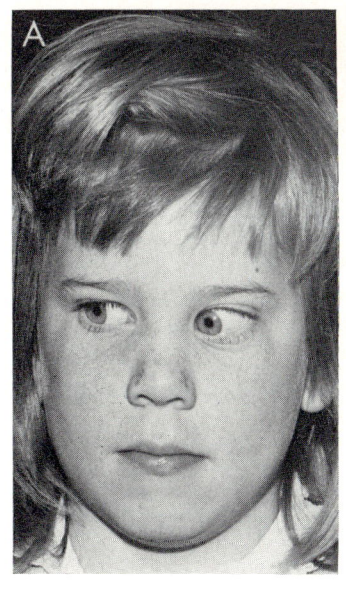

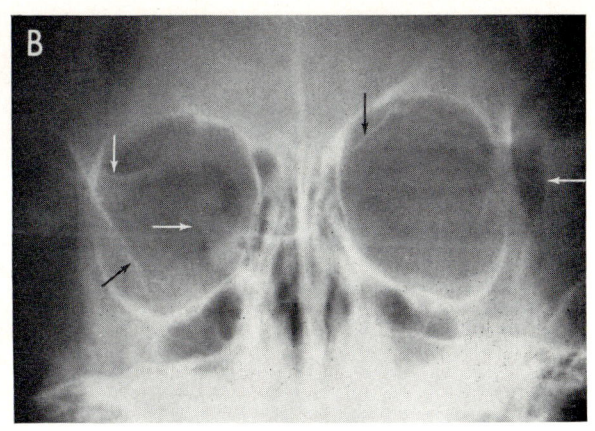

Fig. 13.5.—Extensive defect in sphenoid bone with posterior orbital meningocele and proptosis. **A**, this 6-year-old girl has had facial asymmetry since birth and increasing prominence of the left eye since age 5. She has no neurologic deficit, no stigmata of neurofibromatosis and no diplopia, eye pain, visual deficit, field defects or funduscopic abnormalities. **B**, skull x-rays show an extensive defect in the left sphenoid bone. Note the asymmetry of the orbits: the normal "oblique line of the orbit" is seen on the left (lowest arrow) but is absent on the right; the shadows of the sphenoid ridges are very asymmetrical (vertical arrows), and the anterior clinoids are absent on the right (compare with horizontal arrow on left). Also, note the defect in the calvarium (extreme right arrow) where the sphenoid abuts against the frontal and temporal bones. The proptosis results because the orbital meningocele compresses the globe from above and behind.

it represents a herniated extension of the central nervous system. The masses may be sessile or pedunculated, and they may be covered with normal skin and hair or by parchment-like membrane and no hair. The size of the soft-tissue mass does not indicate accurately the presence or absence of brain tissue within the sac nor does it indicate the extent of the associated intracranial anomalies. Microcephaly, moderate or severe mental defect, spastic motor deficit and seizures are commonly seen in these patients. Congenital blindness, associated with structural defects in the occipital lobes, is not uncommon.

Cranium bifidum without a meningoencephalocele can be associated with all of the clinical manifestations just noted, although hydrocephalus may be less common.

Plain roentgenograms locate the cranial defect accurately. Transillumination and pneumography are helpful in (1) the detection of associated anomalies (Fig. 13.6), (2) the diagnosis of hydrocephalus and (3) the preoperative determination of whether the sac contains cerebrospinal fluid only or brain tissue and a portion of the ventricular system.

Cephalohematomas can be mistaken for encephaloceles, but they can be differentiated by the absence of a cranial defect in cephalohematoma, as well as its restricted parietal location and gradual absorption.

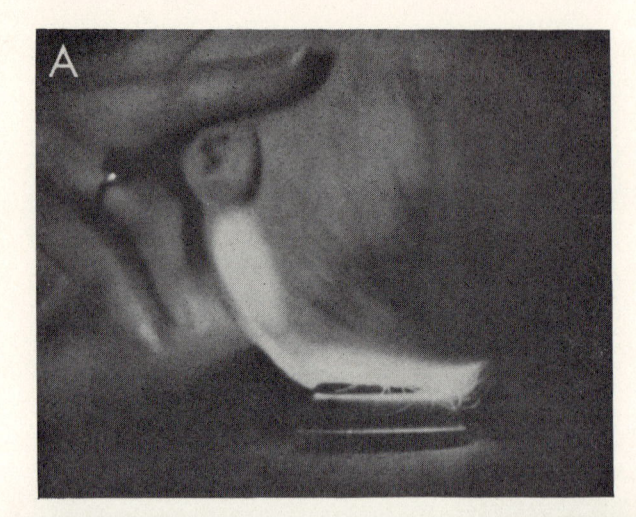

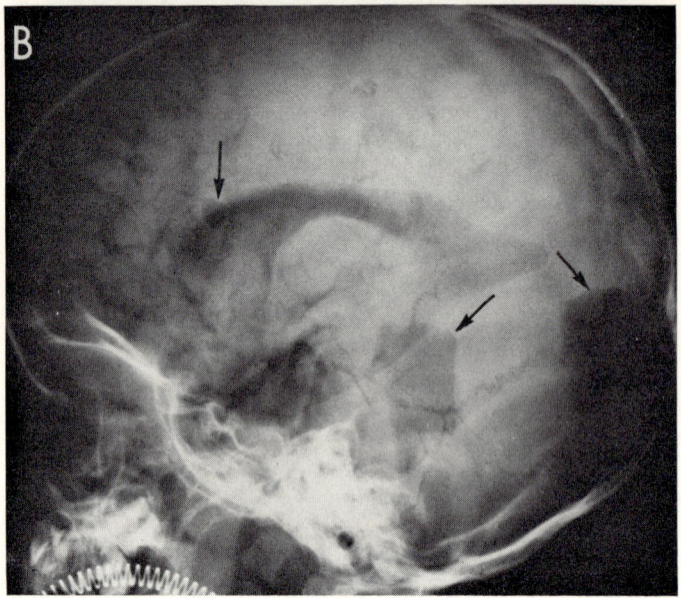

Fig. 13.6.—Transillumination and pneumography in patient with small encephalocele. **A** shows an abnormal degree of transillumination in the posterior fossa. In **B**, note the dilated and deformed fourth ventricle (middle arrow), the abnormal air accumulation in the posterior fossa (right arrow) and the associated epidermoid cyst in the skull (left arrow). An older sibling also had an encephalocele, and both children had cortical blindness, probably due to an occipital lobe anomaly.

MANAGEMENT AND PROGNOSIS.—Operative excision of many encephaloceles is carried out in the first few days or weeks of life because of the imminent danger of rupture of the sac, with secondary meningitis. Except for urgent cases, careful evaluation of the extent of this cerebral anomaly should be carried out to insure the maximum therapeutic value of the operation. When operation is contemplated, one must be prepared for the development of hydrocephalus following removal of the sac, a complication similar to that which often follows repair of a lumbar meningomyelocele.

STRUCTURAL MALFORMATIONS OF OBSCURE ETIOLOGY

In general, the prognosis for life is poor in these patients because of the severity of the primary lesion, the associated occult anomalies of the brain and cord and the threat of hydrocephalus and meningitis.

ANENCEPHALY AND HYDRANENCEPHALY

PATHOGENESIS.—Anencephaly stems from failure of the anterior neural tube to close and results in severe developmental failure in the brain and cranium (Fig. 13.7). Rudimentary brain-stem elements and meningeal coverings are usually present. Hydranencephaly, a condition of less certain origin and possibly of diverse etiology, is characterized by an intact skull, an enlarging head and severe agenesis of cerebral hemispheres.

CLINICAL AND LABORATORY DIAGNOSIS.—Anencephalic babies are often stillborn or die shortly after birth. For this reason they create more embryologic than clinical interest. The obstetrician may suspect an anomaly when he palpates the mother's abdomen and does not feel a normal head. The diagnosis can be established prenatally with x-rays of the mother's pelvis. Infants born with hydranencephaly may appear normal at birth since their movements, nursing habits and reflexes are like those of the normal newborn who functions at a subcortical or brain stem level. The child's nervous system defect is usually suspected because of an abnormal rate of head growth, motor retardation, spastic muscle tone, seizures, poor control of body temperature and episodes of apnea and cyanosis.

Transillumination of the head with a bright flashlight, which can be molded against the scalp with a rubber adapter, produces findings diagnostic of hydranencephaly. The results of this simple examination, which can be used routinely in any infant under suspicion, can be confirmed with a ventriculogram or pneumoencephalogram (Fig. 13.6). Electroencephalograms of these infants show only low voltage, irregular patterns and absence of normal background frequencies. The rapid head growth which is often seen in patients with hydranencephaly raises the diagnostic possibilities of subdural hematoma, congenital hydrocephalus and other unusual causes of excessive head size (Chapter 4).

MANAGEMENT AND PROGNOSIS.—No therapy exists for these conditions. Hy-

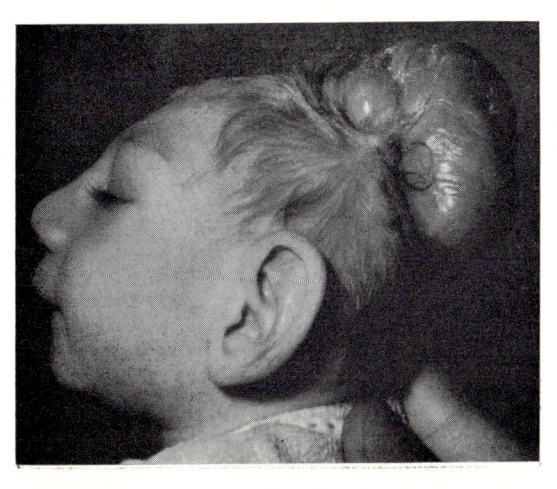

Fig. 13.7.—Anencephaly associated with a large parietal encephalocele.

dranencephalic infants often expire after a few weeks or months, but patients who have lived for several years in a helpless state have been recorded by Hamby and associates.[30]

Anomalies of the Optic and Olfactory Apparatus

PATHOGENESIS.—Anomalies of the optic and olfactory structures often coexist for embryologic reasons, and they are frequently associated with anomalies in the formation of the cerebral hemispheres and ventricular system. Microphthalmia and anophthalmia are often found, along with the severe anomaly, arhinencephaly (absence of the olfactory bulbs and tracts). Centrally these conditions may be associated with fusion of the cerebral hemispheres and a single ventricular cavity. Colobomas (congenital fissures of any part of the eye) represent the ocular embryologic counterpart of cranium bifidum and spina bifida. Recently the association between arhinencephaly and trisomy of a "D" group chromosome has been noted by Miller et al.[53] (p. 169). This same constellation of anomalies also commonly appears in a familial problem and usually behaves as an autosomal dominant trait. Lowe's syndrome (Chapter 21) and the congenital rubella syndrome (p. 173) also exhibit the common vulnerability of the developing eye and nervous system.

CLINICAL AND LABORATORY DIAGNOSIS.—Complete or partial blindness, mental defect, spasticity and failure to thrive are noted clinically in the severe forms of this defect. Colobomas appear as radial defects in the iris, the optic nerve, the retina or the choroid. The degree to which vision is lost in patients with colobomas depends upon the location and the size of the lesion. Isolated congenital aplasia of the optic nerve may appear as a dominant trait and is associated with partial or complete blindness in the affected eye. The clinical diagnosis of these unusual defects rests upon the family history and the eye examination.

Pneumoencephalography may reveal the abnormal ventricular system and the evidence of an absent corpus callosum. Chromosome analysis should also be considered in these patients, especially if the patient exhibits the other clinical signs of an autosomal "D" trisomy.

MANAGEMENT AND PROGNOSIS.—Treatment is symptomatic. The prognosis for longevity depends on the severity of the defect. When major cerebral anomalies occur, the prognosis is poor and care of these patients is often custodial.

Defects in the Development of the Ventricular System
CONGENITAL HYDROCEPHALUS

PATHOGENESIS.—Congenital hydrocephalus almost always results from atresia or incomplete development of some channel in the pathway of cerebrospinal fluid flow. Two general types occur, noncommunicating and communicating. The *noncommunicating* type most frequently results from *atresia* or *forking* of the aqueduct of Sylvius (Fig. 13.8) (well described by Russell[74]), but in a smaller percentage of cases it results from atresia of the foramina of Luschka and Magendie, the Dandy-Walker syndrome[10b, 19b] (Fig. 13.9). *Communicating* hydrocephalus results from a failure in the development of the subarachnoid cisterns, thus preventing the absorption of cerebrospinal fluid by arachnoid villi over the surface of the

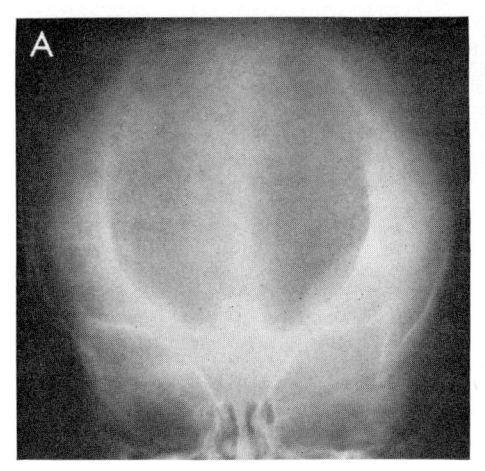

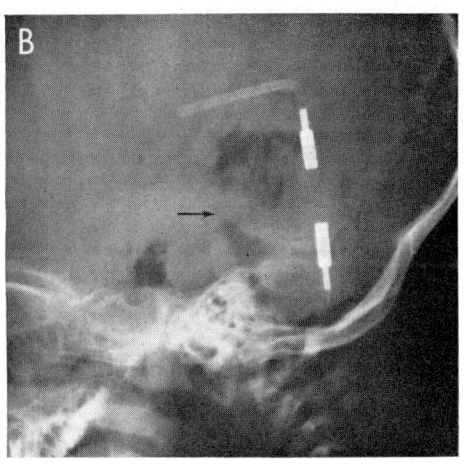

Fig. 13.8.—Congenital hydrocephalus due to aqueductal stenosis. After an unsuccessful attempt at pneumoencephalography, a ventriculogram, **A**, showed the severe obstructive hydrocephalus in this 10-week-old baby. At age 20 months a second pneumoencephalogram, **B**, revealed aqueductal stenosis (arrow). The operators obtained good fourth ventricular filling but, despite much manipulation of the head and further air injection, could not get air to enter the rest of the ventricular system. Note the plastic shunt tube and Holter valve in place.

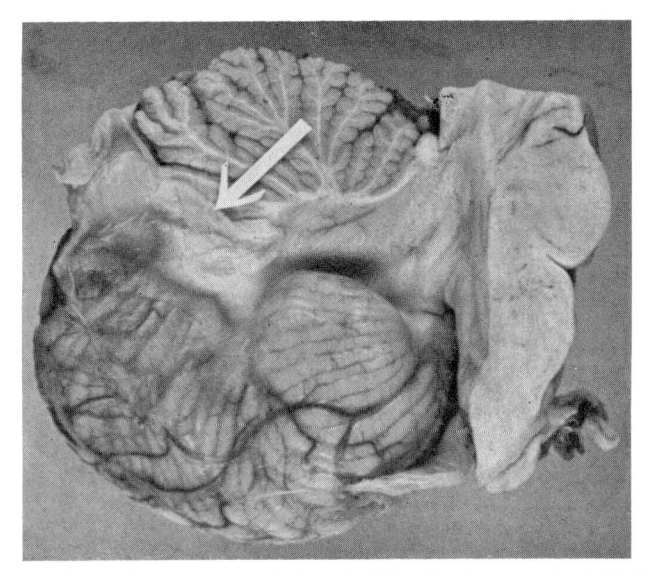

Fig. 13.9.—Dandy-Walker anomaly. Infant had head enlargement at birth, and a pneumoencephalogram with 15 cc. of air showed marked ventricular dilatation. A ventricular-jugular shunt was done for "communicating hydrocephalus." After numerous revisions of the poorly functioning shunt the child died at age 2 years 9 months from increased intracranial pressure. Autopsy revealed dilatation of the fourth ventricle, an abnormal "tongue" of tissue in one midline obstructing the foramen of Magendie (arrow) and a large, thin-walled cystic cavity containing cerebrospinal fluid between the cerebellar hemispheres.

hemispheres after the fluid has left the fourth ventricle. An obscure developmental defect probably causes most cases of communicating hydrocephalus, but inflammation secondary to meningitis or hypoxic intracerebral hemorrhage[27a,46b] (Chapter 16) accounts for some.

CLINICAL AND LABORATORY DIAGNOSIS.—Although most infants with congenital hydrocephalus have normal head size at birth, occasionally head enlargement occurs during intrauterine life and complicates delivery. It is thought that uterine pressure prevents head enlargement in the former, inasmuch as marked ventricular dilatation may be noted early in life. Excessive head growth is usually noted shortly after birth, as are a bulging fontanel, separated sutures, distended scalp veins, irritability and vomiting. In many cases the diagnosis is less obvious, but if head measurements are recorded on charts for normal head growth as a part of routine newborn care, the condition will not be overlooked. Also, percussion of the head in suspected cases may produce a hollow, "cracked-pot" sound rather than the normal flat tone, but this sign is not dependable and is difficult to interpret.

If treatment is delayed, the head enlarges in all directions. Pressure on the orbits from above causes downward displacement of the eyes, giving them a "setting sun" appearance. Papilledema occurs infrequently, but optic atrophy may appear later, along with pendular nystagmus (a sign of early loss of vision) secondary to the generalized increased intracranial pressure or to the direct pressure of the dilated third ventricle on the optic chiasm. Pyramidal tract signs in the form of spastic lower extremities, hyperreflexia and Babinski signs result from a stretching of the corticospinal tracts by the dilating lateral ventricles. Pituitary-hypothalamic signs in the form of sexual precocity and diabetes insipidus often occur later, due to pressure of the dilated third ventricle on the pituitary-hypothalamic structures. Cerebellar ataxia is often seen and is attributed to compression of the cerebellar vermis by a dilated fourth ventricle. Seizures are common in older children.

Occasionally the disorder will not manifest itself until later childhood because of the low-grade nature of the obstruction. In these older children, one must always consider expanding lesions, such as subdural hematomas and neoplasms; however, the pathologic lesion may be identical with that seen in newborn infants, i.e., aqueductal stenosis. Associated anomalies such as the Arnold-Chiari defect, spina bifida, cranium bifidum, absence of the corpus callosum, porencephaly, cerebellar dysgenesis and hydranencephaly may occur and complicate both the clinical picture and therapy.

Plain x-rays of the skull reveal the craniofacial disproportion, increased convolutional markings and bone thinning, suture separation and erosion of the posterior clinoid processes. Plain films on babies with congenital obstruction at the outlets of the fourth ventricle may show (1) disproportionate enlargement and thinning of the occipital area, (2) lambdoid suture separation and (3) a high position of the lateral sinus grooves due to the elevated tentorium.

In infants subdural taps are carefully carried out in all suspected cases. (See Chapter 15 for details of technique.) Generally, a pneumoencephalogram is done first to estimate the degree of hydrocephalus, to locate the obstruction and to rule out other conditions which might mimic hydrocephalus. If the air which is instilled into the lumbar subarachnoid space fails to enter the ventricles, ventriculography may be carried out either through the anterior fontanel or after trephination of the skull. Upside-down and occipital x-ray views are obtained. Sometimes a combined pneumoencephalogram-ventriculogram is necessary in order to locate accurately the point of obstruction (Fig. 13.8). Ingraham and Matson[35] have outlined in detail the use of combined ventricular and spinal pressure measurements as well as phenolsulfonphthalein (PSP) circulation times and absorption rates to locate the point of cerebrospinal fluid obstruction. This more extensive work-up is not employed at present by most workers because "universal shunt" therapy is used in nearly all infants requiring operation.

The differential diagnosis of head enlargement is outlined in Chapter 4.

MANAGEMENT AND PROGNOSIS.—Therapy for hydrocephalus is generally surgical.[49a] However, the surgical treatment must be considered in the light of the fact that the hydrodynamic obstruction in a certain percentage of patients becomes "arrested" or spontaneously corrects itself. Few data are available on untreated groups of patients with hydrocephalus, but in Laurence's[41] series the process was arrested in 45% of the patients, and in 57% of these the IQ values were 75 or above. Data from an anterospective, unselected series of patients treated alternately with operation and observation would help to appraise surgical therapy accurately. At this time there is no way to detect those patients whose obstruction will become "arrested" spontaneously before brain damage develops. Furthermore, it has been pointed out by Schick and Matson[77] that slowly progressive hydrocephalus may be mistaken for arrested hydrocephalus, and they insist that the obstructive process cannot be considered truly arrested until head growth ceases or until it proceeds at a normal rate close to the normal circumferential range. Hence, the physician's general objective is to relieve the obstruction in the cerebrospinal fluid (CSF) pathway until the condition does become arrested or to slow the rate of CSF production.

The treatment for hydrocephalus is directed to the principles of (1) the reduction of CSF production, (2) the shunting of the fluid around the point of obstruction within the CSF circulation or (3) the shunting of the fluid from the ventricular-subarachnoid system to the vascular circulation or another body cavity[69] (Fig. 13.10).

The *first principle,* reduction of CSF production by endoscopic cauterization of the choroid plexuses, has long been used by Scarff[76] to treat communicating hydrocephalus. However, despite its sound theoretical appeal it has not come into widespread use, probably because of the great technical difficulty encountered and the higher mortality rate. More recently Huttenlocher[34] has shown that medical therapy with acetazolamide (Diamox) is beneficial in selected patients, especially those with low-grade "communicating hydrocephalus" (Fig. 4.1, p. 60). This drug is given in a dose of 50–100 mg./kg./day and may be given for months or years provided the physician knows that he can expect to produce a mild metabolic acidosis. Acetazolamide lowers increased intracranial pressure in obstructive hydrocephalus by decreasing the production of cerebrospinal fluid.

The *second principle,* shunting of fluid from the ventricles into another part of the CSF circulation for the treatment of noncommunicating hydrocephalus, has had widespread use, especially with third ventriculostomy and the Torkildsen procedure. Even when the original diagnosis of noncommunicating hydrocephalus is correct, these procedures may fail either because of inadequate development of the surface subarachnoid pathways or because of incisural block caused by downward displacement of the supratentorial structures. The shunting of fluid from the lumbar subarachnoid space into the ureter was popularized by Ingraham and

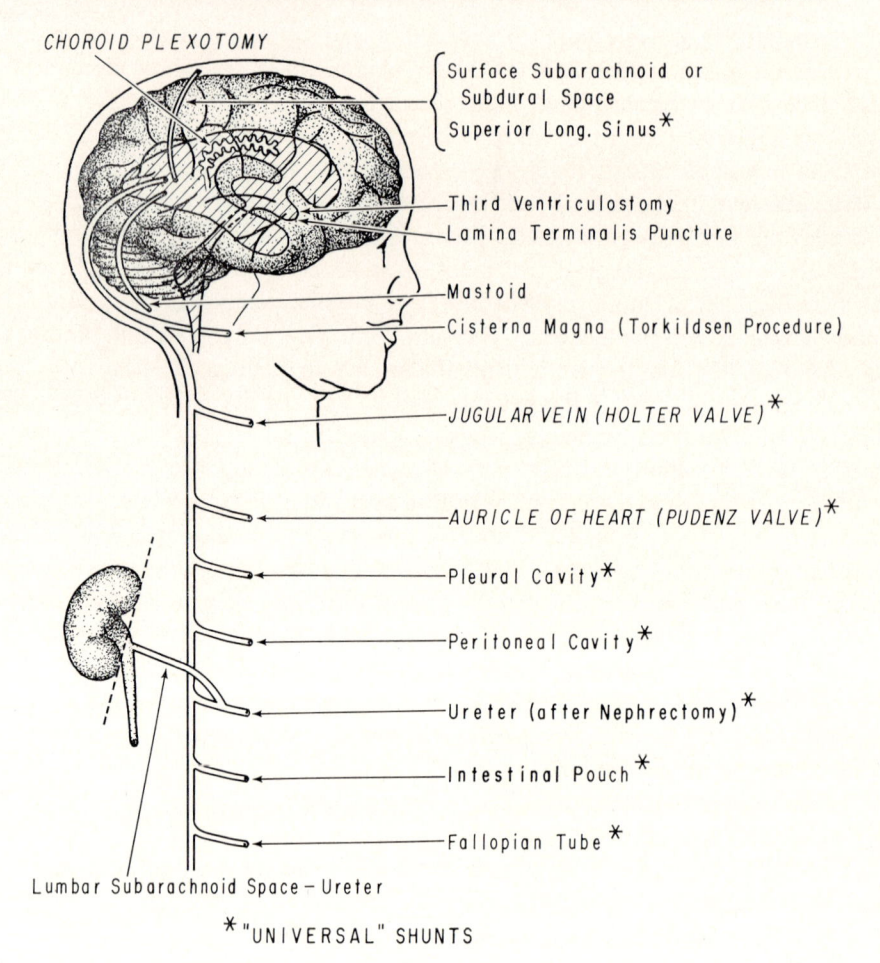

140 CONGENITAL MALFORMATIONS OF THE NERVOUS SYSTEM

Fig. 13.10.—Diagram of several surgical procedures—mostly shunts to bypass obstructions—used in the treatment of hydrocephalus.

Matson[35] for the treatment of communicating hydrocephalus, but the surgeon must be willing to perform a simultaneous nephrectomy with this approach.

The *third principle,* shunting of fluid from the ventricles into the vascular compartment or another body cavity ("universal shunting"), by one technique or another, has entered general use because it theoretically lessens the chance of unsuccessful decompression of the CSF system (Fig. 13.10). The insertion of plastic tubes and valves which allow one-way flow of fluid has led to the successful shunting of cerebrospinal fluid into the jugular vein and right auricle (Fig. 13.8,*B*). Although the mechanical properties of the latter system have worked quite effectively, the complications of bacteremia, bacterial endocarditis, thromboses, embolization and hydrothorax (including chyle accumulation from damage to the thoracic duct) have plagued this form of therapy (Fig. 13.11). One must also be prepared to shunt fluid into other body cavities, such as the pleural space, the ureter (after sacrificing one kidney) and the peritoneal space. Matson[49] has emphasized the need to diagnose and treat the Dandy-Walker syndrome early in order to insure the best prognosis.

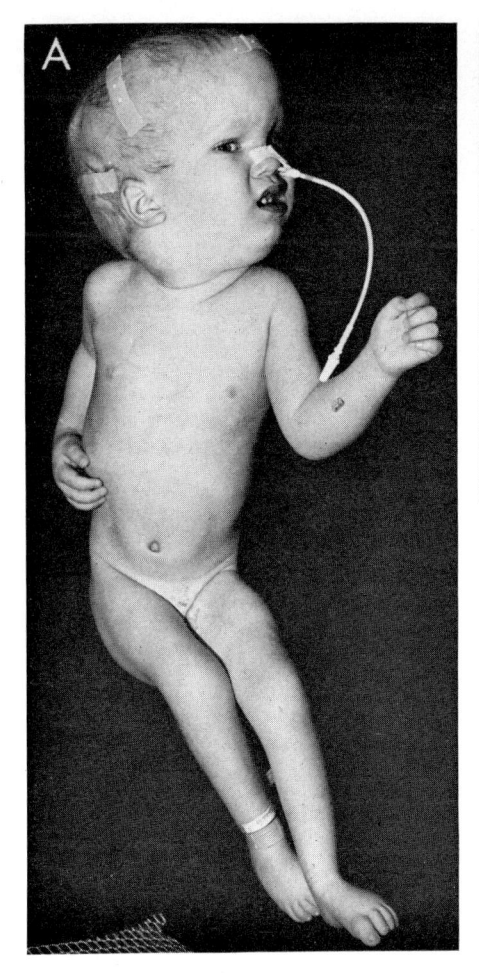

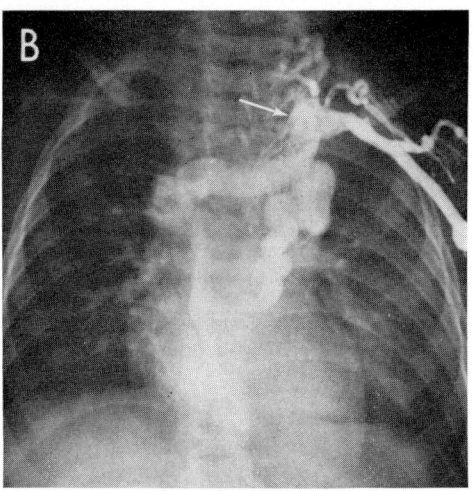

STRUCTURAL MALFORMATIONS OF OBSCURE ETIOLOGY

Fig. 13.11.—Complications of shunt therapy for hydrocephalus. **A**, infant had flaccid weakness of the lower extremities and bilateral corticospinal tract signs. Nasogastric tube feeding was necessary because of secondary pseudobulbar palsy. The infant experienced most of the complications of shunt therapy. In addition to bacterial endocarditis and pulmonary emboli, a retrograde venous thrombosis developed (arrow in venogram, **B**), which extended into the subclavian vein and forced venous blood to return to the heart by a markedly dilated azygous system. After revision of the shunt persistent chylothorax developed due to inadvertent laceration of the thoracic duct when the shunt tube was reinserted.

The surgeon must be prepared to revise the original shunt or switch to an alternative procedure and to treat the medical complications which arise. These include meningitis, thrombosis, embolization, bacteremia, endocarditis and hydrothorax. The variety of different therapeutic procedures indicates that no single surgical approach leads to optimum results, and a review of the literature suggests that the reported results may depend upon the accumulated experience and dedication of the surgeon.

Occult Anomalies of the Brain

PATHOGENESIS.—By definition, these congenital defects can only be suspected on the basis of clinical and laboratory findings because proof of their existence, with a few exceptions, depends upon pathologic study. For these reasons their discussion will be limited, their common features will be grouped and their few distinguishing characteristics will receive special attention. *Agenesis of the corpus callosum*,[51b] *porencephaly* (unilateral or bilateral communication of the lateral ventricles with the surface subarachnoid space), *cerebral atrophy and hypoplasia*,

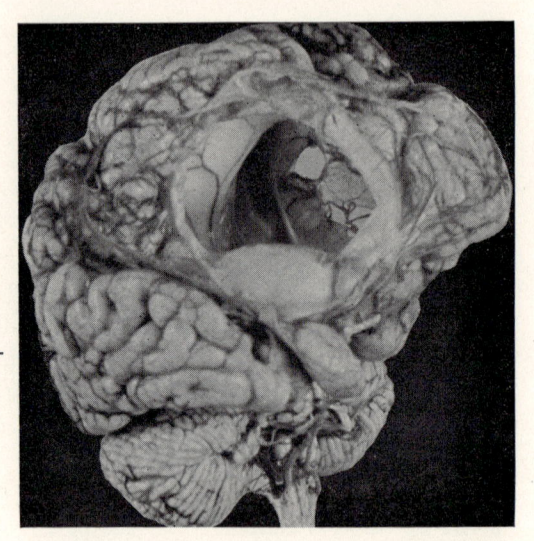

Fig. 13.12.—Bilateral porencephalic cysts (schizencephaly). Pathologic specimen. A definitive diagnosis can often be made clinically with pneumoencephalography.

micropolygyria (gyri which are abnormally small and complex in pattern), *pachygyria* (gyri which are abnormally large and simple in pattern), *heterotopias*[41b] (islands of gray matter which have been misplaced into white matter), *micrencephaly* (small brain size), and *megalencephaly* (brains of excessive weight) appear alone or in combination and result mostly from unknown causes.

Although most of these conditions represent defects in development, cerebral atrophy and unilateral porencephaly may occur as a result of damage (hypoxia, hemorrhage, infection, metabolic abnormality, intoxication) to a normally developed brain. The cerebral atrophies have been reviewed thoroughly from a pathologic viewpoint by Wolf and Cowen[100] and the etiology has been estimated retrospectively. In general, anoxia and metabolic disturbances, either hereditary or secondary, appear to play an important etiologic role in these conditions. The term "porencephaly" should be interpreted to include (1) true developmental defects of the cerebral hemispheres (Fig. 13.12) which are usually bilateral—as described by Yakovlev and Wadsworth[102]—and (2) hemisphere defects, usually unilateral, which result from destructive processses of vascular or traumatic etiology.

CLINICAL AND LABORATORY DIAGNOSIS.—Most patients with one or more of these anomalies exhibit moderate or severe mental deficiency, seizures (grand mal, focal or minor motor) and spasticity.[7] Patients with unilateral defects, e.g., porencephaly, have a spastic hemiplegia and those with bilateral cerebral anomalies exhibit spastic diplegia or quadriplegia. In the latter situations, pseudobulbar palsy with dysphagia dating from birth, dysarthria, drooling and emotional lability are prominent. The syndrome of *atonic diplegia* (a term coined by Ford[19]) or cerebral hypotonia is a strictly clinical constellation of signs and symptoms, characterized by muscle hypotonia, mental defect and incoordination (Chapter 3), and is common in patients with the brain defects listed here. Most of these disorders are characterized by microcrania (abnormally small head size). The exceptions are megalencephaly and those conditions associated with a secondary hydrocephalus, in which abnormal head enlargement is seen.

Pneumoencephalography is usually diagnostic of hypoplasia or *agenesis of the corpus callosum* (Fig. 13.13). The deformed lateral ventricles are widely sep-

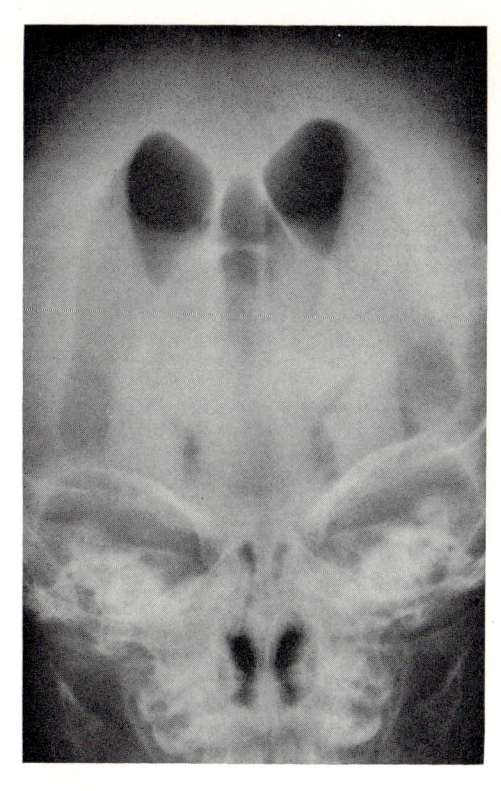

Fig. 13.13.—Partial agenesis of corpus callosum. The typical pneumographic signs of more extensive agenesis of the corpus callosum are described in the text.

arated, their mesial surfaces are concave, and the third ventricle is elevated in the midline to a horizontal plane between the lateral ventricles. In patients with porencephaly, an air encephalogram usually shows ventricular dilatation on the affected side with communication between the ventricle and the subarachnoid space. Patients with *cerebral hypoplasia, micropolygyria, pachygyria* or *focal areas of heterotopia* may show moderate or marked ventricular dilatation as well as an increased quantity of air between the skull and the brain surface (Fig. 13.14). Such pneumographic findings cannot be distingushed from those in patients with cerebral atrophy as a result of infection, hereditary metabolic defect, leukoencephalopathy, etc. The distinction between congenital hypoplasia or agenesis and secondary cerebral atrophy must be made by using all of the available clinical information. The coincidence of developmental brain defects and cystic kidney anomalies has been noted in the literature.[25]

Transillumination of the skull often reveals an abnormal amount of transmitted light, particularly in patients with cerebral or cerebellar atrophy or hypoplasia (Figs. 13.6 and 13.14). Caution must be exercised to avoid overinterpretation of these findings because the amount of light transmitted in normal infants varies considerably, depending upon factors such as the thickness of the skull, the complexion and the quantity and color of hair. In addition, more light is normally transmitted in the frontal and temporal regions, and it is in these same areas that cerebral atrophy may be most marked. Electroencephalography is of little differential diagnostic value, although one may see abnormally slow frequencies and generalized or focal epileptiform discharges.

MANAGEMENT AND PROGNOSIS.—The management of the common manifesta-

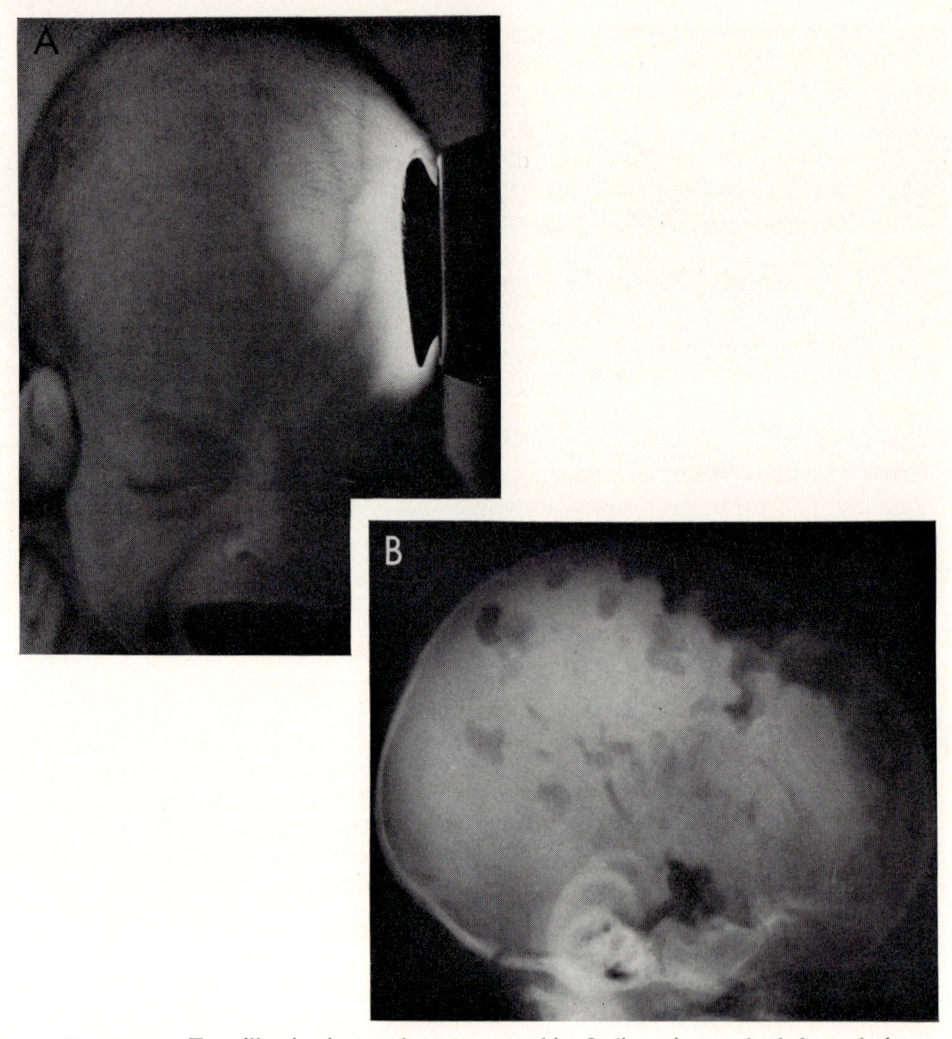

144   CONGENITAL MALFORMATIONS OF THE NERVOUS SYSTEM

Fig. 13.14.—Transillumination and pneumographic findings in cerebral hypoplasia. **A,** this 4½-month-old baby showed developmental retardation and an abnormal amount of transilluminated light. **B,** pneumogram reveals an abnormal accumulation of air in the surface subarachnoid pathways, both over the cerebral convexity and in the basal cisterns.

tions of these anomalies—mental retardation, seizures and spasticity—is covered in Chapters 1–3. Hydrocephalus, if present, is treated in the manner outlined on page 139. Ransohoff and Carter[68] showed that hemispherectomy in carefully selected cases is an effective surgical treatment for those patients with severe spastic hemiparesis, medically uncontrolled seizures and an unmanageable behavior disorder (Chapter 3).

Incontinentia Pigmenti

This rare disorder of unknown etiology manifests itself shortly after birth and causes diffuse central nervous system damage and unusual abnormalities in the skin, teeth, eyes and hair.[51a] Girls are affected much more often than boys (20:1) and a familial incidence sometimes is noted.

In young infants, vesicular lesions often develop, followed by the fixed cutaneous deposition of a brown or blue pigment in a marbling pattern. Microcephaly, retardation, seizures and spasticity may appear prominently. Air encephalography usually shows marked hypotensive hydrocephalus.

Skin biopsy reveals deposition of melanin pigment in the dermis. Results of other laboratory investigations, including chromosome analysis, have been normal.

Treatment is strictly symptomatic (Chapter 1-3), and the prognosis is extremely poor.

Infantile Hypercalcemia Syndrome

Rarely a mentally retarded infant or young child will have a "peculiar facial appearance," anomalies of the heart and great vessels, and hypercalcemia. The etiology of this peculiar clinical constellation is unknown, and we have arbitrarily placed it under congenital malformations. A number of writers[40a,99] have emphasized that patients with supravalvular aortic stenosis exhibit the other signs of this syndrome and that aortic hypoplasia and multiple stenoses of the pulmonary and systemic arteries may be present. What part the hypercalcemia, which may be transient, plays in the pathogenesis is obscure. The unusual combination of an inconstant hypercalcemia, mental retardation and major structural anomalies of the cardiovascular system will be clarified only by further study.

Many of these patients exhibit mental retardation, a "peculiar facies" (this vague term has often included a flat nose bridge, pouting lips and irregular and uneven teeth) and signs of supravalvular aortic stenosis. Hypercalcemia has been noted inconstantly. A surprisingly high incidence of supravalvular aortic stenosis, aortic hypoplasia and stenosis of the pulmonary and systemic arteries has been documented by cardiac catheterization and cineangiographic studies.

Recognition of this constellation of clinical anomalies is important even though thorough understanding and specific treatment are now lacking. The decisions about long-term management of the cardiovascular anomalies can be made only when all the patient's handicaps, including the mental defect, are carefully considered.

Occult Anomalies of the Basal Ganglia, Cerebellum and Brain Stem

PATHOGENESIS.—Defects in any of these parts of the nervous system may occur alone or in combination with the anomalies just described. Their presence is suspected by the proper regional diagnosis of the focal clinical deficit. Care must be exercised in distinguishing true developmental defects from acquired focal damage.

CLINICAL AND LABORATORY DIAGNOSIS.—*Basal ganglia defects* are associated with both movement disorders, such as chorea and athetosis, and rigid muscle tone. The clinical findings may be associated with spasticity and mental defect because of a combination of anomalies. It seems likely that these clinical syndromes can result from pure developmental defects ("status marmoratus") as well as hyperbilirubinemia (hemolytic disease of the newborn), perinatal anoxia and hemorrhage. Laboratory studies are not helpful in the diagnosis of basal ganglia defects.

Cerebellar defects (agenesis or atrophy) are often associated with generalized incoordination, intention tremor, muscle hypotonia and ataxia of the trunk and gait. Such deficits are often mild and become less severe with age. Cerebellar defects are often confused with "atonic diplegia." However, the conditions can usually be distinguished by the more pronounced mental defect in atonic diplegia. The hereditary spinocerebellar degenerations may mimic congenital cerebellar ataxia but can be distinguished by their progressive course and associated sensory and reflex changes. Acute cerebellar disease, including tumor, abscess and encephalitis, usually presents no major problem in differential diagnosis. Clinicopathologic correlation is inconsistent in patients with congenital cerebellar defects since agenesis of a whole cerebellar hemisphere may be found incidentally at autopsy examination in a patient who has had no clinical signs. Pneumoencephalography may reveal hypoplasia, atrophy or agenesis of the cerebellum by an abnormal accumulation of air in the posterior fossa and an enlarged fourth ventricle (Fig. 13.6), but conservative, expert interpretation of such studies is essential.

Congenital defects of the brain stem may involve any of the cranial nerves, alone or in combination, unilaterally or bilaterally. The clinical deficit can result from aplasia of the cranial nerve nuclei in the brain stem or congenital absence of the muscles supplied by the nerves. The oculomotor, abducens, facial and hypoglossal nerves are involved most commonly. The congenital ptosis and the nonreacting pupil seen in third nerve palsy may be associated with the Marcus Gunn phenomenon (opening the jaw causes elevation of the ptotic lid). Congenital facial palsy (Möbius' syndrome) varies in degree and is frequently bilateral. Congenital sixth nerve palsy (Duane's syndrome) causes lateral gaze palsy and retraction of the bulb when the patient attempts to adduct the other eye (Fig. 13.15).

Fig. 13.15.—Bilateral Möbius' and Duane's syndromes in boy, 8. Asked to show his teeth and look to the right, he exhibits (1) bilateral facial weakness and (2) paralysis of abduction on his left with retraction of the right globe when he attempts to look to his right.

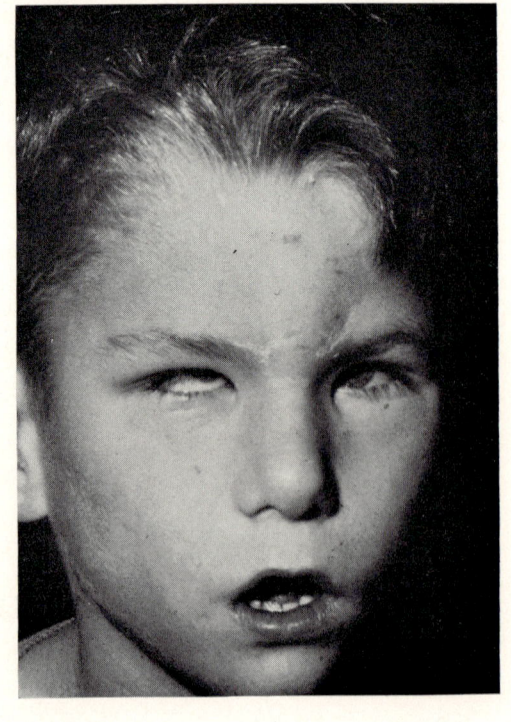

The many variations of Duane's syndrome are described in more detail by Walsh.[93] Less commonly, congenital defects in both the motor and sensory trigeminal branches lead respectively to jaw weakness and ulcerations of the mucous membrane and cornea on the anesthetic side of the face. Congenital paralysis of the palate (vagus nerve) and tongue (hypoglossal nerve) must be distinguished from the more common non-neural anomalies which cause dysphagia and choking—esophageal atresia, tracheoesophageal fistula and compression of the trachea by anomalies of the subclavian artery and aortic arch. Many other anomalies, especially absence of the pectoral muscles, may occur with aplasia of the cranial nerve nuclei. The static nature of these focal neurologic findings and their frequent association with the cerebral symptoms of mental defect and seizures simplify their recognition. Lenz[46a] has pointed out that some of the infants whose anomalies were caused by maternal ingestion of thalidomide have shown defective functioning of the third, fourth, sixth and seventh cranial nerves.

Laboratory findings, except for air encephalography in patients with cerebellar defects, are not valuable in diagnosis.

MANAGEMENT AND PROGNOSIS.—Therapy of the movement disorders and extrapyramidal rigidity with antiparkinsonism agents should be tried,[12] but results are disappointing. Similarly, physical therapy and muscle training should be started early, even though results are not always impressive. The muscle shortening and joint deformities which occur often require tendon lengthening, muscle transplants, peripheral neurectomy and arthrodeses by an experienced orthopedic surgeon. Restricted cortical ablation, anterior and lateral cordotomy and the recently developed procedure of pallidotomy have been used to relieve the athetosis and rigidity. Improvement has been noted in some patients, but since results are inconsistent and benefit is often only transient these procedures should be carried out in only carefully selected cases. Coordination exercises and gait training are used for patients with cerebellar ataxia, but the physician should realize that many patients show spontaneous improvement.

Occult Anomalies of the Spinal Cord and Peripheral Nerves

SYRINGOMYELIA AND SYRINGOBULBIA

PATHOGENESIS.—The terms *syringomyelia* and *syringobulbia* are used to describe tubular cavitations in the spinal cord (Fig. 13.16) and medulla, respectively. These anomalies are often found in association with hydromyelia, a congenital dilatation of the central canal in the cord which does not produce clinical symptoms. Some writers classify syringomeylia as a degenerative or neoplastic process, but its common association with other anomalies such as spina bifida, Arnold-Chiari malformation and platybasia suggests a developmental basis. However, the process in adults is not uncommonly associated with intramedullary glial tumors and neurofibromatosis.[66] Gardner,[24a] who has studied congenital malformations of the hindbrain extensively, postulates a close relationship between syringomyelia and myelocele and suggests that both disorders result from overdistension of the embryonic neural tube. Although any or all segments of the cord may be involved, the cervical, lumbosacral and medullary areas are most frequently affected, in that order.

DORSAL ROOT AND COLUMNS
(Position and Vibratory Sense)

CROSSING SPINOTHALAMIC FIBERS
(Pain and Temperature)

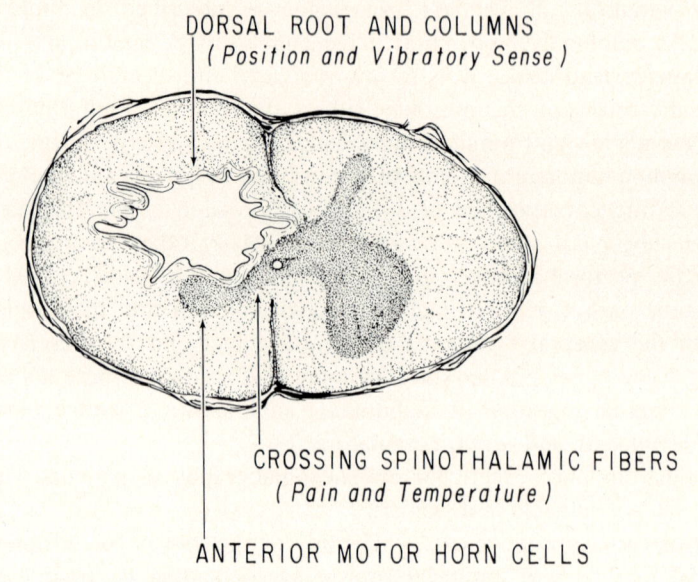

ANTERIOR MOTOR HORN CELLS

Fig. 13.16.—Diagrammatic representation of syringomyelic cavity in spinal cord. Note involvement of the central gray matter, which causes the clinical loss of pain and temperature sense, and the encroachment on the anterior horn cells, which leads to the lower motor neuron signs of flaccid weakness, atrophy and areflexia.

CLINICAL AND LABORATORY DIAGNOSIS.—The fully developed disease picture does not usually appear until adult life, but symptoms and signs often begin in late childhood. An extreme variety of focal neurologic abnormalities is seen in this condition, but the commonest findings are (1) musculoskeletal deformities, (2) disorders of the motor system, (3) disorders of sensation and (4) trophic changes. Scoliosis is the most common deformity (Fig. 13.4), but involvement of the hands and fingers also occurs. Motor manifestations of the disease result from encroachment of the expanding intramedullary cavity on the anterior horn cells. Clinically one sees fasciculations, weakness, atrophy and loss of deep tendon reflexes. Dissociated sensory loss (loss of pain and temperature with preservation of light touch, vibratory and position sense) results from damage to the crossing spinothalamic fibers in the central gray matter of the cord. The distribution of both the motor and sensory deficit is rarely symmetrical and may correspond to a nerve root or to a "glove and stocking" pattern. Characteristically the sensory loss from a cervical syrinx has a capelike distribution over the shoulders. A similar pattern of neurologic deficit is seen much less commonly in patients with a lumbosacral cavitation of the spinal cord. A variety of trophic changes is seen, including edema, cyanosis, ulcerations and a shiny appearance to the skin; these changes probably result from the sensory loss with attendant trauma. Syringobulbia usually produces loss of facial sensation, a Horner's syndrome (ptosis of the lid, a miotic pupil and loss of facial sweating) and weakness of the muscles supplied by the lowest cranial nerves (twelfth, eleventh and tenth). The clinical diagnosis of the incomplete picture presents much greater difficulty, but the physician should remember that the onset of motor disability may precede the sensory loss. If the process is advanced, an experienced radiologist may be able to demonstrate the widened cervical cord with an air myelogram.

A wide range of conditions must be differentiated in the early or rapidly progressing case. Progressive spinal muscular atrophy, poliomyelitis, tumors of the cervical cord and brain stem, Friedreich's ataxia, demyelinating disease, congenital indifference to pain and Raynaud's disease arise most commonly as alternative diagnoses but they can be excluded by the type of sensory deficit, the slow progress of the disease, the normal family history and the random or patchy distribution of the deficit.

MANAGEMENT AND PROGNOSIS.—Medical and radiation therapy offer no relief to patients with syringomyelia. When the pressure within the syringomyelic cavity becomes elevated, cervical laminectomy and decompression of the cord may give considerable temporary relief. Attempts to prevent the subsequent development of increased intramedullary pressure by leaving a wire drain in the cavity have led to considerable temporary improvement in some patients but, unfortunately, little lasting success occurs.

The prognosis is generally poor although the rate of progression varies greatly among patients. When symptoms begin in childhood, the patient's longevity is markedly reduced and a state of helplessness is often reached in early adult life.

CONGENITAL INSENSITIVITY TO PAIN

PATHOGENESIS.—The basic etiology, pathophysiology and anatomic basis for this rare clinical syndrome are poorly understood. The disorder consists of a failure to react normally to ordinarily painful stimuli and is associated in some cases with inability to sweat and with mental defect. Most observers have attributed the condition to an abnormal affective response rather than to truly defective pain perception and have used the term "indifference to pain" to describe the syndrome. The familial occurrence and the association with anhydrosis has led Swanson[86] to postulate a congenital and possibly hereditary defect in peripheral innervation. However, the lack of sufficient pathologic data makes it difficult to reach a consensus about the pathogenesis.

CLINICAL AND LABORATORY DIAGNOSIS.—A failure to react normally to painful stimuli is the hallmark of the syndrome. In many patients this leads to mutilating injuries of the skin, mucous membranes, bones and joints. Some patients manifest the inability to sweat and mental retardation.

One should differentiate the disorder from familial dysautonomia (the Riley-Day snydrome[72]), hereditary ectodermal dysplasia and hereditary sensory radicular neuropathy. Patients with familial dysautonomia show relative indifference to pain but manifest *increased* sweating, absence of tearing, drooling, skin blotching and recurrent pneumonia. Patients with ectodermal dysplasia do not sweat but perceive pain normally and have abnormal hair, teeth and nails. *Hereditary sensory radicular neuropathy* is distinguished from congenital insensitivity to pain by the loss of reflexes and the impairment of all sensory modalities in the former condition. In the latter disorder the tendon reflexes are normal and only pain and temperature sensation are defective.

MANAGEMENT AND PROGNOSIS.—Treatment can be directed only to the prevention of disabling and deforming damage to the bones, joints and soft tissues. Corrective orthopedic measures may be necessary if neurogenic arthropathy (Charcot's joints) develops.

150 CONGENITAL MALFORMATIONS OF THE NERVOUS SYSTEM

The documented affliction of multiple siblings must be borne in mind when discussing the recurrence risk. However, the possibility of multiple etiologies for this syndrome and the paucity of reported hereditary cases call for a cautious attitude in counseling.

Occult Anomalies of the Autonomic Nervous System

Only primary structural malformations of the autonomic nervous system are discussed here. Primary functional or degenerative disturbances in autonomic function are covered in Chapter 21. Although many disease conditions (epilepsy, trauma, tumors, infections, hemorrhage and intoxications) may manifest their effects secondarily via autonomic pathways, they are not discussed separately in this section.

AGANGLIONIC MEGACOLON (HIRSCHSPRUNG'S DISEASE)

PATHOGENESIS.—This state of chronic constipation and abdominal distention results from an absence of the myenteric plexus in a segment of the gut.[88] The involved segment is narrowed and has no peristalsis, giving rise to marked dilatation of the proximal colon.

CLINICAL AND LABORATORY DIAGNOSIS.—Severe abdominal distention and constipation with alternating periods of diarrhea characterize the clinical picture. Visible peristalsis is often noted and the stools are hard and dry.

The diagnosis can be confirmed in some cases by barium enema[6] (Fig. 13.17),

Fig. 13.17.—Congenital aganglionic megacolon. Baby girl with a history of chronic constipation had a barium enema at age 13 months which gave suggestive evidence of a partial obstruction in the lower sigmoid colon. She was treated with enemas and laxatives only to return at age 4½ with vomiting and a severely distended abdomen. A flat plate shows markedly dilated loops of large bowel from an advanced congenital megacolon.

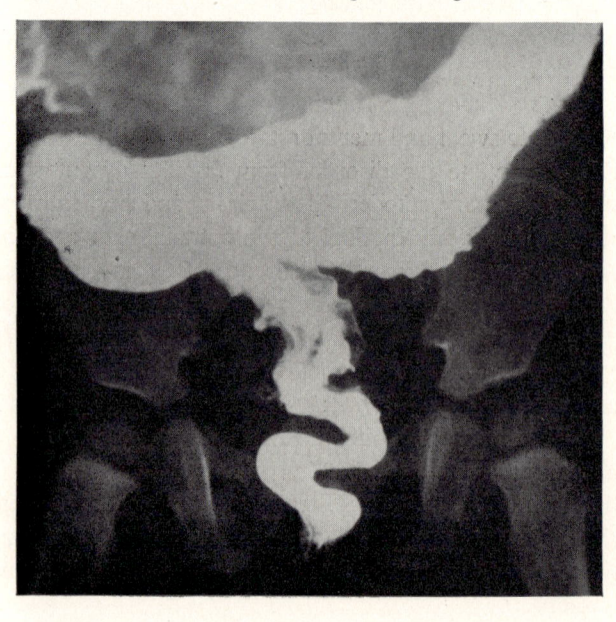

but the interpretation of films requires expert judgment, especially the differentiation from functional megacolon. Swenson and associates[88a] described the diagnostic value of wedge rectal biopsies. Kottmeier and Clatworthy[39] have emphasized the need for full-thickness rectal wall biopsy in questionable cases to avoid (1) unnecessary colon surgery and (2) undesirable and ineffective conservative therapy.

MANAGEMENT AND PROGNOSIS.—Low-roughage diets and stool-softening agents taken orally may control the symptoms in the mild cases. Oil-retention enemas and repeated colonic irrigations with saline may be required to cleanse the bowel before a barium enema or operation. The aganglionic segment of bowel is removed surgically by the "pull-through" procedure as developed by Swenson *et al.*[88] Results of this therapy are good if biopsy at the time of operation reveals that the remaining gut has a normal complement of ganglion cells.

MEGALOURETERS, ACHALASIA AND PYLORIC STENOSIS

Megaloureters have been found in a small percentage of patients with aganglionic megacolon, or they may appear as an isolated finding in patients with urinary retention. The etiology has been attributed to a defect in parasympathetic innervation and a surgical method of treatment recommended.[87] However, this concept and approach to a quite common urologic problem has not received wide acceptance. Many have speculated about the possible etiologic relationship between autonomic nervous system dysfunction and conditions such as achalasia of the esophagus and hypertrophic *pyloric stenosis*. Although conjecture of this sort is quite plausible, most of it lacks factual proof.

FAMILIAL DYSAUTONOMIA

(See Chapter 21.)

Vascular Malformations

Neurologic symptoms resulting from vascular malformations in the nervous system are seen uncommonly during childhood. However, the refinement and application of cerebral angiography suggest that occult vascular malformations must cause more neurologic symptoms and signs in childhood than previously supposed. In addition, improved neurosurgical techniques, induced hypotension and hypothermia have encouraged a more aggressive search for these lesions which can cause progressive neurologic deficit and sudden death from hemorrhage. Congenital vascular malformations of the brain can be divided into two categories: angiomas and arterial aneurysms.

ANGIOMAS

PATHOGENESIS.—Angiomas are tangled masses of abnormal vessels which may lie in the meninges or on the surface or in the depths of the brain. They may or may not be associated with a vascular malformation on the skin or in the retina. Angiomas are sometimes subclassified into *arterial, venous, capillary* and

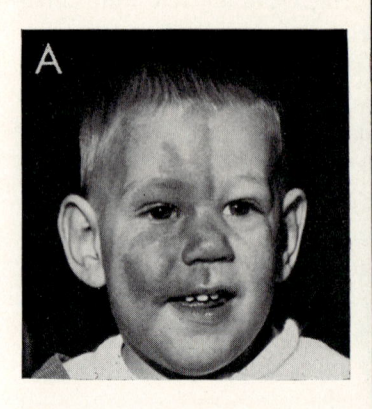

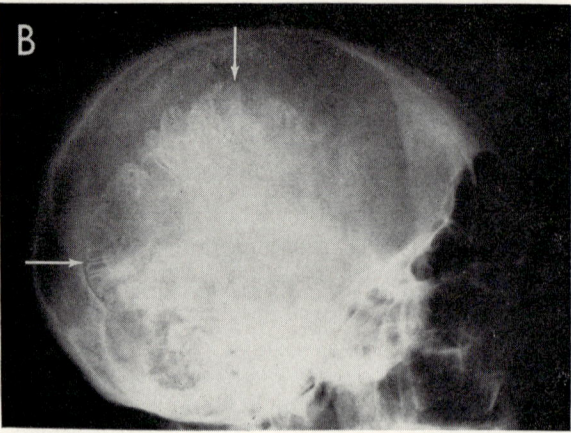

Fig. 13.18.—Sturge-Weber syndrome. **A,** this boy was born with a right, port-wine facial nevus. At 3½ months of age he had a series of left focal motor seizures associated with fever. A left hemiparesis was noted, along with hyperactive behavior and a right-sided epileptiform EEG focus. **B,** lateral view of skull in another patient reveals serpentine or "railroad-track" calcification which is pathognomonic of the capillary angioma seen in Sturge-Weber syndrome.

arteriovenous types. However, with a few exceptions which will be mentioned, the clinical symptoms, signs and syndromes are similar in all types. Obviously congenital and developmental in their nature, they often do not produce symptoms until they have reached sufficient size in late childhood or adult life and until other systemic factors, such as hypertension and atherosclerosis, have been superimposed. They exert their damaging effect by their local irritative and pressure effects and by hemorrhage into the brain or a covering space.

CLINICAL AND LABORATORY DIAGNOSIS.—The usual arterial, venous and capillary angiomas cause focal or generalized seizures and variable degrees of focal neurologic deficit. The patient may have a hemiparesis, a hemisensory deficit, a defect in the visual field and a mental defect. These signs may exist from early infancy, or they may follow a severe focal seizure which, in turn, has resulted from a hemorrhage or thrombosis in the anomalous vessels. Other signs which should suggest the diagnosis of a vascular malformation include vascular nevi on the skin, an intracranial bruit and unexplained subarachnoid bleeding.

Capillary angiomas.—Two special clinical syndromes associated with capillary angiomas can be recognized, although only one should be classified as a congenital malformation. The Sturge-Weber syndrome (encephalotrigeminal angiomatosis) is characterized by (1) a port-wine stain in the area of the upper two divisions of the trigeminal nerve (Fig. 13.18,*A*), (2) a "railroad-track" intracranial calcification which is often most prominent in the occipital area (Fig. 13.18,*B*), (3) contralateral spastic hemiparesis and focal seizures and (4) mental defect. Variations or *formes frustes* of this condition are also seen. The combined involvement of skin and brain can be explained by the common origin of these tissues from ectoderm, but no clear hereditary or familial pattern of occurrence is seen. Capillary angiomas also form an integral part of the ataxia-telangiectasia (Louis-Bar) syndrome (Chapter 21), a condition which is better classed as a metabolic degenerative disorder.

STRUCTURAL MALFORMATIONS OF OBSCURE ETIOLOGY

Arteriovenous angiomas.—These differ not so much in their clinical manifestations as in their size and location. One or more large arteries (most frequently in the middle cerebral but also the anterior and posterior cerebrals) empty into veins by way of a network of thin-walled vessels. Both the patient and the physician, if he auscultates the head, may hear a loud intracranial bruit.

Arteriovenous malformations which involve the posterior cerebral artery are associated with a large aneurysmal dilatation of this vessel (Fig. 13.19,*B*) as it empties into the deep vein of Galen. This anomaly often leads to congestive heart failure in infancy (Fig. 13.19,*A*) and, because of its location near the aqueduct of Sylvius, often causes hydrocephalus.[26] Other common signs include dilatation of the scalp veins, mild cyanosis and papilledema.

The diagnosis of vascular malformations can be established fairly easily if an-

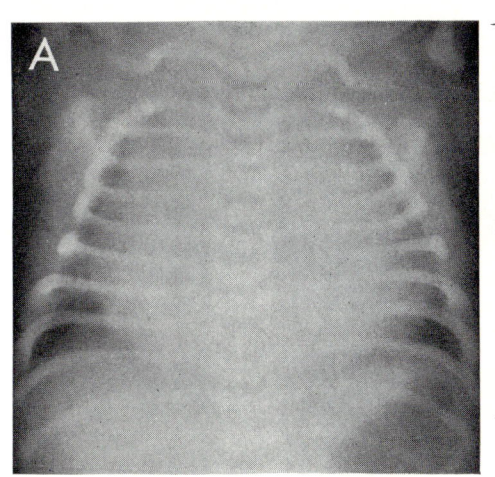

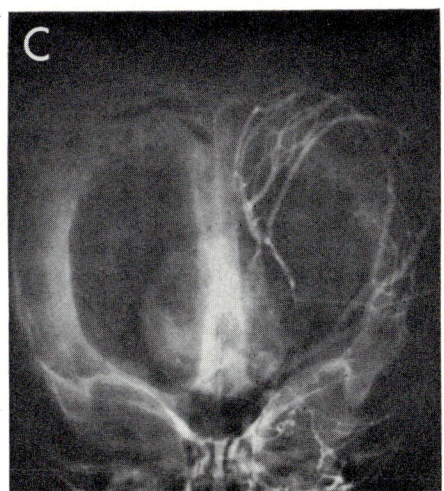

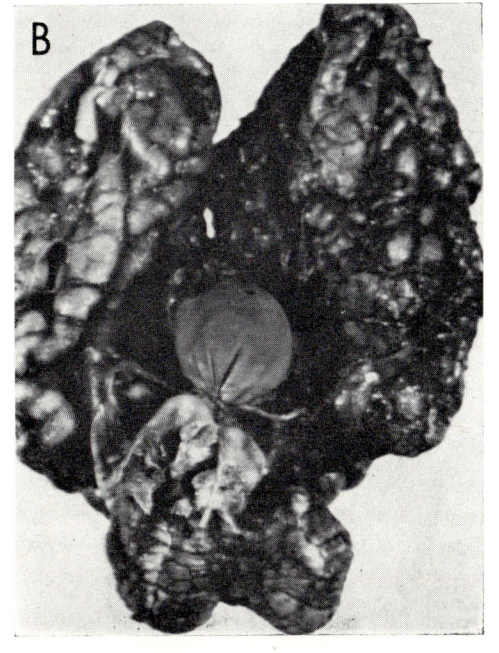

Fig. 13.19.—Aneurysm of vein of Galen. **A,** chest x-ray in newborn infant with dyspnea and cyanosis shows marked cardiomegaly; diagnosis was congenital heart disease. If proper diagnosis is not made and therapy attempted, patients succumb to obstructive hydrocephalus and congestive heart failure. Note the large saccular aneurysm of the vein of Galen in **B.**

C is a frontal projection of a combined pneumoencephalogram-carotid arteriogram in a patient with a vein of Galen aneurysm. The aneurysm is well seen and the obstructive hydrocephalus is also well demonstrated in the form of marked ventricular dilatation. (**C** reprinted from Taveras, J. M., and Wood, E. H.: *Diagnostic Neuroradiology* [Baltimore: Williams & Wilkins Company, 1964.])

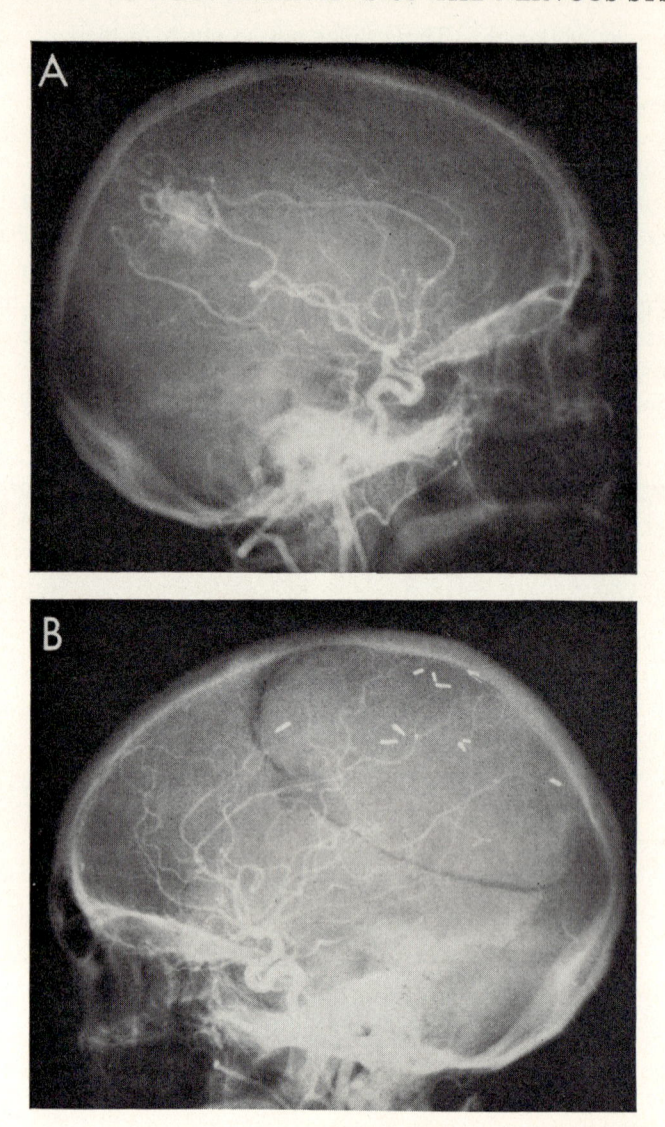

Fig. 13.20.—Arteriovenous malformation. This woman had an episode of status epilepticus when she was 18 and took anticonvulsants periodically thereafter. At age 50 she had a subarachnoid hemorrhage. An arteriogram, **A,** revealed an arteriovenous angioma in the parietal area. After careful surgical ligation of the feeding vessels a postoperative carotid arteriogram, **B,** shows a relatively normal arterial tree on the same side.

giography is performed (Fig. 13.19,*C*). Plain x-ray films of the skull may reveal intracranial calcifications in the area of the vascular anomaly.

MANAGEMENT AND PROGNOSIS.—The therapeutic alternatives, i.e., symptomatic medical management or surgical approach to these lesions, demand critical judgment. Until recent advances in surgical and anesthesiologic technique were developed, operation was not attempted. The size, complexity, location and the threat of fatal hemorrhage influence the decision regarding operation. Ideally, a painstaking and time-consuming resection of all the anomalous vessels with ligation of their feeding arteries is carried out without removal of any brain tissue.[55]

When this approach is impossible, a wedge resection of the vascular malformation and involved brain tissue is performed, and in some cases the operation is limited to strategic ligation of the major feeding arteries. If, in the case of large arteriovenous malformations, surgical resection would increase the patient's neurologic deficit, ligation of the carotid or vertebral vessels in the neck may reduce the threat to life and delay the progression of symptoms. All experienced surgeons stress the need to ligate all of the arterial connections to the anomalous vessels if lasting benefit is to be obtained (Fig. 13.20). Radiation therapy has been applied to small vascular malformations in the hope of shrinking the vessels and preventing hemorrhage, but the results have not been satisfactory. Even the large vein of Galen aneurysms have been managed successfully with benefit to the patient.[89]

Arterial Aneurysms

PATHOGENESIS.—Saccular or "berry" aneurysms are seen rarely in children under age 12 years.[35,50,55,94] They do occur, however, and they behave clinically much the same as in adults. They are seen especially in patients with polycystic kidneys and also in patients with coarctation of the aorta in whom the elevated arterial pressure in the head promotes the development of symptoms and signs.

CLINICAL AND LABORATORY DIAGNOSIS.—The clinical symptoms and signs of saccular aneurysms result either from rupture and hemorrhage or from the direct effects of pressure on adjacent neural structures. The usually sudden symptoms and signs of headache, stupor or coma, meningeal irritation and pre-retinal hemorrhage point to a subarachnoid hemorrhage. If the bleeding is massive, the patient may expire quickly, or a hemiparesis, sensory deficit and a hemianopia may develop. Since aneurysms usually arise from the internal carotid artery or its neighboring vessels in the circle of Willis, pressure of the aneurysm on the second, third, fourth and sixth cranial nerves and ophthalmic division of the fifth cranial nerve

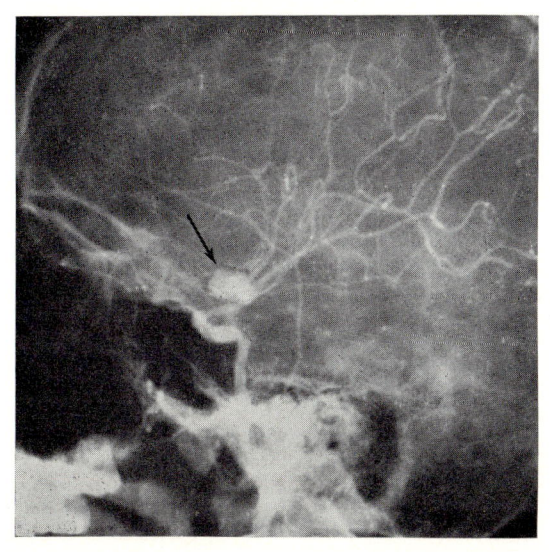

Fig. 13.21.—Berry aneurysm. Girl, 11, had sudden headache, followed by collapse, stupor and convulsions. Lateral arteriographic view shows a large saccular "berry" aneurysm of the left internal carotid artery at its bifurcation. Massive hemorrhage occurred during an attempt to clip the aneurysm. The patient recovered after a stormy postoperative course but four years later exhibits a mild hemiparesis, personality change and mild dementia.

produces pain in the eye, diplopia, absent pupillary light reaction, ptosis, reduced corneal reflex and impaired vision and weakness of the extraocular muscles.

If hemorrhage has occurred, spinal puncture reveals cerebrospinal fluid under elevated pressure. In most cases the fluid is bloody and does not clear as it is collected in three tubes. The supernatant will be xanthochromic if the time interval since the bleeding episode exceeds four hours. Skull x-rays and electroencephalograms usually provide no real diagnostic help, but angiography reveals the size, the location and the number of aneurysms (Fig. 13.21), information which is vital for proper management.

MANAGEMENT AND PROGNOSIS.—A surgical approach to these lesions is generally indicated, as outlined by Mount.[55] The optimal surgical treatment is still a controversial matter. The complex details of proper management of patients with saccular aneurysms falls beyond the scope of this text. In general, clips are placed on the aneurysm itself or on the involved vessel proximal and distal to the aneurysm or on the appropriate neck vessel, if conditions warrant. Sometimes the wall of a large aneurysm is packed with muscle and cauterized. This delicate operation depends for its success on fastidious attention to detail and careful follow-up of the patient.

Skull and Spine Malformations
CRANIOSYNOSTOSIS (CRANIOSTENOSIS)

PATHOGENESIS.—The sutures between the membranous bones of the skull sometimes fuse prematurely. Craniosynostosis can result from primary, premature bony union of the sutures with compression of the brain and the orbits or from microcephaly, a condition in which the slow growth of the brain fails to keep the sutures separated. For therapeutic reasons the distinction between these two broad categories is essential. It is said that craniostenosis results from a developmental mesenchymal defect. This generalization is based upon the common familial incidence of the disorder and the not uncommon coincidence of anomalies in other organ systems. Actually, the precise etiologic mechanism is unknown.

TABLE 13.1.—PHYSICAL FINDINGS WITH DIFFERENT TYPES OF CRANIOSTENOSIS

HEAD DEFORMITY	SUTURE	ASSOCIATED ANOMALIES AND SYNDROMES
Long, narrow head (dolichocephaly, scaphocephaly)	Sagittal	Uncommon
Wide, short head (brachycephaly)	Coronal (bilateral)	Choanal atresia, defects of lip, palate and heart, spina bifida, syndactyly of hands and feet, signs and symptoms of increased intracranial pressure
Wide, conical head (acrocephaly)	Coronal (and frontosphenoidal)	Acrocephalosyndactyly (Apert's syndrome)—similar to premature coronal synostosis (above)
Asymmetry of forehead and face (plagiocephaly)	Coronal (unilateral)	Uncommon
Wide, short head with facial deformities	Coronal, and facial bones	Crouzon's disease (see text)
High, "pointed" head (oxycephaly, turricephaly)	Sagittal and coronal (or all)	Syndactyly
Narrow "keel-shaped" head (trigonencephaly)	Metopic	Orbital hypotelorism, severe brain anomalies (arhinencephaly)

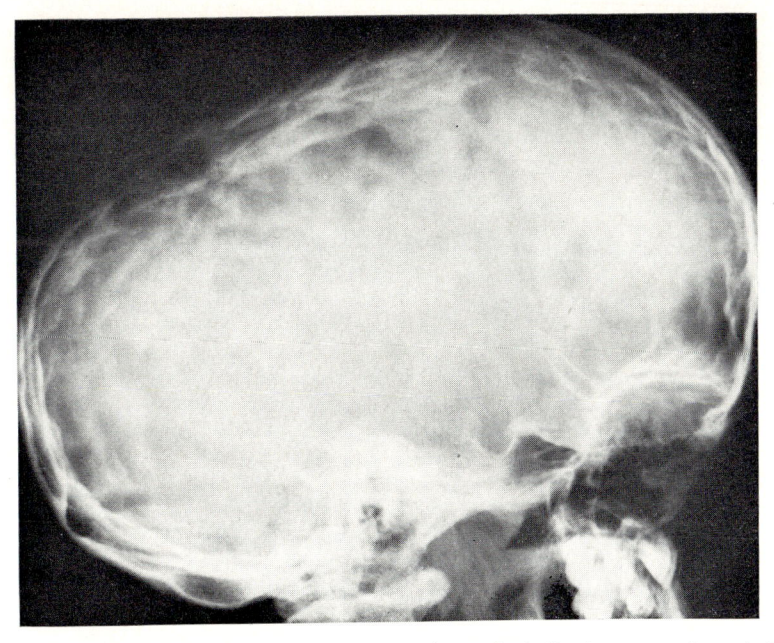

STRUCTURAL MALFORMATIONS OF OBSCURE ETIOLOGY 157

Fig. 13.22.—Sagittal craniostenosis. Lateral view of skull shows scaphocephalic head deformity and abnormally prominent digital markings.

CLINICAL AND LABORATORY DIAGNOSIS.—The craniostenoses can be considered from the standpoint of the suture or sutures which have closed prematurely (Table 13.1) although individual variation can be expected. The severity of the deformity and the danger of neurologic deficit seem to be related to the age of onset. If the condition begins before 1 year of age, while rapid brain growth is taking place, early diagnosis and treatment is especially important.

Each type of craniosynostosis should be considered primarily from the standpoint of the cranial deformity and secondarily with regard to the probability of increased intracranial pressure, eye abnormalities, neurologic deficit and associated congenital anomalies.

In general, when a suture closes too early, head growth is restricted in a plane perpendicular to that suture. The brain then finds growing room in a plane parallel to that suture and the head deformity develops along that parallel axis. Increased intracranial pressure can inhibit normal neurologic development and can cause exophthalmos, papilledema, optic atrophy and ocular squints.

Premature closure of the *sagittal suture* is most common, giving rise to a long, narrow head (scaphocephaly, dolichocephaly) (Fig. 13.22). Although other anomalies, as well as neurologic and eye complications, are seen less frequently in this type of deformity than in others, they do occur. Craniostenosis of the *coronal suture* produces a wide, short head (brachycephaly) (Fig. 13.23). When the coronal suture is involved on one side only, the patient will exhibit asymmetry of the forehead, temple and face (plagiocephaly). The term *acrocephalosyndactyly* (Apert's syndrome) has been applied to the condition of premature closure of the coronal suture in which the widened head has a conical deformity in the region

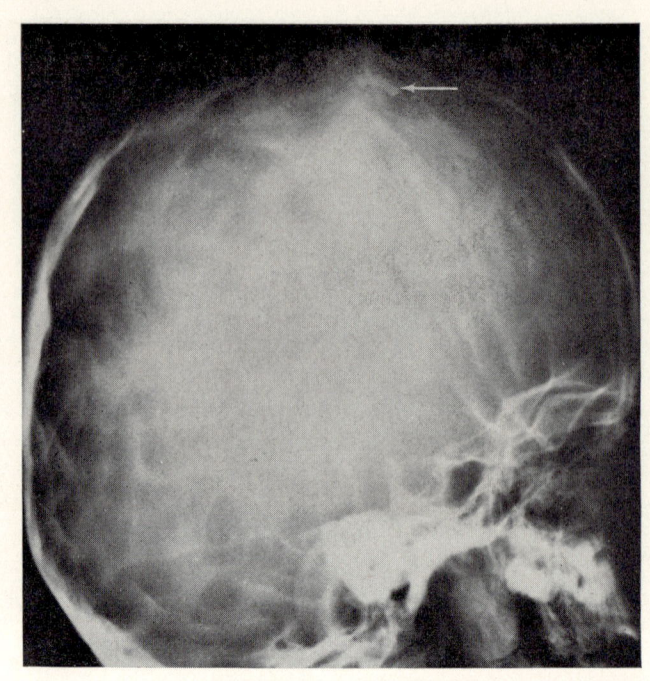

Fig. 13.23.—Coronal suture craniostenosis showing brachycephaly and line of dense bony union (arrow).

of the anterior fontanel and in which the extremities show syndactyly. Other commonly associated anomalies include choanal atresia and defects of the palate and heart.

The clinical signs of increased intracranial pressure are more common in coronal suture craniostenosis. Whether the mental defect and seizures which occur result more commonly from chronic, unrecognized pressure or from associated occult anomalies of the brain is always conjectural unless convincing radiologic or pathologic evidence is collected. *Crouzon's disease* (craniofacial dystosis) represents a special type of coronal synostosis which is inherited as a dominant trait.[11a, 78b] The peculiar facial characteristics—beak nose, prognathism, small maxilla and exophthalmos—result from premature closure of both the coronal suture and the sutures of the facial bones (Fig. 13.24). Despite some reports to the contrary, increased intracranial pressure can also occur in this syndrome.

Oxycephaly (tower skull, turricephaly) is caused by premature closure of most or all of the major sutures. The patient has a high, "pointed" head and the commonly seen increased intracranial pressure causes papilledema, optic atrophy, exophthalmos and visual loss. Headaches, seizures and mental defect often occur if treatment is not prompt and vigorous. Associated anomalies of the skeleton, especially syndactyly and contractures of the elbows and knees, occur frequently.

Trigonencephaly results presumably from premature fusion of the metopic suture and produces a narrow keel-shaped forehead (Fig. 13.25), with narrow-set eyes in some patients. X-rays of the skull in these children often show foreshortening of the anterior fossa, suggesting hypoplasia or compression atrophy of the frontal lobes. We would agree that underlying brain anomaly (arhinencephaly)

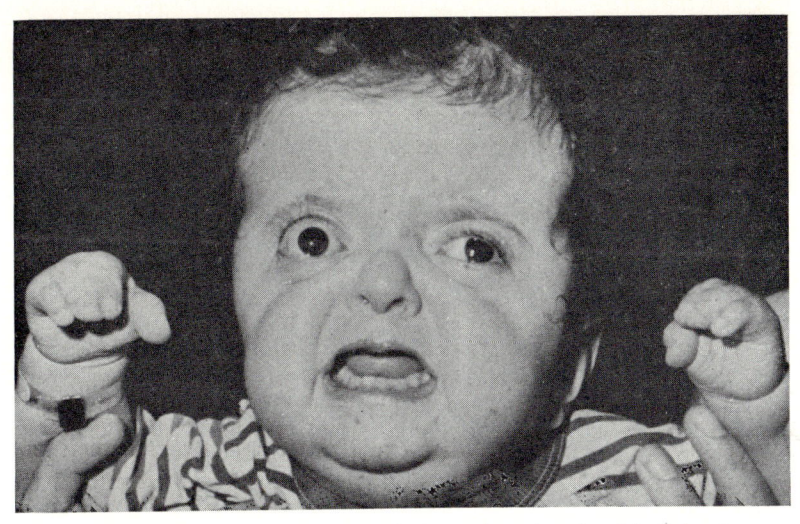

Fig. 13.24.—Crouzon's disease. Grotesque facies and syndactyly of both hands are apparent in this patient. In profile the exophthalmos, beak nose and underdeveloped maxilla are also apparent.

Fig. 13.25.—Trigonencephaly. This 4-month-old boy was studied because of the keel-shaped forehead, A, noted on routine examination. Skull x-rays, B, revealed only a foreshortened anterior fossa.

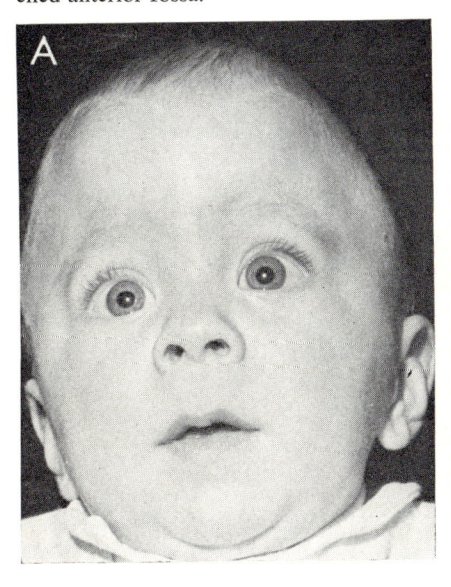

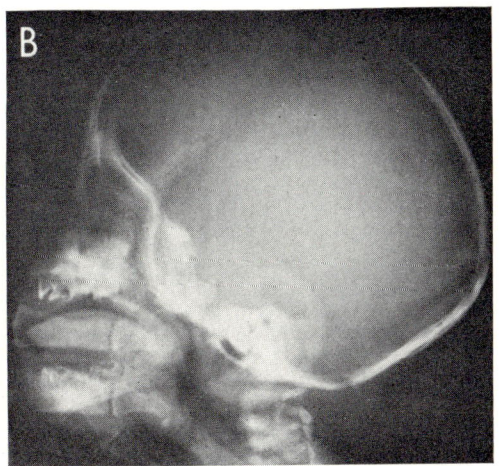

should be considered in these patients, yet some develop quite normally without neurologic deficit. These infants should be followed closely and prognostic statements cautiously made.

Roentgenograms of the skull in patients with craniostenoses may show no visible suture lines if the process is of long standing. Fused sutures will be associated with increased bone density and sometimes mounding up of bone at the line of fusion. The effects of increased pressure are reflected in the prominent digital markings, erosion of the posterior clinoid processes and reduction in the size of the orbits. The head deformity, which is usually obvious clinically, is clearly identified by x-ray (Figs. 13.22 and 13.23), and the coexistent anomalies in the sphenoid, maxillary and nasal bones can often be demonstrated. Air contrast studies are performed in most of these patients to estimate the degree of structural brain damage before a surgical plan is established. Air studies are especially indicated if the patient has neurologic symptoms or any other anomalies. Occasionally the head deformity is recognized during the baby's intrauterine life and can be confirmed with pelvic x-rays, a useful piece of information if the second stage of labor is abnormally prolonged.

The differential diagnosis of craniostenoses should include all causes of abnormal head size and shape (Chapter 4) and the rare hereditary metabolic disorder, hypophosphatasia (Chapter 21).

MANAGEMENT AND PROGNOSIS.—Surgical treatment of these conditions is indicated in most patients provided operation is performed by the age of 3 months.[1c] Whereas a variety of procedures has been used to relieve the pressure on the brain and correct the deformity of the head, truly satisfactory results accrue only when steps are taken to prevent the rapid regrowth of bone. With the technique descibed by Ingraham and Matson,[35] strips of bone are removed along the line of the fused suture, the pericranium is reflected widely and removed, and polyethylene film (or some other inert foreign material) is tied into position over all of the cut cranial edges. Considerable blood loss can be expected at the time of or after operation so that blood transfusion is usually necessary. Accumulation of

Fig. 13.26.—Scaphocephaly, 2½ years postoperatively. This boy had cranioplasties at 7 and 20 months of age for correction of a scaphocephalic head deformity. Subsequent photographs (A and B) at age 4 years 3 months reveal persistent scaphocephaly. At no time has he had any neurologic signs or symptoms.

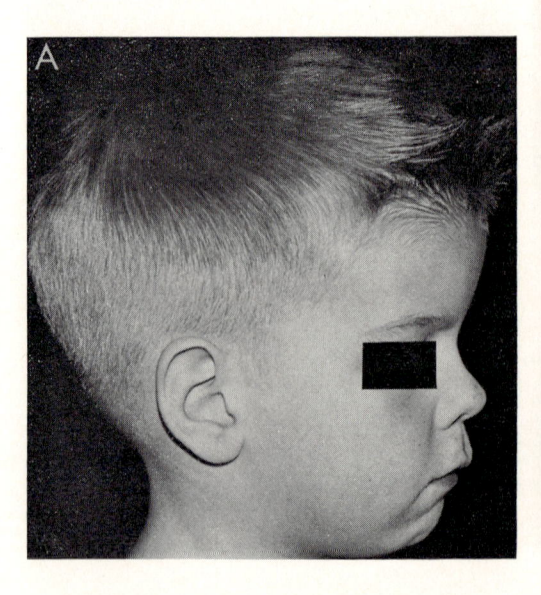

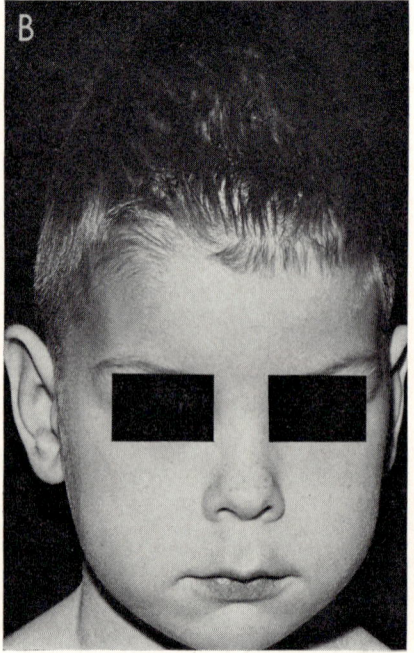

blood and fluid under the scalp occurs frequently and is removed by needle aspiration. When more than one suture is fused, the operation is usually carried out in two stages. Orbital decompression may be necessary to prevent damage to vision, especially in patients with coronal suture fusion.

It has been suggested that in children with premature closure of the sagittal suture often no evidence of brain or orbital compression develops and hence operation is not required. Although such situations undoubtedly occur, one must remember that by the time clinically recognizable neurologic or ophthalmologic problems develop, they are largely irreversible. In addition, many surgeons advocate cranioplasty for the cosmetic benefit which may follow craniectomy. If a good cosmetic result can be obtained, distressing psychologic symptoms in later childhood may be avoided. However, in actual fact, even with extensive and repeated cranioplasties one cannot always prevent significant head deformities with certainty (Fig. 13.26). Also, some patients may be seen so late that considerable brain damage and visual loss are already present, making operation inadvisable.

DIASTEMATOMYELIA

PATHOGENESIS.—This uncommon congenital defect is characterized by a cleft in the lower portion of the spinal cord. A bony spicule and a sheath of dura separate and transfix the two halves of the cord. The lesion may occur anywhere from the fifth thoracic to the fourth lumbar, but it is much more common in the lumbar area and coexists with an occult spina bifida in about half the cases.[35]

CLINICAL AND LABORATORY DIAGNOSIS.—The condition can be suspected by the presence of an overlying skin lesion in most of the cases.[35] The cutaneous defect appears as a tuft of hair, a dimple, a soft-tissue mass or a vascular malformation. Gait disability with lower leg weakness and loss of deep reflexes along with bladder dysfunction and loss of sensation in the saddle area may be present in patients with this anomaly. Pyramidal tract signs may appear in patients with the defect in the thoracic spine.

Anteroposterior roentgen views of the spine confirm the diagnosis in nearly all patients. Pantopaque myelography, though not a diagnostic necessity, outlines the extent of the lesion very well, the stream of dye being separated into two columns.

MANAGEMENT AND PROGNOSIS.—Surgical correction of these lesions in growing children is recommended.[78a] The bony and dural septa are removed to re-establish the normal mobility of the spinal cord within the spinal canal. Established neurologic deficit is not cured by operation, but it is hoped that progress of the deficit will be prevented.

KLIPPEL-FEIL DEFORMITY

PATHOGENESIS.—This rare, random anomaly of the cervical spine is characterized by a failure of segmentation of the cervical vertebrae and is often associated with occult spina bifida. Pathologic studies on a small number of cases have revealed defects in the cervical cord, such as syringomyelia. The diverse clinical signs in these patients should alert one to the likelihood that multiple anomalies in the nervous system can be expected.

CLINICAL AND LABORATORY DIAGNOSIS.—Children with this anomaly have very short necks with limitation of motion and in some cases torticollis, kyphoscoliosis,

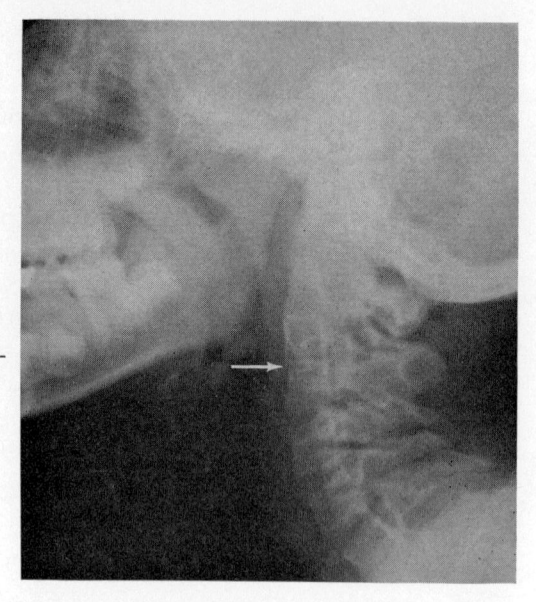

162 CONGENITAL MALFORMATIONS OF THE NERVOUS SYSTEM

Fig. 13.27.—Klippel-Feil deformity. Cervical spine x-rays show (1) the failure of segmentation of parts of the top four vertebrae, (2) fusion of the arches and (3) foreshortening of the bodies of the fused segments adjacent to the disk space where the congenital failure of segmentation has occurred (arrow).

platybasia or Sprengel's deformity (congenital elevation of the scapula). Motor deficit in the form of spastic hemiparesis or quadriparesis may occur, or lower motor neuron deficit with sensory loss may appear in patients with syringomyelia. Mirror movements (unconscious, imitative movements of one hand asociated with intentional movements of the other hand) have been correlated with the Klippel-Feil syndrome and related anomalies of the cervical cord. One must guard against overinterpretation of the significance of this phenomenon because it is seen in some children who otherwise appear normal.

Radiologic examination of the cervical spine (Fig. 13.27) reveals the lack of normal vertebral segmentation, fusion of the arches and anteroposterior foreshortening of the vertebral bodies adjacent to the disk space where the congenital fusion has occurred. Depending on the extent of the clinical problems, a more detailed study of the patient's neurologic status may be indicated, but cervical spine films are diagnostic of this syndrome.

MANAGEMENT AND PROGNOSIS.—No therapy is indicated in uncomplicated cases. In the clinical assessment of the problem one should use caution in predicting the long-range development in view of the common coincidence of other anomalies.

PLATYBASIA

PATHOGENESIS.—This developmental anomaly results from the upward displacement or invagination of the cervical spine causing an elevation of the floor and a reduction in the capacity of the posterior fossa. Compression of the cerebellum with the herniation of the tonsils and an Arnold-Chiari-like deformity with hydrocephalus may occur. Atlanto-occipital fusion, Klippel-Feil syndrome and syringobulbia may coexist with platybasia.

CLINICAL AND LABORATORY DIAGNOSIS.—This condition may be asymptomatic or symptomatic. If symptoms occur, they usually appear in late childhood or early adult life, when a wide variety of signs may develop in a rather insidious fashion.

STRUCTURAL MALFORMATIONS OF OBSCURE ETIOLOGY

Ataxia and nystagmus (from cerebellar compression), lower cranial nerve signs (from stretching), signs and symptoms of increased intracranial pressure (from secondary hydrocephalus) are the most prominent neurologic manifestations. Spasticity of the extremities and signs of syringomyelia may also appear in these patients. The head may appear long in the anteroposterior and short in the vertical diameter.

The radiologic diagnosis usually involves the consideration of several findings on lateral views of the skull and cervical spine. These findings are well demonstrated by Taveras and Wood.[89] The downward slope of the clivus is less steep than normal and the odontoid process projects upward abnormally above Chamberlain's line (Fig. 13.28). Patients may show prominent convolutional markings if hydrocephalus is a complication, and fusion anomalies of the cervical spine and basiocciput may be seen. Pneumography will show ventricular dilatation in patients with hydrocephalus (Fig. 13.28). Lumbar puncture may reveal elevated pressure and evidence of a partial subarachnoid block as measured with cuff manometrics or the Queckenstedt maneuver.

The differential diagnosis must include tumors of the posterior fossa, foramen

Fig. 13.28.—Platybasia and basilar impression with increased intracranial pressure. Young woman, 21, was hospitalized because of primary amenorrhea. Examination showed multiple skeletal deformities (club foot, finger deformities, scoliosis), mild chronic papilledema and borderline intellect. The patient reported intermittent headache (worse when erect) and blurred vision for a year and a half. Skull x-rays and ventriculography (illustrated) revealed (1) basilar impression or invagination. The odontoid process which is poorly seen extends much above Chamberlain's line (dotted line). Note the high position of atlas and odontoid. Chamberlain's line extends from the hard palate to the posterior margin of the foramen magnum. Normally, up to a third of the odontoid process extends above this line but in this case the whole of it lies above. Also note (2) platybasia, (3) suture separation, (4) prominent digital markings, (5) enlargement of the pituitary fossa (2 cm. in greatest diameter) with obliteration of the right anterior clinoid and (6) anomalies of the cervical vertebrae. A ventricular-jugular shunt was performed for extensive hydrocephalus. The patient had a cervical laminectomy a year later and was found to have syringomyelia and an Arnold-Chiari malformation.

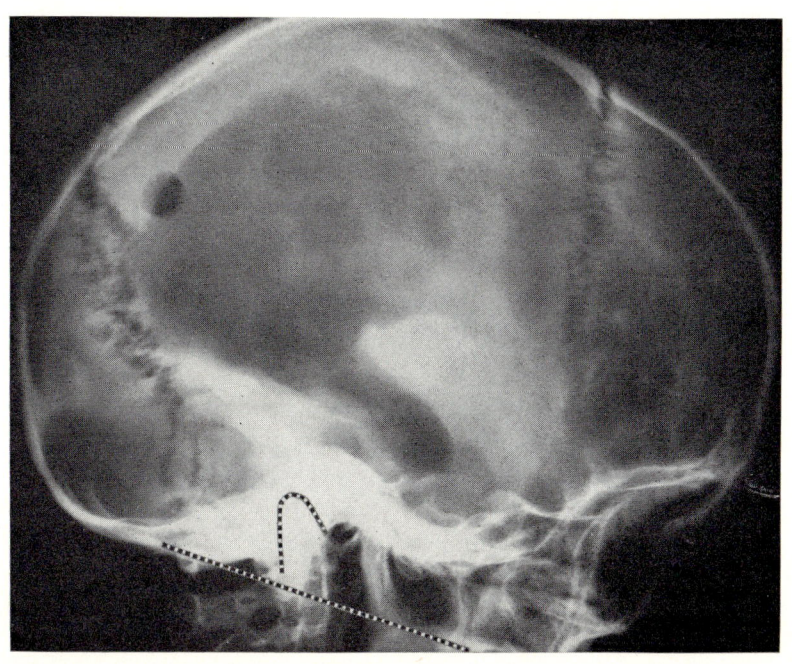

magnum and cervical cord. Also, late-appearing cases of aqueductal stenosis must be considered as well as demyelinating disease and spinocerebellar degenerations.

MANAGEMENT AND PROGNOSIS.—Treatment is directed only at surgical decompression of the posterior fossa and upper cervical canal in selected cases. If hydrocephalus is present, it is managed in the usual manner (p. 139).

CHONDRODYSTROPHY (ACHONDROPLASIA)

PATHOGENESIS.—This generalized disorder of bone formation with dwarfism is usually inherited as an autosomal dominant trait, but kindreds with a recessive inheritance pattern are reported, according to Stern.[83] It begins in prenatal life and is characterized by impaired ossification of cartilage, especially in the long bones of the extremities. Bones of the skull and the vertebrae are involved to a lesser extent. The bones of the base of the skull arise from cartilage and hence are involved, leading to a shortened skull base which presumably can cause an obstruction in the basal cisterns.

CLINICAL AND LABORATORY DIAGNOSIS.—Chondrodystrophic dwarfs typically have short arms and legs, lumbar lordosis and in some cases a large head. Head enlargement, which usually occurs in the transverse and vertical planes with prominence of the forehead, may reflect a low-grade communicating type of hydrocephalus. Paraplegia is seen in some cases as a result of a herniated intervertebral disk or bony compression of the lower dorsal or upper lumbar cord.

Plain spine x-rays may show narrowed interspaces in the area of extreme lordosis and wedging of a low dorsal or upper lumbar vertebra. Pantopaque myelography is useful in confirming the site of subarachnoid block in patients with a developing paraplegia.

MANAGEMENT AND PROGNOSIS.—Patients with progressive paraparesis should have a decompressive laminectomy. The hydrocephalus which occurs in this disorder is usually very indolent and low grade. Its management depends on the total clinical picture and the rate of progression.

In a family with this disorder the affected individuals can expect to pass the trait to a certain number of their offspring since the pattern of inheritance is usually dominant. However, the family pedigree should be studied with care before genetic counseling is offered.

OSTEOPETROSIS

PATHOGENESIS.—This rare disorder of bone formation is characterized by the failure of resorption of partially calcified ground subtsance. This abnormal state leads to thickening of both cortex and trabeculae, with resulting bone brittleness and easy fracture. Eventually, encroachment upon the bone marrow leads to an aplastic type of anemia with a bleeding tendency from thrombopenia. Bony overgrowth at the base of the skull causes foraminal narrowing and encroachment upon cranial nerves entering and leaving the cranial cavity. The possible relationship between this disorder and neurofibromatosis has been considered.

CLINICAL AND LABORATORY DIAGNOSIS.—The diagnosis is usually made incidentally when x-rays are taken to view a fracture. The diffuse bone sclerosis is usually pathognomonic although the skull changes may resemble those in idiopathic hypercalcemia. Subdural hematomas occur in some patients, presumably due to a thrombocytopenia-induced bleeding tendency. Pressure on the cranial nerves may lead to blindness and deafness.

MANAGEMENT AND PROGNOSIS.—Treatment is strictly symptomatic, there being no specific surgical or medical therapy. In the severe and advanced cases multiple fractures, progressive anemia, blindness and deafness can be expected. Life span is generally short.

FIBROUS DYSPLASIA

PATHOGENESIS.—This rare disorder of bone formation can affect localized parts of the skeleton, such as the skull, or it can be polyostotic. Although the exact etiology is not known, the evidence points to an early developmental origin. The possible relationship between this disorder and neurofibromatosis has been discussed.[73a] When the disorder affects the skull, the slow bony overgrowth may compress the optic nerves as they enter the orbits through the optic canals.

CLINICAL AND LABORATORY DIAGNOSIS.—Signs such as facial asymmetry, cranial deformity, proptosis, ptosis and impaired visual acuity appear in middle childhood. Although many cases involving the orbits are unilateral, we have seen patients in whom the disease has progressed to almost total blindness before it was recognized. Occasionally Albright's syndrome, characterized by polyostotic fibrous dysplasia, sexual precocity and large areas of increased skin pigmentation, occurs as a complex. Plain skull x-rays reveal patchy sclerotic zones of increased bone density, sometimes surrounding areas of irregular decreased density. One may also see asymmetry in the whole bony architecture of the orbit, suggesting an early onset. Optic foramen films may confirm the suspicion of encroachment upon the optic nerves. When the process involves the base of the skull, tumors such as meningiomas and chordomas must be considered, although these neoplasms only rarely affect children in the region. Hyperparathyroidism must also be considered, but this disorder is generalized and is associated with hypercalcemia.

MANAGEMENT AND PROGNOSIS.—When there is progressive visual impairment or severe deforming proptosis, the patient may be benefited by operation. Usually the surgeon unroofs the orbit in order to decompress the optic nerve and correct the eye deformity.

The prognosis is reasonably good if the diagnosis is not delayed unduly and if the patient is seen at regular intervals for testing of visual acuity and visual fields as well as serial skull films.

Structural Malformations of Known Etiology

The cause of most nervous system malformations is unknown. Established knowledge about etiology is gradually accumulating, however, and it can be divided arbitrarily into three categories: malformations resulting from (1) chromosome anomalies, (2) maternal infections during pregnancy and (3) other environmental factors which influence the developing embryo and fetus.

Terminology

Chromosomes are the threadlike masses in the nuclei of the cell which bear the genes and which determine the hereditary characteristics. Normally each germ cell (either sperm or ovum) contains 23 chromosomes, half the number found in normal somatic cells (46). Occasionally a mistake in the equal separation of chromosomes to two daughter cells occurs during cell division and this error is called *nondisjunction*. Nondisjunction usually takes place during *meiosis* (germ cell division) but may also occur during *mitosis* (somatic cell division) or early cell multiplication in the embryo. These biologic errors may cause failure of impregnation, miscarriage, birth of viable infants with a limited life expectancy or of babies with malformations. Examination of the normal *karyotype* in a circulating lymphocyte, i.e., the orderly arrangement of the chromosomes which permits systematic analysis, reveals 22 pairs of *autosomes* (the nonsex chromosomes) and one pair of *sex chromosomes* (two X chromosomes in the normal female and one X and one Y in the normal male). Incidentally, a reliable estimate of the number of X chromosomes in a person can be obtained by staining a smear of the buccal epithelial cells and looking for a peripheral sex chromatin "Barr body." The number of X chromosomes is estimated by adding 1 to the number of sex chromatin masses. This technique can be performed in almost any hospital laboratory and has great practical diagnostic value.

Many different anomalies in chromosome number and structure are encountered. *Trisomy* is a condition in which an extra chromosome is found in all somatic cells, i.e., three similar chromosomes are present rather than the normal two. *Monosomy* refers to the presence of only one of an expected pair of chromosomes.

Abnormalities in structure are caused by breakage of chromosomes during meiotic or early mitotic cell division with an altered arrangement of the broken fragments. When chromosomes break and nonhomologous fragments then unite, this is called *translocation*. Small fragments (*deletions*) may be lost because they are nonviable but occasionally they persist in subsequent cell divisions. Sometimes when deletions and translocations occur, the abnormal chromosome will assume a *ring* configuration which may perpetuate itself. The same numbered chromosomes which have been involved in the trisomic state have occurred in the "ring" configuration. The term *partial trisomy* is used frequently in the literature to refer to the presence in triplicate of part of a chromosome. Presumably the trisomic chromosome breaks, the large fragment is *translocated* or *inserted* to another chromosome and a small fragment may be lost or deleted. On rare occasions the chromosome divides horizontally rather than in the usual longitudinal manner, resulting in the formation of *isochromosomes*. The upper and lower segments are usually of approximately equal length. The ability to analyze chromosome constitution of different tissues has revealed that some persons are *mosaics,* i.e., they have cell populations in different parts of the body with different chromosome counts and structures.

TABLE 13.2.—ABNORMALITIES IN CHROMOSOME NUMBER

PHENOTYPE	NO. OF CHROMOSOMES	CLINICAL SYNDROME	REFERENCE
AUTOSOMES			
G (21–22) trisomy	47	Monogolism	Lejeune et al.[43]
		Mental retardation	Ellis et al.[13a]
			Gustavson et al.[20a]
D (13–15) trisomy	47	Multiple congenital anomalies	Patau et al.[61a]
E (16–18) trisomy	47	Multiple congenital anomalies	Edwards et al.[13]
			Smith et al.[81]
SEX CHROMOSOMES			
XXY	47	Phenotypic males with testicular atrophy	Jacobs and Strong[36]
XXXY	48	Phenotypic males with testicular atrophy	Ferguson-Smith et al.[17a]
XXXXY	49	Phenotypic males with testicular atrophy	Fraccaro et al.[22]
XXYY	48	Phenotypic males with testicular atrophy	Carr et al.[8a]
XXXYY	49	Phenotypic males with testicular atrophy	Bray and Sr. Ann Josephine[3]
XXX			Jacobs et al.[37]
XO	45	Phenotypic females with gonadal dysgenesis	Ford et al.[18]
XY Mosaics	46	Phenotypic females with gonadal dysgenesis	Cohen and Shaw[9b]
AUTOSOMES AND SEX CHROMOSOMES			
G trisomy-XXY	48	Mongolism + Kinefelter's syndrome	Ford et al.[17b]
G trisomy-XXX	48	Mongolism + triplo-X syndrome	
E trisomy-XXX	48	E trisomy + triplo-X syndrome	Ricci and Borgatti[71]
D trisomy-XXY			Pergament and Kadotani[63a]
MULTIPLE AUTOSOMES			
D and G trisomies	49	Multiple congenital anomalies	Becker et al.[1e]

Abnormalities in Chromosome Number

PATHOGENESIS.—Established chromosome anomalies are characterized in most cases by structural anomalies in more than one organ system, including the skin.[1,1a,92a] However, neurologic symptoms and signs predominate in some and may be seen in all of the disorders. In general there are two types of chromosome anomalies: abnormalities in the number (more or less than the normal 46) and in the structure (translocations, insertions, deletions and "ring" formations). In view of the fact that new types of cytologic abnormalities and their clinical correlates are accumulating at a steady rate, no attempt will be made here to cover all reported chromosome anomalies. Instead, the commoner abnormalities of number and structure will be described. Only in the years ahead, when the period of data collection is more nearly complete, will a more comprehensive review be possible.

Abnormalities in the number of chromosomes (Table 13.2) result usually from nondisjunction, an error in chromosome separation during meiosis or during

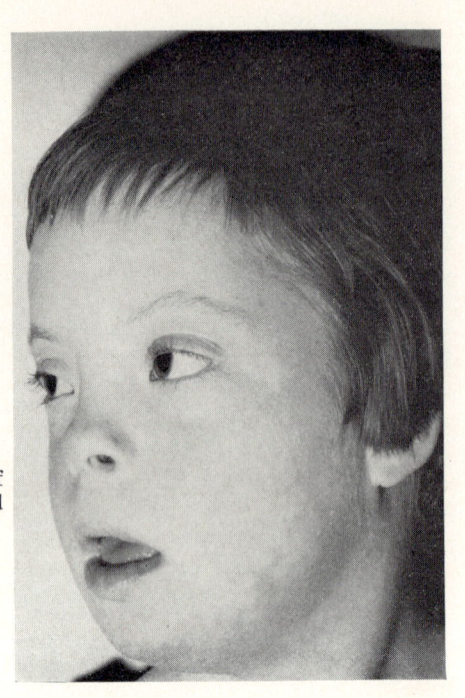

Fig. 13.29.—Mongolism (Down's syndrome). Girl with typical mongoloid facies: small flat nose, mongoloid slant of eyes, epicanthal folds, prominent tongue and brachycephaly. One should look carefully in these patients for anomalies of (1) the heart and (2) the upper small bowel.

earliest mitosis (embryonic cleavage). Clinical observations have shown that nondisjunction occurs more frequently in the older mother regardless of which chromosome is involved, indicating again the combined influence of heredity and environment in the etiology of malformations.

Convincing evidence is accumulating from the study of abortuses and stillborns, such as that of Carr,[8] that chromosomal abnormalities are responsible for a significant amount of embryonic wastage.

CLINICAL AND LABORATORY DIAGNOSIS.—*Autosomes.*—The 21 or G trisomy (mongolism, Down's syndrome) is easily recognized clinically. The children show retarded physical and mental development, small, short heads, slanted eyes with prominent epicanthal folds, a flat nose bridge with noisy respirations, a large, furrowed tongue, blepharitis, characteristic palmar dermatoglyphics[10a] with a simian line, short hands and feet with incurving of the little finger, congenital heart disease with a high incidence of septal defects, and anomalies of the gut with intestinal obstructions resulting from duodenal stenosis (Fig. 13.29). The brains of these patients are low in weight, have a short, round shape and show underdevelopment of certain gyri, but they do not have any severe or consistent microscopic changes, according to Greenfield.[28] This syndrome appears approximately once in every 650 births and is commoner in babies of older mothers. Lejeune and co-workers[43] first demonstrated that the karyotype (the chromosome constitution of a cell) usually shows an extra chromosome (number 21) in the "G" group, and this anomaly is termed a "21 trisomy."

Trisomy in the E group (numbers 16–18) involves chromosome 18. The clinical features include apparent mental defect, overlapping fingers (index over middle) micrognathia, low and malformed ears and dorsiflexion of the great toes.

These patients, like those with the D trisomy, usually die during the first year of life. No detailed neuropathologic studies have been reported yet. These patients show an extra chromosome in the 16–18 group.[13,81] The bulk of cytologic evidence suggests that the number 18 chromosome in the "E" group is trisomic.

The D or 13–15 trisomy is less common, but its incidence is probably underestimated because most of these infants die during the first year of life. The syndrome first described by Patau and associates[61a] is characterized by anomalies in nearly all organ systems, the most distinctive being severe eye defects, cleft palate and lip, hyperextensible thumbs, apparent mental retardation and seizures. The neuropathologic findings in five reported cases[53,61a] show consistent anomalies in the formation of the cerebral hemispheres, the ventricular system and the optic and olfactory apparatus. Despite some individual pathologic variation these findings would suggest a common teratologic basis for the arhinencephaly and the other nonneural anomalies of this syndrome. Karyotype analysis reveals seven large acrocentric chromosomes (instead of the usual six) in the 13–15 or D group.

Monosomy.—Autosomal monosomy is generally a lethal condition. However, recently *21 monosomy* was discovered in a 4-year-old mentally retarded girl.

Sex chromosomes.—Nondisjunction can involve the sex chromosomes and produce a variety of abnormal karyotypes with reasonably similar clinical syndromes. A peculiar constellation of clinical findings, including short stature, amenorrhea, poor breast development, low hair line, valgus deformity of the elbows and occasionally mental defect, is seen in phenotypic females with an absent X chromosome. This XO sex chromosome anomaly and its associated phenotype is called *Turner's syndrome*. The sex chromosome anomaly was first described by Ford et al.[18] In this same clinical picture there may be a combination of a normal X with an isochromosome X,[20] a normal X plus a partially deleted X, XO/XX mosaicism or a normal karyotype. When nondisjunction with trisomy for the X chromosome occurs, it results in a "triplo-X" sex chromosome complement.[37] Although the phenotypic female is usually mentally retarded, sterile and amenorrheic,[38] it is not known whether this anomaly can occur without these clinical deviations inasmuch as most reported cases have been found by screening patients in institutions for the mentally retarded, using the technique of buccal smear for nuclear chromatin.

Phenotypic males with small testes and infertility, gynecomastia, eunuchoid body build and mental retardation in many cases are designated as having *Klinefelter's syndrome*. The karyotype most frequently shows an XXY sex chromosome constitution first described by Jacobs and Strong,[36] but the spectrum of abnormalities has expanded to include XXXY, XXXXY,[22] XXYY, XXXYY[3] and mosaic patterns of the above. It has been suggested that the degree of mental defect and testicular changes is directly proportional to the number of supernumerary X chromosomes, but this remains to be proved. Delinquent or criminal behavior is seen in many of these patients and has been said to be more frequent in those with two Y chromosomes than in those with Klinefelter's syndrome with one Y chromosome.[67] Assuming that this correlation is valid, it is not clear whether the criminal behavior results from the observed large size, impaired intellect, greater innate aggressiveness or a combination of these factors. In one recent study of

129 tall criminal men, one in 11 had sex chromosome anomalies; half had Klinefelter's syndrome and half had XYY anomalies.[89b]

Double trisomies, usually involving autosomal and sex chromosomes, have been reported by a number of workers. These patients have all shown mental deficiency. The double trisomies have included (1) XXY—21 trisomy or Klinefelter's syndrome with mongolism, (2) XXX—18 trisomy or a combination of the clinical features described separately above, (3) XXX—21 trisomy mongolism in a girl with the features of the triplo-X clinical syndrome and (4) a combination of D and G trisomies (Table 13.2).

Despite the similarity in the clinical features of patients with the grossly identical chromosome anomalies described, the reader's attention should be called to certain inconsistencies, lest the problem appear simpler than it is. First, one may see different karyotypes in patients with the same clinical syndrome, e.g., patients with mongolism who have (1) 21 trisomy, (2) translocation or (3) a normal karyotype[65] and patients with Turner's syndrome who have an XO or a normal XX sex chromosome complement.[21a] Conversely, apparently identical chromosome anomalies have been associated with marked differences in clinical appearance, e.g., G, D and E trisomies.

A variety of mosaic chromosome patterns have been described in both autosomal and sex chromosome abnormalities, but this complex and elusive aspect of the problem goes beyond the scope of this discussion.

MANAGEMENT AND PROGNOSIS.—See under Abnormalities in Chromosome Structure.

Abnormalities in Chromosome Structure

PATHOGENESIS.—The etiology of structural chromosome anomalies in human malformations is not understood, but it is known that irradiation, viruses and drugs such as LSD can cause various structural changes in both normal and abnormal dividing human cells. Although most chromosome anomalies originate during or after gametogenesis, occasionally they are inherited and behave like a dominant genetic trait.

CLINICAL AND LABORATORY DIAGNOSIS.—In general, translocations and ring chromosomes are associated clinically with multiple congenital anomalies. A detailed list is given in Table 13.3. Most reported cases present an inconstant constellation of anomalies but some exceptions have been described (see below).

Mongolism.—The commonest type of reciprocal translocation has been found in patients with mongolism in whom the number of chromosomes is 46 instead of the expected 47. Their parents and ancestors have 45 chromosomes, including the "translocated" chromosome, but they are phenotypically normal because the total amount of chromosome material is essentially normal or "balanced." These translocations involve either one chromosome from the large acrocentric (13–15) and small acrocentric (21–22) groups or two chromosomes from the small acrocentric group.

Cri du chat syndrome.—More recently an additional syndrome with rather distinctive clinical characteristics has been described. Infants with a catlike cry or mew, bilateral epicanthi, microcephaly, mental retardation and other malfor-

TABLE 13.3.—ABNORMALITIES IN CHROMOSOME STRUCTURE

PHENOTYPE	NO. OF CHROMOSOMES	CHROMOSOMES INVOLVED*	REFERENCE
TRANSLOCATION			
Mongolism	46	13–15 D/G 21–22	Penrose et al.[63]
	46	21–22 D/G 21–22	Fraccaro et al.[21]
Multiple anomalies of spinal column	45	13–15 D/G 21–22	Turpin et al.[92]
Mental retardation	45	13–15 D/G 21–22	Moorhead et al.[54]
Multiple congenital anomalies	45	2 A/D	Mercer and Darakjian[52]
Mongolism	46	21–22 G/G 21–22	Zellweger et al.[104]
Multiple congenital anomalies	46	4 or 5 B/E 18	Gagnon et al.[24]
Multiple congenital anomalies	46	4 or 5 D/B	Bray and Sr. Ann Josephine[4]
Multiple congenital anomalies	46	A/?	Hsu et al.[32a]
Multiple congenital anomalies	46	4 B/B 5	Shaw et al.[78]
Multiple congenital anomalies	46	2 A/A 3	Lee et al.[42]
deLange's syndrome*†	46	2 A/C	Falek, et al[14]
RING CHROMOSOMES AND DELETIONS			
Cri du chat syndrome*	46	Deletions of short arm #5	Lejeune et al.[44]
	46	Ring-B (5) chromosome	Rohde and Tompkins[73]
Multiple congenital anomalies with mental retardation* (absent thumbs)	46	Ring-D	Sparkes et al.[82]
	46	Ring-E	Wang et al.[95]
	46	Ring-C	Turner et al.[91]
Microcephalic dwarfism*	46	Ring-1	Gordon and Cooke[27]
Mongolism	47	Deletion of trisomic 21	Dent et al.[11]
Cyclops (or multiple anomalies) (see text)	46	Deletion of 18	Nitowsky et al.[61]
Multiple congenital anomalies	46	Partial 21 monosomy	Lejeune et al.[45] Reisman et al.[70]
Multiple congenital anomalies (antimongolism and cri du chat)	46	Deletion of B Deletion of G	Engel et al.[13b]
Mental retardation and multiple congenital anomalies	45	21 monosomy	Al-Aish et al.[1b]

*The exact chromosome or chromosome group involved in the formation of the translocation or ring anomaly is presumptive in most cases.

†These observations have been noted by a number of workers but they have not been found in every case of the syndrome.

mations have exhibited either (1) a deletion of the short arms of chromosome 5 or (2) the formation of a ring chromosome.

Antimongolism.—Lejeune[45] called attention to the fact that partial 21 monosomy (i.e., deletion of one 21 chromosome) is associated with a constellation of anomalies which seem opposite to those described in mongolism. Specifically, these children have very big ears with large canals, a high nose bridge, underdeveloped inner canthi and increased muscle tone.

Chromosome 18-deletion syndrome.—Nitowsky[61] and Lejeune and associates[46] described a number of patients with partial 18 monosomy and a fairly constant clinical picture. These children exhibit microcephaly, deep-set eyes, a poorly developed nose bridge, a well-developed chin with a fish-like mouth and characteristic ear deformities (over-rolled ears with overdeveloped helix, antihelix and antitragus). In some severe cases a cyclops eye deformity has been seen.[61]

The role of chromosome anomalies in such clinical conditions as the deLange,[67a] Sturge-Weber and oral-facial-digital syndromes has not been clarified, but translocations and deletions have been incriminated by some workers (see references in Table 13.3).

MANAGEMENT AND PROGNOSIS.—Therapy for these varied chromosomal anomalies is almost exclusively symptomatic. Surgical correction of congenital heart defects may be considered in certain cases. Replacement sex hormone therapy is used in some patients with Klinefelter's and Turner's syndromes. The reader is referred to texts on pediatrics and internal medicine for details regarding drugs and dosages.

Recurrence Risk in Mongolism

Carter[9,9a] has stated that, from the practical viewpoint of genetic counseling in situations in which chromosome studies are not available, parents who have no other affected close relatives can be told that the risk of recurrence, regardless of maternal age, is of the order of 1–2%. Luzzatti[48] agrees with this generalization. Even though the absolute risk of mongolism in the general population is higher among older mothers, the risk of recurrence in another sibling is higher in the individual case of a young mother who has a child with mongolism, regardless of whether 21 trisomy or a chromosomal translocation is present.

Most workers do not think that chromosome studies are necessary in "old" mothers (over 30 years of age). Instead, parents are counseled on the basis of the incidence of mongolism in the general population. If a mother aged 30–45 has one child with mongolism, the recurrence risk is about 1 in 100 (or 1%). In mothers over 45 the risk is about 1 in 40.

The overall risk in the "young" mother (15–30 years of age) of having one child with mongolism is 1 in 1,200, but after the birth of one mongoloid child the risk increases to 1 in 100. Chromosome studies should be carried out on the child with mongolism who has a "young" mother.[10c,48,63b] If the baby of the young mother exhibits the usual 21 trisomy, the recurrence risk in Luzzatti's experience is 1 in 400. Among 11 selected families with mongolism in more than one member, eight families exhibited standard 21 trisomy,[19a] suggesting an inherited tendency to nondisjunction. If the baby has a translocation anomaly, the parents should have chromosome studies performed. If one of the parents carries a translocation, the recurrence risk is 1 in 3 for a D/21 carrier mother, 1 in 40 for a D/21 carrier father and 1 in 1 for a 21/21 carrier parent. If a translocation is found in the baby but the parents have normal karyotypes, no accurate data on recurrence risk are available but the risk is considered very low.

Recurrence risk predictions for other types of chromosome anomaly syndromes must be based on broad generalizations, such as the increased tendency to nondisjunction in the older mother, because we do not have sufficient data to offer precise predictions.

Malformations Due to Maternal Infections
GERMAN MEASLES (RUBELLA)

PATHOGENESIS.—It has been shown that, if a woman has rubella during the first 12 weeks of pregnancy, her offspring may be born with mental defect and microcephaly, cataracts, deafness, heart disease and dental defects.[29,85] Estimates of the risk of malformation following maternal rubella vary from 5 to 30%.[31]

The exact mechanism of induction of the defects is not understood. It is postulated that qualitative and quantitative variation in the nature of the anomalies depends upon the virulence of the epidemic, the stage of exposure in embryonic life and the genetic complement of both the mother and the fetus.[98] Few pathologic studies on the brains of infants with the maternal rubella syndrome have been carried out, but in two reported cases mild hydrocephalus, a small corpus callosum and moderate gliosis were found.[57]

CLINICAL AND LABORATORY DIAGNOSIS.—Bilateral congenital cataracts and congenital heart disease (especially patent ductus arteriosus and ventricular septal defect) are most common. Neurologic manifestations include deafness, microcephaly, mental defect and spastic diplegia. Achs and co-workers[1a] recently described unusual dermatoglyphics in this syndrome. The deafness, which is usually partial, probably results from the defective development of the organ of Corti. When this constellation of defects is found in association with a history of maternal rubella during the first trimester of pregnancy, the diagnosis is apparent. Occasionally some or all of these anomalies are seen, yet the mother had no rash with her infection. Since it is known that rubella without a rash can damage the embryo, the diagnosis in such questionable cases would be facilitated by an exact diagnostic test for rubella.

MANAGEMENT AND PROGNOSIS.—At present most physicians recommend that young women expose themselves to rubella so that they acquire immunity before they conceive. If such a measure is taken, one should be aware of the rare complication of encephalitis which occasionally accompanies the disease. In the past, gamma globulin and convalescent serum have been given to pregnant women exposed to rubella, but the ability of these agents to confer protection to the embryo is not consistent. Krugman and Ward[40] recommend that pregnant women who have been exposed to rubella should still receive 20 ml. of gamma globulin and that this prophylaxis should be practiced until a vaccine is available. The development of a safe, effective vaccine which will confer lasting immunity to rubella without infecting exposed, susceptible individuals is imminent (Chapter 18), and the vaccine should be available commercially very soon.

TOXOPLASMOSIS, CYTOMEGALIC INCLUSION DISEASE AND SYPHILIS

PATHOGENESIS.—Severe nervous system damage can result from rare prenatal infections with a protozoan (toxoplasma), a virus (the salivary gland virus which causes cytomegalic inclusion disease) and a spirochete (the treponema of syphilis).[101] In all of these prenatal infections maternal sepsis is transferred across the placental barrier to the fetus and a meningoencephalitis ensues. Although these conditions are clearly congenital, they do not generally produce primary structural malformations during the period of organogenesis, with the exception occasionally of cases of cytomegalic inclusion disease.[101]

CLINICAL AND LABORATORY DIAGNOSIS.—*Toxoplasmosis.*—Infants who acquire this infection prenatally may be stillborn or they may manifest signs of the disease shortly after birth. The common neurologic signs include seizures, hydrocephalus, microcephaly, bilateral chorioretinitis (usually in the macular areas), spasticity, microphthalmus and secondary colobomas. The nonneurologic signs of jaundice, hepatosplenomegaly, a maculopapular or hemorrhagic skin rash and fever mimic exactly many other types of sepsis in the newborn. Leukopenia, anemia and xanthochromic cerebrospinal fluid with elevated protein content may be present.

The diagnosis can be established by demonstrating a high titer of toxoplasma antibody in the suspect infant's serum, using the methylene blue dye test. Of great value in the immediate diagnosis is the demonstration of the protozoa in the Giemsa-stained sediment of centrifuged cerebrospinal fluid. The value of newer tests for antibody, namely, tanned red blood cell hemagglutination and the inhibition of fluorescein labeling, remains to be determined.[17] The serologic skin test and complement fixation are less reliable. Intracerebral calcifications were found by Feldman[15] in almost two-thirds of a group of 103 children with the disease.

The coexistence of bilateral chorioretinitis, cerebral defect and intracranial calcifications virtually establishes the clinical diagnosis. However, this constellation of findings has been seen in a few patients with negative results of serologic tests[75] and is termed "Sabin's nontoxoplasmic vascular encephalopathy."

Cytomegalic inclusion disease.—The newborn with this salivary gland virus infection often presents with signs of fulminating sepsis and has disseminated signs of progressive pulmonary, hepatic or renal insufficiency.[60] The diffuse necrotizing encephalitis has a special predilection for the periventricular tissues, and clinically these infants show microcephaly, hydrocephalus, seizures and mental retardation.

The periventricular "shoreline" distribution of calcification seen on roentgen examination appears unique. Exfoliative cytologic examination of epithelial cells in the urinary sediment represents the best diagnostic test. Smears from a fresh, clean urine sediment are fixed immediately and stained with hematoxylin-eosin or according to the Papanicolaou technique. The finding of intranuclear eosinophilic inclusion bodies is diagnostic of salivary gland virus infection.

Congenital syphilis.—Congenital syphilis with nervous system involvement now occurs rarely in most parts of the world. Usually one sees hepatosplenomegaly and lesions of the skin, mucous membranes and bones. Rarely clinical and cerebrospinal fluid evidence of a meningitis will be found. In these patients hydrocephalus and secondary porencephaly and microgyria may later develop.

The diagnostic serologic test for syphilis is often misleading in the newborn period because infants born of treated mothers will often have positive serologic test results for three months. If nervous system involvement has occurred, the CSF serologic test will be positive, the protein will be elevated and a pleocytosis may be present.

Differential diagnosis.—The differential diagnosis of all three conditions just discussed must include bacterial septicemia, hemolytic disease of the newborn due to blood group incompatibility, congenital hydrocephalus, occult nervous system anomalies, herpes simplex encephalitis, congenital hemolytic icterus and congenital leukemia.

MANAGEMENT AND PROGNOSIS.—Although results are difficult to evaluate, toxoplasmosis is usually treated with a combination of sulfadiazine (150 mg./kg.) and pyrimethamine (1 mg./kg.) in divided doses. Treatment is carried out for about two weeks, during which time leukocyte counts are obtained every three or four days. The majority of surviving infants have evidence of cerebral damage. It has been pointed out that offspring of subsequent pregnancies do not have toxoplasmosis.

Treatment of cytomegalic inclusion disease is symptomatic, there being no accepted specific form of therapy. Although survival with the severe neonatal form of the disease does occur, residual brain damage, cirrhosis and fibrotic lung disease can be anticipated.

Congenital syphilis is treated with intramuscular penicillin. A total dose of 50,000 units/lb. of body weight is given over 15 days, with a daily dose of from 75,000 to 150,000 units of procaine G penicillin. Febrile Herxheimer reactions can be expected, but these usually do not justify any change in the planned schedule of therapy.

OTHER MATERNAL VIRUS INFECTIONS

The discovery that rubella could produce congenital malformations aroused speculation that other viral agents might have similar effects. The evidence is largely conflicting and inconclusive. Studies so far suggest that the viruses of mumps, chickenpox, poliomyelitis and ECHO type 9 are not teratogenic, whereas the evidence in the case of the measles and Asian influenza viruses is in dispute. A careful long-term anterospective study, combining clinical and serologic observations, is being conducted by the U.S. Public Health Service, and this should help to answer these important questions.

Malformations Due to Other Environmental Factors
DRUGS

Aminopterin (4-aminopteroylglutamic acid), a folic acid antagonist used primarily to treat tumors of the reticuloendothelial system and also to produce abortion, is a potent teratogen which can cause anencephaly, meningocele, hydrocephalus and cleft lip and palate.[96] Whether quinine, a commonly used abortifacient, can cause congenital deafness is controversial. Obviously, many attempts to effect abortions are not reported, and some workers have speculated that the incidence of congenital defects due to self-administered abortifacient drugs may be higher than suspected.

Anomalies have been attributed to many therapeutic agents including cortisone, myleran and tolbutamide, but the isolated retrospective nature of these observations makes them inconclusive. The teratogenic effect of thalidomide is indisputable, but the only nervous system anomalies reported to date have been the clinical appearance in some patients of defective functioning (probably due to nuclear aplasia) of the third, fourth, sixth and seventh cranial nerves.[46a]

IRRADIATION

Excessive fetal x-irradiation can cause congenital microcephaly, skull defects, spina bifida, blindness, cleft palate, micromelia and clubfoot.[56,64] A correlation has also been demonstrated between babies exposed to atomic bomb fallout while in utero and small head size and retardation in adolescence.[5,101a] The hazard of therapeutic pelvic irradiation has largely been eliminated, but danger from bomb fallout continues.[32,103]

MATERNAL DIABETES, MALNUTRITION AND ANOXIA

Infants born of diabetic mothers are said to have a higher than normal incidence of "soft" neurologic signs on follow-up neurologic examination, but the precise nature of the defects has not yet been documented. Observations on 473 consecutive live-born infants of diabetic mothers have been reported from the Joslin Clinic by Hubbell and associates.[33] The majority of these infants were delivered prematurely at 36 to 37 weeks' gestation. During the neonatal period 35% had hyperbilirubinemia, 27% had the respiratory distress syndromes, 13% had significant congenital malformations and 8% died. These babies behaved much the same as prematures born to nondiabetic mothers and exhibited no unique characteristics. In a large series reported by Pedersen and co-workers[61b] a significantly higher incidence of congenital anomalies was found in the infants of diabetic mothers than in a group of matched controls, but the numbers of anomalies were too small to allow one to judge differences in anatomic distribution. In our opinion the effect of maternal diabetes on the developing infant's nervous system must remain an unanswered question.

Whereas both maternal nutritional deficiency and anoxia can cause malformations in experimental animals, their precise role in the causation of human malformations remains obscure.

Low Birth Weight Infants

Silverman and Sinclair[80] have recently stressed the need to differentiate (1) infants with prematurity (those born before 37 weeks from the first day of the last menstrual period and weighing less than 2,500 Gm.) from (2) infants with "intrauterine growth retardation," a term introduced by Warkany *et al*.[98] to refer to this heterogeneous group of babies (also called "undergrown" babies or "pseudoprematures") who have had a *normal* period of gestation.

Prematurity

PATHOGENESIS.—The reader is referred to Silverman's text[79] for a discussion of the causes and mechanisms of prematurity.

CLINICAL AND LABORATORY DIAGNOSIS.—In this text we are concerned only with the neurologic complications of prematurity. Although there is not complete agreement in the literature on the subject, most workers believe that babies who are born with abnormally low birth weight (1,500–2,500 Gm.) exhibit (1) lower IQ's and (2) a higher incidence of spastic diplegia when compared at a later age with infants of term birth weight. Pneumographic evidence of underlying brain hypoplasia can often be demonstrated (Fig. 13.14). The reader is referred to Silverman's text[79] for a more detailed summary of the evidence in the literature linking prematurity and neurologic deficit.

MANAGEMENT AND PROGNOSIS.—In itself, small size in the newborn certainly does not necessarily imply a gloomy outlook. However, a cautious prognosis must be given to parents until an adequate period of observation has elapsed. Obviously, mildly impaired babies may exhibit no neurologic deficit for many months or even years.

In general, few specific therapeutic measures are available. In recent years Cornblath and his co-workers[10] have emphasized that undergrown infants of low birth weight should be fed early in life to circumvent their tendency to become hypoglycemic.

Intrauterine Growth Retardation

PATHOGENESIS.—In thinking about the causes of intrauterine growth retardation or pseudoprematurity, it is helpful to consider all of the usual mechanisms that cause disease in postnatal life which simply exert their effect upon the fetus. A working etiologic classification follows.

1. Genetic factors[98]
2. Environmental factors
    Congenital malformations (cyanotic heart disease[58])
3. Infections (fetal rubella[59])
4. Trauma (x-irradiation during pregnancy—p. 176)
5. Metabolic defects (maternal phenylketonuria[48a])
6. Vascular insufficiency (small and infarcted placentas secondary to maternal hypertension and toxemia[98])
7. Intoxications (maternal folic acid deficiency secondary to aminopterin therapy[96])
8. Malnutrition
    Prolonged pregnancy ("postmaturity syndrome")
    Multiple pregnancy (twins, etc.[80])

No careful anterospective morphologic study of the brains of these babies has been documented, but circumstantial evidence in selected cases indicates that normal brain growth is seriously impaired.

CLINICAL AND LABORATORY DIAGNOSIS.—In addition to impaired somatic growth these patients often show microcephaly, slow motor and mental development, spasticity, seizures and other signs of chronic neurologic deficit. In the series of 22 surviving babies studied by Warkany and associates,[98] only 5 had normal intellect and 15 had subnormal mental development. Of these 15 patients, 7 had microcephaly, 6 were severely retarded, 2 had borderline intellect, 1 child was deaf and 1 patient's development could not be assessed.

Laboratory manifestations of brain damage are sometimes demonstrable with transillumination, pneumoencephalography (Fig. 13.14), electroencephalography and psychometric study.

MANAGEMENT AND PROGNOSIS.—Therapy and prognosis should be based upon an accurate etiologic diagnosis. It seems quite likely that all or most of the mechanisms which cause disease in postnatal life can affect the fetus also, albeit in a way which results in a somewhat different clinical picture.

In view of the high incidence of neurologic deficit reported by Warkany's group and a similar experience of our own, great caution should be used in prognosticating about neurologic development. It seems probable that more than half the babies with true intrauterine growth retardation as defined here will have brain damage or inadequate brain development.

BIBLIOGRAPHY

1. Achs, R., et al.: Unusual dermatoglyphics associated with major congenital malformations, New England J. Med. 275:1273, 1966.
1a. Achs, R., et al.: Unusual dermatoglyphic findings associated with rubella embryopathy, New England J. Med. 274:148, 1966.
1b. Al-Aish, M. S., et al.: Autosomal monosomy in man, New England J. Med. 277:777, 1967.
1c. Anderson, F. M., and Geiger, L.: Craniostenosis, J. Neurosurg. 22:229, 1965.
1d. Baumgartner, L.: Infant and childhood mortality: 1947, Pediatrics 3:722, 1949.
1e. Becker, K. L., et al.: Double autosomal trisomy (D trisomy plus mongolism), Proc. Staff Meet., Mayo Clin. 38:242, June, 1963.
1f. Bluestone, S. S., and Deaver, G. G.: Habilitation of the child with spina bifida and myelomeningocele, J.A.M.A. 161:1248, 1956.
2. Bradley, W. E., et al.: New method of treatment of neurogenic bladder, Neurology 13:353, 1963.
3. Bray, P. F., and Josephine, Sr. Ann: An XXXYY sex-chromosome anomaly, J.A.M.A. 184:179, 1963.
4. Bray, P. F., and Josephine, Sr. Ann: Partial autosomal trisomy and translocation, J.A.M.A. 187:566, 1964.
5. Burrow, G. N., et al.: Study of adolescents exposed in utero to the atomic bomb, Nagasaki, Japan, J.A.M.A. 192:357, 1965.
6. Caffey, J.: *Pediatric X-ray Diagnosis* (4th ed.; Chicago: Year Book Medical Publishers, Inc., 1961).
7. Carpenter, M., and Druckemiller, W.: Agenesis of corpus callosum diagnosed during life, A.M.A. Arch. Neurol. & Psychiat. 69:305, 1953.
8. Carr, D. H.: Chromosome studies in abortuses and stillborn infants, Lancet 2:603, 1963.
8a. Carr, D. H., et al.: A probable XXYY sex determining mechanism in a mentally defective male with Klinefelter's syndrome, Canad. M. A. J. 84:873, 1961.
9. Carter, C. O.: Personal communication, 1963.
9a. Carter, C. O., and Evans, K. A.: Risk of parents who have had one child with Down's syndrome (mongolism) having another child similarly affected, Lancet 2:785, 1961.
9b. Cohen, M. M., and Shaw, M. W.: Two XY siblings with gonadal dysgenesis and a female phenotype, New England J. Med. 272:1083, 1965.
10. Cornblath, M., et al.: Symptomatic neonatal hypoglycemia: Studies of carbohydrate metabolism in newborn infants, VIII, Pediatrics 33:388, 1964.
10a. Cummins, H., et al.: Palmar dermatoglyphics in mongolism, Pediatrics 5:241, 1950.
10b. D'Agostino, A. N., et al.: The Dandy-Walker syndrome, J. Neuropath. & Exper. Neurol. 22:450, 1963.
10c. Day, R. W., and Wright, S. W.: Down's syndrome at young maternal ages: Chromosomal and family studies, J. Pediat. 66:764, 1965.
11. Dent, T., et al.: A partial mongol, Lancet 2:484, 1963.
11a. Dodge, H. W., et al.: Craniofacial dysostosis: Crouzon's disease, Pediatrics 23:98, 1959.
12. Doshay, L. J.: The therapy of Parkinson's disease, M. Clin. North America 40:5, 1956.
13. Edwards, J. H., et al.: A new trisomic syndrome, Lancet 1:787, 1960.
13a. Ellis, J. R., et al.: An aberrant small acrocentric chromosome, Ann. Human Genet. 26:77, 1962.
13b. Engel, E., et al.: Apparent cri-du-chat and "anti-mongolism" in one patient, Lancet 1:1130, 1966.
14. Falek, A., et al.: Familial deLange syndrome with chromosome abnormalities, Pediatrics 37:92, 1966.

BIBLIOGRAPHY

15. Feldman, H. A.: Congenital toxoplasmosis: Study of one hundred three cases, A.M.A. Am. J. Dis. Child. 86:487, 1953.
16. Feldman, H. A.: Toxoplasmosis, Pediatrics 22:559, 1958.
17. Feldman, H. A.: Toxoplasmosis, in Nelson, W. E. (ed.): *Textbook of Pediatrics* (7th ed.; Philadelphia: W. B. Saunders Company, 1960).
17a. Ferguson-Smith, M. A., *et al.*: Primary amentia and micro-orchidism associated with an XXXY sex chromosome constitution, Lancet 2:184, 1960.
17b. Ford, C. E., *et al.*: The chromosomes in a patient showing both mongolism and the Klinefelter syndrome, Lancet 1:709, 1959.
18. Ford, C. E., *et al.*: A sex-chromosome anomaly in a case of gonadal dysgenesis (Turner's syndrome), Lancet 1:711, 1959.
19. Ford, F. R.: *Diseases of the Nervous System in Infancy, Childhood and Adolescence* (5th ed.; Springfield, Ill.: Charles C Thomas, Publisher, 1966).
19a. Forssman, H., and Lehmann, O.: Chromosome studies in eleven families with mongolism in more than one member, Acta paediat. 51:180, 1962.
19b. Fowler, F. D., and Alexander, E.: Atresia of the foramina of Luschka and Magendie, A.M.A. Am. J. Dis. Child. 92:131, 1956.
20. Fraccaro, M., *et al.*: A new type of chromosomal abnormality in gonadal dysgenesis, Lancet 2:1144, 1960.
21. Fraccaro, M., *et al.*: Chromosomal abnormalities in father and mongol child, Lancet 1:724, 1960.
21a. Fraccaro, M., *et al.*: Further cytogenetical observations in gonadal dysgenesis, Ann. Human Genet. 24:205, 1960.
22. Fraccaro, M., *et al.*: A male with XXXXY sex chromosomes, Cytogenetics 1:53, 1962.
23. Fraser, F. C.: Causes of congenital malformations in human beings, J. Chron. Dis. 10:97, 1959.
24. Gagnon, F., *et al.*: Partial trisomy 18 caused by insertion or translocation 4/18, Union méd. Canada 92:311, 1963.
24a. Gardner, W. J.: Hydrodynamic mechanism of syringomyelia: Its relationship to myelocele, J. Neurol. Neurosurg. & Psychiat. 28:247, 1965.
25. Goldston, A. S., *et al.*: Neonatal polycystic kidney with brain defect, Am. J. Dis. Child. 106:484, 1963.
26. Gomez, M. R., *et al.*: Aneurysmal malformation of the great vein of Galen causing heart failure in early infancy, Pediatrics 31:400, 1963.
27. Gordon, R. R., and Cooke, P.: Ring-1 chromosome and microcephalic dwarfism, Lancet 2:1212, 1964.
27a. Granholm, L., and Radberg, C.: Congenital communicating hydrocephalus, J. Neurosurg. 20:338, 1963.
28. Greenfield, J. G.: *Neuropathology* (London: Edward Arnold & Co., 1958).
29. Gregg, N. M.: Congenital cataract following German measles in mother, Tr. Ophth. Soc. Australia 3:35, 1942.
29a. Gustavson, K. H., *et al.*: An apparently identical extra autosome in two severely retarded sisters with multiple malformations, Cytogenetics 1:32, 1962.
30. Hamby, W. B., *et al.*: Hydranencephaly: Clinical diagnosis, Pediatrics 6:371, 1950.
31. Hill, A. B., *et al.*: Virus diseases in pregnancy and congenital defects, Brit. J. Prev. & Social Med. 12:1, 1958.
32. Hollingsworth, J. W., *et al.*: Seminar on the Use of Vital and Health Statistics for Genetic and Radiation Studies (sponsored by the U.N. and W.H.O.). Medical findings and methodology of studies by the Atomic Bomb Casualty Commission on atomic bomb survivors in Hiroshima and Nagasaki (New York: United Nations, 1962).
32a. Hsu, L. Y. F., *et al.*: Mosaicism of an abnormally long B chromosome in a boy with physical and mental retardation, Pediatrics 39:68, 1967.
33. Hubbell, J. P., *et al.*: The newborn infant of the diabetic mother, M. Clin. North America 49:1035, 1965.
34. Huttenlocher, P. R.: Treatment of hydrocephalus with acetazolamide, J. Pediat. 66:1023, 1965.
35. Ingraham, F. D., and Matson, D. D.: *Neurosurgery of Infancy and Childhood* (Springfield, Ill.: Charles C Thomas, Publisher, 1961).
36. Jacobs, P. A., and Strong, J. A.: A case of human intersexuality having possible XXY sex-determining mechanism, Nature, London 183:302, 1959.
37. Jacobs, P. A., *et al.*: Evidence for the existence of the human "super female," Lancet 2:423, 1959.
38. Johnston, A. W., *et al.*: The triple-X syndrome: clinical, pathological, and chromosomal studies in three mentally retarded cases, Brit. M. J. 2:1046, 1961.
39. Kottmeier, P. K., and Clatworthy, H. W.: Aganglionic and functional megacolon in children—a diagnostic dilemma, Pediatrics 36:572, 1965.

40. Krugman, S., and Ward, R.: Rubella: Demonstration of neutralizing antibody in gamma globulin and re-evaluation of rubella problem, New England J. Med. 259:16, 1958.
40a. Kurlander, G. J., et al.: Supravalvar aortic stenosis; roentgen analysis of twenty-seven cases, Am. J. Roentgenol. 98:782, 1966.
41. Laurence, K. M.: The natural history of hydrocephalus, Lancet 2:1152, 1958.
41a. Laurence, K. M.: The natural history of spina bifida cystica: Detailed analysis of 407 cases, Arch. Dis. Childhood 39:41, 1964.
41b. Layton, D. D.: Heterotopic cerebral gray matter as an epileptogenic focus, J. Neuropath. & Exper. Neurol. 21:244, 1962.
42. Lee, C. S. N., et al.: Familial chromosome-2,3 translocation ascertained through an infant with multiple malformations, New England J. Med. 271:12, 1964.
43. Lejeune, J., et al.: Les chromosomes humaines en culture de tissues, C. R. Acad. Sci. (Paris) 248:602, 1959.
44. Lejeune, J., et al.: Trois cas de délétion partielle du bras court d'un chromosome 5, C. R. Acad. Sci. (Paris) 257:3098, 1963.
45. Lejeune, J., et al.: Mosaique chromosomique, probablement radio-induite in utero, C. R. Acad. Sci. (Paris) 259:485, 1964.
46. Lejeune, J., et al.: La délétion partielle du bras long du chromosome 18: Individualisation d'un nouvel état morbide, Ann. Human Genet. 9:32, 1966.
46a. Lenz, W.: Proceedings, Second International Congress on Congenital Malformations, New York, July 14-19, 1963, Lancet 2:189, 1963.
46b. Lourie, H., and Berne, A. S.: A contribution on the etiology and pathogenesis of congenital communicating hydrocephalus, Neurology 15:815, 1965.
47. Low, N. L., et al.: Brain tissue in the nose and throat, Pediatrics 18:254, 1956.
48. Luzzatti, L.: Personal communication, 1966.
48a. Mabry, C. C., et al.: Mental retardation in children of phenylketonuric mothers, New England J. Med. 275:1331, 1966.
48b. Malpas, P.: The incidence of human malformations and the significance of changes in the maternal environment in their causation, J. Obst. & Gynaec. Brit. Emp. 44:434, 1937.
49. Matson, D. D.: Prenatal obstruction of the fourth ventricle, Am. J. Roentgenol. 76:499, 1956.
49a. Matson, D. D.: Hydrocephalus, New England J. Med. 271:1360, 1964.
49b. Matson, D. D., and Ingraham, F. D.: Intracranial complications of congenital dermal sinuses, Pediatrics 8:463, 1951.
50. McDonald, C. A., and Korb, M.: Intracranial aneurysms, Arch. Neurol. & Psychiat. 42:298, 1939.
51. McIntosh, R., et al.: The incidence of congenital malformations: A study of 5,964 pregnancies, Pediatrics 14:505, 1954.
51a. McPherson, A., and Auth, T. L.: Bloch-Sulzberger syndrome (incontinentia pigmenti), Arch. Neurol. 8:332, 1963.
51b. Menkes, J. H., et al.: Hereditary partial agenesis of the corpus callosum: Biochemical and pathological studies, Arch. Neurol. 11:198, 1964.
52. Mercer, R. D., and Darakjian, G.: Apparent translocation between chromosome 2 and an acrocentric in group 13-15, Lancet 2:784, 1962.
53. Miller, J. Q., et al.: A specific congenital brain defect (arhinencephaly) in 13-15 trisomy, New England J. Med. 268:120, 1963.
54. Moorhead, P. S., et al.: A familial chromosome translocation associated with speech and mental retardation, Am. J. Human Genet. 13:32, 1961.
54a. Morales, P. A., et al.: Urological complications of spina bifida in children, J. Urol. 75:537, 1956.
55. Mount, L. A.: Intracranial Vascular Malformations, in Jackson, I. J., and Thompson, R. K.: Pediatric Neurosurgery (Springfield, Ill.: Charles C Thomas, Publisher, 1959).
56. Murphy, D. P.: Ovarian irradiation and the health of the subsequent child, Surg. Gynec. & Obst. 48:766, 1929.
57. Mutrux, S., et al.: Contribution á l'étude clinique et anatomo-pathologique des troubles cérébraux de l'embryopathie rubeoleuse, Schweiz. Arch. Neurol. u. Psychiat. 64:369, 1949.
58. Naeye, R. L.: Unsuspected organ abnormalities associated with congenital heart disease, Am. J. Path. 47:905, 1965.
59. Naeye, R. L., and Blanc, W.: Pathogenesis of congenital rubella, J.A.M.A. 194:1277, 1965.
59a. Neel, J. V.: A study of major congenital defects in Japanese infants, Am. J. Human Genet. 10:398, 1958.
60. Nelson, J. S., and Wyatt, J. P.: Salivary gland virus disease, Medicine 38:223, 1959.
61. Nitowsky, H. M., et al.: Partial 18 monosomy in the cyclops malformation, Pediatrics 37:260, 1966.

BIBLIOGRAPHY

61a. Patau, K., et al.: Multiple congenital anomaly caused by an extra autosome, Lancet 1:790, 1960.
61b. Pedersen, L. M., et al.: Congenital malformations in newborn infants of diabetic women, Lancet 1:1124, 1964.
62. Penrose, L. S.: Genetics of anencephaly, J. Ment. Defic. Res. 1:4, 1957.
63. Penrose, L. S., et al.: Chromosomal translocations in mongolism and in normal relatives, Lancet 2:409, 1960.
63a. Pergament, E., and Kadotani, T.: A new double aneuploid: XXY D-trisomy, Lancet 2:695, 1965.
63b. Petersen, C. D., and Luzzatti, L.: The role of chromosome translocation in the recurrence risk of Down's syndrome, Pediatrics 35:463, 1965.
64. Plummer, G.: Anomalies occurring in children exposed in utero to the atomic bomb in Hiroshima, Pediatrics 10:687, 1952.
65. Polani, P. E., et al.: A mongol girl with 46 chromosomes, Lancet 1:721, 1960.
66. Poser, C. M.: *The Relationship Between Syringomyelia and Neoplasm* (Springfield, Ill.: Charles C Thomas, Publisher, 1956).
67. Price, W. H., et al.: Criminal patients with XYY sex-chromosome complement, Lancet 1:565, 1966.
67a. Ptacek, L. J., et al.: The Cornelia de Lange syndrome, J. Pediat. 63:1000, 1963.
68. Ransohoff, J., and Carter, S.: Hemispherectomy in the treatment of convulsive seizures associated with infantile hemiplegia, A. Res. Nerv. & Ment. Dis., Proc. 34:176, 1954.
69. Ransohoff, J., et al.: Hydrocephalus: A review of etiology and treatment, J. Pediat. 56:399, 1960.
70. Reisman, L. E., et al.: Anti-mongolism: Studies in an infant with a partial monosomy of the 21 chromosome, Lancet 1:394, 1966.
71. Ricci, N., and Borgatti, L.: XXX 18-trisomy, Lancet 2:1276, 1963.
72. Riley, C. M., et al.: Central autonomic dysfunction with defective lacrimation: I. Report of five cases, Pediatrics 3:468, 1949.
73. Rohde, R. A., and Tompkins, R.: "Cri du chat" due to a ring-B (5) chromosome, Lancet 2:1075, 1965.
73a. Rosenberg, R. N., et al.: The interrelationship of neurofibromatosis and fibrous dysplasia, Arch. Neurol. 17:174, 1967.
74. Russell, D.: *Observations on the Pathology of Hydrocephalus*. Medical Research Council Special Report Series no. 265 (London: His Majesty's Stat. Off., 1949).
75. Sabin, A. B., and Feldman, H. A.: Chorioretinopathy associated with other evidence of cerebral damage in childhood, J. Pediat. 35:296, 1949.
76. Scarff, J. E.: Evaluation of treatment of hydrocephalus, Arch. Neurol. 14:382, 1966.
77. Schick, R. W., and Matson, D. D.: What is arrested hydrocephalus? J. Pediat. 58:791, 1961.
78. Shaw, M. W., et al.: A familial 4/5 reciprocal translocation resulting in partial trisomy B, Am. J. Human Genet. 17:54, 1965.
78a. Sheptak, P. E., and Susen, A. F.: Diastematomyelia, Am. J. Dis. Child. 113:210, 1967.
78b. Shiller, J. G.: Craniofacial dysostosis of Crouzon, Pediatrics 23:107, 1959.
78c. Shopfner, C. E., et al.: Craniolacunia, Am. J. Roentgenol. 93:343, 1965.
79. Silverman, W. A.: *Dunham's Premature Infants* (New York: Paul B. Hoeber, Inc., 1961).
80. Silverman, W. A., and Sinclair, J. C.: Infants of low birth weight, New England J. Med. 274:448, 1966.
81. Smith, D. W., et al.: A new autosomal trisomy syndrome: Multiple congenital anomalies caused by an extra autosome, J. Pediat. 57:338, 1960.
82. Sparkes, R. S., et al.: Absent thumbs with a ring D2 chromosome: New deletion syndrome, Am. J. Human Genet. 19:644, 1967.
83. Stern, C.: *Principles of Human Genetics* (San Francisco: W. H. Freeman and Co., 1960).
84. Stevenson, A. C., and Warnock, H. A.: Observations on the results of pregnancies in women resident in Belfast, Ann. Human Genet. 23:382, 1959.
85. Swan, C., et al.: Final observations on congenital defects in infants following infectious diseases during pregnancy, with special reference to rubella, M. J. Australia 2:889, 1946.
86. Swanson, A. G.: Congenital insensitivity to pain with anhydrosis, Arch. Neurol. 8:299, 1963.
87. Swenson, O., and Fisher, J. H.: New techniques in the diagnosis and treatment of megaloureters, Pediatrics 18:304, 1956.
88. Swenson, O., et al.: Hirschsprung's disease: A new concept in etiology, New England J. Med. 241:551, 1949.

88a. Swenson, O., et al.: Rectal biopsy in diagnosis of Hirschsprung's disease: Experience with 100 cases, Surgery 45:690, 1959.
89. Taveras, J. M., and Wood, E. H.: *Diagnostic Neuroradiology* (Baltimore: Williams & Wilkins Company, 1964).
89a. Teng, P., and Papatheodorou, C.: Arnold-Chiari malformation with normal spine and cranium, Arch. Neurol. 12:622, 1965.
89b. Telfer, M. A., et al.: Incidence of gross chromosomal errors among tall criminal American males, Science 159:1249, 1968.
90. Thiersch, J. B.: Therapeutic abortions with folic acid antagonist, 4-aminopteroylglutamic acid (4-amino P.G.A.) administered by oral route, Am. J. Obst. & Gynec. 63:1298, 1952.
91. Turner, B., et al.: A self-perpetuating ring chromosome, M. J. Australia 49:56, 1962.
92. Turpin, R., et al.: Aberrations chromosomiques et maladies humaines: la polydysspondylie à 45 chromosomes, C. R. Acad. Sci. (Paris) 248:3636, 1959.
92a. Uchida, I. A., and Soltan, H. C.: Evaluation of dermatoglyphics in medical genetics, Pediat. Clin. North America 10:409, 1963.
93. Walsh, F. B.: *Clinical Neuro-ophthalmology* (2d ed.; Baltimore: Williams & Wilkins Company, 1957).
94. Walton, J. N.: *Subarachnoid Hemorrhage* (Edinburgh: E. & S. Livingstone, Ltd., 1956).
95. Wang, H. C., et al.: Ring chromosomes in human beings, Nature, London 195:733, 1962.
96. Warkany, J., and Kalter, H.: Congenital malformations, New England J. Med. 265:1046, 1961.
97. Warkany, J., et al.: Attempted abortion with aminopterin (4-amino-pteroylglutamic acid); malformations of the child. A.M.A. Am. J. Dis. Child. 97:274, 1959.
98. Warkany, J., et al.: Intrauterine growth retardation, Am. J. Dis. Child. 102:249, 1961.
99. Wiltse, H. E., et al.: Infantile hypercalcemia syndrome in twins, New England J. Med. 275:1157, 1966.
100. Wolf, A., and Cowen, D.: The cerebral atrophies and encephalomalacias of infancy and childhood, A. Res. Nerv. & Ment. Dis., Proc. 34:199, 1954.
101. Wolf, A., and Cowen, D.: Perinatal infection of the central nervous system, J. Neuropath. & Exper. Neurol. 18:191, 1959.
101a. Wood, J. W., et al.: In utero exposure to the Hiroshima atomic bomb, Pediatrics 39:385, 1967.
102. Yakovlev, P. I., and Wadsworth, R. D.: Schizencephalies: Study of congenital clefts in the cerebral mantle, J. Neuropath. & Exper. Neurol. 5:116, 169, 1946.
103. Yamazaki, J. N., et al.: Outcome of pregnancy in women exposed to atomic bomb in Nagasaki, A.M.A. Am. J. Dis. Child. 87:448, 1954.
104. Zellweger, H., et al.: An unusual translocation in a case of mongolism, J. Pediat. 62:225, 1963.

14

Idiopathic Epilepsy

Minor Seizures   Major Seizures
Petit Mal   Focal   Grand Mal

THE TERM "epilepsy" refers to recurrent cerebral seizures or convulsions and is often used to connote either a genetic or an acquired etiology. In this chapter the term is restricted to genetic or familial epilepsy. We consider most cases of "centrencephalic" epilepsy and many cases of "idiopathic" epilepsy to have a primary genetic basis.

The fundamental etiology of centrencephalic or idiopathic epilepsy is considered hereditary even though the clinical incidence of seizures in any case may be increased by extrinsic, environmental factors as well as intrinsic, constitutional factors. A discussion of symptomatic seizures, those which clearly result from discrete structural or biochemical factors (such as congenital malformations, metabolic defects, infections, tumors, trauma, intoxications or anoxia), is covered in Chapter 2 and under the respective categories of disease in other chapters of Part II.

PATHOGENESIS

The actual fundamental mechanism which triggers seizures in patients with idiopathic or centrencephalic epilepsy is not known. A significant body of work leaves no doubt that the incidence of seizures is greater in some families than it is in others. Furthermore, workers who have employed their own control groups have reached the unanimous conclusion that the incidence of epilepsy in near relatives of affected persons is significantly higher than one would expect in a control population. In 1940 Lennox and co-workers[20] suggested that the "cerebral dysrhythmia" underlying epilepsy (as measured with the electroencephalogram) is inherited as a mendelian dominant trait. Later Lennox[19] indicated an incidence of clinical epilepsy 7.2 times higher in relatives of patients with "essential" epilepsy and 3.6 times higher in relatives of patients with "symptomatic" epilepsy than in the control population. If the reader considers these two figures carefully, he will see that both indicate a hereditary factor in the etiology of cerebral seizures.

Summarizing data from four different studies, Metrakos[24] reported the incidence of epilepsy in 350 twin pairs. Among the monozygotic, or genetically identical, twin pairs a 60% concordance for epilepsy was found, whereas among the dizygotic, or genetically dissimilar twins, a 10% concordance for epilepsy was found. In a subsequent report the Metrakoses[26] selected index cases with centrencephalic epilepsy—i.e., seizures of varying clinical appearance associated with paroxysmal, diffuse, bilaterally synchronous spike-wave EEG abnormalities—and studied the electroencephalograms of close relatives. Bray and Wiser[1a] conducted a similar controlled study, selecting epileptic patients on the basis of focal epileptiform discharges in midtemporal or temporal-central regions. Both studies showed that these disorders are genetically determined and probably operate as a single, dominant trait with variable, age-dependent penetrance.[2,26] In other words, successive generations are affected with epilepsy of varying severity which reaches its peak incidence in middle childhood. On the basis of long-term EEG sampling of families with both types of electrographic abnormalities, Bray and Wiser[3] have proposed a unifying concept of idiopathic epilepsy in which the spectrum of EEG abnormalities varies from a consistently focal spike discharge to shifting focal spike discharges to petit mal-type abnormalities. Although the biochemical mechanism which causes this trait is unknown, experimental and clinical evidence accumulated by Jasper[14] and Penfield[29] indicates that the physiologic defect has its anatomic foundation in the reticular formation and its projections upward and downward from the brain stem and thalamus—hence the term "centrencephalic" epilepsy (Fig. 2.1,*A*, p. 26). The over-all incidence of epilepsy in the general population has been estimated at 0.5%, but this figure should be interpreted cautiously since it probably includes many patients with recurrent seizures of varying etiologies.

For over a century the significance of the pathologic findings in the brains of patients with idiopathic epilepsy has been debated. In general the nature of the lesions and their location resemble closely those seen in persons who have suffered from anoxia. Hence, it seems most likely that the findings are secondary to anoxia and not primarily pathognomonic of idiopathic or centrencephalic epilepsy. Cortical cell loss (cerebral and cerebellar), subpial gliosis and Ammon's horn (hippocampal-uncal-amygdaloid) sclerosis are commonly found as pointed out in Greenfield's text in neuropathology.[12] The fact that the last abnormality can occur in patients who have never had a cerebral seizure and that it may result from increased intracranial pressure from other causes (Chapters 8 and 16) suggests strongly that it is the result and not the cause of major convulsive seizures. Neither can there be any doubt that such lesions can give rise secondarily to "psychomotor" seizures.

Clinical and Laboratory Diagnosis

From a practical standpoint, idiopathic epilepsy (usually genetic) can be divided into three clinical categories or syndromes: *petit mal, focal* and *grand mal.*

Petit Mal

Petit mal epilepsy is characterized electroencephalographically by paroxysmal bilaterally synchronous 2–4 cycles/second spike and wave discharges (Fig. 14.1)

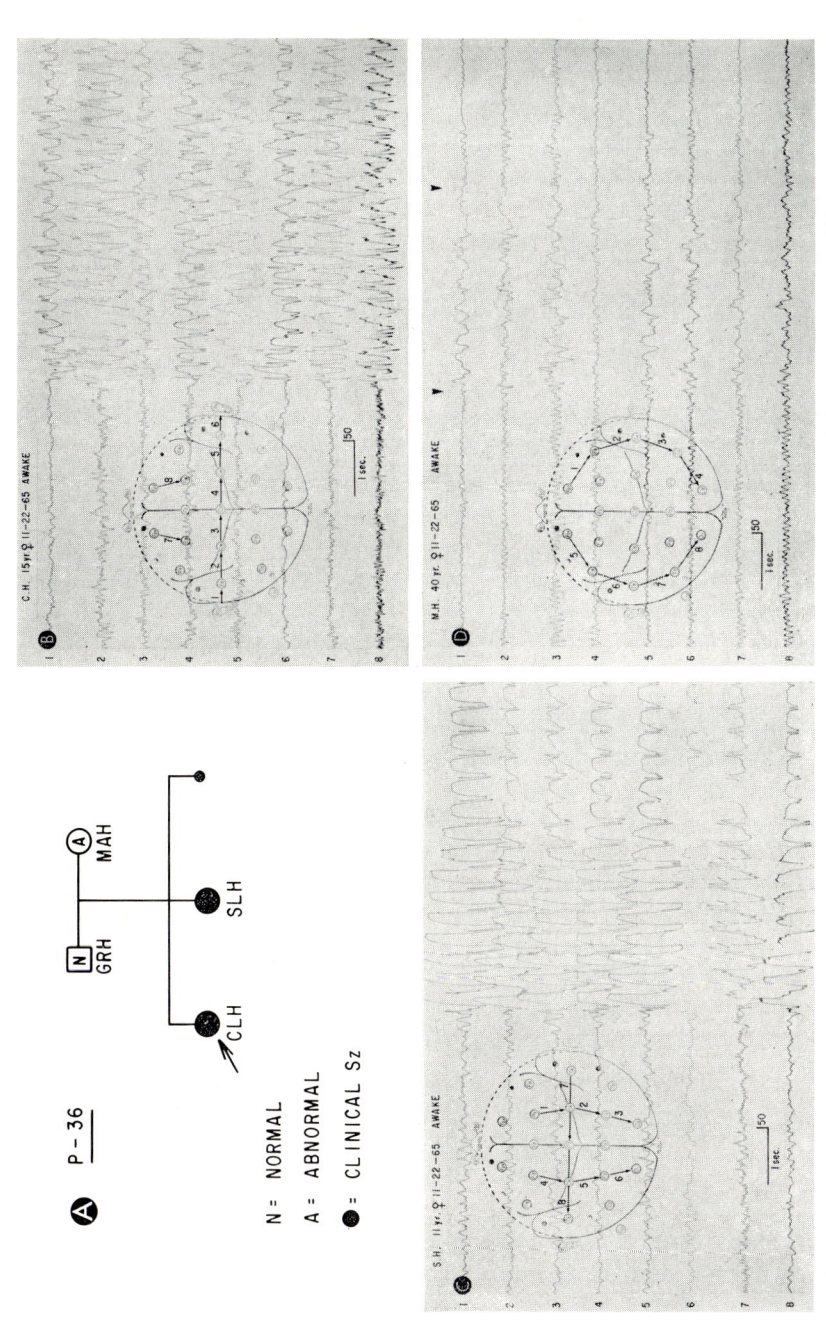

Fig. 14.1.—Familial petit mal or centrencephalic epilepsy. A, kindred diagram of family with the trait for centrencephalic epilepsy. One daughter, the index case C.H., has had uncontrollable "absence" attacks with occasional generalized seizures. A sister, S.H., likewise has both minor "absence" and major attacks. B and C, the electroencephalograms of both girls show fairly typical, diffuse rhythmic spike wave activity throughout. The mother, M.H., reports that she has never had a seizure, but D shows recurrent generalized EEG bursts (between arrows) of irregular slow activity mingled with some diffuse, synchronous sharp waves (arrow). The latter bursts do not represent a stage of drowsiness.

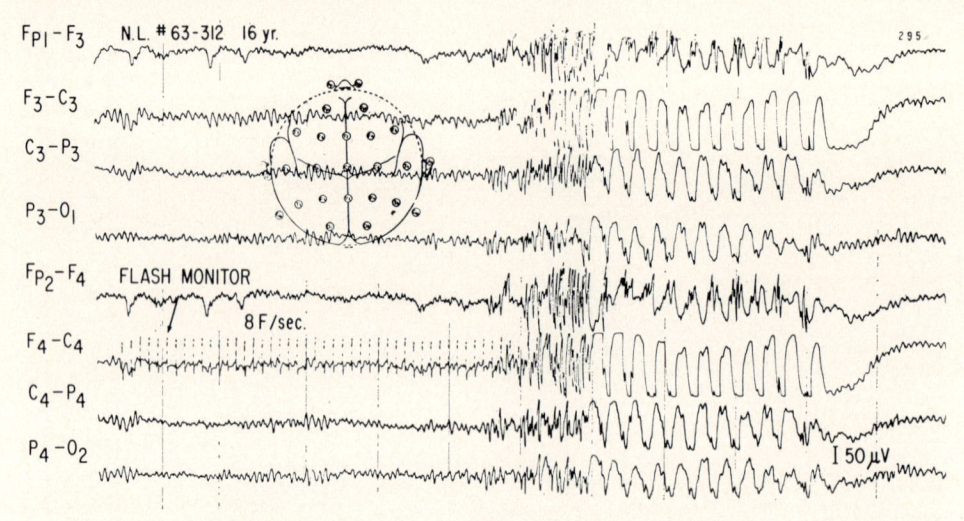

Fig. 14.2.—Light-sensitive petit mal epileptiform EEG abnormalities in 16-year-old boy. He had a history of five mild, generalized seizures over a five-year period. When questioned carefully, relatives reported that he also had occasional fluttering movements of the eyelids when forced to look into bright sunlight. Note the polyspike and spike wave EEG abnormalities in response to flashing light. This EEG response occurred at all flicker frequencies.

and clinically by "absence" seizures (i.e., momentary lapse of consciousness with cessation of activity except for blinking of the eyelids and staring). However, one must realize the great variation in both the EEG abnormality and the clinical seizures.[26] Specifically, in patients with petit mal and in their close relatives, the diffuse 3 cycles/second spike wave EEG classic abnormality is seen less frequently than "atypical" bursts of high voltage slow wave and spike intermixtures. Also, much variation is seen in the types of clinical seizures which are experienced. When one sees enough such cases the character of the attack runs the full gamut of all seizure types, as pointed out by Daly and Klass[8] (including "psychomotor" episodes with lip smacking, automatisms, etc.).

Both the EEG abnormality and the clinical seizure can be evoked in many of these patients by hyperventilation or by flickering light. Advantage is taken of these characteristics by making hyperventilation and photic stimulation part of the routine EEG activation repertoire in every patient[1,9,13a] (Fig. 14.2). The recently reported seizures induced by the viewing of faulty television sets[6,28] are probably produced via the same mechanism as the diffuse spike and wave discharges activated by flickering light in the laboratory.

Focal

The focal motor form of idiopathic epilepsy is also seen commonly in middle childhood, as emphasized by the Gibbses.[10] The clinical attacks in these patients appear as generalized motor (grand mal) episodes or as focal motor attacks which begin on one side of the face and spread to involve the arm and leg on the same side. Some of these patients will have attacks in which they will remain conscious but will be unable to speak. The attacks occur most often in sleep, especially in the hours just after retiring or just before arising. However, as in the case of pa-

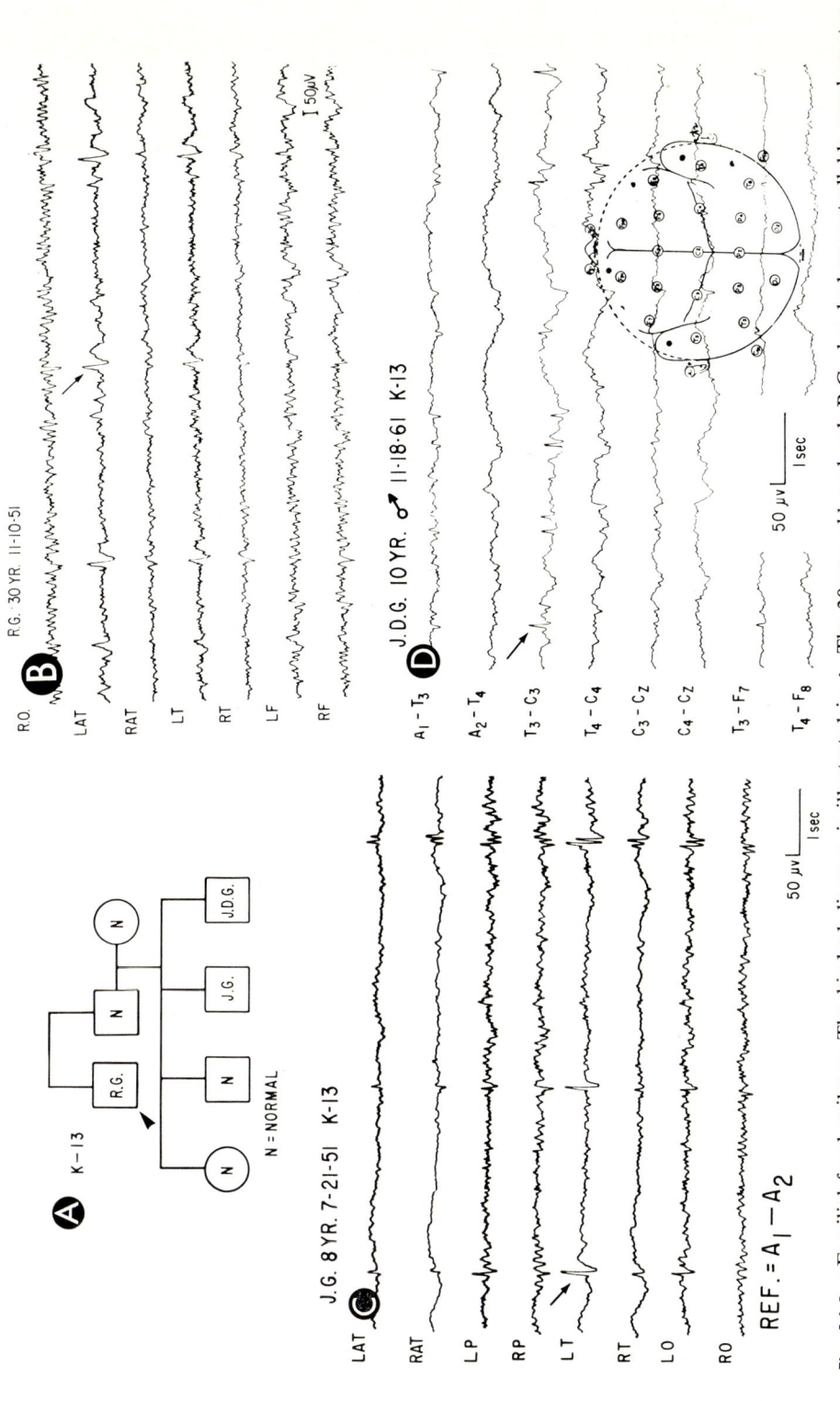

CLINICAL AND LABORATORY DIAGNOSIS   187

Fig. 14.3.—Familial focal epilepsy. The kindred diagram is illustrated in **A**. The 30-year-old proband, R.G., has had uncontrollable psychomotor automatisms since childhood, together with occasional generalized seizures; **B** shows a consistent spike focus in the left anterior temporal (LAT) area. A nephew, J.G., had generalized seizures during childhood in association with a frequent left hemisphere EEG spike discharge, maximal in the left midtemporal region (**C**). Another nephew, J.D.G., who is free of neurologic symptoms has a frequent spike or sharp wave discharge in the left temporal-central area (**D**).

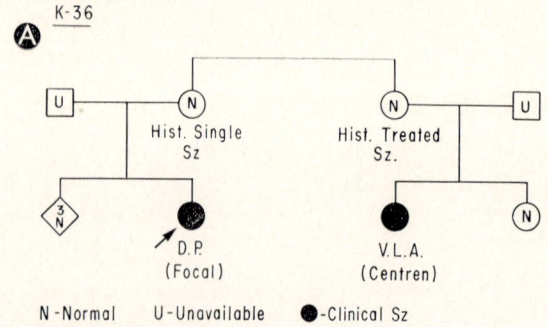

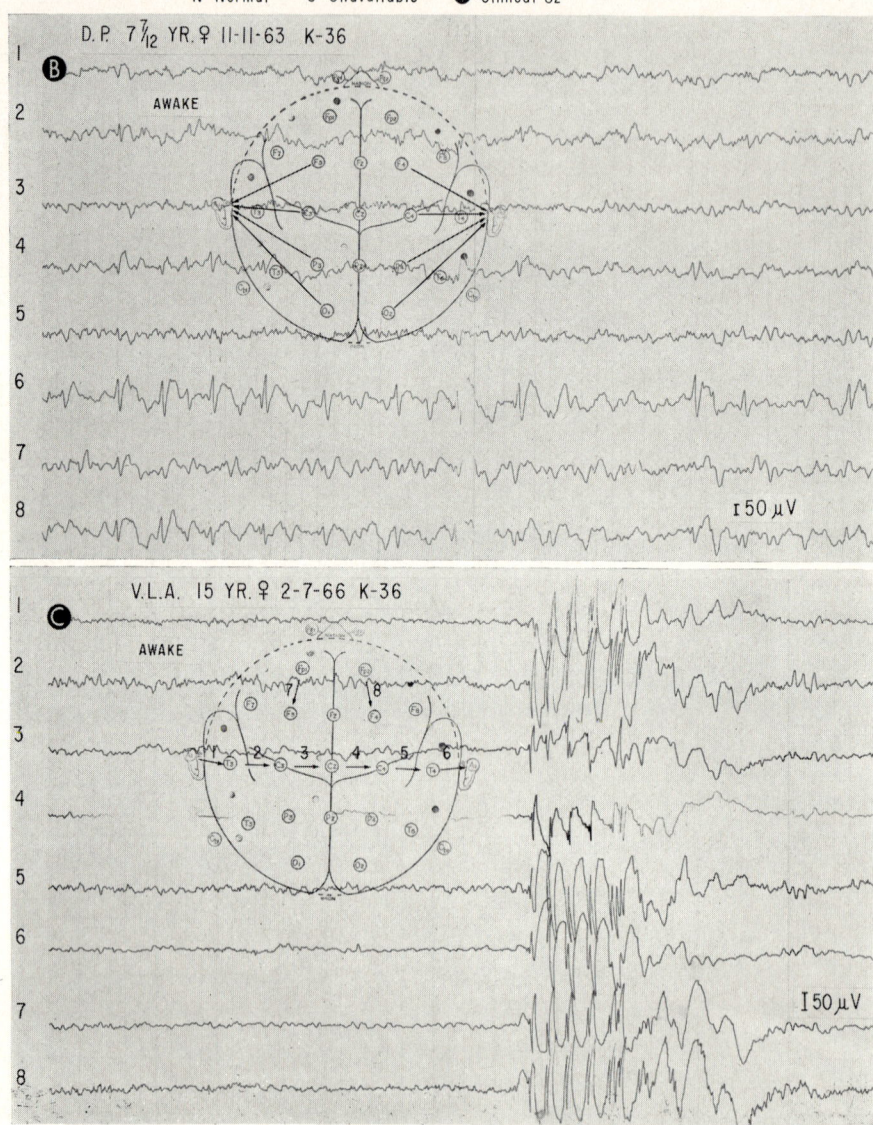

Fig. 14.4.—Familial petit mal and focal epilepsy in close relatives. In this family (A), the proband, D.P., suffered from generalized seizures; B shows an epileptiform spike discharge emanating from the right central area (channel 6). A first cousin, V.L.A., has had typical "absence" attacks and several generalized convulsions, which are associated with typical petit mal EEG activity (C). The 38-year-old mother of V.L.A. is taking anticonvulsant drugs for seizures which began at age 13, whereas the mother of the proband reported a single convulsion at age 6.

tients presenting with a petit mal type of electroencephalogram, the spectrum of clinical seizure types varies widely from generalized (grand mal) to focal motor and, much less commonly, to "psychomotor" or "absence" attacks.[1a] Electrical recording from the scalp in these patients reveals a contralateral midtemporal or temporal-central sharp wave or spike focus that is usually restricted to one side (Fig. 14.3) or that may appear independently from the homologous areas of both hemispheres. Although these abnormal brain waves may be seen with the patient at rest, their frequency and amplitude are often magnified during light sleep. Evidence accumulated by Bray and Wiser[3] in the EEG study of families who have a focal motor type of epilepsy suggests that their disorder may be closely related to if not identical with centrencephalic epilepsy (Fig. 14.4).

Grand Mal

Seventy-five to 80% of patients with petit mal or focal seizures have generalized or grand mal seizures,[21,25] and many have myoclonic jerks (single or multiple brief jerking movements of the arms or legs) or akinetic attacks (sudden loss of postural tone with a fall to the floor, often with only momentary lapse of consciousness). Some patients with idiopathic epilepsy (with either a focal spike or a diffuse spike and wave EEG abnormality) have only generalized clinical seizures.

DIFFERENTIAL DIAGNOSIS.—The diagnosis of idiopathic or centrencephalic epilepsy can be made *only* by exclusion because of the fact that the clinical type of seizure and the commonly associated brain wave abnormalities can be seen in patients with a variety of structural, metabolic and neoplastic brain disorders. Generally speaking, in patients with this disorder the onset of regularly recurring seizures is not until age 4 or 5 and the disorder tends to disappear in adolescence or early adult life (Fig. 14.5). It must be understood, however, that this disease, which reaches an overall peak incidence in middle childhood (9–10 years), may first manifest itself in the form of recurrent or severe febrile convulsions in infancy[17] or as an intractable form of generalized (grand mal) seizures in adulthood. It is helpful for the reader to remember that the threshold for seizures in all persons varies with normally operating neural and non-neural physiologic mech-

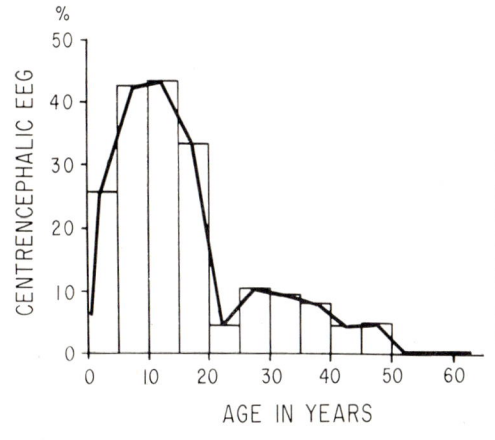

Fig. 14.5.—Age-distribution curve of petit mal EEG abnormality. In a large study of close relatives of patients with petit mal, the Metrakoses found the diffuse spike and wave epileptiform abnormality much more commonly in relatives between the ages of 4 and 16. Under 4 and over 20 years the abnormal electrographic discharge occurred infrequently.

anisms, such as fever, sleep, states of alkalosis produced by hyperventilation and hormonal shifts which accompany menstruation. These mechanisms may suffice to cause an attack in persons whose hereditary or constitutional threshold for seizures is low.

We would like to stress emphatically that the diagnosis of idiopathic or centrencephalic epilepsy can be made only after excluding all other etiologies for the syndrome, especially tumors. A number of workers have reported brain tumors[22,23] in patients who exhibit electroclinical findings indistinguishable from the petit mal or focal motor forms of idiopathic epilepsy.

Management

GENERAL CONSIDERATIONS.—The total care of patients with seizures requires a full understanding of anticonvulsant drug therapy and the rare need for special diet therapy. In addition, the psychologic well-being of the patient must be considered carefully. The patient and the family should be educated to the medical problem so that they understand the need for careful record keeping and regular administration of drugs, the side effects of drugs and the prognosis. In general, patients should be encouraged to live as complete an existence as possible. However, sensible restrictions must be placed on driving automobiles, working around machinery with moving parts, and nearness to water, fire and heights.

Much sociolegal controversy surrounds the question of driving licensure for patients with epilepsy. Although a detailed discussion of the subject lies beyond the scope of this text, we believe that the physician in the case should evaluate the findings carefully and present his honest medical opinion (which should include a careful history of seizure control, need for medication and serial EEG findings) to the local department of motor vehicles for final judgment. We deplore the practice of permitting patients with epilepsy to drive on the ground that driving a car is critical for their psychologic well-being or for earning a living.

DRUG THERAPY.—Details of anticonvulsant drug therapy are covered in Chapter 2. Seizures are discussed in the same way that they are treated medically—according to clinical type.

SURGICAL THERAPY.—In general, patients with genetically determined idiopathic epilepsy are not considered candidates for operative therapy.

Prognosis

DURATION OF DISEASE AND SEIZURE CONTROL.—Before drug therapy is begun the patient or the family should be told what to expect concerning the probable duration of the disorder and the chances for complete seizure control (Table 14.1). Before making any predictions or prognostications, the physician must eliminate from consideration as fully as possible any progressive, neoplastic, chemical, degenerative or structural etiology for the disorder. In patients with petit mal and in those with focal types of centrencephalic epilepsy the prognosis for disappearance of the clinical seizures and the associated brain wave disorder is fairly good.[11] Similarly, good seizure control can be achieved in 66–75% of patients. Most patients recover from the disorder, have intellect within the average range and are

TABLE 14.1.—CENTRENCEPHALIC (PETIT MAL) EPILEPSY: PROGNOSIS AND RECURRENCE RISK

	NO. OF PATIENTS	Incidence of Major Seizures	Seizure Control Good	Seizure Control Fair	Seizure Control Poor	Intelligence Normal	Intelligence Defective	RECURRENCE RISK IN ANOTHER SIB
Lennox[18]	137	54%	?	?	?	83%	17%	—
Livingston et al.[21]	117	54%*	78.6%	—	21.4%	89%	11%	—
Holowach et al.[13]	88	61%	63%	17%	17%†	76%	24%	—
Metrakos and Metrakos[25]	211	78%‡	—	—	—	—	—	1 in 12
Needham et al.[27]	43	79%§	—	—	—	73%	27%‖	1 in 11¶
Charlton and Yahr[5]	117	50%**	—	—	—	70%	30%‖	—
Keith[15]	62	—	—	—	—	65%	35%	—
Currier et al.[7]	32	38%	44%	—	56%	—	—	—

*Livingston et al.[21] emphasize that major seizures occur frequently (80.5%) when only "petit mal drugs" are used, but occur infrequently (35.6%) when a combination of a "major motor anticonvulsant" and a "petit mal drug" is given.

†Presumably another 3% of patients were lost to follow-up.

‡Major seizures or convulsions occurred in 54% of patients with typical centrencephalic EEG abnormalities and in 78% of patients with atypical centrencephalic patterns.

§This includes patients with both typical and atypical petit mal EEG abnormalities in families where at least one other member has a similar type of EEG.

‖An IQ value of 80 (WISC, WAIS and Stanford-Binet) was used to divide patients with "normal" and "defective" intellect.

¶Unpublished data.

**Only nonfebrile grand mal seizures are included.

able to lead normal lives. Having conceded this optimistic outlook in the majority of cases, one must realize that some patients remain refractory to medical therapy and that a small percentage of patients do not "outgrow" their seizures in adult life.[13,16]

MENTAL COMPETENCE.—A review of the literature reveals a variety of opinions regarding the predictions about intelligence in these patients. Many of the expressed opinions have been based upon uncontrolled observations and personal clinical impressions[5,7,14,18,21,26] (Table 14.1). Unfortunately, many people, both laymen and physicians, have found it difficult to consider dispassionately either the influence of epilepsy upon intellectual performance or the possible inheritance of the disorder. We have recently completed a study of intellectual functioning in 73 patients with idiopathic epilepsy and compared the results with the IQ scores of their close nonepileptic relatives (parents and siblings).[27] Approximately 70% of the patients with epilepsy scored significantly lower than did their close relatives. However, the *mean* IQ scores were within or near the average ranges. One-fourth to one-third of the patients had scores within the borderline and defective categories. We would like to emphasize that these data refer only to patients with idiopathic epilepsy of the familial type and not to the large heterogeneous epileptic population.

PREDICTION OF RECURRENCE RISK.—Reliable data about the recurrence risk of idiopathic epilepsy are only now being accumulated. It has been pointed out that the disorder is inherited as an autosomal dominant trait, which means that both sexes are affected equally and one can expect relatives in succeeding generations to be involved.

Parents often want to know the risk of having another child with the disorder when one is already affected. It can be safely stated that in general the likelihood is quite low. In the studies of the Metrakoses[25] and of Bray and Wiser[4] the recurrence risk for the petit mal syndrome is approximately 1 in 12 (8%) (Table 14.1). Therefore, these data justify a general attitude of optimism, especially when one considers the generally good prognosis in the patient actually affected. Despite this recommendation for optimism for most patients and their families, the need for caution must be remembered. In given families, for example, the disorder can affect several siblings, and affected patients can be clearly retarded either in terms of absolute IQ scores or in comparison with their siblings. What has not yet been established is whether the defective intelligence in these selected cases is (1) secondary to the disease, epilepsy, (2) secondary to drug therapy, (3) another manifestation of gene action or (4) a combination of these factors.

BIBLIOGRAPHY

1. Bray, P. F.: Electroencephalography, in Brennemann-Kelley: *Practice of Pediatrics* (Hagerstown, Md.: W. F. Prior Company, Inc., 1964), vol. IV.
1a. Bray, P. F., and Wiser, W. C.: Evidence for a genetic etiology of temporal-central abnormalities in focal epilepsy, New England J. Med. 271:926, 1964.
2. Bray, P. F., and Wiser, W. C.: Hereditary characteristics of familial temporal-central epilepsy, Pediatrics 36:207, 1965.
3. Bray, P. F., and Wiser, W. C.: The relation of focal to diffuse epileptiform EEG discharges in genetic epilepsy, Arch. Neurol. 13:223, 1965.
4. Bray, P. F., and Wiser, W. C.: Unpublished data.
5. Charlton, M. H., and Yahr, M. D.: Long-term follow-up of patients with petit mal, Arch. Neurol. 16:595, 1967.
6. Charlton, M. H., and Hoefer, P. F. A.: Television and epilepsy, Arch. Neurol. 11:239, 1964.
7. Currier, R. D., et al.: Prognosis of "pure" petit mal, Neurology 13:959, 1963.
8. Daly, D. D., and Klass, D.: Personal communication.
9. Gastaut, H., et al.: Diagnostic value of electroencephalographic abnormalities provoked by intermittent photic stimulation (abstract), Electroencephalog. & Clin. Neurophysiol. 10:194, 1958.
10. Gibbs, E. L., and Gibbs, F. A.: *Atlas of Electroencephalography* (Reading, Mass.: Addison-Wesley Publishing Co., Inc., 1952), vol. 2.
11. Gibbs, E. L., and Gibbs, F. A.: Good prognosis of mid-temporal epilepsy, Epilepsia 1:448, 1960.
12. Greenfield, J. G.: *Neuropathology* (2d ed.; Baltimore: Williams & Wilkins Company, 1963).
13. Holowach, J., et al.: Petit mal epilepsy, Pediatrics 30:893, 1962.
13a. Hughes, J. R.: Usefulness of photic stimulation in routine clinical electroencephalography, Neurology 10:777, 1960.
14. Jasper, H. H., and Drogleever-Fortwin, J.: Experimental studies on the functional anatomy of petit mal epilepsy, A. Res. Nerv. & Ment. Dis., Proc. 26:272, 1947.
15. Keith, H. M.: *Convulsive Disorders in Children* (Boston: Little, Brown & Company, 1963).
16. Lees, F., and Liversedge, L. A.: The prognosis of "petit mal" and minor epilepsy, Lancet 2:797, 1962.
17. Lennox, M. A.: Febrile convulsions in childhood: Their relationship to adult epilepsy, J. Pediat. 35:427, 1949.
18. Lennox, W. G.: *Epilepsy and Related Disorders* (Boston: Little, Brown & Company, 1960).
19. Lennox, W. G.: The heredity of epilepsy as told by relatives and twins, J.A.M.A. 146:529, 1951.
20. Lennox, W. G., et al.: Inheritance of cerebral dysrhythmia and epilepsy, Arch. Neurol. & Psychiat. 44:1155, 1940.
21. Livingston, S., et al.: Petit mal epilepsy, J.A.M.A. 194:227, 1965.
22. Madsen, J. A., and Bray, P. F.: The coincidence of diffuse electroencephalographic spike-wave paroxysms and brain tumors, Neurology 16:546, 1966.
23. Marsan, C. A., and Lewis, W. R.: Pathologic findings in patients with "centrencephalic" electroencephalographic patterns, Neurology 10:922, 1960.

24. Metrakos, J. D.: Heredity as an Etiological Factor in Convulsive Disorders, in Fields, W. S., and Desmond, M. M. (eds.): *Disorders of the Developing Nervous System* (Springfield, Ill.: Charles C Thomas, Publisher, 1961).
25. Metrakos, J. D., and Metrakos, K.: Childhood epilepsy of subcortical ("centrencephalic") origin, Clin. Pediatrics 5:536, 1966.
26. Metrakos, K., and Metrakos, J. D.: Genetics of convulsive disorders: II. Genetic and electroencephalographic studies in centrencephalic epilepsy, Neurology 11:474, 1961.
27. Needham, W. E., *et al.*: Intelligence and EEG studies in families with idiopathic epilepsy, J.A.M.A. 207:1497, 1969.
28. Pantelakis, S. N., *et al.*: Convulsions and television viewing, Brit. M. J. 1:633, 1962.
29. Penfield, W., and Jasper, H.: Highest level seizures, A. Res. Nerv. & Ment. Dis., Proc. 26:252, 1947.

15

Trauma

| *Pathologic Effects* | *Clinical Signs and Complications* |

Postnatal Injury (Direct)
  Head
    Brain
      Avulsion of axons and neuronal disintegration   Concussion (confusion, stupor, coma, vomiting, vertigo and shock)
      Contusion
      Edema   Seizures
      Laceration   Acute focal deficit
            Chronic motor deficit

    Vascular Accidents
      Epidural hematoma
      Subdural hematoma   Mental and behavior disturbances
      Subarachnoid hemorrhage   Hypothalamic damage
      Intracerebral hemorrhage
      Subdural hygroma
      Arteriovenous aneurysm

    Skull Fractures
      Linear   Leptomeningeal cyst formation
      Basal   Infections (meningitis and wound infections)
      Diastatic
      Depressed   Rhinorrhea, otorrhea
      Compound   Aerocele formation

    Scalp
      Avulsion of scalp and meninges

  Spine and Spinal Cord
    Sprain, subluxation, fracture-dislocation

  Peripheral Nerves
    Mechanical trauma
    Postinjection trauma

Natal (Birth) Injury
- Head
  - Vascular Accidents
    - Subarachnoid hemorrhage
    - Intracerebral hemorrhage
    - Subdural hematoma
    - Death
    - Spastic "cerebral palsy"
    - Choreoathetosis
    - Seizures
    - Behavior disorders
    - Mental retardation
  - Brain
    - Herniation
  - Skull
    - Fracture
  - Scalp
    - Caput succedaneum
    - Cephalhematoma
    - Necrosis
- Spinal Cord and Spine
  - Obstetric stretching injury
- Peripheral Nerves
  - Brachial plexus
  - Facial nerve
  - Motor deficit

Other Physical Injuries to the Nervous System
- Radiation
- Electric Current

Postnatal Injury (Direct)

Head

INJURIES TO THE HEAD and brain are common at all periods of life. Their severity varies greatly and is related to many factors, including (1) the force of mechanical impact, (2) the speed of head movement (acceleration or deceleration) at the time of impact, (3) the resilience or rigidity of the impact object, (4) the thickness of the skull (injury is often greater in infants and children because of the thin skull), (5) the site of skull fracture and (6) the adherence of the dura to the inner table (greatest in infancy and old age). Head injuries are often classified as *closed* or *open,* depending on whether the dura mater remains intact or is lacerated. In general, closed injuries are milder than open ones, but there are so many exceptions to this rule that the classification at the beginning of the chapter, which is based upon clinical and pathologic findings, seems preferable.

Pathogenesis
Brain

The immediate effects of head injury are brought about by (1) disintegration of neurons and shearing or tearing of axis cylinders due to movement of the brain within the skull, (2) contusion of brain substance, (3) development of cerebral edema and (4) laceration of brain substance. The importance of cerebral edema is controversial, but its clinical significance in certain cases is indisputable, as emphasized by Evans.[13]

The term "concussion" has a strictly clinical connotation and is discussed under Clinical and Laboratory Diagnosis. Accompanying cerebral contusion or laceration one finds varying types and degrees of hemorrhage, both into the subarachnoid space and into the brain substance. Hemorrhage often results from tearing of blood vessels or degeneration of vessel walls a short time after injury. Contusions or lacerations may occur on the opposite side of the brain (*contrecoup*), damaging the poles of the frontal and temporal lobes in cases of severe or repeated head injury. Occasionally thrombotic lesions develop in either arteries or superficial veins, and these may cause secondary infarction of brain tissue.

Vascular Accidents

Epidural (extradural) hematoma.—Usually, but not invariably, epidural hematomas result from a direct injury to the temporal bone which causes rupture of the middle meningeal artery or vein. This problem is often, but not always, associated with a skull fracture which crosses the path of the middle meningeal vessel (artery or vein). The bleeding which ensues is extensive and continuous and acts as a rapidly expanding intracranial mass. Of practical importance is the fact that this complication is uncommon in infancy and old age because at these times the dura is firmly adherent to the inner table of the skull. During the intervening years of childhood and adult life the dura and inner table are readily separated and permit the accumulation of large collections of blood.

Subdural hematoma.—These hematomas always result from venous bleeding into the subdural space due to tearing of veins which traverse the space between the brain substance and the draining sinuses. The acute subdural collection of blood is usually seen after a moderate or severe head injury and causes neurologic symptoms and signs quite promptly. In chronic subdural hematomas, more common in infants and the elderly, clinical signs usually appear only after a considerable interval, during which the clot organizes, becomes encapsulated, develops a liquid center and eventually acts as an irritative, compressive intracranial mass.

Usually the hemorrhage is widely distributed over the convexity of the hemispheres (Fig. 15.1), but occasionally the clot is confined to the middle, the posterior or the anterior fossa. If the clot reaches sufficient size, intracranial hypertension develops and uncal herniation ensues, with false localizing hemiparesis, homonymous hemianopia, sixth nerve palsy and third nerve palsy (Fig. 8.1, p. 85).

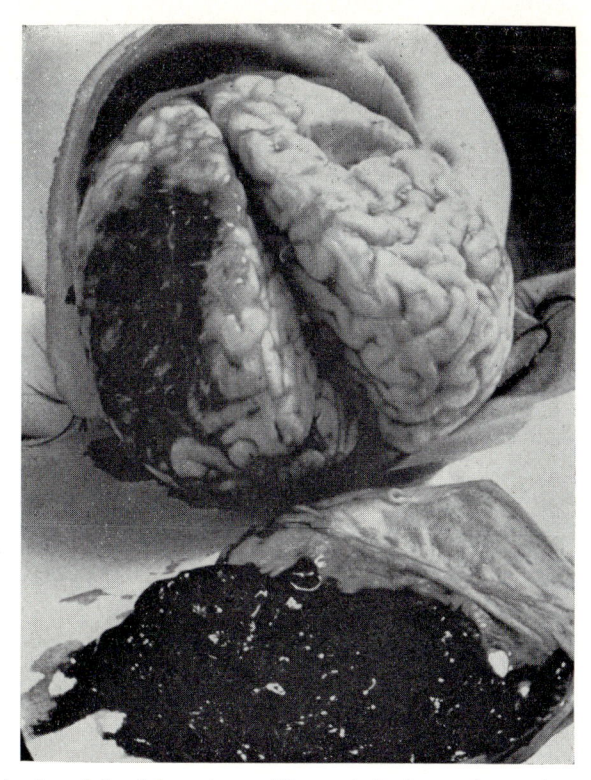

Fig. 15.1.—Acute subdural hematoma. The pathologic specimen shows a large subdural hematoma (below). Note the compressive indentation over the convexity as a result of the clot.

At one time a certain amount of mystery surrounded the etiology of this condition since a history of trauma or clinical or x-ray evidence of head trauma is found in only the minority of cases. Most workers are now agreed that some type of trauma accounts for all but a small handful of cases, in which the diagnosis of a true bleeding disorder must be considered. Some have suggested that bridging veins are torn or sheared when a small child is shaken by an angry parent or custodian. The fact that babies with subdural hematomas more often come from economically deprived families suggests not that they are suffering from malnutrition and hence are more prone to bleeding with injuries, but that the complex psychologic and social disturbances in their environment more commonly lead to violence.

If an excessive dose of hypertonic urea is given or if the dose is given too rapidly to reduce cerebral edema, subdural bleeding can result. We have seen this complication of urea administration in an infant with Eastern equine encephalomyelitis, and similar cases have been reported.[26a]

Subarachnoid hemorrhage.—Hemorrhage into the subarachnoid space occurs whenever an injury is severe enough to cause a contusion or laceration with bleeding near the surface of the brain. In general, this type of bleeding alone does not cause serious consequences, although many believe it can lead to obstructive hydrocephalus by blocking the CSF outflow at the foramina of the fourth ventricle.

Intracerebral hematoma.—Intracerebral hemorrhages appear commonly as multiple small petechiae in the white matter of patients dying of injury. Larger hematomas may result from laceration of vessels, especially in the frontal and temporal lobes. These occasional solitary collections of blood must be borne in mind in the clinical evaluation and management of the patient.

Subdural hygroma.—Rarely fluid with the appearance and composition of the cerebrospinal fluid in the subarachnoid space accumulates in the subdural space. The existence of this process as a disease entity and the exact nature of its pathogenesis are subjects of continuing controversy. Most experienced workers think that subdural hygromas result from a tear in the arachnoid membrane which permits fluid to leave the subarachnoid space and collect in the subdural space.[7,15] If blood is intermixed with the fluid, the process is called a hematoma, but if the fluid is clear it is considered a hygroma. Most hygromas occur in infants as a result of head trauma, but they may also complicate the treatment of hydrocephalus.

Arteriovenous fistula.—A rare complication of head injury, arteriovenous fistula results from laceration of the internal carotid artery as it passes through the cavernous sinus. The arterial laceration is brought about either by a penetrating missile or by fracture of the sphenoid bone.

Focal neurologic deficits, seizures, mental and personality disturbances, as well as diabetes insipidus, are later complications of head injury. These complications are discussed under Clinical and Laboratory Diagnosis.

Skull Fracture

The immediate effects of uncomplicated *linear skull fractures* are negligible, their ill effects being attributable only to associated vascular accidents and brain injury. *Depressed fractures* damage the underlying meninges, blood vessels and brain substance if the fragments are driven inward far enough to cause laceration and hemorrhage. Depressed fractures which lacerate major vessels such as the longitudinal sinus can cause rapidly fatal hemorrhage. *Compound fractures* carry the threat of secondary wound infection, meningitis, thrombophlebitis and abscess formation. *Basal skull fractures* represent a special type of problem because of (1) the tendency to lacerate cranial nerves, (2) the special *complications* of compound basal fractures (rhinorrhea, otorrhea, pneumatocele or leptomeningeal cyst formation and meningitis) and (3) damage to the hypothalamus, the pituitary gland or their connecting tracts. With hypothalamic or pituitary damage there may be pathologic metabolism of water, salt and sugar as well as abnormal sleep patterns and sexual development. The complications of different types of fractures are discussed on page 210.

CLINICAL AND LABORATORY DIAGNOSIS

The common occurrence of head injuries in children and the labile response of children to the injury complicate the immediate clinical evaluation of the episode. The injury may be followed promptly by intense crying, vomiting, pallor, sweating and drowsiness. Whether these signs herald the development of more ominous neurologic signs or will disappear without sequelae in an hour or two can be determined only by careful observation.

Concussion

This term implies alteration or loss of consciousness, which in mild cases is characterized by confusion, disorientation, drowsiness and stupor and in severe cases by coma and unresponsiveness. The depth and duration of coma are related to the extent and location of the associated contusion, laceration and edema. Prolonged coma may occur in severe contusions of the hemispheres, but a persistent state of coma suggests either direct contusion and hemorrhage into the brain stem or hemorrhage into the stem secondary to increased intracranial pressure from a large supratentorial hematoma (Chapter 8).

When consciousness is regained, the patient commonly complains of headache and dizziness, the latter due in many cases to direct trauma to the vestibular end-organ in the middle ear. Vertigo is usually transient although in exceptional cases it may be a prolonged, disabling complaint. In infants and young children who do not verbalize complaints, vertigo is manifested by the assumption of a fixed position in bed, resistance to movement and the development of nystagmus and vomiting on forcible movement. Surgical shock often complicates the clinical picture, especially when the patient has suffered extensive injuries to other parts of the body.

Seizures

Conclusions in the literature about the incidence of post-traumatic epilepsy (P.T.E.) in different types of head injuries vary a great deal, so the following comments are restricted to some attitudes in which there appears to be consensus. The incidence of post-traumatic epilepsy varies from 1 to 50% according to the type of head wound and the extent of brain damage, in the experience of Walker[38] (739 cases), Caveness and Liss[5] (407 cases), Evans[12] (422 cases), Jennett[21] (over 500 cases) and Russell[31a,31b] (1,166 cases). The incidence of post-traumatic epilepsy rises in patients with depressed fractures, unconsciousness which lasts more than two hours,[38] hematoma formation,[21] penetrating injuries from objects such as missiles[12] and open head injuries associated with a hemiparesis.[38] A seizure sometimes occurs promptly at the time of head trauma (more commonly in closed than in open injuries). This should not be considered a serious event if the patient does not have focal neurologic deficit, signs of a hematoma or prolonged unconsciousness.[38] Generalized seizures several hours after the acute injury may carry a grave prognosis,[28a] but focal seizures are less ominous and may reflect hematoma formation. In general, the incidence of post-traumatic epilepsy, according to Walker,[38] is 1–5% in patients with closed head injuries and 20–50% in patients with open wounds. About 50% of these patients have the first attack within six months after the injury and 80% before the end of the second year.[4a,38] Patients with closed injuries rarely have onset of attacks after two years, but 1% of patients with open injuries develop attacks each year until the tenth post-traumatic year, after which new cases are rarely seen.

Acute Focal Deficit

A wide assortment of focal deficits may be exhibited, depending upon the location of the traumatic lesion. Among these are cranial nerve signs, hemiparesis, focal cortical sensory deficit, aphasia and other specific language disabilities.

Olfactory nerve.—Loss of the sense of smell commonly occurs in head injuries associated with basal skull fractures or in situations in which the olfactory filaments are sheared off where they pass through the cribriform plate. Patients may also report some loss of taste since the two sensations are interdependent. Olfactory hallucinations may result from trauma but only as a manifestation of temporal lobe epilepsy.

Optic nerve.—Avulsion of the optic nerve can result from severe head trauma and leads to optic atrophy. When visual symptoms and optic nerve swelling or pallor follow a head injury of questionable severity, a careful differential diagnosis must be considered.

Oculomotor, trochlear and abducens nerves.—Trauma to these nerves produces certain general symptoms and signs including diplopia, paralysis of eye movement, ptosis of the upper lid, dilated fixed pupil and a deviated eyeball.

Trigeminal nerve.—Fifth nerve trauma causes loss of facial sensation and loss of the corneal reflex as well as paralysis of the muscles of mastication. Opening the mouth causes the jaw to deviate toward the paralyzed side.

Facial nerve.—The deficit accompanying damage to the seventh nerve depends on the site of injury. If the injury is near the nerve's exit from the brain stem, all functions are affected. There will be loss of movement of all facial muscles on that side, partial loss of taste and defective lacrimation and salivation. Injury to the nerve at the stylomastoid foramen causes only facial muscle paralysis. Intermediate injury still causes muscle weakness, but preservation of autonomic gland function and taste depends on how far distally the nerve is traumatized.

Acoustic nerve.—Partial damage to the eighth nerve causes the irritative symptoms of vertigo and tinnitus, whereas more severe injury results in hearing loss, equilibratory ataxia and nystagmus. Audiometric and caloric tests give more objective information about eighth nerve deficit.

Glossopharyngeal, vagus, accessory and hypoglossal nerves.—Lesions of these lowest cranial nerves are rarely due to the trauma of head injuries but do occur in a variety of disease processes (see Chapter 8).

Chronic Motor Deficit

See Chapter 3.

Mental and Behavior Disturbances

Restlessness, irritability and mental confusion are common in the acute stage of the injury, as is an intolerance for loud sounds and bright lights. Amnesia often occurs, especially for events immediately before the injury and for those occurring shortly after consciousness is regained. The duration of the memory loss is related to the severity of the injury and may be for weeks.

Changes in personality and behavior commonly follow more severe injuries and vary from mild, transient accentuations of the child's pretraumatic personality to severe sociopathic activity requiring continuous supervision or institutionalization. Whereas altered behavior and personality patterns in adults are sometimes motivated by a desire for compensation through litigation, these considerations generally do not arise directly in children but may originate with parents. Common behavioral changes include emotional instability, temper tantrums, a restless, destructive, combative behavior and an abbreviated attention span. Significant intellectual deficit in the strict sense does not occur very often. Psychometric and psychologic testing, which help considerably in defining the nature and extent of mental changes, can be used to follow the patient's progress and has some value in prognosis.

These signs and symptoms are discussed in more detail in Chapter 1.

Hypothalamic Damage

That head trauma can cause certain hypothalamic syndromes is indubitable. However, the time lag between the injury and the vegetative signs, the common occurrence of mild head trauma and the danger that results from incorrect diagnosis should make the physician very cautious before attributing any of these syndromes to trauma. It is generally assumed that hypothalamic damage results more often with basal skull fractures, the latter diagnosis often being made presumptively on the basis of blood or cerebrospinal fluid leaking from the ears or nose rather than by x-ray demonstration of fracture. As in other lesions of the hypothalamic area, there may be evidence of pituitary overactivity (presumably on the basis of the irritative effect of the lesion) or underactivity (presumably due to the destructive action of the injury). The hypothalamic syndromes and their etiologies are described in Chapter 11.

Vascular Accidents

Increased intracranial pressure.—The results of repeated neurologic examinations and observations of vital signs should be recorded carefully in patients with severe head injury. Only in this way can early signs of increased intracranial pressure, uncal herniation and cerebral decompensation be detected. Progressive obtundation, papilledema, pupillary dilatation on the side of the hematoma or the herniating temporal lobe and a contralateral hemiparesis demand immediate medical and operative therapy. Skull x-rays may reveal a fracture across the path of the middle meningeal artery and signs of intracranial hypertension. Lumbar puncture is not recommended in this clinical situation, but pressure elevation is recorded if a diagnostic tap is carried out. If the diagnosis is in doubt and if the patient's condition warrants the inevitable delay, definitive diagnostic information can often be obtained with angiography. Angiographic demonstration of transtentorial uncal herniation is difficult, but subtle changes in the position of the anterior choroidal, anterior cerebral and posterior cerebral arteries may be found.[36]

Epidural (extradural) hematoma.—In uncomplicated epidural hematoma the usual sequence of events consists of (1) initial injury with concussion (this may vary from a temporary confused or dazed condition to brief loss of consciousness), (2) a subsequent lucid interval of several hours during which the child or adult may appear to have recovered completely except for headache and (3) gradual progression into a state of stupor and coma, during which time the patient may vomit, the pulse rate slows and the systolic blood pressure becomes elevated. This ominous sequence of events is due to increasing intracranial pressure and herniation of the uncus through the tentorial notch. These lead to an ipsilateral (sometimes contralateral) dilated fixed pupil, contralateral or sometimes ipsilateral hemiparesis, deepening coma and failing vital signs (slow pulse, respiratory irregularities and hypotension), the result of secondary brain stem compression and hemorrhage. Convulsions and papilledema occur infrequently. Posterior fossa epidural hematomas following fractures of the occipital bone run a course similar to those in the middle and anterior fossae, but they may be associated with nuchal rigidity and cerebellar signs.

Skull x-rays should be taken whenever the clinical events suggest the possibility of an epidural clot. Fractures which cross the groove of one of the meningeal arteries alert one to the diagnosis. Electroencephalography is of value only if it points to consistent suppression of the electrical activity coming from one hemisphere or if it clearly shows a slow wave focus. A normal electroencephalogram or one with diffuse abnormalities has little diagnostic value. Echoencephalography provides valuable evidence of an intracranial clot in some cases. Definitive diagnosis can be made in suspected cases by a carotid angiogram, and the findings are identical with those seen in patients with subdural hematoma (see below). The presence of a hematoma may be manifested in older patients by a shifted pineal gland, when it is calcified. Spinal puncture may reveal clear fluid (or bloody fluid if the injury is accompanied by brain contusion or laceration) under increased pressure, but lumbar puncture is not recommended if an epidural hematoma is strongly suspected.

Subdural hematoma.—These lesions are often classified as acute or chronic, depending upon the interval between the injury and the onset of clinical symptoms. The signs are quite similar in the two types. The chronic form represents a delay in diagnosis because of the insidious development of symptoms and signs in both infants and older patients and the nonspecific nature of the clinical signs in infancy. One cannot insist upon a history of an impressive head injury before suspecting the diagnosis, regardless of the age of the patient.

The disorder in infants is distinctive because of (1) its common occurrence, (2) its many nonspecific clinical symptoms and signs (Table 15.1), (3) the major threat of permanent damage to the developing nervous system, (4) the presence of bilateral bleeding in about 85% of patients, (5) the ease with which diagnosis can be made with subdural taps and (6) the high incidence of large fluid-filled cavities surrounded by newly formed membranes. The classical clinical description of subdural hematomas in children was made by Ingraham and Matson[18] in 1944. Despite the emphasis placed upon the importance of early diagnosis, most consultants see several patients each year in whom earlier diagnosis may have improved the long-term prognosis.

Head enlargement, commonly in the young child, should immediately suggest the diagnosis of subdural hematoma, not congenital hydrocephalus. Seizures are

TABLE 15.1.—CLINICAL SIGNS OF SUBDURAL HEMATOMA

SYMPTOMS

INFANCY	CHILDREN AND ADULTS
Convulsions	Headache
Vomiting	Irritability
Irritability	Mental confusion, depression, psychosis
Infection	Somnolence or stupor
Stupor	Convulsions (rare)
History of trauma	

SIGNS

Fever	Hemiparesis and facial weakness
Hyperreflexia	Aphasia (rare)*
Bulging fontanel	Hemianopia (rare)*
Anemia	Ocular squint
Head enlargement	
Abnormal fundi	
Paralysis	
Skull fracture	
Abnormal transillumination	

*These signs generally do not develop unless contusion or hemorrhage in the brain substance occurs concurrently.

frequently noted in infants, along with such nonspecific symptoms as vomiting, irritability, frequent infections and somnolence or stupor. However, a history of head trauma (natal or postnatal) is obtained in less than half the cases. The physician should maintain a constantly low threshold of suspicion for this diagnosis in the light of both the symptoms and the signs. Fever and anemia are common (Table 15.1), as are neurologic signs such as head enlargement, bulging fontanel, hyperreflexia, retinal hemorrhages, occasional papilledema and paresis (hemiparesis and eye muscle paralysis[30a]). The heads of young infants with large, liquid, subdural accumulations will often transilluminate abnormally well (Figs. 13.6 and 13.14, pp. 134 and 144). In rare cases, localized thinning and enlargement of the cranium occur, especially in patients with middle fossa subdural hematoma[5a] (Fig. 15.5,B). Although skull fractures are found in only a small percentage of cases, Caffey[4] showed that skeletal surveys of these patients reveal a surprisingly high incidence of fractures and other signs of trauma which had previously been unsuspected or unrecognized (Fig. 15.2). Such observations over the past 20 years have led to an enhanced awareness of the "battered-child" syndrome[23,33,40] (see Management). At the present time in the United States most states have laws which provide the physician with professional immunity when he reports suspected cases of child abuse to the juvenile police authorities.

Technique of subdural tap.—Whenever the diagnosis is suspected, subdural taps should be carried out promptly, with all necessary precautions. Although the procedure is simple, it should be done with great care and with proper attention to asepsis (Fig. 15.3). The baby is "mummified" with a sheet and given a sugar nipple (sometimes preoperative sedation in small amounts is advisable). The anterior half of the head is then shaved completely, prepared thoroughly and draped. A sharp but short, beveled, 1½ in. no. 20 lumbar puncture needle with the stylet in place is inserted through a Novocain scalp wheal either at the extreme lateral angle

204   TRAUMA

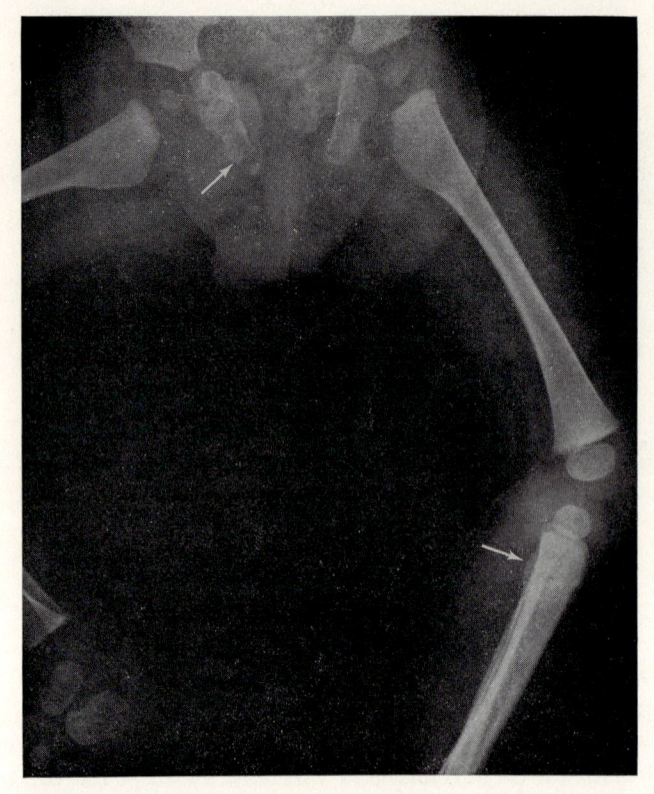

Fig. 15.2.—Chronic subdural hematoma with skeletal trauma. Year-old infant was hospitalized and studied for several weeks because of fever and failure to thrive. Eventually the diagnosis of subdural hematoma was considered and easily proved with subdural taps. Note the fractured pelvis and the healing callus on the tibia. The baby's mother was a "lady wrestler."

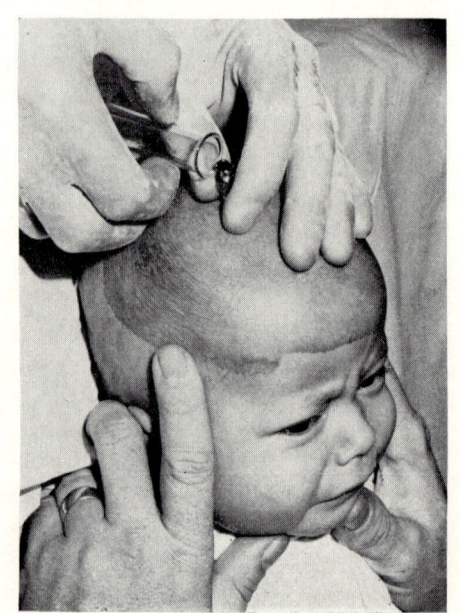

Fig. 15.3.—Subdural tap in progress. Note the prominent "square" appearance of the forehead in this infant with bilateral subdural hematomas. Note also that the operator failed to drape the posterior half of the head properly.

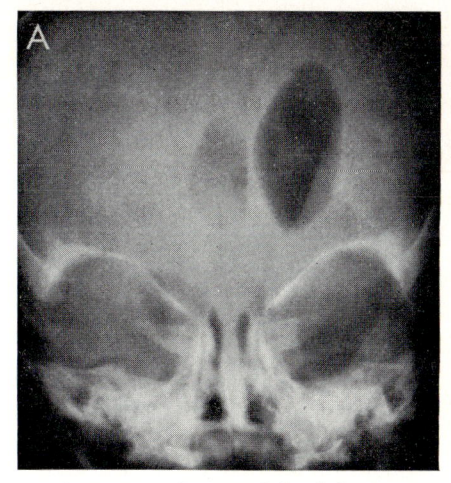

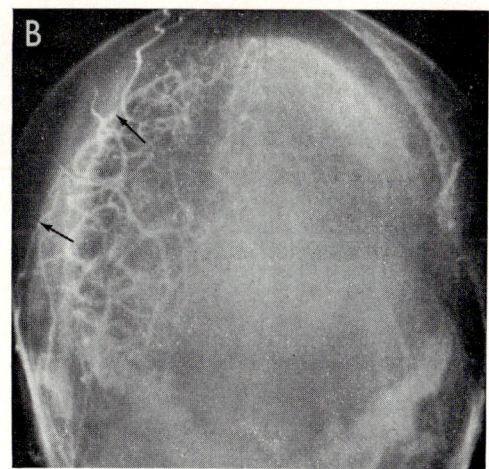

Fig. 15.4.—Acute subdural hematoma. On the second day of life, following a breech delivery, this infant had convulsions and vomiting; the right pupil became dilated and fixed. Examination also revealed bilateral ankle clonus and a bulging fontanel. Subdural taps yielded only 2 cc. of bloody fluid on the right and 1 cc. on the left. The baby was anemic (hematocrit 38), and lumbar puncture showed over 8,000 red blood cells. **A,** ventriculogram shows bilateral ventricular dilatation with depression of the body of the right lateral ventricle. **B,** right carotid arteriogram reveals displacement of the middle cerebral branches away from the inner table (arrows). The vessels seen near the inner table are probably filled from the external carotid circulation. A right-sided craniotomy was performed and a large, solid hematoma evacuated. The clinical syndrome was that of uncal herniation. Ventricular dilatation is a common finding with subdural hematomas.

of the anterior fontanel (if the angle measures no less than 3 cm. from the midline) or at the coronal suture lateral to the fontanel. After the scalp is penetrated, the advancing tip of the needle should be controlled with great care so that when the dura is perforated the needle is not allowed to plunge any deeper.

Normally one may get only a wet needle or a few drops of clear fluid, but occasionally one gets several cubic centimeters of fluid, the composition of which is identical to that of cerebrospinal fluid in the lumbar subarachnoid space. In the latter event the possibility of subdural hygroma (p. 198) must be considered. In the case of a fresh, recent hematoma red, bloody fluid with xanthochromic supernatant will be recovered, whereas later the uncentrifuged fluid takes on a clear xanthochromic or greenish tint and contains fewer red blood cells.

X-ray contrast studies.—Most neurologists and neurosurgeons like to have the information provided by an arteriogram or a pneumoencephalogram before trephination or craniotomy. In the older child or young adult whose fontanel and sutures are closed, either procedure may provide evidence for the diagnosis. Most patients with moderate-sized or large subdural hematomas have some degree of hydrocephalus, due to partial obliteration of the absorptive surface pathways, an incisural block or cerebral contusion and atrophy. Pneumoencephalography tells (1) whether the ventricular system is dilated, (2) how much cerebral atrophy has occurred from the chronic effects of pressure and (3) whether to expect a solid or organized clot on one or both sides of the head (Fig. 15.4,*A;* compare with Fig. 15.1).

Electroencephalography sometimes helps by demonstrating (1) the suppressive effect of a hematoma on the normal alpha pattern (flattening of the amplitude on the affected side) or (2) a slow wave focus over the hematoma.[30b] No pathognomonic findings are found on skull x-rays unless the hematoma is calcified, and this happens only rarely and in chronic, unrecognized cases. There may be evidence of acute or chronic increased intracranial pressure in the form of suture separation, prominent digital markings or erosion of the posterior clinoids or dorsum sellae. Lumbar puncture in these patients may reflect elevated pressure, the fluid may be clear or xanthochromic, and the protein concentration may be increased. Angiography is discussed below.

Convexity subdural hematoma.—The air study usually demonstrates a depression of the lateral ventricle on the side of the clot and a shift of the whole ventricular system to the side opposite the lesion (Fig. 15.4,*A*). Angiography in the typical case reveals significant displacement of the middle cerebral branches (an avascular clear space) 2–3 cm. away from the inner table of the skull in the frontal projection (Fig. 15.4,*B*). The findings in angiograms taken in the lateral projection are discussed below.

Anterior, middle and posterior fossa subdural hematoma.—Although most subdural collections are demonstrated best on the frontal angiographic view because of their common location over the convexity of the temporal or parietal lobe, the lateral angiographic film is the view of choice to demonstrate a subdural mass located over the frontal or occipital pole. The tendency for unrecognized subdural hematomas in infancy to loculate in the middle fossa (the syndrome of chronic relapsing juvenile subdural hematoma described by Davidoff and Dyke[11]) can be suspected strongly in some cases on the basis of clinical examination and plain films (Fig. 15.5,*A* and *B*). Additional contrast studies are valuable in confirming the diagnosis. Pneumoencephalography may show compression of the ipsilateral ventricle and shift to the opposite side, and arteriography illustrates elevation of the middle cerebral artery in the frontal projection (Fig. 15.5,*C*). Subdural collections in the posterior fossa occur rarely and have few distinctive clinical or roentgen findings.[31] Clinically a history of trauma to the occiput may be elicited, and patients may show incoordination, stiff neck and signs of increased intracranial pressure. X-rays show only ventricular dilatation and obstruction and anterior displacement of the aqueduct of Sylvius in the upside-down lateral view.

INTRACEREBRAL HEMORRHAGE.—Collections of blood within the brain substance which result from injury are usually small and clinically silent except for signs of meningeal irritation and blood in the cerebrospinal fluid. Large, solitary hematomas are seen rarely (usually in older patients) and are manifest clinically by contralateral hemiparesis, ipsilateral pupillary dilatation, deepening stupor or coma and noisy respirations. These clinical signs are indistinguishable from those produced by acute epidural or subdural clots. One must also remember that intracerebral bleeding disorders in children with conditions such as acute leukemia or hemophilia and in adults with hypertension may easily be confused with bleeding of traumatic etiology, especially if clinical symptoms are ushered in by a fall and a head injury.

Plain skull x-rays and electroencephalograms do not differentiate epidural, subdural and intracerebral hemorrhage. The diagnostic procedure of choice, angiography, may show displacement and distortion of vessels, findings which closely

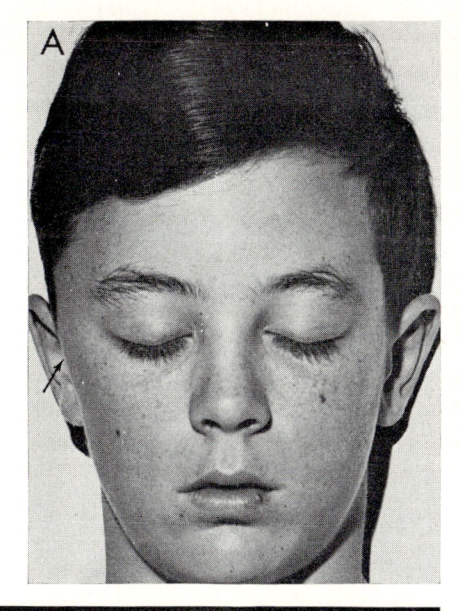

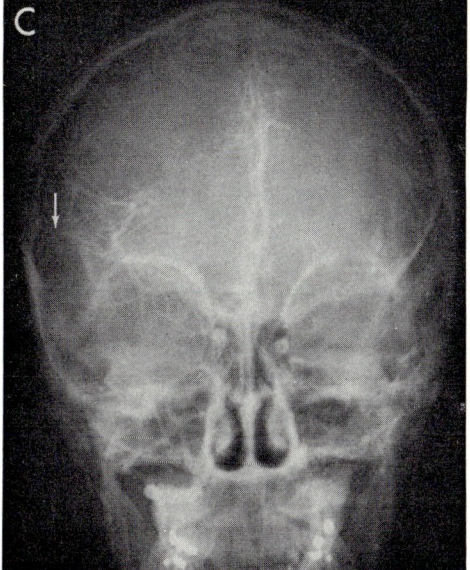

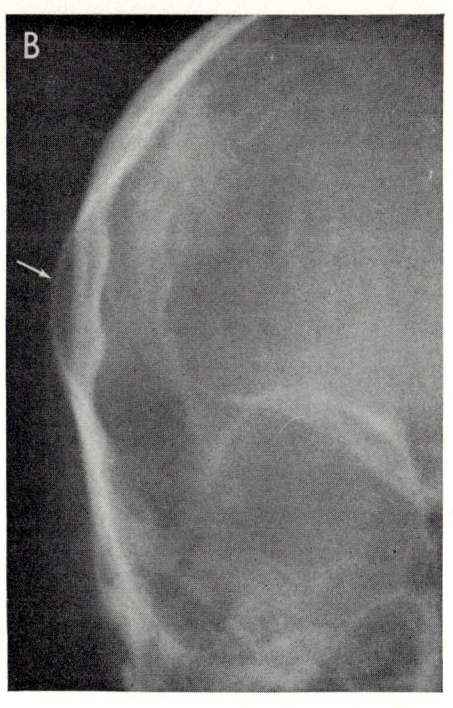

Fig. 15.5.—Chronic middle fossa (relapsing juvenile) subdural hematoma. Boy, 12, was well until 6 weeks before when severe, bifrontal headache with intermittent diplopia and vomiting developed. **A,** prominence of the right temple area (arrow) compared to the left had been noted since birth. Except for moderate bilateral papilledema and subjective diplopia the patient had no neurologic signs. **B,** skull x-ray reveals thinning of the inner table and localized bulging of the temporal bone. **C,** right carotid arteriogram shows elevation of the right middle cerebral artery with displacement of its branches away from the inner table. At right temporal craniotomy a large, old, subdural hematoma was evacuated. The highly vascular inner membrane was attached intimately to the pia arachnoid and could not be removed. The cyst was aspirated repeatedly but adequate decompression was finally accomplished only with a ventriculojugular shunt. The patient has remained asymptomatic for four years.

resemble those in patients with diffuse edema of the hemisphere. If the patient's condition is deteriorating or fails to improve, diagnosis of intracerebral or intracortical clot must be considered, especially if epidural or subdural hematoma has been satisfactorily excluded. In addition, it must be remembered that finding a subdural or epidural hematoma on angiography or by surgical exploration in no way eliminates the possibility of coexisting intracerebral hematoma.

SUBDURAL HYGROMA.—The clinical and x-ray findings in patients with a hygroma are identical to those described for subdural hematoma. Definitive diagnosis is made by analysis of the fluid obtained by aspiration or trephination.

ARTERIOVENOUS FISTULA.—The clinical diagnosis is usually suspected early because of the prompt onset of dramatic symptoms and signs. If the patient is old enough, he reports an audible bruit in his head; this is associated with exophthalmos, edema and congestion of the lids and conjunctivas. When the latter signs appear in patients of any age, listening to the head (over the temples and the orbits) may elicit a loud bruit, which is synchronous with the pulse. The intraorbital hypertension eventually causes extraocular muscle paralysis, papilledema, glaucoma, loss of vision and optic atrophy. Manual pressure on the carotid artery in the neck will reduce or obliterate the audible bruit. The fistula is easily demonstrated with angiography. The contrast substance fills the cavernous sinus and ophthalmic veins during the early phases of injection, and the jugular vein and carotid artery are opacified together on some of the seriograms.

Skull Fracture

It is well known that the presence or absence of a skull fracture does not necessarily provide an accurate index to the severity of a head injury. Fatal injuries can take place without a fracture as a result of severe brain contusion and intracranial hemorrhage and, conversely, many linear skull fractures are associated with only mild clinical signs of concussion. Nevertheless, the presence of a fracture gives a rough idea about the force of the impact and should alert one to complications which accompany different types of fractures. The fact that fracture is used as evidence of severity of injury when litigation is involved falls outside the scope of this discussion, except to say that x-rays which show the fracture simply provide a permanent visible record of an injury. In some cases fractures cause cranial nerve palsies, meningitis, rhinorrhea, otorrhea, leptomeningeal cysts and aerocele formations.

LINEAR.—Linear fractures of the cranial vault are usually seen with ease on x-ray examination, but basal fractures are notoriously difficult to demonstrate. In a general way, fractures tend to follow a vertical or horizontal course. The location of linear fractures has special significance in that they can lead to complications which require special management.

> *Fractures which tear vascular channels.* Linear fractures of the temporal or parietal bones near the path of the middle meningeal artery or its branches account for many cases of epidural hematoma.
>
> *Fractures into air sinuses.* Linear fractures can also open into the paranasal or mastoid air cells and become internal compound fractures.
>
> *Basal skull fractures.* These are usually not visualized on x-ray examination. A presumptive diagnosis of basilar fracture is often made because of the following signs: (1) cranial nerve palsies, especially the olfactory, optic, oculomotor, first and second divisions of the trigeminal, the abducens, the facial and the acoustic, (2) bleeding from the ear or blood behind the tympanic membrane, (3) leakage of cerebrospinal fluid and

blood from the nose (rhinorrhea) or the ear (otorrhea), (4) radiologic opacification of the paranasal air sinuses from bleeding into them, (5) tenderness and ecchymosis behind the ear over the mastoid process (Battle's sign), (6) aerocele or traumatic pneumocephalus and (7) the late development of diabetes insipidus and other hypothalamic syndromes.

Diastasis. Diastasis of the sutures (usually the lambdoid) as a result of trauma and without a visible fracture occurs occasionally in children and young adults. More often the suture diastasis is seen as a continuation of an adjacent fracture line. At times the roentgen findings, together with the clinical picture, may raise the question of suture separation due to increased intracranial pressure. However, with traumatic diastasis there is an abrupt change in width between the normal suture line and the line of diastasis.

DEPRESSED (AND COMMINUTED).—Injuries of greater severity cause depression and fragmentation of bone (Fig. 15.6). A depressed fracture exerts its dam-

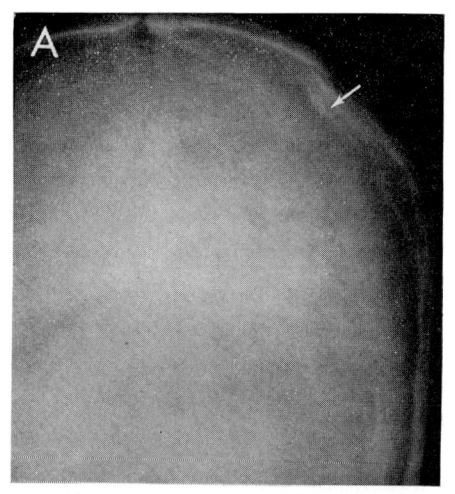

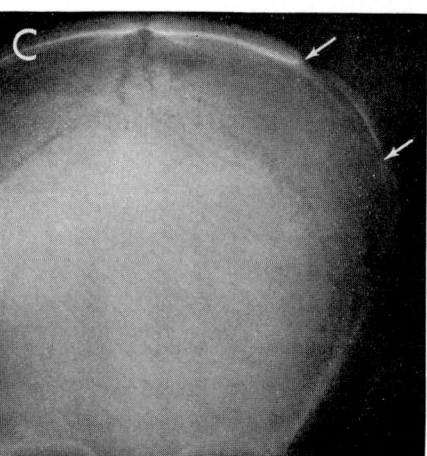

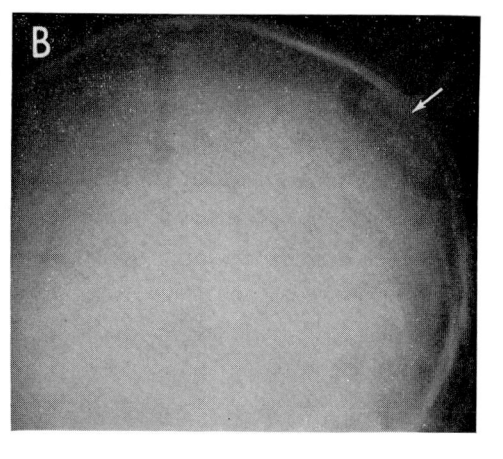

Fig. 15.6.—Depressed fracture with leptomeningeal cyst formation. Boy, 3, was struck by a truck and suffered a depressed fracture of the left parietal bone (arrow in **A**). The depressed fragments were elevated immediately but, because of laceration and avulsion of the dura, it was not possible to approximate the edges of the dura closely. Repeat x-rays eight days later showed good elevation of the bone fragments (**B**). Follow-up examinations revealed persistence of the bony defect on palpation. Repeat films showed not only inadequate bony healing but resorption and thinning of the adjacent margins of the skull (arrows in **C**). On reoperation, a small leptomeningeal cyst was noted beneath the site of the old fracture. A tantalum plate was inserted and the patient has done well. This case illustrates the need to demonstrate proper healing of skull fractures with follow-up films.

age by (1) direct contusion and laceration of nerve tissue and (2) tearing of the superior longitudinal or lateral sinuses with venous bleeding and thrombosis.

COMPOUND FRACTURES.—These should be considered from two viewpoints: (1) external compound fractures, i.e., those associated with a scalp laceration and (2) internal (occult) compound fractures, which are those contaminated from the outside by way of fractures into the air sinuses and through the tympanic membrane.

Complications of Skull Fracture

Formation of a leptomeningeal cyst.—Occasionally, instead of bony healing, follow-up x-ray examination shows progressive rarefaction of the skull adjacent to the fracture site. Taveras and Ransohoff[35] have discussed in detail the pathogenesis and management of seven patients with this complication. Presumably, a tear in the dura occurred with the initial injury and the arachnoid membrane is caught or pinched between the two edges of broken bone. Continuous pulsation of the brain gradually leads to bony resorption and "enlargement" of the fracture. These cysts in the subarachnoid space may enlarge and cause sizable defects in the skull and secondary pressure atrophy of the underlying brain substance. Occasionally these patients present with the complaint of head pain.[25] This complication alone emphasizes the need for serial x-ray examination at about three-month intervals to make certain of complete healing of skull fractures in children (Fig. 15.6).

Infections.—Compound fractures may be contaminated from the outside with bacteria. Infections limited to the extradural space may present as simple wound infection or as osteomyelitis of the skull. Diagnosis is established by wound infection, appropriate cultures and x-ray examination. Infection in the subarachnoid space (meningitis) often complicates compound skull fractures. Subdural empyema is rare and presents the same signs as subdural hematoma but is accompanied by clinical signs of infection. The signs and symptoms usually develop during the week after injury and differ in no way from those of hematogenous purulent meningitis. One should watch closely for meningitis in patients who have cerebrospinal fluid rhinorrhea and otorrhea. Intracerebral infection (abscess formation) is seen only rarely, especially after penetrating missile injuries. Diagnosis is made according to the criteria used for any brain abscess. The syndrome of recurrent meningitis is discussed in Chapter 18.

Rhinorrhea.—Bleeding from the nose is common in head injuries of varying severity. Always watch closely for persistent, clear discharge (of cerebrospinal fluid) after the bleeding has ceased. This complication results from a fracture through the cribriform plate and a tear in the dura and arachnoid which permits ready drainage of fluid to the outside. A persistent rhinorrhea per se represents no serious threat, but the almost inevitable secondary meningitis can pose an extremely difficult problem in accurate localization and management.

Cerebrospinal fluid rhinorrhea can be differentiated from ordinary nasal discharge by testing for glucose content, using filter paper impregnated with Benedict's solution (Clinistix). The cerebrospinal fluid will contain reducing substance, whereas ordinary nasal discharge will not. Contrast substances can be instilled into the lumbar subarachnoid space; with proper manipulation the material can be run into the head along the basal cisterns into the anterior fossa where the material may find an exit at the site of fracture. Sterile fluorescein (0.25 cc. of 5% fluorescein) can be instilled in the lumbar sac and its course followed with an ultraviolet (Wood's) lamp in a dark room.[24] A yellowish fluorescent glare in the region of the tympanic membrane, the nasal cavity or the paranasal sinuses can sometimes be demonstrated with the use of routine ENT instruments. Alternatively, Lipiodol can be used and the procedure carried out in the manner of myelography.

Otorrhea.—Bleeding from the ear usually indicates a compound fracture of the base which has caused a tear in the tympanic membrane. Persistent CSF otorrhea occurs much less commonly than rhinorrhea, but the diagnosis and management are the same and equally difficult.

Aerocele (pneumatocele) formation.—Rarely aerocele formation is a delayed complication of compound fracture. The cause is either (1) entry of air from a sinus (especially the frontal) when the patient sneezes or blows his nose or (2) gas formation from the growth of a contaminating anaerobic organism. The air or gas can be pocketed in the subarachnoid, intracerebral or intraventricular space. As a general rule, skull x-rays in this complication are interpreted erroneously as (1) bony rarefaction, (2) intracranial lipoma or (3) nonrecognition of the air contrast shadow.

Of interest is the fact that the value of diagnostic cerebral pneumography was discovered by accident in 1912.[26] The air-filled ventricles were noted on x-rays of the skull which were taken when a patient who had suffered an injury continued to complain of headache. A frontal aerocele which communicated with the ventricles accounted for the discovery which led to the technique of diagnostic pneumography in 1918.[10]

Scalp

AVULSION OF SCALP AND MENINGES.—Laceration and avulsion of the scalp and meninges present no serious diagnostic problem but do represent a major problem in first-aid and later repair for the plastic surgeon or neurosurgeon.

MANAGEMENT AND PROGNOSIS

The treatment of head injuries is tabulated in Table 15.2.

No Loss of Consciousness

The physician is frequently asked for advice in the proper management of head injury in a child when the patient does not lose consciousness but does exhibit vigorous crying, pallor, vomiting and drowsiness or inactivity. A judgment must be made, often over the telephone, about the need for medical examination and hospitalization. If the injury seems mild and consciousness is not lost, the following advice is suggested: (1) the parents should observe the child carefully and note the degree of responsiveness; (2) they should be instructed to wake the child every three hours during the first night to be sure that the child is in a normal sleep state and not in deepening stupor or coma; (3) the parents should

TABLE 15.2.—Treatment of Head Injuries

Type of Injury	Observations and Special Studies	Clinical Signs and Complications	Nonoperative Treatment	Operative Treatment
A. No loss of consciousness (mild closed injury)	1. Careful observation by parents 2. Wake from sleep every 3 hr. on first night 3. Seek medical examination for increasing headache, somnolence, paresis or unequal pupils		Aspirin in small amounts	
B. Loss of consciousness (moderate or severe injury)	1. Immediate, rapid survey for associated injuries 2. Portable x-rays of chest and abdomen 3. Record vital signs	1. Lacerations 2. Fractures 3. Pneumothorax Hemothorax 4. Ruptured spleen Ruptured viscus 5. Noisy, labored respirations 6. Hemorrhagic shock* 7. Restlessness, confusion, anxiety, pain	Oral airway Nasal oxygen Position patient on side I.V. blood, plasma, plasma substitutes* Glucose-electrolyte solutions* Warmth Small doses of rectal paraldehyde, I.M. sodium phenobarbital, codeine, Demerol Reassurance (Therapeutic hypothermia)	Suture lacerations Splint or cast fractures Closed chest drainage Abdominal laparotomy Tracheostomy Bronchoscopy Ligate bleeding vessels

C. Increased intracranial pressure
1. Hematoma formation
  a) Epidural
  b) Subdural
  c) Intracerebral
	Repeated neurologic examination
	Skull x-rays
	Echoencephalogram
	Angiogram
		Progressive stupor
		Papilledema
		Signs of uncal herniation
		Separated sutures
		Elevated CSF pressure
				a) Trephination with ligation of bleeding vessel
				b) Bilateral trephination, membrane re-

TABLE 15.2.—TREATMENT OF HEAD INJURIES—CONTINUED

TYPE OF INJURY	OBSERVATIONS AND SPECIAL STUDIES	CLINICAL SIGNS AND COMPLICATIONS	NONOPERATIVE TREATMENT	OPERATIVE TREATMENT
2. Cerebral edema		Progressive stupor Papilledema Signs of uncal herniation Separated sutures Elevated CSF pressure	a) I.V. 30% urea b) I.V. 20% mannitol c) I.V. and oral dexamethasone	moval and possible shunt in chronic cases c) Trephine opening and evacuation of clot (in selected cases)
D. Depressed fracture	Skull x-rays			Surgical elevation of depression
E. Compound fracture (including all basal fractures)	Skull x-rays	Rhinorrhea Otorrhea		Complete cleansing and debridement of wound Suture laceration Cranioplasty (usually deferred)

1. Infection
  a) Wound infection
  b) Meningitis
  c) Subdural empyema
  d) Brain abscess
  e) Osteomyelitis of skull
	Vital signs
	Cultures
	Lumbar puncture
	Angiogram
		Fever
		Meningitis
		Seizures
		Focal neurologic signs
			Antibiotics (see Appendix 5)	Surgical drainage

2. Rhinorrhea and otorrhea	Glucose test on fluid Locate CSF leak with fluorescein or Lipiodol	Rhinorrhea Otorrhea Meningitis (subarachnoid space)		Surgical repair and grafting
3. Aerocele	Skull x-rays	Headache (meningitis is a rare complication)	Antibiotics Avoid straining	

*See Appendices 3 and 4.

call the physician if the child manifests increasing headache, drowsiness, focal weakness, a seizure or unequal pupils.

Loss of Consciousness

Every person losing consciousness as a result of a head injury should be examined by a physician. An immediate, rapid survey should be carried out in a search for (1) evidence of active bleeding, (2) fractures elsewhere in the body, (3) lacerations, (4) chest injuries with signs of rib fractures, pneumothorax or hemothorax and (5) abdominal trauma with rupture of the spleen or a hollow viscus.

Adequate ventilation should be established immediately using an oral airway, mechanical suction and oxygen by way of a nasal catheter. If the patient is deeply stuporous or comatose and if secretions are pooling and respirations are persistently noisy and labored, a tracheostomy should be performed without delay. This will help prevent aspiration pneumonia, obstructive atelectasis and hypoxic cerebral edema. The patient should be placed on his side (unless some other injury contraindicates this position) so that both secretions and vomitus will drain out of the mouth by gravity.

Although hemorrhagic or hypovolemic shock does not commonly occur without intracranial hemorrhage or severe injury elsewhere in the body, one should be alert to signs of shock—rapid pulse, falling blood pressure and cool, sweaty skin. Therapy includes whole blood, plasma, plasma substitutes or glucose and electrolyte solutions (Appendices 3 and 4). Patients in shock should be kept warm. They should be given small doses of analgesics (codeine and Demerol) and reassurance. In general, sedatives should be used with caution in order not to aggravate restlessness and confusion and not to depress the respiratory center. Small doses of paraldehyde given rectally and sodium phenobarbital given intramuscularly may be used judiciously to control anxiety and restlessness and as prophylactic anticonvulsants in patients wtih cortical lacerations.

Use of a cooling mattress or ice-filled plastic bags has been advocated in patients with severe head injury. The purpose of such therapeutic hypothermia is to lower intracranial pressure and to reduce cerebral metabolism and in this way increase the brain's tolerance for anoxia. As yet this form of therapy has not received general acceptance because convincing proof of its value is lacking. Moreover, its use involves more vigilant nursing care and monitoring of vital signs because the necessary adjunctive use of chlorpromazine to prevent shivering enhances the risk of hypotension. Prolonged use of therapeutic hypothermia may mask the signs of intracranial hemorrhage and increase the incidence of pneumonia. The management of cerebral edema is discussed in Chapter 8 and Appendix 2.

Active hemorrhage should be arrested by ligating the bleeding vessels and applying direct pressure to prevent traumatic shock. If physical or x-ray examination reveals signs of a ruptured spleen or abdominal viscus, the patient should have a celiotomy to stop the bleeding and repair the ruptured organ. Patients with loculated air or blood in the pleural cavity may require closed chest drainage. Persistent respiratory distress in a patient whose upper airway is clear and who has been tracheostomized may require bronchoscopy to relieve obstructive atelectasis.

Patients who have contusions or lacerations of the brain as a result of head injury may develop post-traumatic epilepsy. A major epidemiologic problem, neurologic sequelae of head injuries have received much study and attention because the seizures are often quite intractable to anticonvulsant therapy and because mental changes may lead to major problems in social adjustment.[5]

Increased Intracranial Pressure

EPIDURAL HEMATOMA.—This diagnosis, if established or even strongly suspected, is an indication for exploratory burr holes to be made as soon as possible. An infusion should be started promptly, blood should be added as soon as it is cross-matched, and the patient should be taken to the operating room. The surgeon usually locates the clot without difficulty and he then identifies and ligates the bleeding vessel or vessels.[6]

SUBDURAL HEMATOMA.—Treatment consists of (1) subdural aspiration of liquid blood, (2) bilateral trephinations to remove clots and to look for the formation of fibrous membranes, (3) craniotomy for complete clot and membrane removal (when possible) and (4) a "universal shunt" if necessary in the rare case.

Subdural aspiration establishes the diagnosis in infants and also provides a simple way to remove liquid blood and fluid until the clot organizes and can be completely removed surgically. Generally 20–30 cc. of fluid is removed at a time. In the presence of bilateral fluid accumulations, it is recommended that the two sides be tapped on alternate days after the increased intracranial pressure has been relieved. When the spaces are tapped dry or if large quantities of fluid are still obtained after a week, plans for bilateral burr holes should be made.

Bilateral trephinations may be carried out as a separate procedure or as the first step before turning a craniotomy flap. In patients with large chronic subdural masses a burr hole may be made to explore for a membrane, and a major procedure for membrane removal is then carried out on the same side. At a later date the same steps can be taken on the opposite side. In patients with acute subdural hematomas the condition is often discovered before membranes have had time to develop. In these, the hematoma may be removed by suction and irrigation through one or more enlarged burr holes. Drainage of bloody, yellow cerebrospinal fluid can be expected, sometimes for weeks.

Craniotomy is done when complete removal of clots and membranes cannot be achieved through the trephine openings. Often a thick outer membrane is densely adherent to the dura and can be removed without risk to the patient. The inner membrane generally adheres to the pia so that its removal often cannot be effected without causing fresh bleeding and possible damage to the cortex. Small transfusions may be necessary to compensate for blood loss during these procedures.

Shunt procedures must be considered in those unusual cases of chronic subdural hematoma or hygroma in which there is evidence of much brain atrophy in addition to persistent copious accumulation and drainage of cerebrospinal fluid, and a fistulous connection between the subarachnoid and subdural spaces is suspected. Such a communication probably results from an arachnoid tear and accounts for the rapid reaccumulation in the subdural space of relatively clear fluid which may act as a compressive mass leading to further brain atrophy.

Calcified subdural hematoma.—Chronic subdural hematomas calcify in rare instances and become obvious on plain skull x-rays. Surgical removal of the calcified clots is not usually indicated because the associated neurologic deficit is not benefited.[26b]

Prognosis.—In our opinion the long-term prognosis in these patients must

216   TRAUMA

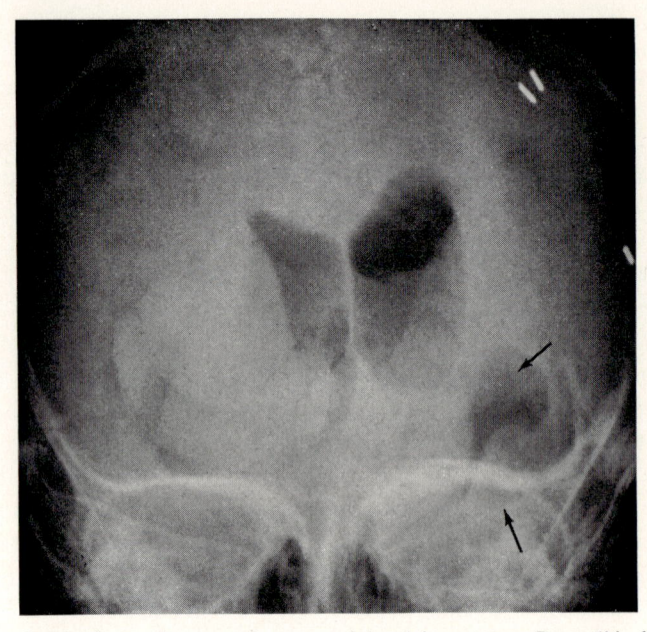

Fig. 15.7.—Cerebral atrophy secondary to subdural hematoma. Boy, 5½, had a series of convulsions at age 3 months. Head enlargement was noted, and a left subdural hematoma was evacuated surgically. At present he is moderately retarded and has bilateral corticospinal tract signs, greater on the right than on the left. The pneumoencephalogram shows marked dilatation of the left lateral ventricle, including the temporal horn (upper arrow), underdevelopment of the left hemicranium with elevation of the left sphenoid ridge (lower arrow). This syndrome of retardation, hemiparesis and potential seizure disorder occurs commonly with large subdural hematomas unless they are detected and treated early.

be guarded. Acute symptoms and signs are readily relieved by the foregoing procedures but irreversible deficit may become apparent only after months or years of observation.[11a]

When the diagnosis is made reasonably promptly, the prognosis for life is very good. However, in our experience the neurologic morbidity in these patients is high. Residual deficits include mental retardation, seizures, spastic hemiparesis or quadriparesis and behavior disorders (Fig. 15.7).

INTRACEREBRAL HEMATOMA.—This complication should be considered in any patient with head injury that takes a progressive course or in which the other findings (especially subdural) do not seem sufficient to account for the severity of the clinical signs. Such patients should have burr holes and exploratory subcortical needling of the brain substance. If an intracerebral clot is encountered, craniotomy is usually necessary to evacuate the clot and debride the necrotic brain satisfactorily.

Depressed Fractures

All depressed skull fractures should be elevated surgically. This policy is especially important in infants and young children in whom the rapidly growing brain may be compromised by depressed bone fragments, thereby creating a potentially epileptogenic focus in the cerebral cortex. Although elevation of the depressed fragments may be delayed until the patient's general condition has improved, the procedure should be carried out before the patient leaves the hospital. No attempt should be made in the early first-aid care of the wound to elevate bone fragments, since one must be prepared to encounter and control new bleeding, especially in the area of the large venous sinuses.

Compound Fractures

Compound fractures are common in middle childhood and should be treated definitively by thorough debridement and removal of all foreign material, bone fragments and necrotic tissue. Although this operative therapy should be carried out promptly, it should be delayed long enough to transport the patient to a hospital with facilities large enough for the job to be done completely. In the event of such delay, the patient should have (1) emergency shock therapy, (2) proper provision for adequate ventilation, (3) prophylactic antibiotic therapy and (4) a sterile dressing applied over the scalp wound which has been widely shaved and cleansed.

INFECTIONS.—Contaminated wounds of the scalp, meningeal spaces and brain may cause wound infections, meningitis, extradural or subdural empyema, osteomyelitis of the skull and brain abscess. The principles of management of all these infections are covered in Chapter 18 and Appendix 5.

CEREBROSPINAL FLUID RHINORRHEA OR OTORRHEA.—The discharge usually stops spontaneously without operative intervention, but if the condition persists, it carries with it the threat of repeated bouts of meningitis. Once the diagnosis of either of these difficult and persistent conditions is established (p. 210 f.) and the point of leakage localized, a craniotomy should be performed. After the dural tear and the fracture line are identified the surgeon must decide whether to close the tear primarily or to cover the defect with a dural flap or a graft of fascia lata. Until there has been sufficient time for healing, antibiotic therapy should be given and the patient should be instructed to avoid excessive straining and forceful nose blowing.

AEROCELE FORMATION.—Usually the air enters through a fracture into a paranasal sinus and the air pocket is absorbed spontaneously without complications. However, one must be prepared to treat secondary intracranial infections and to repair the dural defect as in the case of rhinorrhea or otorrhea.

Avulsion of Scalp and Dura

In patients who have severe compound fractures with loss of bone and soft tissue (scalp and dura), the wound is closed as tightly as possible. In most cases, however, plastic procedures designed to repair the defect in the bone or in the avulsed scalp or dura are carried out at a later time. Grafts of bone, periosteum and dura and pedicle skin flaps may be needed to provide adequate protection to the brain and to achieve the best cosmetic end result.

Spine and Spinal Cord

Sprain, Subluxation, Fracture and Dislocation

PATHOGENESIS.—Most spine injuries are caused by vehicular accidents, falls or diving. Simple sprains of the neck or lower back can result from contusion or laceration of the supporting spinous ligaments without bony or cord injury. Severe sprains in the same areas may cause abnormal alignment or mobility of the vertebral column, i.e., subluxation, with nerve root compression and muscle spasm. In violent injury, especially with a whiplash component, fracture and fracture-dislocation can occur with degrees of damage to nerve roots and spinal cord varying from minor compression of a root to complete cord transection.

CLINICAL AND LABORATORY DIAGNOSIS.—At the time of the accident it may be difficult to assess accurately the extent of the injury because of the acute pain and fright, the condition of spinal shock and the common coincidence with head injury. In sprain and subluxation there are local pain and tenderness, limitation of motion, muscle spasm and symptoms of nerve root irritation. Objective findings may include diminished or altered sensation in one or more dermatomes (Fig. 15.8) as well as depressed reflexes and an altered pattern of sweating. Fractures and dislocations in the cervical region may cause flaccid paralysis and anesthesia of the arms, trunk and legs, leading to a flail chest and exclusively diaphragmatic breathing. Urinary incontinence appears, bladder emptying becomes automatic and the deep tendon reflexes are lost. Injury to the dorsal or lumbar spine causes the same signs except that the arms and chest are not involved. When the period of spinal shock has cleared in a few days or weeks, much of the neurologic deficit may disappear if cord transection has not taken place.

After necessary first-aid measures have been taken, the whole spine should be x-rayed if the patient's condition permits his being moved to the x-ray department. Films should be inspected for signs of subluxation (Fig. 15.8, *A*) and linear or compression fractures of the laminae, pedicles and vertebral bodies. One may find an atlantoaxial dislocation with or without a fractured odontoid process. Cervical spine dislocations may occur at any level, but compression fractures are most common in the dorsolumbar spine, especially involving the tenth to twelfth dorsal vertebrae.

As in the case of severe head injuries, one should look for x-ray damage to other parts of the skeleton. One should also look for air in the peritoneal cavity if the patient's clinical condition suggests a ruptured viscus.

MANAGEMENT.—Great care should be taken in moving any child with a suspected spine injury. Excessive twisting, flexion or extension must be avoided. In general, patients should be placed carefully on a stretcher in the supine position and a blanket or folded coat put under the shoulders in the case of a neck injury or under the site of injury if the trauma has occurred in the thoracic or lumbar area. General measures aimed at the treatment of shock—adequate airway, oxygenation, control of hemorrhage, sedation and restraints—are used as soon as the patient is admitted to the hospital.

Definitive medical and surgical treatment.—The severity of the bony injury and of the neurologic deficit determines the mode of management. Isolated linear fractures of a vertebra without neurologic deficit can be managed with rest on a firm bed, a cervical collar or a body cast for four to eight weeks. Compression fractures and dislocations in the cervical region are treated initially with halter head traction and slight extension. Subsequently, direct skull traction with Crutchfield tongs in older children (Fig. 15.8, *B*) and with metal bands passing between bilateral burr holes in infants and younger children must be applied for eight to 10 weeks, followed by the use of a brace or cast for several months. Cervical subluxations which do not respond to traction may require surgical fusion (Fig.

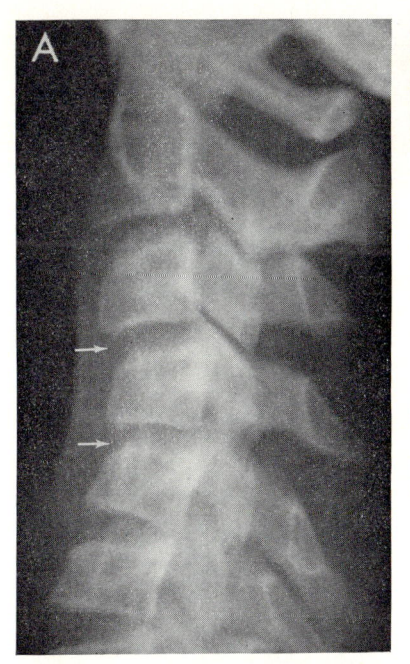

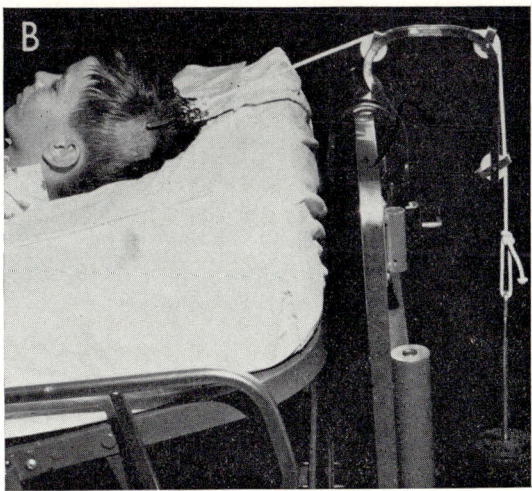

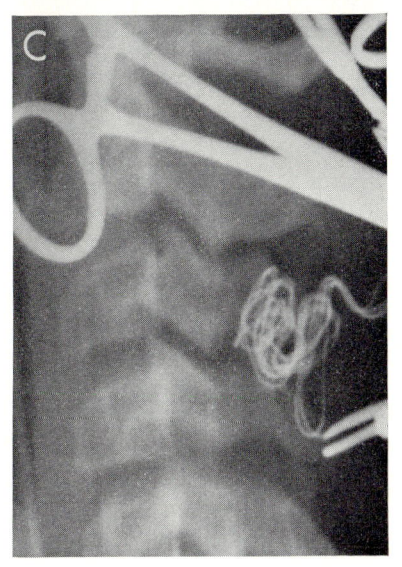

Fig. 15.8.—Subluxation injury to cervical spine. Two weeks after an auto accident this 13-year-old boy sought medical help because of neck pain. Examination revealed local tenderness of the upper cervical spine, marked muscle spasm, a discrete C_4 dermatome sensory loss on the left side and no other deficit. A revealed a subluxation of C_3 on C_4 and C_4 on C_5. The patient was placed in traction with Crutchfield tongs (B) for 10 days and then a fusion of the spinous processes of C_{3-4} and C_{4-5} was carried out, bringing about reduction of the subluxation (C).

15.8, C). Thoracic and lumbar compression fractures are treated with a hyperextension cast and a Stryker frame when necessary.

When the diagnosis of cord compression is established without doubt by clinical and x-ray evidence, open reduction and decompression should be performed, followed by spinal fusion. Nasogastric tube feeding may be required at first. Later, intensive nursing care is essential to prevent the formation of decubitus skin lesions. It may be necessary to place an indwelling catheter in the bladder. The catheter should be removed periodically until the patient is able to void spontaneously or automatically at regular intervals.

PROGNOSIS.—In patients with sprain, subluxation and fracture not associated with significant neural damage the prognosis is good provided satisfactory nursing care and physical therapy are added to proper medical and surgical support. However, with cord transection, the outlook depends upon the location and the severity of the lesion. High cervical transection may lead to death immediately by causing paralysis of all muscles of respiration. Transection below the level of the fifth cervical does not interfere with diaphragmatic breathing, but in these patients one must prevent or treat complications such as pneumonia, urinary tract infections and decubitus ulcers. When incomplete transection occurs, strength, sensation and bladder function return in varying degrees over a period of many months. The patient may be left with an automatic bladder, flexor spasms of the legs and the threat of chronic renal infection and insufficiency.

Peripheral Nerves

Mechanical and Postinjection Trauma

Mechanical trauma to cranial nerves occurs most frequently in association with head injury. Damage to large, single nerves, although uncommon in children, can result from deep lacerations, fractures or penetrating wounds. Most often seen are lacerations of the median and ulnar nerves at the wrist and injury to the sciatic nerve in the buttock or the radial nerve in the upper arm due to faulty intramuscular injections.

Table 15.3 lists the clinical signs which aid in the diagnosis of the more common peripheral nerve injuries. The reader is referred to other sources for more details.[22,27,28]

MANAGEMENT AND PROGNOSIS.—If a peripheral nerve has been partially or completely severed and the wound is clean and recent, the severed ends should be sutured together primarily and without tension. Splinting of the extremity may be necessary to avoid tension on the suture line. Repair of an injured nerve is delayed when the wound is contaminated or when the nerve injury is associated with much soft-tissue injury or fracture. The decision to carry out exploration, neurolysis and nerve suture is made only if spontaneous regeneration is not anticipated. During the period of waiting electromyographic and nerve stimulation studies may help in deciding whether to explore the nerve or to wait longer for spontaneous recovery of function. Occasionally autogenous nerve grafts may be required to approximate normal function in an extremity, but such an approach requires expert judgment and experience. Physiotherapy also has an important role in restoring the part to a normal level of functioning.

Postinjection sciatic neuropathy is managed with early exploration and neurolysis in some clinics,[19] despite the fact that full recovery may occur in three to six months without surgical intervention.[2,9] Early sciatic nerve neurolysis can be justified by (1) the rationale of avoiding what may appear later as unwarranted delay and (2) the relatively simpler technical problems with a procedure in this area. In the series of Combes et al.,[8] recovery of function was incomplete in most cases, but the average period of follow-up was relatively short and most of the patients were newborn infants. In our opinion, the value of operation in this condition has not been clearly established, and the decision to operate or to follow the patient without operation must depend upon the physician's judgment as well as the skill and experience of the neurosurgical consultant.

TABLE 15.3.—DIAGNOSTIC SIGNS OF PERIPHERAL NERVE INJURIES

NERVE	USUAL TYPE OF INJURY	ABNORMAL POSTURE or DEFORMITY	MAJOR MUSCLE WEAKNESS	AREA OF ABSOLUTE SENSORY DEFICIT
Radial	Humerus fracture, especially supracondylar; injection into lower deltoid	Wristdrop	Triceps, dorsiflexors of wrist and fingers	Dorsum of hand between thumb and forefinger
Median	Laceration at wrist	Extension of first two fingers and flexion of other fingers	Flexors of thumb and index fingers; Opposition of thumb	Volar aspect of index finger
Ulnar	Laceration of wrist and humeral fracture	Clawhand	Flexion of ring and 5th fingers	Volar aspect of 5th finger
Sciatic	Faulty injections or lacerations of buttocks; postdislocation of hip	Foot drop	Dorsiflexors of foot; Flexors of leg	Sole of foot; Plantar aspects of toes
Peroneal	Fracture of upper fibula	Foot drop	Dorsiflexors of foot	Dorsum of foot between great and second toes
Long thoracic	Pressure of straps or heavy weights on the shoulder	Winging of scapula on anterior elevation of arm	Elevators of arm above horizontal plane	—

Traumatic neuropathies which result from the injection of therapeutic or prophylactic drugs and biologicals are at least theoretically preventable. Injections into the buttocks and deltoid area have been abandoned and even prohibited by many hospitals and clinics, being replaced by injections into the midanterior thigh. This policy is applied to all age groups in many units despite the greater frequency of sciatic complications in premature infants and small children.

Facial palsies which appear in infants delivered by forceps nearly always disappear spontaneously because the nerve injury is partial.

The prognosis depends upon the type of peripheral nerve injury, its severity and its location. Some general comments have already been made about birth injuries to the facial nerve and what one can expect with postinjection neuropathies. In traumatic mononeuropathies in the extremities, good return of function may be expected if the injury is mild or if primary suturing is carried out. However, if the injury is severe and is associated with retraction of severed nerve ends, neuroma formation and other soft-tissue damage, recovery is often incomplete despite optimal surgical and physical therapy. Diagnostic nerve conduction studies may aid in prognostication.

Natal (Birth) Injury

Head

The over-all incidence of intracranial birth injuries is not well documented and, unless one restricts a study to fatal birth injuries, it seems unlikely that completely satisfactory clinical studies of neurologic morbidity can be carried out with

TABLE 15.4.—LOCATION OF NEONATAL INTRACRANIAL HEMORRHAGE DUE TO
BIRTH TRAUMA AND ANOXIA[17]

MECHANICAL TRAUMA	ANOXIA

1. Rupture of superior cerebral veins
   a) Convexity subdural hematoma (Fig. 15.4)
   b) Middle fossa subdural hematoma (Fig. 15.5)
2. Tentorial lacerations involving the vein of Galen and the large venous sinuses
   a) Subtentorial hemorrhage
   b) Generalized subarachnoid and subdural hemorrhage
	1. Terminal veins
	   a) Subarachnoid hemorrhage (Fig. 16.6)
	2. Veins in pia mater
	   a) Isolated subpial hemorrhages (Fig. 16.6)
	3. Subependymal veins
	   a) Subependymal hemorrhage
	   b) Intraventricular hemorrhage (Fig. 16.7)

real accuracy. Nonetheless, a long-term anterospective collaborative study of this problem has been in progress in the United States for 10 years under the auspices of the U.S. Public Health Service (the Perinatal Research study) and useful data may accrue eventually.

PATHOGENESIS.—Intracranial damage at birth results from hemorrhage or ischemic damage to brain tissue. The hemorrhage in turn results either from direct trauma (more frequent in the full-term infant) or in certain cases from asphyxia (more common in the premature infant) (Table 15.4). Often, of course, mechanical trauma and anoxia act jointly to cause bleeding, and a single causative mechanism cannot be identified clinically. Damage to the nervous system which is considered anoxic is covered in Chapter 16 and is not discussed further here.

Occasionally in newborn infants depressed skull fractures are a result of either digital or forceps trauma. "Ping-pong ball" fractures may be depressed without comminution, fragmentation or damage to the brain or blood vessels by virtue of the elastic quality of membranous bone at this age. Blood clots which accumulate beneath the pericranium and which are confined within the limits of the suture lines are called cephalhematomas. They are due to the trauma of prolonged or difficult labors and their course is usually benign. We have seen several complications from overzealous obstetric use of vacuum extractors. Complications resulting from the use of these devices include severe subgaleal hemorrhage, herniation of the brain and ventricular system,[1] scalp trauma[29] and skull fracture.

CLINICAL AND LABORATORY DIAGNOSIS.—The diagnosis of intracranial hemorrhage (or anoxic neuronal damage) is difficult because the clinical signs are nonspecific and may be a reflection of a serious anomaly of the nervous system, an intrauterine infection, cardiopulmonary disease, intoxication from maternal analgesics and anesthetics or an inherited metabolic defect. The common signs include (1) irregular respirations or apnea, (2) a weak, high-pitched cry, (3) poor suckle or vomiting, (4) cyanosis or pallor, (5) restlessness or inactivity, (6) an incomplete Moro reflex and (7) seizures or opisthotonus. In some infants abnormal eye movements, ptosis of an eyelid and focal paresis point more specifically to intracranial hemorrhage (Fig. 15.4).

Examination of the cerebrospinal fluid is often carried out, especially if it is thought that the diagnosis of neonatal meningitis must be differentiated. It is known, however, that the normal birth process is traumatic to the extent that slight

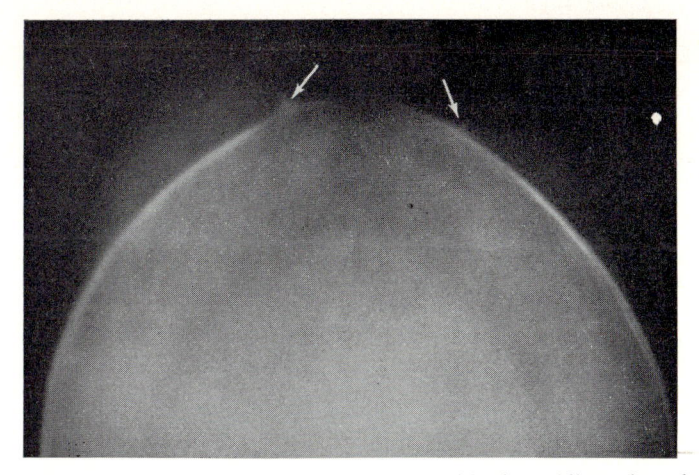

Fig. 15.9.—Bilateral cephalhematomas. Note that with these bilateral cephalhematomas the soft-tissue mass stops at the line of the sagittal suture. Also note the peripheral rims of calcification (arrows). To palpation, these often feel like a depressed fracture.

intracranial bleeding may occur without clinical signs. Routine lumbar puncture in normal newborn infants may reveal an increased number of erythrocytes, xanthochromia and elevated total protein content of the cerebrospinal fluid. Consequently, the diagnosis of significant subarachnoid bleeding may be difficult.[30,34,39]

Subdural taps are useful, as is pneumoencephalography. Angiography may be needed to establish a diagnosis which is in doubt. Serial hematocrit determinations have been employed in clinical research as a tool in the diagnosis of intracranial hemorrhage in prematures. Although it is impractical to recommend them as a matter of routine, the physician should be encouraged to utilize repeated hematocrit readings in any newborn infant with suspected bleeding.

Cephalhematomas may be confused at times with encephaloceles, caput succedaneum and depressed skull fractures. About half of the cephalhematomas are associated with linear skull fractures. They are distinguished by their restricted parictal location, but they may resemble a depressed skull fracture because of the firm peripheral rim surrounding the organizing liquid clot. In some cases, only a skull x-ray will distinguish a cephalhematoma from a depressed fracture (Fig. 15.9). Caput succedaneum, a diffuse scalp swelling, involves that segment of the soft tissues which presents through the mother's dilating cervix. It may be confused with encephalocele over the cranial vault, but the latter lesion is associated in all cases with a defect in the skull, cranium bifidum, which can be seen on x-ray.

MANAGEMENT AND PROGNOSIS.—The patient's general condition must be stabilized with general supportive newborn care, blood transfusion, reduction of increased intracranial pressure and, if necessary, repeated subdural taps. If the baby's vital signs are stable and the cardiopulmonary status is satisfactory, it may be advisable to evacuate a clot surgically (Fig. 15.4), contrary to the conservative stand recommended by some workers. This procedure should be undertaken with much caution, however, since these babies often have subarachnoid and subpial hemorrhage as well as damage or disease in other organ systems.

Vitamin K prophylaxis (0.5 mg. intramuscularly within one hour after birth) appears to protect premature and medium-sized infants against large hemorrhages over the brain convexities but has no influence on asphyxial hemorrhages.[16]

Cephalhematomas should always be treated conservatively, and the temptation to aspirate or drain a large fluctuant clot must be resisted because of the high risk of producing a serious soft-tissue infection. Caput succedaneum likewise requires no specific therapy and should be managed conservatively.

Depressed "ping-pong ball" fractures in the newborn should be elevated surgically when the baby's condition is stable. The procedure is usually not difficult because comminution of the bone is uncommon. Such fractures are operated upon since they will not reduce themselves spontaneously in spite of the fact that there may be no real break in the continuity of the bony cortex.

The prognosis in the newborn with intracranial hemorrhage must be very guarded. The physician should be neither too gloomy nor too optimistic in predicting the neurologic outcome until he has sufficient evidence upon which to base his decision. Without a doubt, many of these infants will have permanent motor deficit of the spastic type, as well as seizures, mental retardation and behavior disorders, but predicting such sequelae in the individual case is extremely difficult. Repeated neurologic examinations are most helpful and only in the minority of cases do electroencephalograms and pneumoencephalograms aid clinical predictions in the early months of life.

Spinal Cord and Spine

PATHOGENESIS.—Obstetric injuries to the spinal cord almost always occur during difficult breech deliveries or version and extraction maneuvers. Byers[3] has focused special attention on this clinicopathologic entity. Traction on the baby's

Fig. 15.10.—Severe cord avulsion and hematoma formation from a birth injury. (Reprinted from Towbin, A.: Arch. Path. 77:620, 1964.)

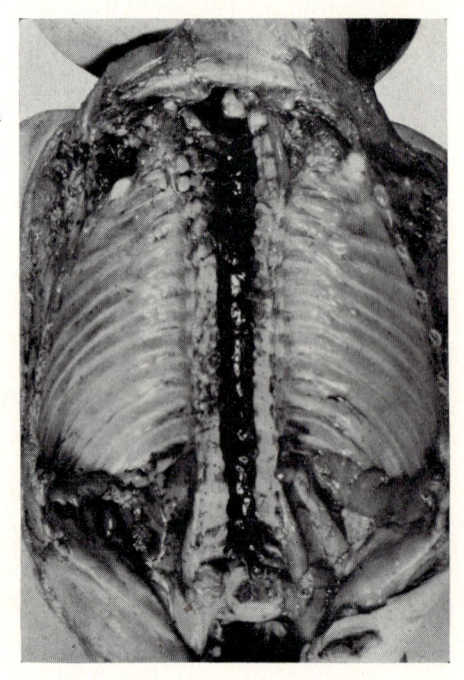

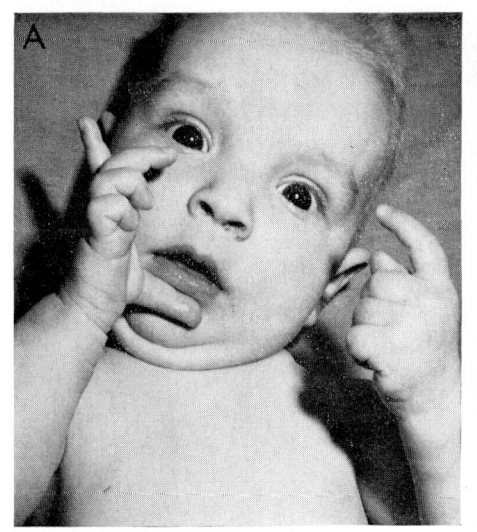

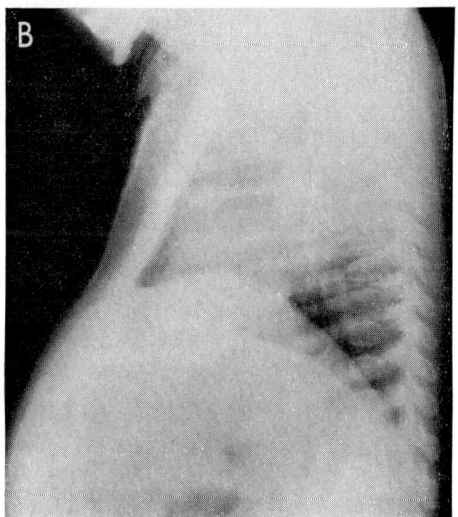

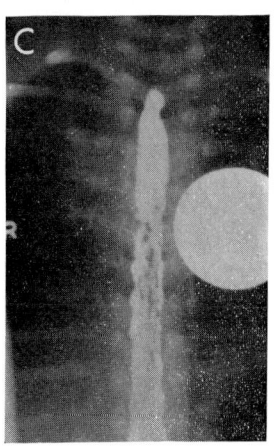

Fig. 15.11.—Cord avulsion from breech delivery. **A**, 2½-month-old infant was delivered by breech and had considerable respiratory distress and cyanosis. Initially the diagnosis of congenital heart disease was considered, but several weeks later the peculiar posturing of the hands was noted along with weakness and hyporeflexia in the arms. There were mild spasticity in the legs and ankle clonus. The chest moved poorly, the breathing being almost entirely diaphragmatic (see lateral chest x-ray, **B**). Lumbar puncture showed xanthochromic fluid with a high protein value. A myelogram, **C**, revealed a complete block at T_1. Contusion, avulsion and hematoma formation of the lower cervical cord as a result of difficult breech delivery caused this sequence of events.

trunk with fixation of the aftercoming head in the pelvis leads to excessive hyperextension of the neck. The latter maneuver causes stretching of the spinal cord to the point where there is contusion, subarachnoid hemorrhage, hematomyelia or, in some cases, complete rupture (Fig. 15.10). The focal damage to the cord usually occurs in the upper thoracic or lower cervical area. Fracture and/or dislocation is seen only rarely with birth injuries in contrast to spine trauma in older children and adults. Towbin[37] has pointed out that, in addition to direct trauma to the cord, autopsy frequently shows avulsion of the spinal roots and brachial plexus as well as hemorrhage into the brain stem.

CLINICAL AND LABORATORY DIAGNOSIS.—The clinical picture varies with the severity of the injury and at times may offer some diagnostic difficulty. In the severe case the infant may appear acutely ill and may resemble infants with the respiratory distress syndrome or with intracranial hemorrhage. Ford[14] has pointed out that in some cases the subarachnoid bleeding is sufficient to cause cerebral symptoms. The neurologic basis for the signs may remain obscure for several days until limited movement and impaired sensation in the legs are noted. Arm movement may seem quite good, but hand weakness occurs in nearly all cases (Fig. 15.11, *A*) and sensation is lost below the clavicles. The high thoracic site of the lesion causes intercostal paralysis, so that the respiratory effort is diaphragmatic (Fig. 15.11, *B*). Initially the tendon reflexes in the legs may be hypoactive due to spinal shock, but later hyperreflexia and spasmodic reflex movements appear. In early stages urinary retention or constant dribbling may occur, succeeded in rare instances by the pattern of an automatic bladder which discharges at regular intervals, often in response to sensory skin stimuli. In a minority of cases one may find focal clinical signs of injury to the brachial plexus (see below). Injury to the brain stem is usually proved only in fatal cases but should be suspected in infants with severe respiratory distress and apnea.

When traction damage or avulsion of the cord is suspected, a lumbar puncture may disclose bloody or xanthochromic cerebrospinal fluid with an elevated protein content. If myelography is necessary for diagnosis, 3–4 ml. Pantopaque may reveal an obstruction in the lower cervical or upper dorsal region, especially if the injury is associated with hematoma formation (Fig. 15.11, *C*).

Peripheral Nerves

PATHOGENESIS.—*Brachial plexus injuries.*—Stretching or avulsion birth injuries of the brachial plexus represent the commonest examples of peripheral nerve trauma in childhood. Two types of injury occur. Upper arm (Erb) palsy, involving the fifth and sixth cervical roots or the upper trunk of the plexus, results either from difficulty in breech delivery of the aftercoming head or from excessive traction on the shoulders in difficult vertex delivery. Lower arm (Klumpke) palsy, involving the lower cervical roots, results from any obstetric maneuver which causes hyperabduction of the arm at the shoulder. Occasionally there are associated fractures of the clavicle or the humeral neck. The lower arm type of palsy is occasionally seen also in young children as a result of rough play or of swinging a child by one arm with all of his weight suspended at the shoulder. Fortunately, in most such injuries the clinical signs reflect only edema and contusion, but occasionally avulsion and complete rupture of the roots or nerves occur.

Facial nerve injuries.—Compression of the facial nerve at birth by obstetric forceps or by pressure of the face against the sacral prominence is quite common, but fortunately the dysfunction is usually only temporary and full recovery takes place. Hepner[17a] found that in 6.4% of 875 consecutive births the infants had facial paresis which did not seem related to the use of forceps. However, the side of the weakness did seem related to the side of the head which lay next to the sacral prominence.

The clinical findings associated with the important nerve injuries of the upper and lower extremities are outlined in Table 15.3.

MANAGEMENT AND PROGNOSIS.—One finds a general consensus about the inadvisability of exploring brachial plexus injuries not only because of the technical difficulties involved but because of the generally good prognosis for recovery with conservative management. If no return in function is noted and there is a history of hematoma formation and residual thickening in the supraclavicular area, exploration is carried out by some surgeons as pointed out by Ingraham and Matson.[19]

Other Physical Injuries to the Nervous System

In addition to direct head trauma, the brain, cord and peripheral nerves can be injured physically by excessive irradiation and electric current. Physical factors such as severe burns, sunstroke, decompression sickness and ultrasound will not be discussed here because of their extreme rarity in children.

Radiation Injury

PATHOGENESIS.—The effects of excess prenatal irradiation on the nervous system are covered in Chapter 13 (p. 176). In postnatal life damage to the nervous system occurs most frequently as a result of excessive roentgen therapy for tumors or chronic skin eruptions[15] or by accident. The potential danger to the nervous system of atomic bomb fallout radiation is still fortunately only a theoretical problem. Death usually results from the blast injury or systemic factors.

CLINICAL AND LABORATORY DIAGNOSIS.—Excessive irradiation of the head causes acute and chronic reactions. In the acute reaction, which is often fatal, symptoms consist of nausea and vomiting, drowsiness and stupor and finally convulsions, ataxia and death. These symptoms may not reach a peak until a month after exposure, whereas in the chronic reaction symptoms appear from one to seven years later. Scholz and Hsu[32] described patients with dementia, seizures, focal deficit and death. Ford[15] observed a patient who received roentgen therapy for ringworm of the right side of the scalp several years before a left hemiparesis, cortical sensory loss and refractory focal fits developed. Operative exploration revealed extensive atrophy and scarring of the cortex beneath the area of alopecia on the scalp.

The syndrome of myelomalacia secondary to irradiation of neoplasms in the spinal cord and spinal canal is now well documented. Itabashi and associates[20] reported a series of cases in which the neurologic deficit was clearly related to radiotherapy and the clinical findings were those of a partial transverse myelopathy (the Brown-Sequard syndrome). These patients exhibit loss of proprioception and pyramidal tract signs on the side of the radiation-induced cord lesion, with contralateral loss of pain and temperature. Our experience is similar to that of Itabashi *et al.* Radiation damage to nerve roots and peripheral nerves is rarely seen but can cause slowly progressive lower motor neuron deficit (both sensory and motor signs).

MANAGEMENT AND PROGNOSIS.—Obviously, in the case of radiation injury, the best treatment is prevention. Acute injury requires good supportive care, including (1) careful asepsis, (2) antibiotic therapy for established infections, (3) transfusions of fresh blood and platelet-rich plasma and autologous bone marrow transplantation in imminently fatal cases and (4) proper fluid and electrolyte therapy. The management of the chronic effects of radiation is the same as that of any chronic neurologic deficit (see Part I).

Electric Current

PATHOGENESIS.—Accidental electric shocks are due to contact with high-tension currents used in industry or to lightning. Most patients either die promptly as the result of ventricular fibrillation or they recover completely. Rarely patients survive an episode of near-electrocution. The neurologic damage occurs in the spinal cord and peripheral nerves more often than in the brain itself.

CLINICAL AND LABORATORY DIAGNOSIS.—In the acute stage of injury, the patient loses consciousness and has convulsive seizures. Death results either from ventricular fibrillation or from anoxic respiratory arrest secondary to circulatory collapse. Transient paraplegia with anesthesia affects some patients, a phenomenon which is poorly understood. Late signs of electrical damage to the nervous system rarely produce permanent deficit. Evidence of peripheral nerve damage occurs most often as a sign of chronic neurologic damage. Obviously, it is often difficult to differentiate late cerebral signs of injury (dementia, hemiplegia, subjective sensory symptoms) from other organic diseases and hysteria. Electroshock therapy, commonly used in adults for the treatment of severe mental depression, regularly causes transient loss of memory and change in personality.

MANAGEMENT AND PROGNOSIS.—Immediate therapy is directed at cardiopulmonary resuscitation. Most general hospitals have intensive care units which are elaborately equipped and able to handle such problems. In emergency situations, where first-aid is needed, artificial respiration, closed-chest cardiac massage and intracardiac administration of epinephrine may be necessary.

As previously indicated, patients who survive the initial shock will, in most cases, have no residual deficit.

BIBLIOGRAPHY

1. Bajwa, R.: An unusual complication of vacuum extraction, Lancet 1:630, 1965.
2. Bray, P. F.: Unpublished data.
3. Byers, R.: Cerebral Palsy, in Brennemann-Kelley: *Practice of Pediatrics* (Hagerstown, Md.: W. F. Prior Company, Inc., 1965), vol. IV.
4. Caffey, J.: Multiple fractures in the long bones of infants suffering from chronic subdural hematoma, Am. J. Roentgenol. 56:163, 1946.
4a. Caveness, W. F.: Onset and cessation of fits following craniocerebral trauma, J. Neurosurg. 20:570, 1963.
5. Caveness, W. F., and Liss, H. R.: Incidence of post-traumatic epilepsy, Epilepsia 2:123, 1961.
5a. Childe, A. E.: Localized thinning and enlargement of the cranium, Am. J. Roentgenol. 60:1, 1953.
6. Clare, F. B., and Bell, H. S.: Extradural hematomas, J.A.M.A. 177:887, 1961.
7. Clark, D. B.: Subdural Hygroma, in Nelson, W. E. (ed.): *Textbook of Pediatrics* (8th ed.; Philadelphia: W. B. Saunders Company, 1964).
8. Combes, M. A., et al.: Sciatic nerve injury in infants, J.A.M.A. 173:1336, 1960.
9. Curtiss, P. H., and Tucker, H. J.: Sciatic palsy in premature infants, J.A.M.A. 174:1586, 1960.
10. Dandy, W. E.: Ventriculography following the injection of air into the cerebral ventricles, Ann. Surg. 68:5, 1918.
11. Davidoff, L. M., and Dyke, C. G.: Relapsing juvenile chronic subdural hematoma: Clinical and roentgenographic study, Bull. Neurol. Inst., New York 7:95, 1938.
11a. Echlin, F. A., et al.: Acute, subacute and chronic subdural hematoma, J.A.M.A. 161:1345, 1956.
12. Evans, J. H.: Post-traumatic epilepsy, Neurology 12:665, 1962.
13. Evans, J. P.: Advances in the understanding and treatment of head injury, Canad. M. A. J. 95:1337, 1966.

14. Ford, F. R.: Breech delivery in its possible relations to injury of the spinal cord, Arch. Neurol. & Psychiat. 14:742, 1925.
15. Ford, F. R.: *Diseases of the Nervous System in Infancy, Childhood and Adolescence* (5th ed.; Springfield, Ill.: Charles C Thomas, Publisher, 1966).
16. Gröntoft, O.: Intracranial hemorrhage and blood-brain barrier problems in the newborn: Pathologico-anatomical experimental investigation, Acta path. et microbiol. scandinav., supp. 100, 1954.
17. Haller, E. S., et al.: Clinical and pathologic concepts of gross intracranial hemorrhage in perinatal mortality, Obst. & Gynec. Surv. 11:179, 1956.
17a. Hepner, W. R.: Some observations on facial paresis in the newborn infant: Etiology and incidence, Pediatrics 8:494, 1951.
18. Ingraham, F. D. and Matson, D. D.: Subdural hematoma in infancy, J. Pediat. 24:1, 1944.
19. Ingraham, F. D. and Matson, D. D.: *Neurosurgery of Infancy and Childhood* (2d ed.; Springfield, Ill.: Charles C Thomas, Publisher, 1961).
20. Itabashi, H. H., et al.: Postirradiation cervical myelopathy, Neurology 7:844, 1957.
21. Jennett, W. B.: *Epilepsy after Blunt Head Injuries* (Springfield, Ill.: Charles C Thomas, Publisher, 1962).
22. Johnson, E. W.: Examination of muscle weakness in infants and small children, J.A.M.A. 168:1306, 1958.
23. Kempe, C. H., et al.: The battered-child syndrome, J.A.M.A. 181:17, 1962.
24. Kirchner, F. R.: Use of fluorescein for the diagnosis and localization of cerebrospinal fluid fistulas, Surg. Forum 12:406, 1961.
25. Low, N. L., and Correll, J. W.: Head pain due to leptomeningeal cysts, Brit. J. Surg. 53:791, 1966.
26. Luckett, W. H.: Air in the ventricles of the brain following a fracture of the skull, Surg., Gynec. & Obst. 17:237, 1913.
26a. Marshall, S., and Hinman, F.: Subdural hematoma following administration of urea for diagnosis of hypertension, J.A.M.A. 182:813, 1962.
26b. McLaurin, R. L., and McLaurin, K. S.: Calcified subdural hematomas in childhood, J. Neurosurg. 24:648, 1966.
27. Medical Research Council: War Memo No. 7. *Aid to the Investigation of Peripheral Nerve Injuries* (2d ed.; London: Her Majesty's Stationery Office, 1943).
28. Merritt, H. H.: *Textbook of Neurology* (4th ed.; Philadelphia: Lea & Febiger, 1967).
28a. Mock, H. W.: *Skull Fractures and Brain Injuries* (Baltimore: Williams & Wilkins Company, 1950).
29. Munsat, T. L., et al.: A comparative clinical study of the vacuum extractor and forceps: II. Evaluation of the newborn, Am. J. Obst. & Gynec. 85:1083, 1963.
30. Otila, E.: Studies on the cerebrospinal fluid in premature infants, Acta path. et microbiol. scandinav., supp. 100, 1954.
30a. Pevehouse, B. C., et al.: Ophthalmologic aspects of diagnosis and localization of subdural hematoma, Neurology 10:1037, 1960.
30b. Rodin, E. A., et al.: Electroencephalographic findings associated with subdural hematoma, A.M.A. Arch. Neurol. & Psychiat. 69:743, 1953.
31. Rothballer, A. B.: Traumatic cerebellar hematoma in the newborn, J. Neurosurg. 19:913, 1962.
31a. Russell, W. R.: Disability caused by brain wounds: Review of 1166 cases, J. Neurol. Neurosurg. & Psychiat. 14:35, 1951.
31b. Russell, W. R., and Whitty, C. W. M.: Studies in traumatic epilepsy, J. Neurol. Neurosurg. & Psychiat. 15:93, 1952.
32. Scholz, W., and Hsu, Y. K.: Late damage from roentgen irradiation of the human brain, Arch. Neurol. & Psychiat. 40:928, 1938.
33. Silverman, F. N.: The roentgen manifestations of unrecognized skeletal trauma in infants, Am. J. Roentgenol. 69:413, 1953.
34. Silverman, W. A.: *Dunham's Premature Infants* (3d ed.; New York City: Paul B. Hoeber, Inc., 1961).
35. Taveras, J. M., and Ransohoff, J.: Leptomeningeal cysts of the brain following trauma with erosion of the skull, J. Neurosurg. 10:233, 1953.
36. Taveras, J. M., and Wood, E. H.: *Diagnostic Neuroradiology* (Baltimore: Williams & Wilkins Company, 1964).
37. Towbin, A.: Spinal cord and brain stem injury at birth, Arch. Path. 77:620, 1964.
38. Walker, A. E.: Post-traumatic epilepsy, World Neurol. 3:185, 1962.
39. Widell, S.: On the cerebrospinal fluid in normal children and in patients with acute abacterial meningo-encephalitis, Acta paediat. (supp. 115) 47:1, 1958.
40. Woolley, P. V., and Evans, W. A.: Significance of skeletal lesions in infants resembling those of traumatic origin, J.A.M.A. 158:539, 1955.

16

Hypoxia

Etiology	CNS Pathology
Prenatal Disease	
Placental "Insufficiency"	Necrosis of cortical neurons
Placenta Previa	Diffuse
Premature Separation of Placenta	Focal (hippocampal, occipital, basal ganglia)
Torsion of Umbilical Cord	
Neonatal Disease (Respiratory Distress Syndrome)	Periventricular leukomalacia
	Hemorrhage
Prematurity	Subarachnoid
Hyaline Membrane Disease	Subependymal
Pulmonary Hypoperfusion	Intraventricular
Maternal Oversedation	Uncal herniation (see also Chapter 8)
Intracranial Disease (Hemorrhage, Anomaly)	
Postnatal Disease	
Near Drowning	
Strangulation	
Toxic Respiratory Arrest (Chapter 20)	Necrosis of cortical neurons
Poisoning with Carbon Monoxide (Chapter 20)	Diffuse
	Focal (hippocampal, occipital)
Cardiac Arrest	
Congenital heart disease with arrhythmia	
Severe seizures	
Fever	
Cerebral scar (birth anoxia)	
Congenital anomaly (e.g., microgyria)	
Metabolic defect (e.g., hypoglycemia)	
Hereditary degenerative disease (e.g., tuberous sclerosis)	Cerebral edema
Intoxication (water, lead, etc.)	
Hypertensive encephalopathy (acute glomerulonephritis and hyperadrenocorticism)	
Supratentorial Mass with Uncal Herniation (Ischemia)	
Status epilepticus—swollen hemisphere	

Hematoma (subdural or epidural)
Cerebral hemisphere tumor
Toxic cerebral edema (water, lead, hyponatremia)
Hippocampal infarction—sclerosis
Calcarine infarction—sclerosis
Pontine hemorrhage
Arterial or venous thrombosis

Pathogenesis

HYPOXIC DAMAGE to the brain induces pathologic changes which can be distributed diffusely or focally. Four general categories of anoxia cause disease of the brain: (1) *Anoxic anoxia* in which normal hemoglobin is not adequately saturated with oxygen. This type causes essentially all types of prenatal and postnatal anoxic tissue damage. (2) *Ischemic anoxia* in which occlusive disease of the blood vessels causes tissue anoxia. This type, in conjunction with hemorrhage, causes most postnatal anoxia. (3) *Stagnant anoxia* in which arrest of heart action (from congenital heart disease or general anesthesia) causes nerve tissue damage. (4) *Anemic anoxia* in which the brain is supplied with insufficient oxygen as a result of abnormal hemoglobin binding (carbon monoxide poisoning) or hemoglobin deficiency (severe anemia).

Unfortunately, the accurate assessment of anoxia as a primary etiologic factor in brain damage (which can be well established on clinical grounds) poses a major scientific epidemiologic problem. This is especially true in the unborn and newly born infant. Obviously, in the child who is clinically normal before an anoxic insult and then abruptly shows neurologic impairment, there is no significant diagnostic problem. However, one may never be certain (unless the infant dies) whether severe asphyxia in the newborn infant is due to a primary anoxic brain insult or has resulted from (1) an occult cerebral anomaly, (2) a small intracranial hemorrhage, (3) an obscure metabolic disturbance, such as vitamin B_6 dependency, (4) an intoxication from maternal oversedation during delivery or (5) undiagnosed intrauterine sepsis. Despite the difficulties of accurate clinical diagnosis in a given case, the various etiologies of hypoxia and the resulting neuropathologic states are quite well known. These are shown in the outline at the beginning of this chapter.

Prenatal Hypoxia

In the opinion of many workers vascular accidents involving the placenta and cord, such as placenta previa, premature separation of the placenta, "placental insufficiency" (Fig. 16.1) and torsion of the umbilical cord, cause many cases of anoxic brain damage.[3a] However, until adequately controlled, statistically significant, anterospective studies are performed (such as the long-term perinatal research study being conducted by the U.S. Public Health Service), the evaluation of etiologic factors in any given case will remain extremely difficult and at present is largely speculative. In one recent series by Banker and Larroche[2] nine of 51 infants who died with evidence of anoxic encephalopathy had "placental abnormalities." This finding was more common in premature than in full-term infants.

Neonatal Hypoxia

Anoxia occurs far more frequently in the newborn premature than it does in the full-term infant and usually results from apnea. The apnea in turn may be due

232 HYPOXIA

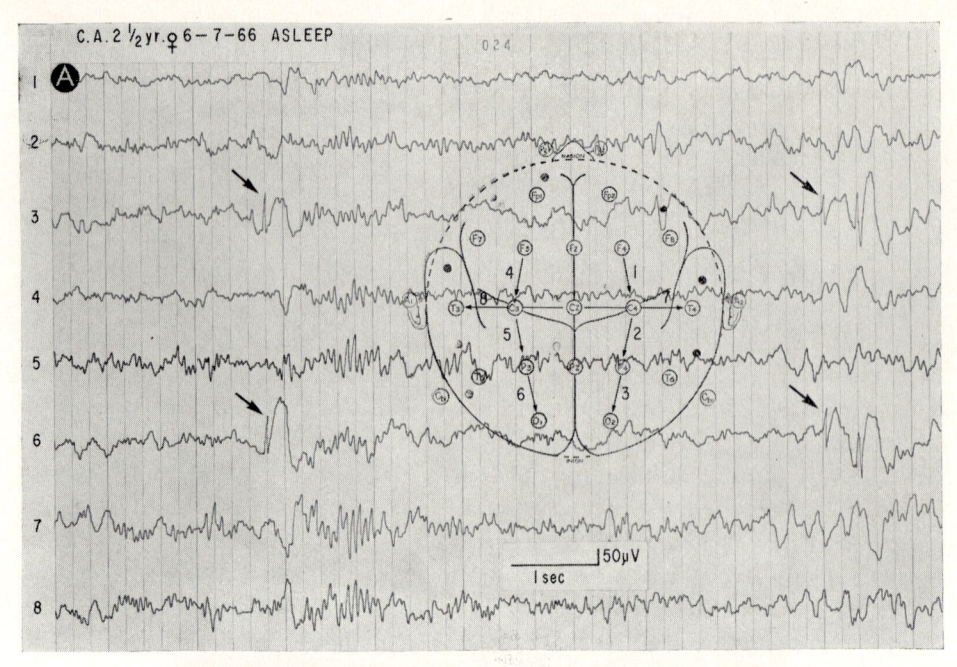

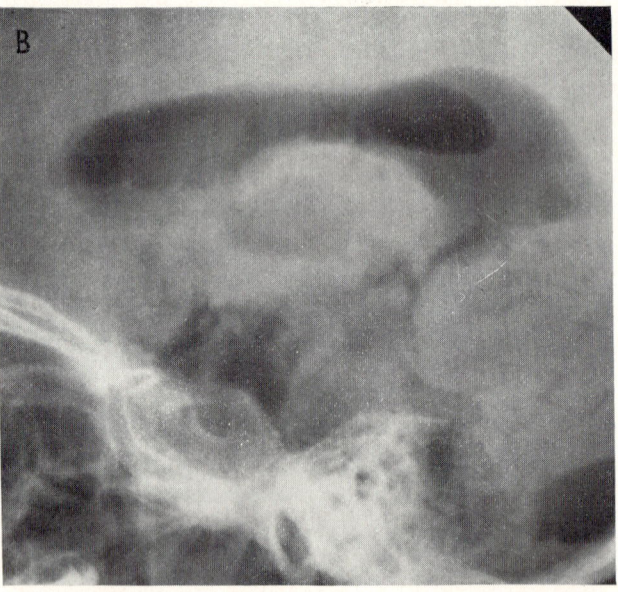

Fig. 16.1.—Placental insufficiency—anoxic brain damage. The 18-month-old girl was the product of a *45-week* pregnancy. Labor was induced, the birth was uncomplicated (birth weight, 8 lb.), but the cord and placenta were "discolored and degenerated" and the amniotic fluid was meconium-stained. The baby appeared normal until 5 hours of age when generalized seizures began. After much initial difficulty with seizure control, only occasional seizures subsequently occurred. At 18 months microcephaly, motor and mental retardation were noted. **A,** epileptiform EEG record shows frequent, bilaterally synchronous, brief spike wave discharges, most prominent in bioccipital regions. **B,** a pneumoencephalogram reveals generalized ventricular dilatation which was more marked in the atria and occipital horns. Diagnosis was placental insufficiency with prenatal cerebral anoxia. EEG and PEG findings suggest that the occipital lobes may have suffered preferentially from the atrophic process. (Compare with Fig. 16.9.)

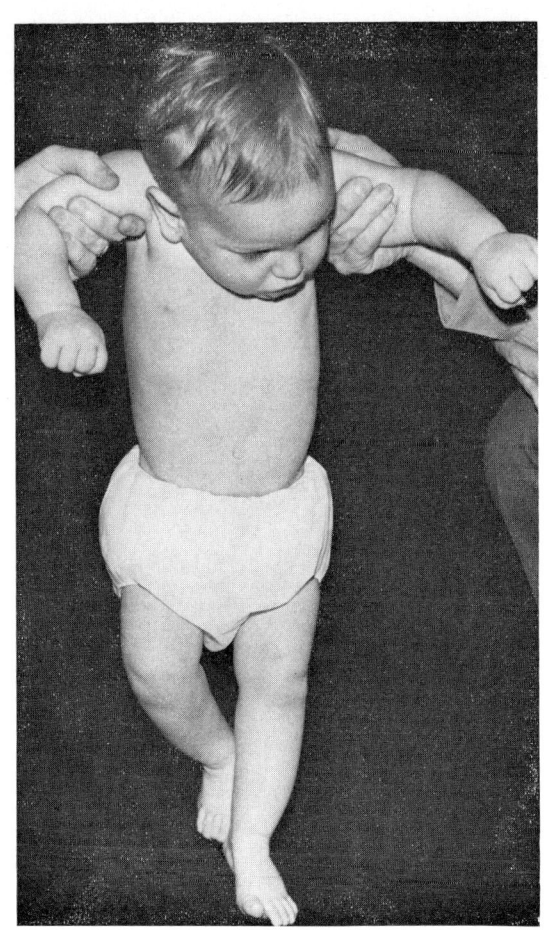

Fig. 16.2.—Neonatal apnea with diffuse anoxic cerebral damage secondary to breech delivery. This 13½-month-old baby boy, the product of a normal pregnancy, had severe respiratory distress following a prolonged breech delivery. After 12 minutes of apnea, during which he required intubation and artificial respiration, he began to breathe. Shortly after, spasticity was noted. He did not hold his head up until 8 months of age and at 13 months he could not sit. He has a moderate spastic quadriparesis, bilateral "cortical" hands (held fisted) and persistent grasp reflexes. He smiles frequently and inappropriately (probably due to pseudobulbar palsy with emotional incontinence). Note the poor head support, the tendency for the legs to "scissor" and the clenched fists.

to the respiratory distress syndrome—an incompletely understood multifactorial problem associated with a diminished amount of the intra-alveolar enzyme surfactant, vascular underperfusion of the lungs, systemic metabolic acidosis and pulmonary atelectasis. Apnea may also be secondary to congenital heart disease or maternal oversedation during delivery. Extremely rarely, newborn infants will become anoxic as a result of primary muscle weakness, in conditions such as neonatal myasthenia gravis.

Anoxia occurring in the prenatal or neonatal period causes three basic types of pathologic change in the brain: (1) loss of cortical neurons which may be diffuse or focal (Figs. 16.2 and 16.3), (2) periventricular leukomalacia[2] (Fig. 16.4) and (3) hemorrhage—subarachnoid, subependymal or intraventricular—in the premature[5,10] (Figs. 16.5–16.7). For years the concept of hippocampal-uncal-amygdaloid sclerosis has been attributed to local ischemia of the inferior mesial aspect of the temporal lobe as the result of circulatory compromise of the anterior choroidal and posterior cerebral arteries at the time of birth.[3] The high incidence of this lesion at operation or autopsy in patients with epilepsy has intensified interest in this concept. Localized areas of cortical infarction and atrophy (or sclerosis or ule-

234   HYPOXIA

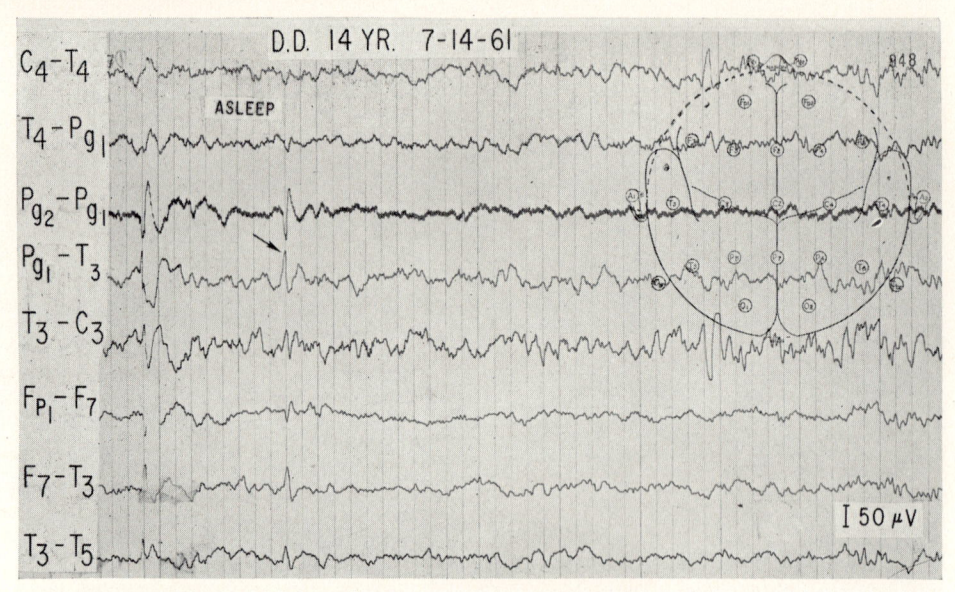

Fig. 16.3.—Temporal lobe epilepsy secondary to prematurity with neonatal anoxia. Boy, 14, had had seizures since infancy. The product of a 7-month pregnancy (birth weight, 4 lb.), he was kept in the hospital for six weeks after birth because of cyanosis and respiratory distress. Generalized seizures with fever in the first two years were followed by psychomotor episodes (dizziness, confusion, swallowing movements and incoherent speech) which have never been fully controlled with anticonvulsant drugs. In addition he is withdrawn and quiet, has very few friends and differs strikingly from his siblings in personality. Intellectual functioning is good (Full Scale IQ 116) but some subtest scores are in the brain-injured range. Repeated electroencephalograms have shown a left temporal spike focus, most active in recordings from the left pharyngeal area. A pneumoencephalogram and a left carotid arteriogram were normal. Clinical diagnosis was hippocampal sclerosis (secondary to neonatal anoxia and prematurity) with psychomotor epilepsy.

Fig. 16.4.—Hypoxia in a premature with presumed periventricular leukomalacia. The patient, a 3-month-old boy, who was born prematurely (weight 3 lb. 10 oz.), had recurrent episodes of apnea with cyanosis and tachycardia and bilateral pulmonary infiltrates, presumably due to aspiration pneumonia. Examination showed a feeble, irritable baby with poor suckle and swallow. Fundi were normal and subdural taps were dry. Spinal tap revealed water-clear fluid which contained 1 lymphocyte and *113 mg./100 ml. protein*. The pneumogram reproduced here reveals slight but definite ventricular dilatation. Clinical diagnosis was mild hypotensive hydrocephalus. The presumptive clinical diagnosis of anoxic cerebral damage (periventricular leukomalacia) is based upon the course of events, the CSF protein, the ventricular dilatation and the absence of other diagnostic evidence. Definitive diagnosis of this entity can be made only with tissue examination.

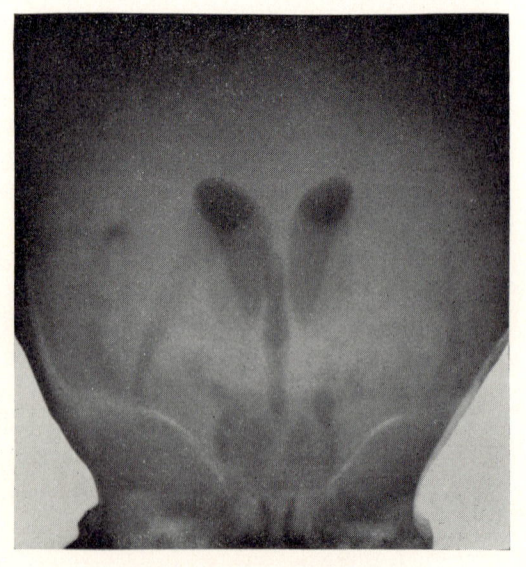

PATHOGENESIS 235

CLINICAL CONSIDERATIONS

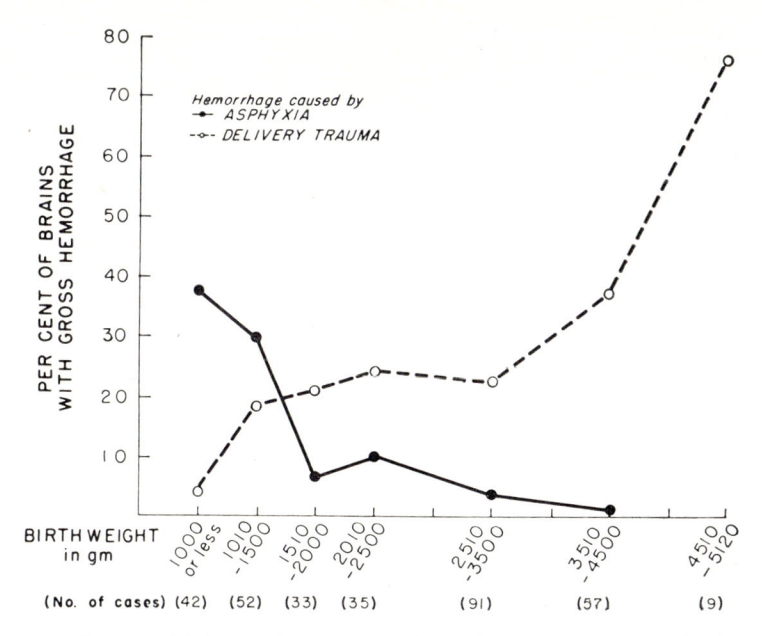

Fig. 16.5.—Intracranial hemorrhage due to hypoxia and trauma. Asphyxia caused 43 hemorrhages, 27 from the terminal subependymal veins, 12 from the leptomeningeal veins, 3 in the parenchyma and 1 from the choroid plexus. (From Silverman, W. A.: *Dunham's Premature Infant* [3d ed.; New York City: Paul B. Hoeber, Inc., 1961].) Modified from Gröntoft.[5]

Fig. 16.6.—Hypoxic subarachnoid hemorrhage in premature. Boy was born at 26 weeks as a footling breech, weighing 1,075 Gm. No spontaneous respiration occurred. Intubation, suction and mouth-to-mouth resuscitation gradually brought about irregular respirations with much cyanosis. X-rays showed atelectasis, and he died 18 hours after birth. The autopsy specimen shows subarachnoid and subpial hemorrhages. Also, the simple gyral architecture of the premature can be seen.

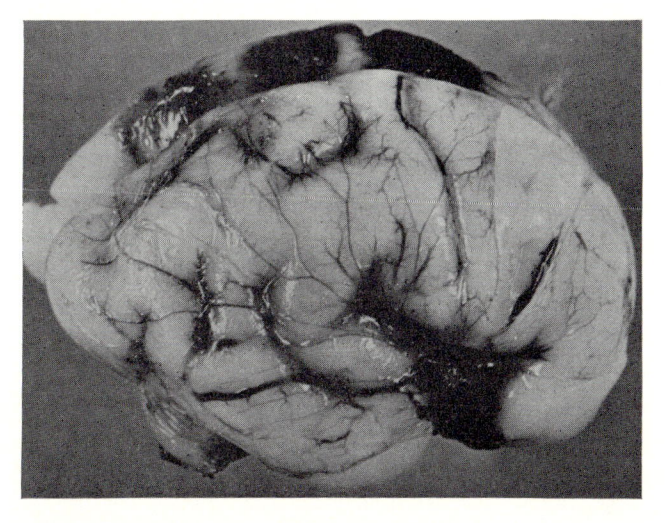

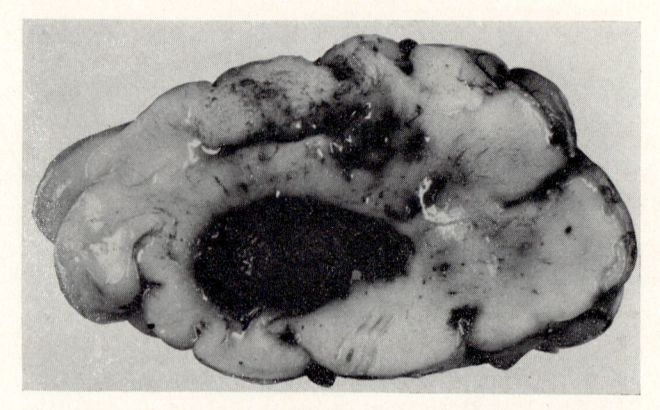

Fig. 16.7.—Hypoxic intraventricular hemorrhage in premature. Premature infant (4 lb. 11 oz.) was the product of a pregnancy complicated by polyhydramnios and a midforceps delivery. Apnea was present at birth along with cyanosis and flaccidity. Artificial respiration was continued until death at 32 hours. At autopsy much fluid blood covered the ventral surface of the cerebrum, brain stem and cerebellum. The sagittal section reveals a blood-clot cast filling the ventricular system. The latter finding, common in prematures, is due to anoxic subependymal venous bleeding which ruptures into the ventricle.

gyria) can occur, as can a peculiar change in the basal ganglia referred to as *état marbré*.[4]

An extensive neuropathologic study of 13 brains showing cerebral atrophy and encephalomalacia was reported by Wolf and Cowen.[13] The authors believe that anoxia played a major role in the etiology and pathogenesis of the severe, diffuse brain damage.

Postnatal Hypoxia

Anoxia which occurs after the neonatal period can have a wide variety of causes (p. 239). Basically the brain is damaged via one of two mechanisms: primary cortical neuron anoxia or secondary tissue anoxia from uncal herniation. Primary anoxia can cause diffuse damage to the neurons of the cerebral cortex or localized anoxia of the cells in the hippocampus, the cerebellar cortex and the basal ganglia. To a lesser extent, the subcortical white matter in infants (Fig. 16.4) is the site of ischemic lesions. The direct type of hypoxia results from a severe or prolonged seizure or series of seizures. Such severe seizures may result from a high fever in an infant, a cortical "scar" secondary to birth anoxia (Fig. 16.8), a congenital anomaly acting as an epileptogenic focus, a metabolic disorder such as hypoglycemia or phenylketonuria, a degenerative disease such as tuberous sclerosis or toxic factors such as water and lead. Other causes of hypoxia include (1) cardiac arrest secondary to an arrhythmia induced by congenital heart disease or a general anesthetic, (2) respiratory arrest from a variety of drugs (e.g., barbiturates) and, more commonly, (3) near drowning, (4) strangulation and (5) hypertensive encephalopathy.

Secondary anoxia can cause tissue damage as a result of *uncal herniation*. The need for an awareness of this concept is stressed in this text because we believe that many physicians do not appreciate the frequency with which this mechanism

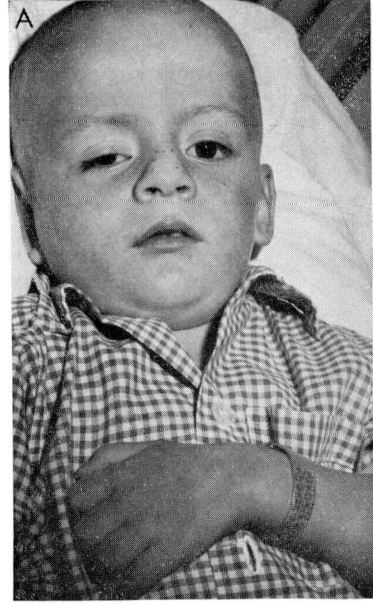

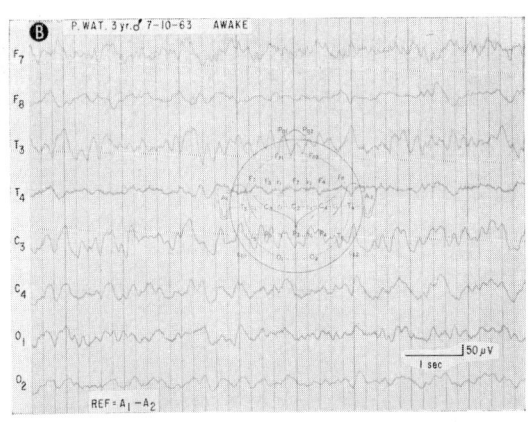

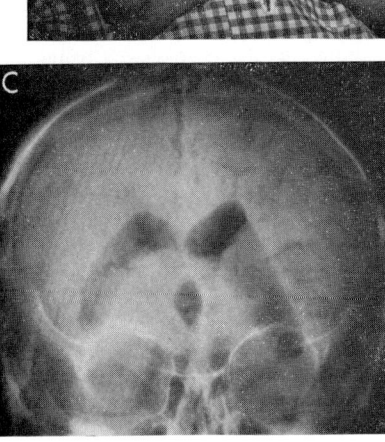

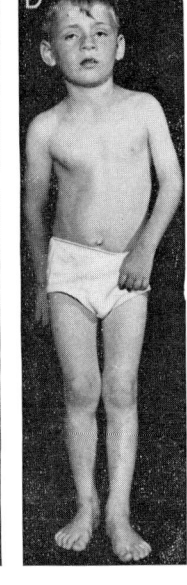

Fig. 16.8.—Status epilepticus (acute toxic encephalopathy) with residual hemiparesis and mental retardation. The patient weighed 4 lb. 10 oz. at birth and had marked neonatal asphyxia with apnea and cyanosis. Although he developed more slowly than his siblings, he reached the developmental milestones at a normal age. Febrile seizures began at 14 months, with recurrences at 20 and 29 months. At age 3 he had an episode of left focal motor status epilepticus associated with coma, papilledema, a left hemiparesis and a right third-nerve palsy (note right-sided ptosis in A), with some right-sided EEG flattening (compare F_8 and T_4 with F_7 and T_3 in B). A ventriculogram (C) showed moderate ventricular dilatation, absence of air over the right hemisphere and slight depression of the body of the right lateral ventricle. At the current age of 6 (D), he exhibits moderate mental retardation, a left hemiparesis, markedly hyperactive, unmanageable behavior and a seizure disorder that is well controlled.

This sequence of events and this syndrome occur commonly in children, emphasizing the importance of preventing recurrent convulsions in infancy, regardless of the cause (see text). In retrospect, this boy had recurrent febrile seizures which resulted eventually in status epilepticus. The episode of status led to the clinical picture of acute toxic encephalopathy and resulted in a persistent left hemiparesis. The ventriculogram and clinical findings are compatible with acute cerebral edema with evidence of diffuse cerebral atrophy. Whether the atrophy resulted from neonatal anoxia, recurrent febrile seizures, or both, is conjectural. That the hemiparesis resulted from the episode of status seems probable.

occurs and the damage which it can produce. The uncus of the temporal lobe herniates through the incisural notch as a consequence of numerous factors which can raise the supratentorial pressure. Among these are hypoxic cerebral edema secondary to status epilepticus (Fig. 16.8), subdural or epidural hematoma, toxic cerebral edema from excessive water, lead or hyponatremia and a tumor of the cerebral hemisphere. The herniation damages brain tissue by (1) compromising the anterior choroidal blood supply to the hippocampus with residual scar formation

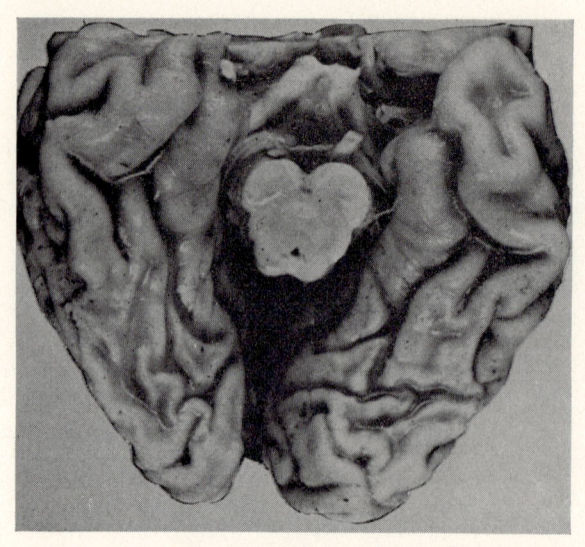

Fig. 16.9.—Occipital lobe atrophy secondary to status epilepticus in patient with phenylketonuria. Following a normal pregnancy and birth the patient did well until age 3 months when slow motor development was noted along with eczema. At 6½ months she had an ictal episode associated with prolonged cyanosis (10–15 minutes). In the hospital, recurrent generalized and left focal motor seizures were noted as well as slight microcephaly, motor retardation and typical infantile eczema. The mother volunteered that, following the seizure and severe cyanosis, the infant seemed less alert and appeared not to see. The retardation subsequently became more apparent and the diagnosis of phenylketonuria was made. The patient died at age 13. A 17-year-old brother has the same disorder but is less severely affected. Autopsy showed bilateral occipital ulegyria (compare the shrunken occipital gyri with the normal-sized temporal gyri). This type of atrophic process is commonly seen in this region as the result of compromised circulation of the posterior cerebral arteries secondary to severe seizures, anoxia and uncal herniation. These major pathologic brain changes were attributed to anoxia—not to phenylketonuria.

which is potentially epileptogenic,[8] (2) compromising the posterior cerebral blood supply to the calcarine cortex, resulting in ulegyria with residual cortical blindness[12] (Fig. 16.9) and sometimes hemiparesis, (3) venous or arterial thrombosis with secondary infarction and (4) venous hemorrhages into the brain stem from back pressure, often causing death by damage to the vital centers (Fig. 8.1, p. 85).

Clinical and Laboratory Diagnosis

The physician may be asked to evaluate the evidence of anoxic brain damage at the time of the asphyxic episode or at some later date.

Prenatal and Neonatal Hypoxia

Clinical signs shortly after an episode of asphyxia are notoriously nonspecific in the neonate: weak cry, poor suckle, lethargy, inactivity, abnormal Moro response, opisthotonus and in some cases seizures.[2] This constellation of clinical signs strongly suggests serious brain damage, but no positive confirmatory diagnostic tests are available to differentiate an anoxic etiology from other causes. An occult cerebral anomaly is suspected if the infant's head transilluminates an abnormal amount of light (Fig. 13.6, p. 134, and Fig. 13.14, p. 144), and an intracranial hemorrhage can be considered if the hematocrit is low or failing, if a subdural clot is found or if there is gross evidence of bleeding in the lumbar cerebrospinal fluid. However, the fact that many normal newborn infants have numerous erythrocytes, xanthochromia and elevated CSF protein for days and weeks following delivery makes cautious interpretation of CSF findings mandatory. A metabolic disturbance such as neonatal hypoglycemia, neonatal hypocalcemia or vitamin B_6 dependency or an intrauterine infection of the fetus causing sepsis or meningitis can usually be recognized with proper chemical and bacteriologic studies. A Tensilon test to rule out neonatal myasthenia gravis should be performed on any hypotonic newborn with respiratory distress if there is no good alternative explanation for the difficulty.

Over a century ago Little[7] made a major contribution to our understanding of natal anoxia when he pointed out that some birth complications result in mental retardation and bilateral spasticity (viz., Little's disease). The multiplicity of symptoms and signs (motor and mental retardation, seizure disorders[8] (Fig. 16.3), spasticity, intention or action myoclonus,[6] choreoathetotic cerebral palsy, language disturbances, behavior disorders, microcephaly and cortical blindness[12]) calls for a broad and thorough study of such chronically, neurologically handicapped children. In Part I the differential diagnosis of these syndromes is considered at length.

In summary, one must differentiate anoxic neonatal brain damage from (1) congenital malformations, (2) transient or hereditary metabolic or degenerative disorders, (3) trauma (subdural hematoma), (4) inadequately treated meningitis, (5) primary muscle diseases and in some cases idiopathic epilepsy. Examples of patients in whom brain damage was undoubtedly due to prenatal and neonatal anoxia are shown in Figures 16.1 and 16.2. Laboratory studies useful in the thorough study of late effects of anoxia include (1) head measurements, (2) psychometric examination, with special attention to tests which measure visual-motor disturbances, (3) electroencephalography and (4) pneumoencephalography.

Postnatal Anoxia

Regardless of the basic disease etiology and the pathologic mechanisms involved, the clinical and laboratory sequelae of hypoxia are similar. The symptoms and signs which develop in the acute stage are described in detail in Chapter 2 under Postseizure Hemiplegia. Chronic deficits resulting from severe hypoxia include dementia (mental retardation), seizures (generalized and "psychomotor" or temporal lobe attacks), hyperactive behavior disorders, aphasia or retarded speech development, hemianopia or cortical blindness, and astereognosis with poor hand use.

Abnormalities in the electroencephalogram, the pneumoencephalogram and plain skull x-rays, in measurements of head circumference and in psychometric performance nearly always provide documentary evidence of the organic structural basis of these clinical syndromes. In rarer instances one has the opportunity to confirm clinical suspicions with autopsy evidence.

Management and Prognosis

Prenatal and neonatal hypoxia.—The asphyxiated newborn infant should be treated with whatever resuscitative efforts are necessary to maintain optimal oxygenation. The reader is referred to Silverman[11] and McKay and Smith[9] for a discussion of (1) methods of resuscitation, (2) airway maintenance, (3) oxygenation, (4) respiratory stimulants, (5) antibiotics, (6) bicarbonate therapy for metabolic acidosis and (7) newer agents to counteract the basic mechanical and chemical cardiopulmonary disturbances. Occasionally asphyxiated newborn infants will have generalized or focal seizures, which are best treated with small doses of parenteral phenobarbital (8 mg. two to three times a day). In trying to control seizures, one must of course guard against aggravating an existing state of respiratory depression. Other than these steps, general supportive care and careful attention to differential diagnosis represent the only therapy.

Inasmuch as nobody knows exactly how much clinical anoxia is damaging, great caution must be used in prognosticating to families. The more severe and prolonged the acute signs of aspyhxia and the lower the Apgar score,[11] the graver is the outlook. It is difficult, if not impossible, to predict eventual intellectual performance (as measured by the Gesell adaptive performance or the Stanford-Binet test) on the basis of the severity of neonatal anoxia.[1]

Many infants die in this state of medical emergency (Figs. 16.6 and 16.7), and an unknown percentage of those who live have permanent neurologic deficit.

Postnatal hypoxia.—The reader is referred to appropriate sections of Part I for discussions of the symptomatic management of the signs of chronic brain damage mentioned in this chapter. Treatment of status epilepticus and cerebral edema are outlined in Appendices 1 and 2.

BIBLIOGRAPHY

1. Apgar, V., et al.: Neonatal anoxia, Pediatrics 15:653, 1955.
2. Banker, B. Q., and Larroche, J.: Periventricular leukomalacia of infancy, Arch. Neurol. 7:386, 1962.
3. Earle, K. M., et al.: Incisural sclerosis and temporal lobe seizures produced by hippocampal herniation at birth, A.M.A. Arch. Neurol. & Psychiat. 69:27, 1953.
3a. Freytag, E., and Lindenberg, R.: Neuropathologic findings in patients of a hospital for the mentally deficient, Johns Hopkins M. J. 121:379, 1967.
4. Greenfield, J. G.: *Neuropathology* (2d ed.; London: Edward Arnold & Co., 1963).
5. Gröntoft, O.: Intracranial hemorrhage and blood-brain barrier problems in the newborn: Pathologico-anatomical experimental investigation, Acta path. et microbiol. scandinav., supp. 100, 1954.
6. Lance, J. W., and Adams, R. D.: The syndrome of intention or action myoclonus as a sequel to hypoxic encephalopathy, Brain 86:111, 1963.
7. Little, W. J.: The influence of abnormal parturition, difficult labours, premature birth and asphyxia neonatorum on the mental and physical condition of the child, especially in relation to deformities, Tr. Obst. Soc. London 3:293, 1861.
8. Malamud, N.: The epileptogenic focus in temporal lobe epilepsy from a pathological standpoint, Arch. Neurol. 14:190, 1966.
9. McKay, R. J., and Smith, C. W.: The Newborn Infant, in Nelson, W. E. (ed.): *Textbook of Pediatrics* (8th ed.; Philadelphia: W. B. Saunders Company, 1964).
10. Ross, J. J., and Dimmette, R. M.: Subependymal cerebral hemorrhage in infancy, Am. J. Dis. Child. 110:531, 1965.
11. Silverman, W. A.: *Dunham's Premature Infant* (3d ed.; New York City: Paul B. Hoeber, Inc., 1961).
12. Weinberger, H. A., et al.: Prognosis of cortical blindness following cardiac arrest in children, J.A.M.A. 179:126, 1962.
13. Wolf, A., and Cowen, D.: The cerebral atrophies and encephalomalacias of infancy and childhood, A. Res. Nerv. & Ment. Dis., Proc. 34:199, 1955.

17

Tumors of the Nervous System

INTRACRANIAL TUMORS

General Discussion
    Incidence
    Pathogenesis, Location and Histopathology
    Clinical Diagnosis
    Laboratory Diagnosis
    Differential Diagnosis
    Management and Prognosis
Subtentorial or Posterior Fossa Tumors
    Cerebellar Tumor (Astrocytoma)
    Fourth Ventricle Tumors
        Medulloblastoma
        Ependymoma
        Choroid plexus papilloma
    Brain Stem Glioma
    Extra-axial Tumors
Supratentorial Tumors
    Tumors of the Cerebral Hemisphere
    Parasellar Tumors
        Craniopharyngioma
        Optic glioma
    Posterior Third Ventricle Tumors (Pinealoma)
    Intraventricular Tumors
        Choroid plexus papilloma
        Ependymoma
        Colloid cyst
Metastatic Intracranial Tumors
    Leukemia or Lymphosarcoma
    Neuroblastoma
    Wilms' Tumor (Hypernephroma)

INTRASPINAL TUMORS

General Discussion
    Incidence and Pathogenesis
    Clinical Diagnosis
    Laboratory Diagnosis
    Differential Diagnosis
    Management

Intramedullary Tumors
    Gliomas (Astrocytoma, Ependymoma)   Syringomyelia (Chapter 13)
Extramedullary Intradural Tumors
    Meningioma   Gliomatous "Seeding" (Medulloblastoma) and Other Gliomas
    Neurofibroma   Congenital Tumors (Dermoid, Teratoma)
Extradural Tumors
    Spinal Epidural Leukemia   Sarcoma
    Neuroblastoma (Sympathicoblastoma)   Chordomas

TUMORS OF THE SKULL

Congenital Tumors (Dermoid, Epidermoid, Teratoma)   Orbital Tumors (Chapter 6)
Primary Neoplasms (Osteoma, Sarcoma)

Intracranial Tumors

General Discussion

Before the steps in diagnosis and management of specific types of tumors are discussed, some *general* considerations are presented here to give the reader proper orientation and perspective.

INCIDENCE.—Brain tumors occur uncommonly in children, but as refinements in diagnostic techniques have taken place, it has become clear that tumors occur more frequently than was supposed years ago.[1,6,11,18,19,30] Tumors are rarely seen in infants, the peak incidence being in midchildhood (5–6 years), the time that cerebellar astrocytoma and brain stem glioma occur most commonly. The peak incidence of the cerebellar medulloblastoma comes at about age 4. The sex incidence is discussed according to tumor type.

PATHOGENESIS.—The location and the dominant histologic tumor types make it easier to understand the usual clinical picture, the preferred approaches to diagnosis, the natural history of the disease and the problems of treatment and prognosis. About two-thirds of brain tumors in children develop in the posterior fossa, in contrast to a reverse ratio in adults. Of the remaining one-third, approximately half occur in or near the midline. This predilection for the posterior fossa and midline causes the early development of increased intracranial pressure and also complicates surgical removal in many cases. Approximately 75% of brain tumors in children are gliomas, two-thirds of these being cerebellar medulloblastomas and astrocytomas. Next in frequency are brain stem gliomas, ependymomas, hemisphere gliomas and craniopharyngiomas. Less common are sarcomas, meningiomas, dermoids, hamartomas and hemangiomas. The common adult brain tumors—pituitary adenoma, meningioma and acoustic neurinoma—are seen only rarely in children.

CLINICAL DIAGNOSIS.—Symptoms of increased intracranial pressure often are a result of obstructive hydrocephalus. Nausea, vomiting and headache are seen, often after the child arises in the morning. A change in personality, with irritability and somnolence, frequently heralds the onset of this clinical syndrome. However, the nonspecific nature of the symptoms and the tendency for parents and physicians to attribute them to psychogenic causes in an otherwise healthy child often lead to a delay in their correct evaluation.

In infancy and early childhood the cranial sutures usually separate to relieve the increased pressure temporarily, and this mechanism leads in turn to clinically measurable head enlargement. Even when there is an ocular squint from unilateral or bilateral sixth cranial nerve palsies (false localizing signs induced by pressure), the child may complain of visual impairment rather than diplopia. In the early stages increased intracranial pressure does not actually impair visual acuity, but it may cause subjective blurring of vision. Such complaints often lead the parent to suspect a refractive error and again, if the physician is not alert, further delay may ensue.

Although generalized convulsions and minor or focal seizures can certainly result from supratentorial hemisphere tumors in children, they occur rarely from this cause compared to other, more common etiologies of seizures in childhood. Tumor should be suspected if a parent or a physician notes that the child holds the head cocked to one side. The head tilt usually results from the child's attempt to avoid diplopia or from the pain caused by early herniation of the cerebellar tonsils into the cisterna magna. The signs of focal neurologic deficit which are so important in making proper regional diagnosis with any neurologic disorder are described under the specific tumors and in Chapter 9.

LABORATORY DIAGNOSIS.—Steady progress in the development of useful diagnostic tools now permits accurate localization of nearly all intracranial tumors. Especially helpful have been the new studies employed by the radiologist. These and other procedures are discussed in Chapter 12. Although pneumography and angiography have enjoyed wide popularity for many years, newer, technically simpler and medically safer procedures such as radioisotope scans and echoencephalography will undoubtedly be used more widely if they can provide as much or more information. Neurologists and neurosurgeons sometimes make the mistake of condemning a procedure because of their limited experience with it or because of its allegedly high morbidity and mortality risks. As a result they may attempt to select a procedure with which they are more familiar in a situation in which the clinical facts would indicate they could not expect to obtain diagnostic information. This attitude can lead to diagnostic procedures of limited value with the attendant morbidity and mortality risks, not to mention the economic burden to the patient. Table 17.1 gives in a general way the indications and the contraindications (or relative uselessness) for various diagnostic procedures.

DIFFERENTIAL DIAGNOSIS.—The differentiation of intracranial neoplasms from other disorders which present with focal deficit will be considered under the discussion of individual tumor types. In this section on differential diagnosis of increased intracranial pressure only a listing of those conditions which should be considered will be given. One must consider: subdural hematoma (especially large bilateral effusions), congenital hydrocephalus, status epilepticus with anoxic cerebral edema (secondary to fever, hypocalcemia, hypoglycemia, areas of scarring or inborn errors of metabolism such as phenylketonuria), acute head trauma (with epidural hematoma, intracerebral hematoma and rarely cerebral edema), meningitis (espe-

TABLE 17.1.—Diagnostic Procedures for Localization of Brain Tumors

Procedure	Indications	Contraindications
Plain skull x-rays	Any patient suspected of having an intracranial tumor, regardless of location	none
Electroencephalography	Patients (with signs of pressure, unlocalized) suspected of having a supratentorial mass	none
Echoencephalography	same	none
Radioisotope scans	Supratentorial posterior fossa or parasellar neoplasms	
Angiography	Patients suspected of having hemisphere tumors and those with marked pressure and no localizing signs	
Ventriculography (Pantopaque)	Patients suspected of having posterior fossa tumors in whom air studies (including combined PEG and ventriculogram) have not been diagnostic	Any case in which diagnostic information can be obtained by the use of air
Ventriculography (air)	Markedly increased intracranial pressure Nondiagnostic angiography Nonfilling of the ventricles on PEG	Any case in which another procedure is indicated and is reasonably safe
Lumbar pneumoencephalography (PEG)*	Clinical signs of brain stem tumor or suprasellar tumor Increased intracranial pressure, unlocalized (without evidence of midline shift), especially patients *with* pseudotumor cerebri Clinical evidence of hemisphere masses without signs of pressure	Clinical signs of tumor with signs of severe pressure

*This decision should be made only by an experienced neurologist or neurosurgeon.

---

cially chronic granulomatous infections such as tuberculosis and cryptococcosis which develop insidiously), degenerative diseases (Schilder's disease, acute multiple sclerosis) and intoxications (lead, vitamin A, water). The differentiating clinical and laboratory characteristics of these disorders are considered under their separate headings.

Special attention is called to the need for a continued alertness for patients with slow-growing gliomas which may cause neither pressure symptoms nor focal deficit for many years. These patients often present with seizures and are carried with the diagnosis of idiopathic epilepsy after a series of contrast studies give normal results.

MANAGEMENT AND PROGNOSIS.—As techniques of early diagnosis, improved methods of neurosurgery and advances in radiation and chemotherapy have become established, an increasingly optimistic attitude has developed toward the problem of treating intracranial tumors in children. Complete surgical removal and cure can be achieved best in the cystic astrocytoma of the cerebellum. However, in certain cases of intraventricular ependymoma, choroid plexus papilloma, colloid cyst, congenital tumors (dermoids and teratomas) and neurofibroma and in some cases of craniopharyngioma and optic nerve glioma surgery can be expected to produce long-term, symptom-free survival and in some cases permanent cure. Similarly, radiation has a definitely beneficial place in the treatment of some tumors. Included in this group are medulloblastoma, brain stem glioma, optic glioma, craniopharyngioma, central nervous system leukemia, neuroblastoma and Wilms' tumor. Bouchard[2] has documented a rather extensive experience with a literature review on the value of radiation therapy.

Drug therapy of cerebral edema (Appendix 2) has become an important tool, especially for the management of supratentorial masses and metastatic tumors and to reduce the procedural risks in some patients who are having x-ray contrast studies. Drug therapy is used frequently not only by the neurosurgeon but as a palliative medical measure. Therapy of intracranial gliomas with oncolytic agents has been reported recently,[22,34,38] but the precise value of this approach is still uncertain.

The physician should avoid a hopeless attitude in speaking with relatives at the outset unless he is certain of an early, fatal outcome. Furthermore, the defeated, nihilistic attitude on the part of the physician often leads to an incomplete and inadequate diagnostic study in patients for whom cure or long-term survival can be expected. Accurate regional diagnosis and, in nearly all cases, histologic definition of the tumor type by biopsy are indicated.

Subtentorial or Posterior Fossa Tumors
CEREBELLAR TUMOR (ASTROCYTOMA)

PATHOGENESIS.—The second commonest brain tumor in children[27] is the cerebellar astrocytoma. It can develop as a cystic or solid tumor in the cerebellar hemisphere or in the midline. Its exact etiology is unknown and, as in many other tumors in children, a possible developmental or embryonic origin has been considered. Most common during childhood, it reaches a peak incidence between 5 and 8 years of age.

CLINICAL AND LABORATORY DIAGNOSIS.—Increased intracranial pressure is present in the vast majority of these patients and causes headache, vomiting, papilledema and head enlargement (in the younger child). Ataxia, usually causing an unsteady or wide-based gait at first, is seen in nearly all patients. Incoordination of the extremities on the side of the lesion occurs later, especially if the tumor is in the cerebellar hemisphere. The patient may seem generally "weak," but this is usually a reflection of cerebellar hypotonia rather than true paresis and is associated with hyporeflexia.

The patient may present early with an ocular squint or strabismus and, if he is old enough, may report diplopia or blurred vision. The squint is usually attributable to external rectus weakness from increased intracranial pressure and is not a true localizing sign of sixth nerve nucleus involvement in the brain stem. Third nerve palsy as a result of pressure is much less common. Horizontal nystagmus is often present and may be accentuated on gaze toward the side of a lateralized tumor. Papilledema is noted in almost all these patients, though occasionally optic nerve pallor due to atrophy develops by the time the diagnosis is made.

Head enlargement, especially in young children, results from pressure-induced suture separation. Head tilt, stiffness of the neck and suboccipital tenderness are seen as a result of herniation of the cerebellar tonsils from the growing tumor.

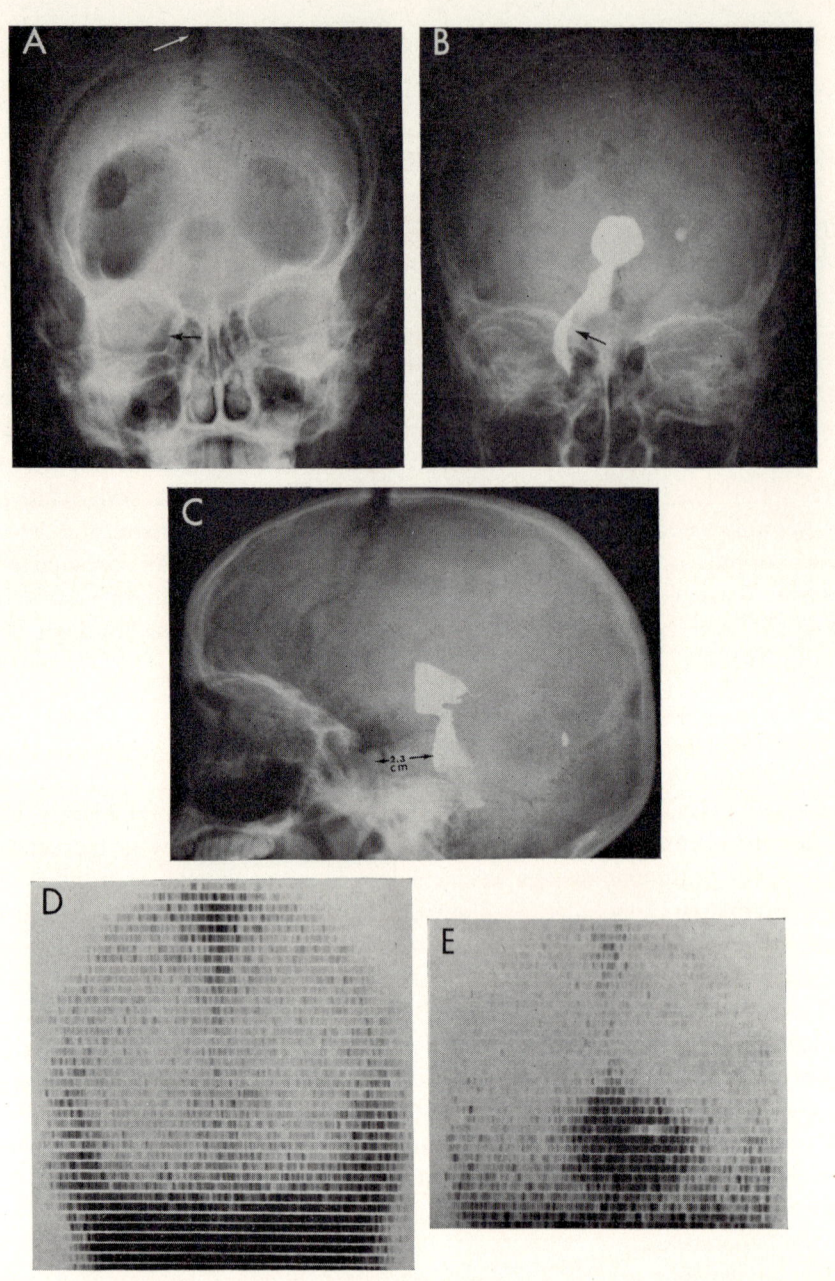

Fig. 17.1.—Cystic cerebellar astrocytoma—value and limitation of contrast studies. Boy, 10½, had "fainting spells," vomiting, a tremor of the right hand and gradually increasing gait ataxia. Examination showed bilateral papilledema, nuchal rigidity, obtundation and a preference to hold his head to the right. Bilateral Babinski signs were found with generalized hypotonia, left more than right. Skull x-rays revealed striking suture separation (upper arrow in A) and a ventriculogram showed generalized dilatation, but initial films were not considered diagnostic in terms of localizing the mass. In retrospect, one can see the fourth ventricle (lower arrow in A) shifted from left to right on the frontal projection; this was proved with the Pantopaque ventriculogram (B). In C, note the upper anterior displacement of the fourth ventricle (compare with normal measurements in Appendix 9). Exploration of the posterior fossa revealed a large cystic astrocytoma in the left cerebellar hemisphere which was removed totally. Postoperative course was uneventful.

Value of isotopic scan. Girl, 11, had symptoms and signs of increased intracranial pressure and mild incoordination in the left hand. A technetium-99m brain scan revealed no abnormalities in the anteroposterior projection (D), but a definite area of increased uptake in the reverse Towne's projection to the left of the midline (E). A large cystic astrocytoma of the cerebellum was removed totally via suboccipital craniotomy.

Only in exceptional cases in which the tumor infiltrates the brain stem do cranial nerve or corticospinal tract signs develop. Tonic "cerebellar fits" are rare and usually represent episodes of decerebrate rigidity from tonsillar herniation. Herniation may be accompanied by irregularities of pulse, respiration and state of consciousness, and occasionally true ictal attacks occur.

Plain skull x-rays often show suture separation or other radiologic signs of pressure (Fig. 17.1,*A*), including thinning of the occipital bone in long-standing cases. Also, as a result of pressure the electroencephalogram may show diffuse bilateral slowing which is sometimes more prominent posteriorly. Generally speaking, because of the dangers of lumbar pneumoencephalography, ventriculography should be carried out to localize the lesion. The difficulties in obtaining definitive radiologic evidence of the tumor location and the need for a somewhat flexible approach is illustrated in Figure 17.1.

Ventriculography usually shows symmetrical dilatation of the lateral and third ventricles as well as the upper portion of the aqueduct. If the tumor is located in the cerebellar hemisphere, the aqueduct and fourth ventricle are usually displaced to the opposite side on the frontal pneumogram (Fig. 17.1,*A* and *B*). In the lateral pneumogram or Pantopaque ventriculogram the aqueduct and fourth ventricle are usually displaced forward and the height of the fourth ventricle is reduced (Fig. 17.1,*C*). When one has occasion to measure the CSF protein level, it may be normal with slow-growing cystic lesions of the hemisphere or moderately elevated when the tumor invades the areas adjacent to the ventricle. Pneumoencephalography can safely be done on some of these patients, but nonfilling of the ventricles may result and necessitate a further definitive diagnostic procedure. Although radioisotopic scans have most value in supratentorial lesions, occasionally these studies will localize a mass in the posterior fossa[51] (Fig. 17.1,*D* and *E*).

MANAGEMENT AND PROGNOSIS.—Treatment of this tumor is entirely operative and the prognosis is generally good. Cystic astrocytomas confined to the hemisphere can be removed totally, whereas invasive midline lesions may be only partially resectable. Even in the latter case the slow-growing nature of the lesion often leaves the patient symptom free for many years, at which time a second operation may be indicated. Roentgen therapy cannot be expected to benefit the patient much, but it is sometimes used with the invasive nonresectable lesion.

Fourth Ventricle Tumors
Cerebellar Medulloblastoma

PATHOGENESIS.—This malignant tumor, the commonest brain tumor of childhood, arises from the cerebellar vermis in the midline. It affects boys about twice as often as girls, and the peak incidence is at age 3–4 years. This rapidly growing tumor may invade the cerebellar hemispheres asymmetrically. It nearly always grows into the lumen of the fourth ventricle, sometimes extending rostrally into the aqueduct, into the lateral recesses of the fourth ventricle through the foramina and into the cisterna magna. This tumor may "seed" itself throughout the spinal subarachnoid space, compressing nerve roots or spinal cord.

CLINICAL AND LABORATORY DIAGNOSIS.—Obstructive symptoms of increased pressure, such as headache, vomiting, unsteady gait and head enlargement, ap-

248 TUMORS OF THE NERVOUS SYSTEM

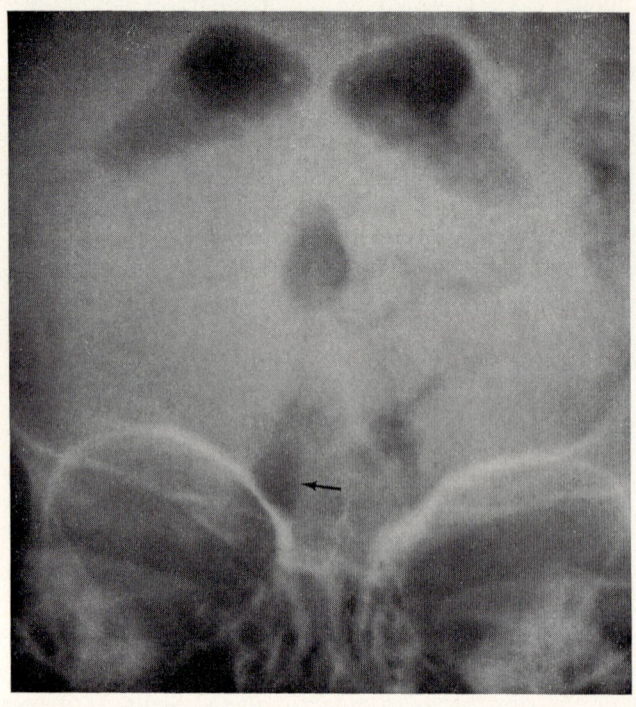

Fig. 17.2.—Cerebellar medulloblastoma arising from the left side of the fourth ventricular floor in a 3-year-old. Note the displacement from left to right of the fourth ventricle (arrow) on frontal projection.

pear early. Papilledema often occurs as do truncal ataxia and nystagmus. Cranial nerve and pyramidal tract signs are seen uncommonly and signify invasion of the brain stem. Neck stiffness, tenderness and head tilt are often seen and suggest tonsillar herniation. Lower motor neuron signs (root pain, flaccid weakness, atrophy and hyporeflexia) may appear during the terminal stages when the tumor has seeded extensively.

Plain skull film changes and EEG abnormalities are similar to those seen with other cerebellar neoplasms (p. 247). A ventriculogram usually shows angulation and forward displacement of the lower aqueduct as well as displacement of the fourth ventricle (if it fills) forward and upward. In addition, the fourth ventricle may be displaced laterally in the frontal projection (Fig. 17.2). The CSF protein content is not measured routinely because of the dangers of lumbar puncture, but when this measurement is made the protein level may be over 100 mg./100 ml. and the fluid may be xanthochromic or bloody.

MANAGEMENT AND PROGNOSIS.—Partial surgical removal of the tumor is not difficult, but complete removal has so far proved impossible. Biopsy of the lesion should always be carried out, along with suboccipital decompression. Since the medulloblastoma is a very radiosensitive tumor, most patients who survive operation can be offered striking symptomatic relief with a course of deep radiation therapy. A tumor dose of 3,000 r to the posterior fossa is started about a week after operation. An additional 2,000–3,000 r is delivered fractionally to the rest of the cerebrospinal fluid axis to prevent growth of seeded tumor.[18] Repeated courses of radiation therapy are sometimes given, but the patient's tolerance (limited by leukopenia and vomiting) and longevity limit what benefit can be expected. Although a few long-term survivals following radiation therapy have been seen by us and reported by others,[18] most patients die within a year or two after diagnosis. Isolated efforts to treat this tumor with intrathecal chemotherapeutic agents have been made, but this approach cannot yet be recommended for practical use.[21]

Ependymoma

This tumor in children usually arises from the floor of the fourth ventricle, often filling the latter cavity and extending outward and downward like the medulloblastoma. It often causes obstructive hydrocephalus.

The clinical picture resembles closely that of the medulloblastoma with symptoms and signs of pressure, ataxia and severe vomiting. Because of its somewhat slower growth and invasive character, it may produce varying signs of compression of structures in the brain stem. When the cerebrospinal fluid can be examined, it usually shows markedly elevated protein content.

Diagnosis can sometimes be made by ventriculography if air can be moved into the fourth ventricle. In both the frontal and lateral pneumogram one may see a dilated fourth ventricle indented from below by a lobulated tumor mass.

Partial but not complete surgical removal of tumor can be effected. Too-vigorous operative efforts will damage vital structures in the brain stem and will heighten the mortality risk. The surgeon usually must settle for decompression of the ventricular fluid pathway, which often requires upper cervical laminectomy. A tumor dose of approximately 3,000 r is then given to the posterior fossa in all cases. The radiation therapy can only be considered palliative.

Choroid Plexus Papilloma

This very rare tumor arises either in the fourth ventricle or in the atrium of the lateral ventricle. Grossly it resembles a pink cauliflower. It produces clinical signs by obstructing the flow of the cerebrospinal fluid in the fourth ventricle.

The clinical picture is characterized only by symptoms and signs of increased intracranial pressure. Similarly, plain x-rays of the skull reveal signs of pressure, and ventriculography reveals evidence of an expanding mass in the fourth ventricle, similar to the picture seen with an ependymoma in this area.

Complete excision is usually attempted and is usually more feasible than with other tumors arising inside the fourth ventricle. Operative removal is complicated by the need to dissect into the lateral recesses of the fourth ventricle, and this carries a significant risk. Survival time with this rare lesion varies greatly.

BRAIN STEM OR PONTINE GLIOMA

PATHOGENESIS.—A relatively common intracranial tumor of childhood, glioma of the brain stem typically grows slowly by infiltrating the pons, medulla and occasionally the midbrain (Fig. 17.3,*B*). Spongioblastoma polare and astrocytoma represent the commonest tumor types, but glioblastomatous transformation can occur

250   TUMORS OF THE NERVOUS SYSTEM

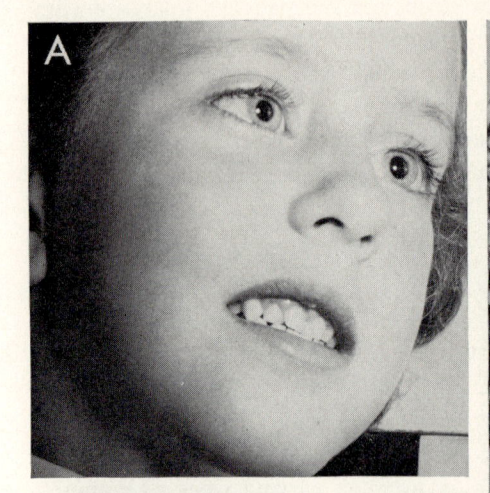

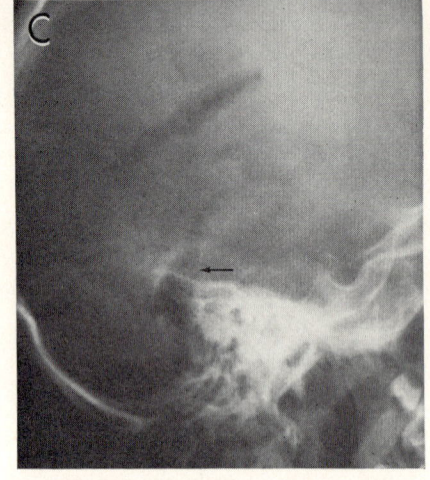

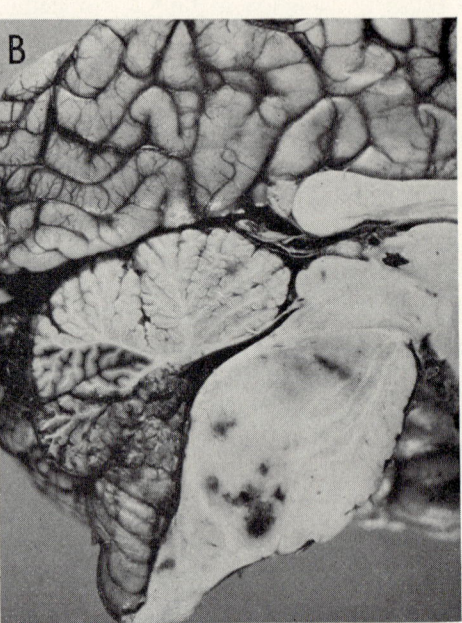

Fig. 17.3.—Brain stem glioma—clinicopathologic features. In this 5-year-old girl head tilt gradually developed, followed by diplopia and a squint for which she had a corrective eye muscle operation. Three months later constant headaches developed, together with a right-sided limp, ataxia, personality changes, hearing loss and dysarthria. Examination revealed an expressionless face with facial diplegia (she is being asked to show her teeth in **A**), bilateral facial sensory loss, a squint with right abducens palsy, bilateral hearing loss and left palatal weakness. Truncal ataxia, bilateral horizontal nystagmus and a left hemiparesis were also noted. Pneumoencephalography was attempted but no air entered the ventricles. A careful posterior fossa exploration revealed a brain stem glioma. The patient died within 24 hours of respiratory failure despite the fact that no tissue was removed at the time of craniotomy. **B**, a sagittal section through the brain stem shows the large, diffusely infiltrating tumor containing some small hemorrhages.

Radiologic diagnosis and therapy. Girl, aged 6 years, 8 months, had symptoms and signs very similar to those described above. **C**, initial pneumoencephalogram revealed slight "bowing" of the aqueduct and the distance from the dorsum sellae was at the upper normal limits (3.8 cm.). Six weeks later this measurement was unequivocally abnormal (4.5 cm.). The CSF protein was 18 mg./100 ml. and opening lumbar puncture pressure was 430 mm. H_2O. Diagnosis of brain stem glioma was made and a 5,000 r tumor dose was given with significant improvement in personality, gait, and right-hand strength and less drooling. When signs of progression later appeared she received intrathecal Methotrexate and Vincristine without any improvement.

and may be associated with seeding locally and in distal parts of the spinal subarachnoid space. This tumor does not usually produce severe obstructive hydrocephalus. The peak incidence is noted in 6-year-old children without sex preponderance.

CLINICAL AND LABORATORY DIAGNOSIS.—Detailed descriptions of series of these tumors[3,18] indicate that the lesion is typified by multiple cranial nerve deficits (eventually involving bilateral nuclei), ataxia, corticospinal tract signs and only occasionally by sensory deficit. Although all cranial nerves with nuclei in the stem can be affected, sixth, seventh and tenth nerve deficit is noted most frequently. Gait disturbance, squint, vomiting, headache, dysarthria, facial weakness, personality change and dysphagia, in that order, are common presenting symptoms (Fig. 17.3,*A*). Papilledema is noted at some time during the course of the illness in only about one-third of the patients and rarely at the time the patient is first seen. Vomiting, which is common, probably represents involvement of the medullary vomiting center rather than reflecting an increase of intracranial pressure. In the later stages of the disease the patient often shows unilateral or bilateral weakness of eye abduction, nystagmus (horizontal and vertical), facial diplegia, impaired facial sensation and corneal reflexes, absent gag reflex, ataxia of the trunk and extremities and spastic hemiparesis or quadriparesis. Less commonly partial deafness and impaired deep sensation are found. Terminally, patients may enter a state of decerebrate rigidity associated with a state of continuous sleep (presumably secondary to tumorous involvement of the brain stem reticular formation).

Lumbar puncture usually shows normal cerebrospinal fluid without elevation of pressure or protein content. Pneumoencephalography is the preferred diagnostic procedure. It is extremely important to get films promptly after instillation of the first 10–15 cc. of air, since the critical areas (fourth ventricle, aqueduct and basal cisterns) are usually filled early. The diagnosis is confirmed by demonstrating in the lateral pneumoencephalogram that the aqueduct of Sylvius and floor of the fourth ventricle are displaced or "bowed" upward and backward (Fig. 17.3,*C*; Appendix 9). The height of the fourth ventricle is reduced and the pontine cistern is narrowed or obliterated. Large tumors will sometimes elevate the posterior floor of the third ventricle. In the frontal pneumogram the fourth ventricular air shadow is measurably widened by the compressive mass. Getting air into the basal cisterns is important in order to differentiate intramedullary from extra-axial tumors. Obviously, extra-axial tumors are much less common in children, but visualization of the pontine cistern should be attempted in all cases.

If lumbar pneumoencephalography fails to fill the fourth ventricle and aqueduct, a combined ventriculogram and pneumoencephalogram must be perfomed to obtain diagnostic evidence. If evidence is still lacking, it is necessary to carry out a posterior fossa exploration, realizing that in patients with this lesion the mortality rate is high with this procedure (Fig. 17.3). Needless to say, biopsy of the lesion is contraindicated unless one can take tumor which has extended or seeded outside of the stem. Slight to moderate dilatation of the lateral ventricles is present in about two-thirds of the cases.

Occasionally one sees a child with typical signs of a brain stem tumor which disappear in a week or two under observation. The diagnosis of "pontine encephalitis" is made in such cases, usually without good laboratory evidence. Caution and careful observation as well as normal pneumograms serve to separate these cases from true tumors.

MANAGEMENT AND PROGNOSIS.—Once a satisfactory diagnosis is made, preferably on clinical and radiologic grounds, the patient is treated with one or more courses of x-ray therapy.[3] Although few long-term survivals and no definite cures have been seen, temporary remission of the patient's symptoms and signs can often be achieved. However, the remission is usually short-lived, and only a limited amount of radiation can be given because of its damaging effects on normal nerve tissue. Despite the clear-cut reversal of the signs with this therapy, the longevity of the patients has not been shown to differ significantly from that in untreated cases. Most parents appreciate the temporary improvement which permits them to gain a little time and to accept the emotional catastrophe better.

Extra-axial Tumors

Extra-axial posterior fossa mass lesions include the neurofibromas, meningiomas and congenital tumors (dermoid, teratomas and chordomas). These are rare in children, and their discussion goes beyond the scope of this text.

Supratentorial Tumors
Tumors of the Cerebral Hemisphere

PATHOGENESIS.—Primary tumors of the cerebral hemisphere account for 10–15% of all intracranial neoplasms in childhood. In a recent series of 123 cases analyzed by Low et al.[25] a histologic diagnosis was made in 115, and a wide variety of different tumor types was found. Pure astrocytomas or astrocytomas mixed with other types of gliomas accounted for 46% of the cases; two-thirds of all the astrocytomas were cystic. The other common types of tumors in this series are listed in Table 17.2. No striking peak-age incidence has been noted and no consistent sex preponderance has been found.

CLINICAL AND LABORATORY DIAGNOSIS.—Unlike posterior fossa tumors in children, clinical evidence of pressure does not appear early in these patients. Often in retrospect the parents will recall a change in personality with irritability, inactivity and listlessness. Unfortunately, these complaints are so nonspecific that they are attributed to other common childhood illnesses or to a psychologic response to environmental factors. Headache is a common and vomiting an uncommon early complaint. Seizures occur in 30–40% of the patients. Motor weakness (a limp or impaired hand use) is commonly noted as a presenting complaint, and on examination it may coexist with a mild spastic hemiparesis, a one-sided reflex preponderance and a Babinski sign. Rarely tumors of the cerebral hemisphere present clinically with extrapyramidal signs.[37] Tremor is most common but other manifestations such as athetosis, torsion spasm, posturing, rigidity and slowness of movement are also seen. By the time patients are examined carefully, two-thirds have papilledema. Subtle signs of impaired cortical and hemisphere function (aphasia, astereognosis, apraxia, disorders of mentation and visual field defects), which are so valuable for early diagnosis of tumors in adults, do not have diagnostic value very often in the young child. In older children and adults with psychiatric symptoms one should think seriously of tumors involving the limbic system of the brain.[26]

We believe that the type of clinical seizure (i.e., generalized vs. focal motor or "psychomotor") does not help differentiate tumors from other causes of ictal or convulsive episodes. Similarly, the type of EEG abnormality (focal spike, focal slow wave or even diffuse spike wave abnormality) is not a dependable means of

TABLE 17.2.—CEREBRAL HEMISPHERE TUMORS IN CHILDREN: A SERIES
OF 115 HISTOLOGICALLY PROVED CASES*

HISTOLOGIC TYPE	No.	%
Astrocytoma	53	46
Glioblastoma	14	12
Oligodendroglioma	14	12
Ependymoma	9	8
Meningioma	7	6
Sarcoma	5	4
Others	13	12
Total	115	100

*Modified from Low, N. L., et al.: Arch. Neurol. 13:547, 1965.

differentiating tumors from other causes of seizures, including genetically determined epilepsy (Fig. 17.4,*A* and *B*). Admittedly, a slow wave focus or consistent amplitude suppression in a patient with a consistently focal clinical seizure refractory to anticonvulsant therapy (Fig. 17.5,*A*) should alert one to the possibility of an underlying mass lesion. This is especially true if focal neurologic deficit and evidence of pressure are associated. The situation which should and does haunt the alert pediatrician or neurologist is the child with persistent seizures which are poorly controlled and are associated with a focal spike or focal spike wave EEG abnormality. Some such patients have normal pneumographic and angiographic findings when they are first studied only to turn up later with abnormal studies and a tumor. Slow-growing gliomas, especially cystic lesions, may cause this sequence of clinical events (Fig. 17.4,*C*)

Whenever a supratentorial neoplasm is suspected, plain skull films, electroencephalography and a visual field examination (if possible) should be carried out. If these studies and a careful physical examination do not reveal serious evidence of pressure, a brain scan and/or echoencephalography can be performed without any risk. The decision to carry out other procedures (angiography and pneumography) must be made with great care and is usually delegated to the neurosurgeon or neurologist. Angiography accurately localizes some mass lesions and is helpful in demonstrating shifts across the midline (Fig. 17.5,*B*) or distinctive vascular patterns in some tumors. In patients without serious signs of pressure or midline shift, a lumbar pneumogram will provide useful diagnostic information, but this procedure must be used with caution. A detailed description of the angiographic and pneumographic abnormalities found in children with supratentorial masses falls beyond the scope of this text and the reader is referred to other good sources[43] as well as the illustrations. When and if the cerebrospinal fluid is examined, the protein content may be found to be elevated, but a normal value in no way rules out a tumor. In fact, a normal lumbar CSF protein value was found in over a third of the patients in one sizeable series.[25]

MANAGEMENT AND PROGNOSIS.—Gliomas of the cerebral hemispheres should be completely excised if at all possible. Unfortunately, most of these neoplasms are so large, so invasive and so close to vital areas which control speech, movement, sensation and vision that only a limited resection is possible. To avoid additional

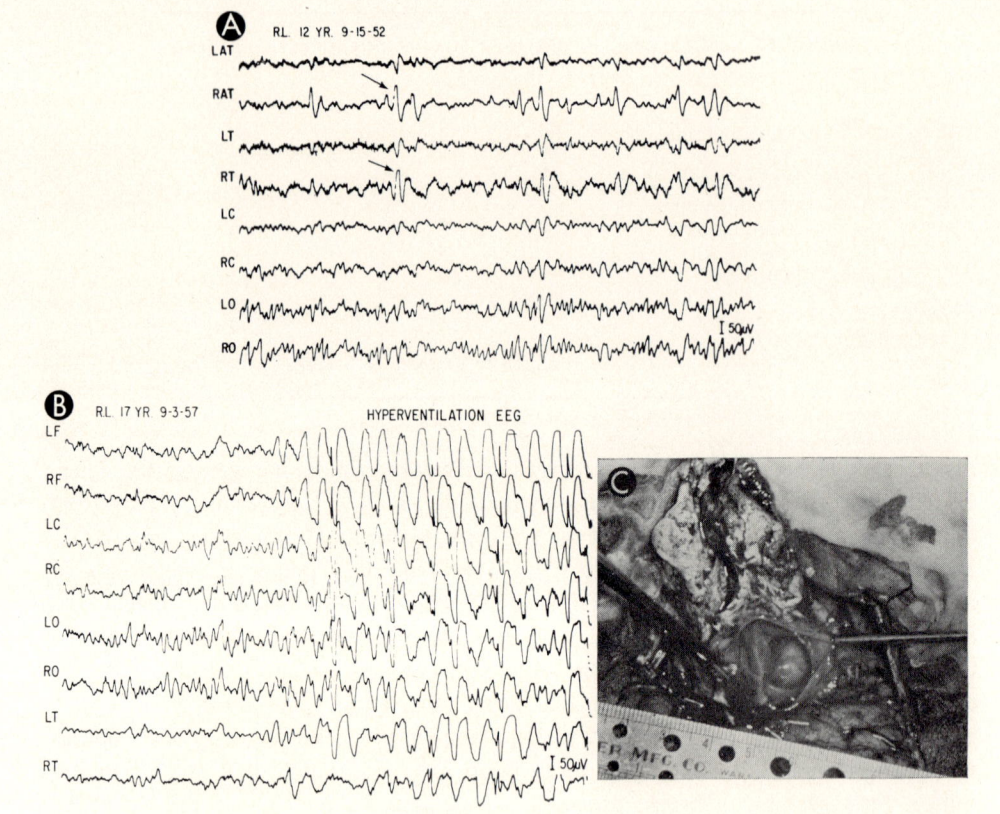

Fig. 17.4.—Cystic astrocytoma—temporal lobe. At age 11 this boy had onset of prolonged psychomotor attacks (inability to speak and auditory hallucinations) followed by headache and fatigue. When he was 13, he experienced left-sided focal motor attacks which became generalized. Despite intensive anticonvulsant therapy the seizures increased in frequency and severity. The patient had two normal skull x-ray series, two normal pneumoencephalograms and negative findings on neurologic examinations. Electroencephalograms showed a consistently well-localized spike and slow wave focus (A) in the right anterior temporal region. On some occasions, with hyperventilation, a diffuse, irregular spike wave abnormality resembling that in petit mal was seen (B). At craniotomy a cystic astrocytoma in the right anterior temporal lobe (C) was found and removed totally. Postoperatively the patient improved greatly, but he has required maintenance anticonvulsant therapy for persistent seizures of an acute confusional type without motor manifestations.

loss of neurologic function, some surgeons have advocated staging the procedure in an effort to effect more complete resection of the marsupialized tumor at the time of reoperation.[18] Refined surgical techniques, better anesthesia, improved control of cerebral edema as well as proper fluid and electrolyte therapy have made radical glioma excision more feasible. However, the overall outlook remains gloomy. In contrast, the more benign tumors (especially cystic astrocytomas in the temporal lobe of the minor hemisphere) can be removed totally and cure can be expected (Fig. 17.4,C). All patients who have undergone operation for a cerebral glioma should be placed on anticonvulsant therapy for an indefinite time. The decision to discontinue drug therapy should be made only after follow-up of at least two years and the evaluation of serial electroencephalograms.

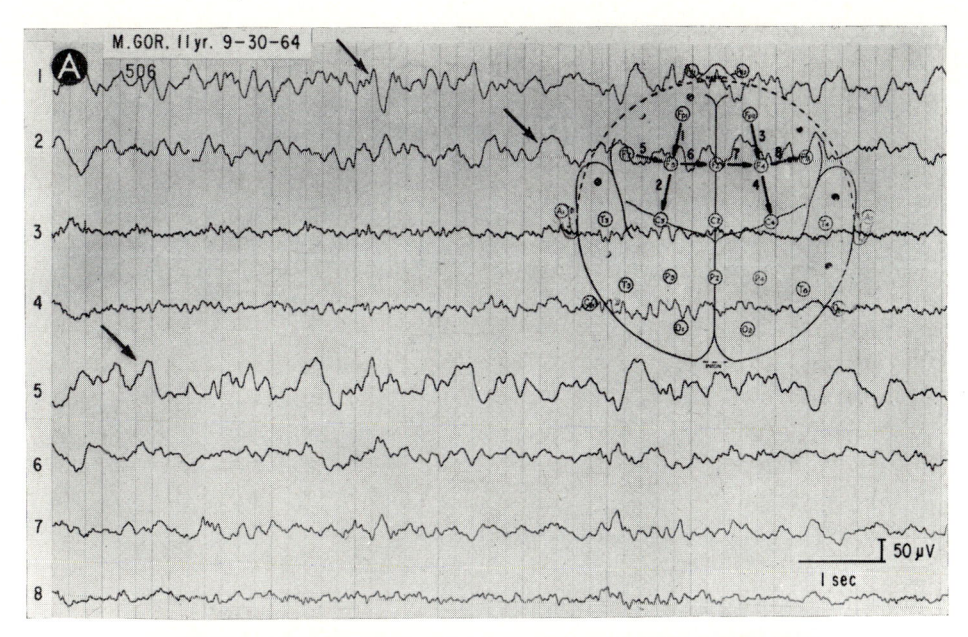

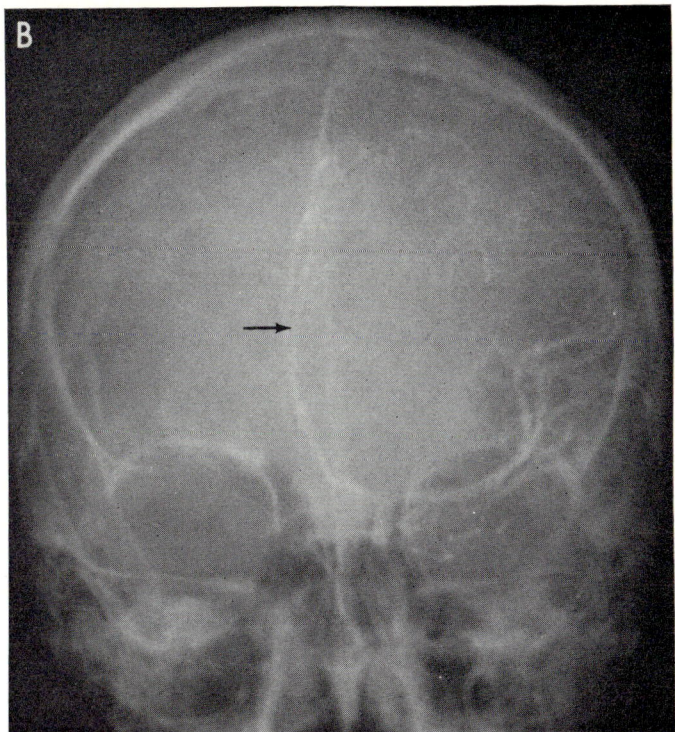

Fig. 17.5.—Malignant tumors of the cerebral hemisphere—value of electroencephalography and arteriography. This boy started to have generalized seizures when he was 8, followed a year later by increasing headache and vomiting. At age 10 bilateral papilledema and a mild right hemiparesis were found. An electroencephalogram (A) showed a large delta focus in the left frontal area. Visual fields were normal except for enlarged blind spots due to papilledema. Arteriograms showed a mass in the left frontal lobe displacing the anterior cerebral artery across the midline (arrow in B). At craniotomy a large, deep necrotic tumor (giant cell sarcoma) was partially removed. The patient died 9 months later.

Although radiation therapy is used frequently in patients who have undergone subtotal resection of a glioma, the results are difficult to interpret. It seems likely that this therapy benefits some patients temporarily, but the uncertain effect on longevity must be balanced against such undesirable side effects as vomiting, bone marrow suppression and alopecia.

Parasellar, Chiasmatic or Anterior Third Ventricle Tumors

Craniopharyngioma

PATHOGENESIS.—This neoplasm, also called a suprasellar cyst, Rathke's pouch cyst, adamantinoma, cholesteatoma and hypophyseal duct tumor, falls into the category of congenital tumors which originate, according to Russell and Rubinstein,[35] as the result of perverted embryogenesis. It accounts for about 5–6% of intracranial tumors in childhood and it is the most common nonglial tumor in that age group. It can, however, occur at any age, including the newborn. The neoplasm is primarily a solid tumor but often is partially cystic (Fig. 17.6,*E*). The mass exerts its damaging effect by compressing the optic chiasm anteriorly, the pituitary-hypothalamic structures below and the third ventricle above. Extensive upward or lateral growth of the tumor commonly causes obstructive hydrocephalus by distorting the foramen of Monro and blocking the flow of fluid in the third ventricle. Histologically the tumor is composed of solid masses of squamous epithelium and cystic areas containing cholesterol, keratin and cellular debris.

CLINICAL AND LABORATORY DIAGNOSIS.—The presenting symptoms vary with the patient's age. In childhood there is usually evidence of pressure (headache, vomiting, papilledema and suture separation). Compression of the optic chiasm often causes impaired visual acuity, optic nerve pallor and, in patients old enough to cooperate with visual field examination, temporal field cuts which progress classically to a bitemporal hemianopia. Not uncommonly in young children partial blindness from optic atrophy occurs before one can check the visual fields.

Most patients manifest striking evidence of pituitary and hypothalamic damage in the form of dwarfed stature (Fig. 17.6,*A*), diabetes insipidus, cold intolerance, obesity (Fig. 17.6,*C*), pathologic somnolence, lassitude and smooth skin with fine hair. The term "Froehlich's syndrome" has been misused by applying it loosely to that large group of fat, feminine-appearing boys who have no endocrinopathy. Strictly speaking, use of the eponym should be restricted to patients with a hypothalamic lesion, obesity and sexual infantilism—a rare clinical complex.[49]

Plain skull x-rays usually show abnormalities—and these may be diagnostic—or nonspecific and misleading signs of generalized increased intracranial pressure. Enlargement or distortion of the sella turcica and suprasellar calcification are seen in about 75% of cases[43] (Fig. 17.6,*B* and *D*). The lateral pneumogram (either lumbar air study or ventriculography, depending upon the degree of pressure) usually shows ventricular dilatation and obliteration of the suprasellar and prechiasmatic cisterns. In many cases the tumor indents the floor of the third ventricle and the advancing edge of the mass is clearly outlined. Then, deformities of the lateral ventricle(s) may develop from compression by a large mass. Occasionally in the frontal pneumogram the inferior portion of the third ventricular air shadow is tilted laterally.

INTRACRANIAL TUMORS 257

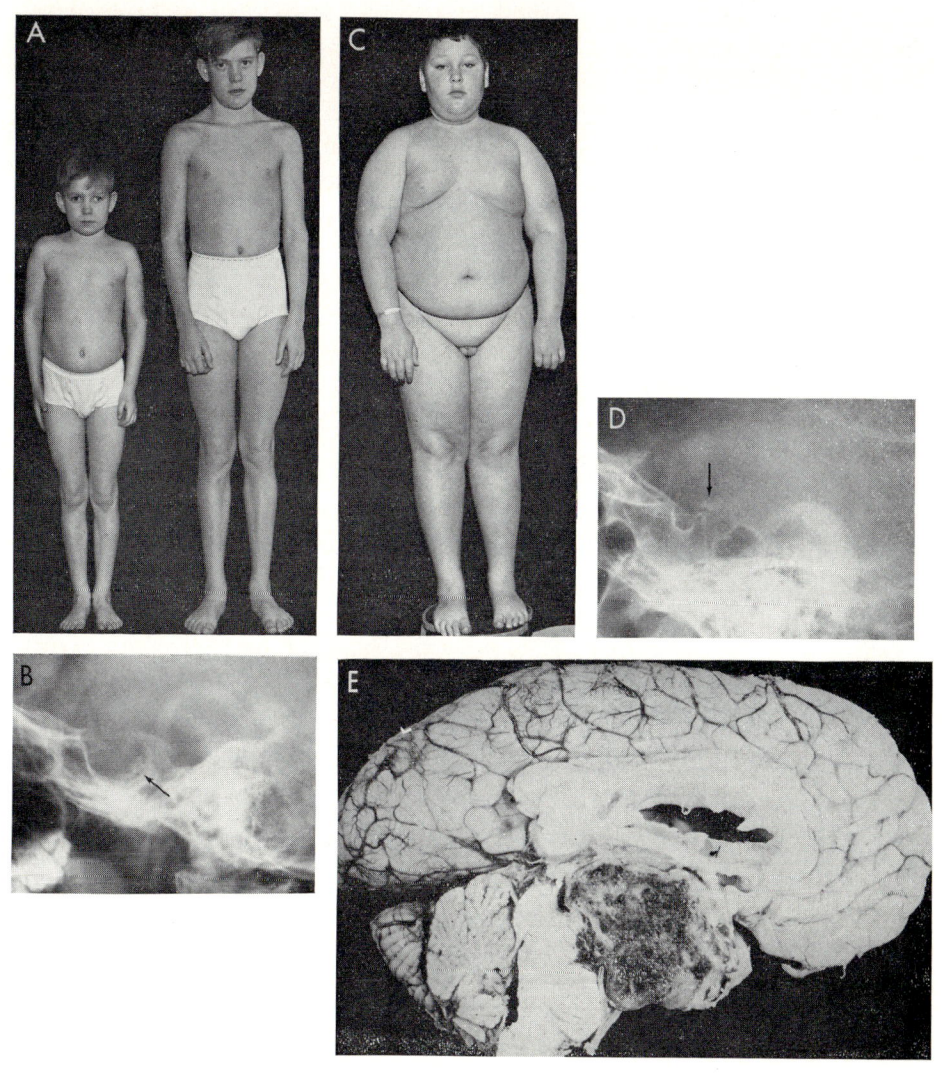

Fig. 17.6.—Craniopharyngioma with hypothalamic syndromes. A, boy, 14, is shown (on the left) with his *identical twin* brother. He was well until age 6 when he complained constantly of being cold, even in summer, and became listless. At 7, the lag in growth was noted, along with polydipsia and polyuria. At 8, poor school work and failing vision led him to a physician. Examination revealed a dwarfed boy with bilateral optic atrophy and mild mental retardation. Skull x-rays (B) showed an enlarged sella turcica with greatest anteroposterior diameter of 19 mm. (compare with 17 mm. in Appendix 11) and a few flecks of calcium posteriorly (arrow). Diagnosis of craniopharyngioma was confirmed at craniotomy and the tumor was resected partially. Postoperatively the patient was placed on pitressin therapy for *diabetes insipidus* and on desiccated thyroid for secondary *hypothyroidism*.

This 9-year-old boy (C) had onset of severe frontal headache at age 5. Plain skull films and a pneumoencephalogram showed suprasellar calcification (arrow in D) and dilatation of the lateral ventricles from an anterior third ventricle obstruction. Craniotomy revealed a craniopharyngioma which was not resectable. A ventricular-jugular shunt was performed to relieve the obstruction and cobalt therapy was given. Over the ensuing four years the patient has had occasional mild headaches, failing vision, progressive obesity (Froehlich's syndrome), marked loss of energy and a tendency to sleep much of the time. At present there is marked obesity (C) with bilateral optic atrophy and generally constricted visual fields on tangent screen study. Note the normal-sized sella in this case (D).

E, pathologic specimen of a craniopharyngioma.

Fluid from a large cyst is sometimes encountered at the time of ventriculography or at operation. This fluid has a golden brown appearance, an oily consistency and on examination is found to contain cholesterol crystals. Other abnormal laboratory studies include evidence of secondary hypothyroidism (low protein-bound iodine), hypoadrenocorticism (low 17-ketosteroids, high eosinophil counts and low fasting plasma levels of cortisol) and impaired carbohydrate metabolism (hypoglycemia and a flat glucose tolerance curve).

MANAGEMENT AND PROGNOSIS.—Most neurosurgeons find it impossible to achieve total removal of the tumor because of the great risk of damage to the pituitary gland and hypothalamus as a result of overzealous dissection in this area. Consequently, they usually drain the cystic portion of the tumor and remove the cyst wall and those solid portions which they can remove safely. In some cases a ventriculoatrial shunt is used to bypass an obstructing mass but this is not often necessary. At the time of operation *the patient should be given adrenal corticosteroids parenterally*. Later the patient may receive other forms of replacement hormone therapy, such as thyroid, pitressin or a synthetic analogue, as well as cortisone or a derivative. The value of radiation therapy is difficult to assess, but some radiologists believe it should be used and may be especially helpful in preventing reaccumulation of cyst fluid.

Patients who have been managed conservatively (as outlined here) can expect many comfortable years of life, provided good supportive care is given. However, it is difficult to promise total cure, and the operative mortality is significant even though it has decreased since the advent of cortisone therapy.

Anterior Third Ventricle Gliomas

Gliomas may arise in the subfrontal area or in the glial tissue near the hypothalamus and infundibulum. The pneumoencephalographic findings (Fig. 17.7) resemble those described for craniopharyngioma. The peculiar constellation of symptoms and signs, referred to as the "diencephalic syndrome," is occasionally seen in patients with tumors in this region (Fig. 17.7 and Chapter 11).

Optic Gliomas

PATHOGENESIS.—This unusual tumor of childhood arises within the optic nerve or chiasm and slowly infiltrates along the course of the nerve, often reaching a very large intracranial size. This tumor, which is composed of astrocytes and oligodendroglia, can occur as a solitary glioma or as one manifestation of neurofibromatosis. Not uncommonly the chiasmal glioma expands to cause obstructive hydrocephalus by blocking the foramen of Monro. In a series of 56 patients with a proved diagnosis,[4] tumor was present at birth in six, and the peak age incidence was reached in the preschool child, i.e., between 2 and 6 years of age.

CLINICAL AND LABORATORY DIAGNOSIS.—Most patients present with symptoms of impaired visual acuity, exophthalmos or strabismus (Fig. 17.8,*A*) or with symptoms of increased intracranial pressure. In Chutorian's series[4] the diagnosis was reached more quickly when patients had exophthalmos than when they had any other complaint and, as one might expect, the tumor in the vast majority of these

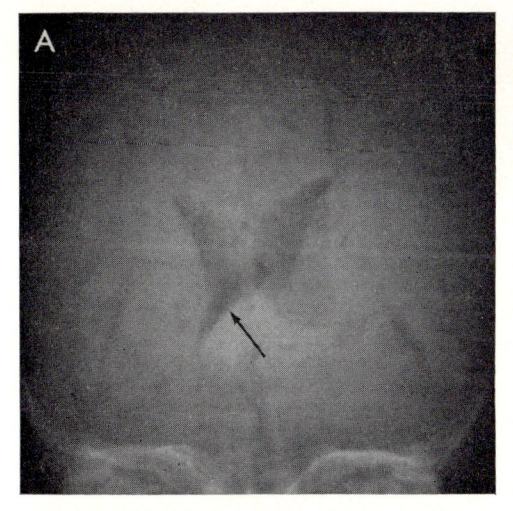

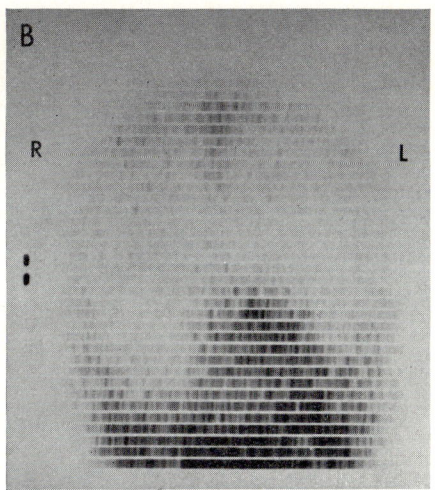

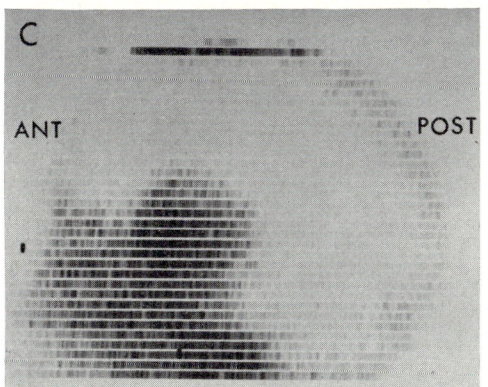

Fig. 17.7.—Left subfrontal astrocytoma with aphasia and diencephalic syndrome. The parents of the patient noticed nystagmus when he was 3, and the referring physician found signs of optic atrophy. The parents had also noted unsatisfactory speech development, a tendency to stumble and bump into objects and apparent weight loss. Examination revealed a very thin boy with bilateral optic atrophy, more marked on the left. He said only single words and exhibited pendular nystagmus with the eyes in the primary position as well as horizontal and rotary nystagmus on left lateral gaze. He also had a mild right hemiparesis. A, pneumoencephalogram shows displacement of the third ventricle (arrow) on the frontal projection from left to right. This finding was confirmed by a 5 mm. shift of the midline to the right on the echogram (upper normal limit is 3 mm.). B and C, brain scan (Tc 99m) confirmed the presence of a left parasellar mass lesion. Views of the optic foramina were normal. Biopsy of this subfrontal tumor revealed a grade II astrocytoma. The patient received 5,000 r postoperatively and showed definite improvement in gait and in general activity but no benefit to his speech.

patients was confined to the optic nerve. Examination usually reveals unilateral or bilateral loss of visual acuity, measurable exophthalmos, pallor or blurring of the discs and an ocular squint. Evidence of neurofibromatosis in the form of multiple cafe-au-lait spots was found in 22% of the 56-patient series.

Plain skull x-rays with special views of the optic foramina often provide the best confirmatory diagnostic evidence. One should consider an optic foramen enlarged if it exceeds 6.5 mm. in its greatest diameter (Fig. 17.8,C) and, even though some size asymmetry between the two sides is common, an abnormality should be suspected if the difference is 2 mm. or more.[43] A pear-shaped (also called J- or mandolin-shaped) deformity of the anterior aspect of the sella turcica (Fig. 17.8,B) commonly occurs, often asymmetrically, as a result of deepening and lengthening of the chiasmatic groove. One must remember that some normal children without disease have a pear-shaped sella and that it may occur in gargoylism or congenital hydrocephalus. Either translumbar pneumography or ventriculog-

260   TUMORS OF THE NERVOUS SYSTEM

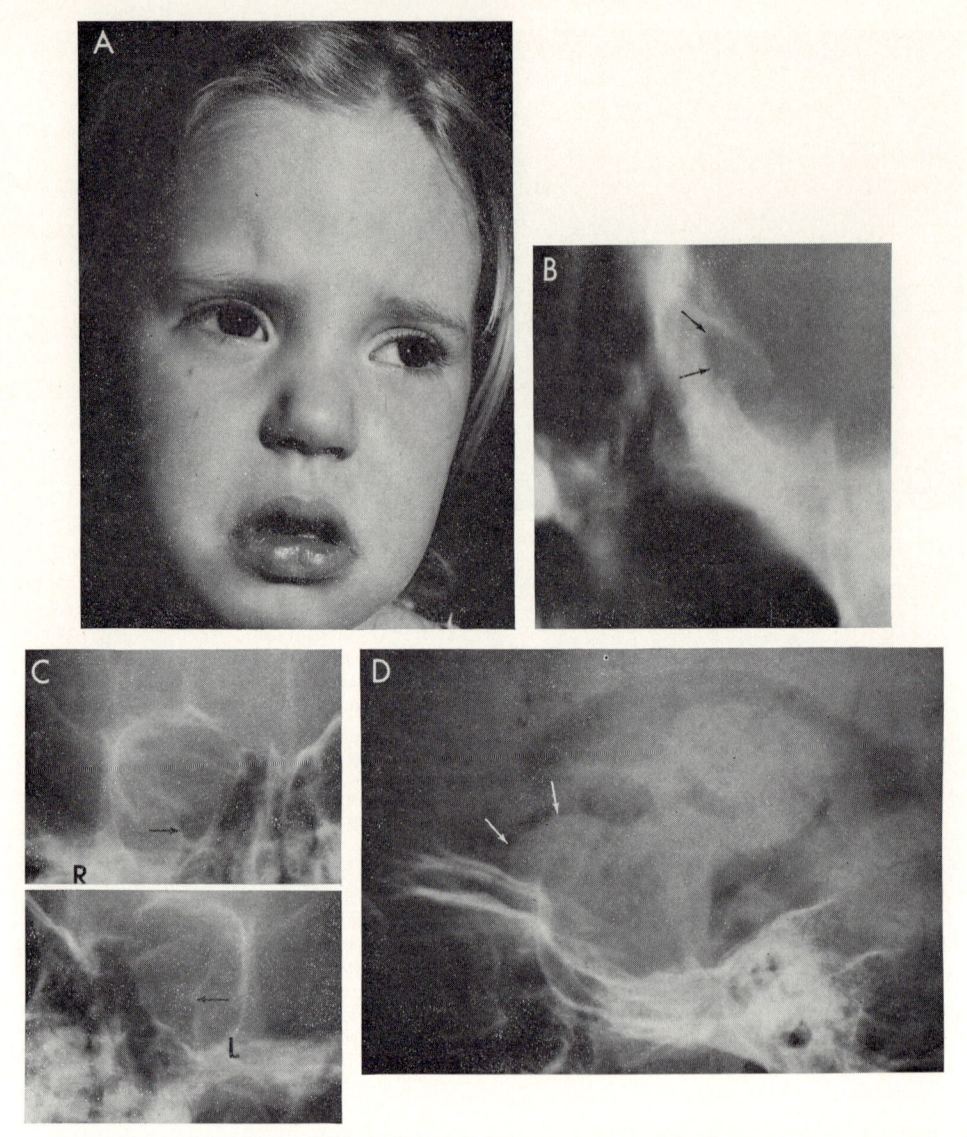

Fig. 17.8.—Optic glioma with typical x-ray abnormalities. The parents of this girl noted a left exotropia at age 1 year. No medical diagnosis was made until age 3½ when bilateral optic atrophy was noted by an ophthalmologist. Examination four months later revealed a left exotropia (**A**), bilateral optic atrophy and marked bilateral visual loss but no exophthalmos. Skull x-rays revealed an abnormal sella turcica with asymmetrical elongation and flattening in the region of the tuberculum sellae and the chiasmatic groove (arrows in **B**). **C**, optic foramen view shows marked enlargement (arrows) with indistinct optic canal margins despite repeated films. **D**, a pneumoencephalogram reveals a large mass above the sella obliterating normal cisterns and producing a curvilinear shadow (arrows) of subarachnoid gas outlining the mass. The mass had not caused ventricular obstruction. Craniotomy and biopsy confirmed the diagnosis of optic glioma and the patient received deep radiation therapy.

raphy reveals evidence of a suprasellar mass with obliteration of the basal cistern air shadows and elevation of the anterior floor of the third ventricle. Sometimes a curvilinear subarachnoid air shadow outlines the tumor anteriorly (Fig. 17.8,*D*). When the clinical and roentgen findings do not lead to a conclusive diagnosis, biopsy of the mass is necessary to rule out the presence of resectable lesions such as meningioma and neurofibroma.

MANAGEMENT AND PROGNOSIS.—Evaluation of any therapy for this lesion is difficult because of the variable and slow-growing character of the tumor and the relatively benign course in many patients who had only subtotal surgical removal of the tumor.[16] However, the threat of blindness and obstructive hydrocephalus compels the physician to offer any reasonably hopeful therapy to these otherwise healthy children. Most workers are convinced, as are we, that radiation therapy[44] should be employed after a reasonably certain diagnosis has been made. When a course of radiation therapy leads to (1) improved visual acuity, (2) a reduction in proptosis and (3) a reduction in the size of the optic canal on x-ray, one has no difficulty in justifying this type of therapy. Although subtotal surgical removal of an obstructive intracranial mass may be indicated, radical efforts at removal of tumor involving the optic nerve and chiasm are clearly contraindicated. In some cases bypass shunts are needed to manage obstructive hydrocephalus.

When the tumor is confined to one optic nerve, the prognosis for vision and survival is much better than when there is chiasmal involvement. In individual cases accurate prognostication is difficult, but many patients who have been followed enjoy symptom-free living for periods up to 20 years.

POSTERIOR THIRD VENTRICLE TUMORS

PATHOGENESIS.—A variety of histologically different tumors is found in this area, including (1) pinealomas, (2) teratomas, (3) gliomas and (4) dermoid cysts. Because of the rarity of the lesions, their similar clinical picture and their similar management, they will be considered together here.

Fig. 17.9.—Pinealoma causing obstructive hydrocephalus. Boy, 15¼, was hospitalized because of a divergent squint and recent marked change in personality. Examination revealed bilateral papilledema, right sixth nerve palsy, paralysis of upward gaze, bilateral horizontal nystagmus and bilateral pyramidal tract signs. Plain skull films showed all the usual signs of increased intracranial pressure. A ventriculogram showed lateral ventricular dilatation, a posterior third ventricle mass indenting the air shadow (horizontal arrow) and calcification in the region of the pineal gland (vertical arrow). At craniotomy a posterior third ventricle mass (pinealoma) was found. A Torkildsen procedure relieved the obstructive hydrocephalus.

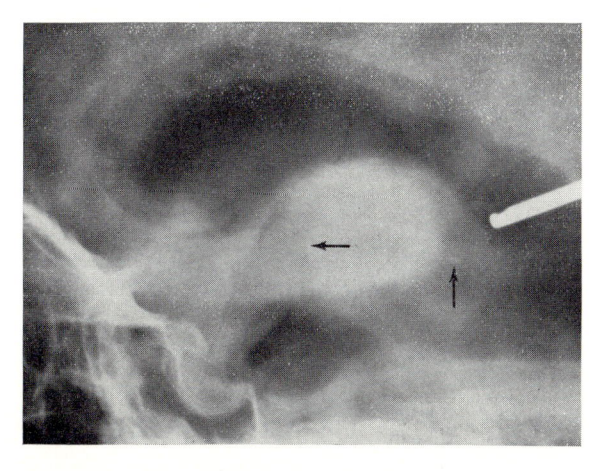

CLINICAL AND LABORATORY DIAGNOSIS.—In patients with tumors in this area symptoms and signs of obstructive hydrocephalus develop early in the course. If the mass arises in or near the pineal gland, it compresses the quadrigeminal plate of the midbrain from above and produces the Parinaud syndrome, i.e., paralysis of conjugate upward eye movements without paralysis of convergence. The pupils may be dilated and respond poorly to light. Ataxia and pyramidal tract signs often develop because of pressure or direct involvement of long tracts in the midbrain and basal ganglia.[5] In boys with pineal tumors, sexual precocity is said to occur frequently. When it does, it is probably caused by involvement of hypothalamic nuclei and not by any real pineal endocrinopathy.

Plain skull x-rays often show signs of increased pressure and abnormal calcification in the area of the pineal gland. Ventriculography usually reveals dilatation of the lateral and anterior third ventricles as well as a mass indenting the air shadow in the posterior third ventricle (Fig. 17.9). Surgical biopsy of the lesion is often necessary to identify accurately the nature of the tumor and its extent.

MANAGEMENT AND PROGNOSIS.—Surgical excision of masses in this area presents serious technical problems. Therefore, procedures are often limited to exploration, biopsy and shunting to bypass obstructive lesions. Radiation therapy is often used but without impressive results.

Longevity for patients with lesions in this area is usually limited, but conservative management with relief of pressure offers the greatest hope.

Cummins et al.[5] recommend radiotherapy and shunt procedures for obstructive hydrocephalus, and they report a 61% five-year survival rate. This is in contrast to a very high mortality rate when surgical excision is attempted.

Intraventricular Tumors

Choroid Plexus Papilloma

These rare tumors usually arise in the atrial portion of the lateral ventricle or in the fourth ventricle. In gross shape they resemble a cauliflower and they have a dark pink color. They are associated with a communicating hydrocephalus which may result from overproduction of cerebrospinal fluid.

These tumors usually cause symptoms and signs of increased intracranial pressure. Focal long-tract signs rarely develop and then only late in the course of the disease. Plain skull films reflect evidence of intracranial hypertension, and pneumography usually provides a striking demonstration of an intraventricular mass.

These tumors can usually be totally excised when they develop in the lateral ventricle. If this can be accomplished without excessive hemorrhage, patients may be cured.

Colloid Cyst of the Third Ventricle

This mass lesion, which is seen very rarely in childhood, arises from the anterior third ventricle. It produces clinical disease by obstructing the flow of cerebrospinal fluid. It has the gross appearance of a small, round cyst attached to the walls of the ventricle and it contains mucoid material of uncertain origin.[40]

The lesion has the notorious reputation of causing intermittent or paroxysmal pressure symptoms, presumably precipitated by a shift in head position or by straining. Even though this clinical picture may be accurate, it certainly does not differentiate this rare lesion from other common intracranial masses. Pressure signs are only rarely accompanied by later evidence of compression of adjacent long-tract or hypothalamic structures.

In addition to plain roentgen evidence of pressure, ventriculography shows marked dilatation of the lateral ventricles and an obvious mass in the anterior portion of the third ventricle.

Accurate and early diagnosis is important because it makes total surgical removal feasible. Not without its technical difficulties, the success of operation is made more certain if the obstruction is not too severe and if extensive pressure damage to adjacent neural structures has not occurred.

Ependymomas

Tumors of this type in children arise less commonly above the tentorium than in the fourth ventricle or the central canal of the spinal canal. The supratentorial lesions can project into the lumen from the wall of the ventricle or occasionally arise from ectopic ependyma within the brain substance.

As in other intraventricular masses ependymomas create problems by giving rise to obstructive hydrocephalus. Their location is identified by the ventriculographic demonstration of a space-occupying mass.

If the ependymoma in this portion of the ventricular system is encapsulated and pedunculated, it may be excised completely. Often, however, the tumor will have grown to a huge size and its total removal will not be feasible.

Metastatic Intracranial Tumors

Because of the low incidence of carcinoma, metastatic tumors in the intracranial cavity are uncommon in children compared to the situation in adults. Discussion will be confined here to the relatively common problems of leukemia, Wilms' tumor (nephroblastoma) and neuroblastoma.

LEUKEMIA

PATHOGENESIS.—During the past 10–15 years, as chemotherapeutic drugs and adrenocortical steroids have entered widespread use and prolonged the life of children with *acute leukemia* (the most common malignancy of childhood), the incidence of nervous system involvement has shown a startling rise.[17] The disease produces clinical neurologic signs by (1) leukemic infiltration of the leptomeninges, nerve roots (Fig. 17.10), spinal cord and brain substance, (2) circulatory insufficiency by leukemic infiltration of blood vessel walls and by occluding the vessel lumen and (3) direct compression of neural structures by leukemic tissue (Fig. 17.10). In addition, of course, leukemia in relapse can have a devastating indirect effect upon the nervous system by causing intracerebral hemorrhage, secondary to thrombopenia.[29] Experience indicates that most standard oral and parenteral therapy for systemic leukemia has little effect upon "CNS leukemia." In fact, in our experience two-thirds of the patients in whom neurologic symptoms and signs developed were in relapse and were receiving standard antileukemic therapy. Of interest is the fact that the remaining third had evidence of nervous system involvement while they were in complete hematologic remission. Presumably this phenomenon results from the fact that none of the standard antifolic acid, antimetabolite drugs (viz., Methotrexate, 6-mercaptopurine or vincristine) crosses the blood-brain barrier in significant concentrations. Although prednisone does cross the barrier to some extent, it may fail to prevent the development of neurologic deficit.

CLINICAL AND LABORATORY DIAGNOSIS.—The clinical syndromes of "CNS leukemia" can be divided arbitrarily into the *cranial* and *spinal* forms. Most frequently patients with intracranial disease have symptoms and signs of increased intracranial pressure (headache, vomiting, papilledema and sixth nerve palsy). Occasionally, however, other cranial nerves (facial and optic) are affected (Fig. 17.10), seizures occur and pyramidal tract signs (hemiparesis) appear. An exact interpretation of the clinical picture is usually difficult. However, one may be aided if CSF pressure is elevated. In addition the fluid often contains varying numbers (100–4,000) of mononuclear cells (lymphocytes and lymphoblasts). Although no consistently striking abnormality has been found in the CSF protein and sugar, in

Fig. 17.10.—Leukemic infiltration of the optic nerve. Boy, 6½, was treated successfully for acute lymphoblastic leukemia over a two-year period. Then failing vision developed and he showed signs of chronic papilledema with impaired acuities (20/200 and 4/200) and leukemic infiltrate of one retina. He was placed on 6-mercaptopurine orally and Methotrexate intrathecally; the papilledema subsided, leaving evidence of optic atrophy but fair vision. Special x-ray views of the optic foramina showed definite bilateral enlargement (arrows), which indicated that the visual loss resulted from leukemic infiltration of the optic nerves rather than increased intracranial pressure. The foramina measured 8 mm. and 9 mm. (arrows), the upper normal limit being 6.5 mm.

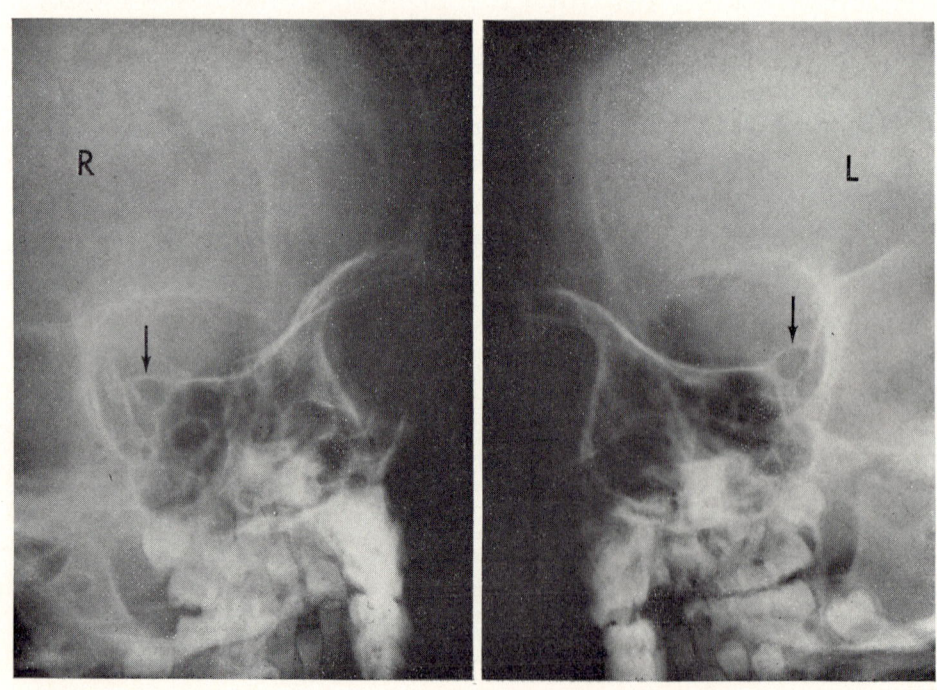

a number of patients the sugar content is significantly depressed (30–35 mg./100 ml. on the average) and protein is slightly elevated (50–75 mg./100 ml.). On rare occasions these chemical values deviate markedly from normal. Autopsy examination usually confirms the extensive infiltration of the leptomeninges, the cortex and the blood vessels.

The spinal syndromes are discussed in the following section.

MANAGEMENT AND PROGNOSIS.—The neurologic signs (which often usher in the terminal stage of the illness) are best treated with (1) oral and parenteral adrenal steroids, (2) irradiation to the cranium and (3) intrathecal Methotrexate.[7,9,23,33,39,41,47] Prednisone is used initially in the dose of one mg./lb./day until benefit occurs. If it fails to produce improvement, the patient is given a course of radiation; a tumor dose of about 1,000 r given through wide anterior, posterior and bilateral portals usually brings about benefit. If these methods have been used and the patient is still symptomatic, Methotrexate (0.3–0.5 mg./kg.) is instilled into the lumbar subarachnoid space. Initially this treatment is repeated twice a week and later at monthly intervals or less depending upon the patient's course.

WILMS' TUMOR (NEPHROBLASTOMA)

PATHOGENESIS.—Wilms' tumor is the commonest abdominal neoplasm in children. In most patients with this tumor symptoms develop before age 3. These tumors arise within the limits of the kidney parenchyma and they tend to metastasize widely to the lungs, bone and brain.[32] Miller et al.[28] pointed out the provocative and puzzlingly high coincidence of congenital anomalies in a series of 440 children with Wilms' tumor.

CLINICAL AND LABORATORY DIAGNOSIS.—The neurologic picture is usually characterized by symptoms and signs of increased pressure, and the focal deficit depends upon the location of the metastatic nodule. Most lesions become lodged in the substance of the cerebral hemisphere and behave like any other neoplasm in the same areas. The physician should not only conduct a careful search for a primary focus elsewhere in the body but he should consider whether the intracranial signs are due to single or multiple lesions. These factors may influence strongly the way the problem is managed. If one is dealing with a primary Wilms' tumor, a firm nontender abdominal mass is usually felt easily. It may be associated with hematuria and the intravenous pyelogram often provides diagnostic evidence of an intrarenal mass. The intracranial lesion (or lesions) is defined best by unilateral or bilateral angiography.

MANAGEMENT AND PROGNOSIS.—When the primary diagnosis is established, nephrectomy should be performed immediately and without further abdominal palpation if the metastatic survey is negative. Some workers start a course of actinomycin D preoperatively and complete it postoperatively, along with a course of radiation therapy.[45] If signs of a metastatic cerebral lesion develop, no further surgical procedure should be performed unless the physician is convinced that the lesion has a reasonable chance of being a solitary one. Effective therapeutic programs for patients with widespread metastases have not yet been developed. However, Farber[10] has recently summarized his results which point out the value of combined nephrectomy, actinomycin D and radiotherapy. Efforts to relieve pressure symptoms with drugs that reduce cerebral edema (Appendix 2) are certainly indicated.

Neuroblastoma

See Intraspinal Tumors.

Intraspinal Tumors

General Discussion

A few generalizations about intraspinal tumors will be made before the individual tumors are discussed according to location.

INCIDENCE AND PATHOGENESIS.—The rarity of intraspinal neoplasms in childhood accounts for the lack of extensive literature on the subject.[15,18] The text by Rand and Rand[31] treats the subject comprehensively. Our experience and that of others suggest that (1) intramedullary gliomas, (2) extradural sarcomas and metastatic tumors and (3) extradural congenital tumors (teratomas and dermoid cysts), in that order, comprise the most common lesions in childhood. In contrast to adults, meningiomas and neurofibromas are found infrequently in children, and then often in association with neurofibromatosis. When series are compared, one finds that these lesions affect all age groups without any consistent peak incidence. As indicated in the preceding section on Metastatic Tumors, the incidence of "CNS leukemia," both cranial and spinal forms, is mounting with the increasing survival times of children with this common disorder. Intraspinal tumors are distributed anatomically along the whole neuraxis, but some workers have recorded a higher incidence of "congenital" tumors in the cervical and lumbar areas, similar to the prevailing distribution of congenital malformation of the spine and cord.

CLINICAL DIAGNOSIS (Table 17.3).—Diagnosis is often delayed because of the general rarity of the problem and because symptoms and signs develop insidiously. In addition, the infrequent complaint by children of paresthesias and of pain (because of low incidence of nerve root and meningeal tumors) delays the diagnosis. In order of frequency, patients or parents usually report (1) disturbance of gait or posture, (2) back or abdominal pain and (3) weakness or incontinence appearing later.

LABORATORY DIAGNOSIS.—A discussion of spine x-rays and myelography is presented in Chapter 12.

DIFFERENTIAL DIAGNOSIS.—A detailed description of the clinical differentiation is given for the individual intraspinal tumors. As mentioned before, delay in diagnosis of cord tumor represents the rule and not the exception. Patients are often carried for long periods with other diagnoses: (1) static orthopedic deformities, such as idiopathic scoliosis, (2) primary spinal cord degenerations, e.g., poliomyelitis, progressive neural muscular atrophy, transverse myelitis, syringomyelia, (3) muscular dystrophy, (4) occult spina bifida with neurologic deficit and (5) cerebral palsy. A reasonable attempt should be made to distinguish on a clinical basis whether the lesion can be classified as intramedullary or extramedullary. However, the general rules which have been applied often fail to hold in an individual case

TABLE 17.3.—DIAGNOSIS OF INTRASPINAL TUMORS

		CLINICAL		CSF		X-RAY ABNORMALITIES			MYELOGRAPHY
	Pain	Pyramidal Tract Signs	Lower Motor Neuron Signs	Block	Protein	Canal Widening	Bone Erosion	Foramen Enlargement	
Intramedullary	Uncommon	Late	Common	Late	Low or slightly elevated	3–4+	3–4	0	Fusiform cord swelling; Pantopaque diverted laterally
Extramedullary intradural	Common	Early and marked	Uncommon	Early	4+	Present late	Present late	±	Clearly outlined mass indenting dye column and compressing cord
Extradural	Common	Early and marked	Uncommon	Late	Normal or slightly elevated	Uncommon	Minimal	Common	Sweeping arclike indentation of dye column or a tapering to a point medially

and for this reason the neurologic evidence must be combined with the roentgen findings and lumbar puncture studies to reach an accurate diagnosis.

MANAGEMENT.—Optimal therapy depends upon early clinical suspicion, accurate radiologic study and prompt surgical intervention. Prompt and proper therapy lessens the number of patients with permanent neurologic deficit. In Rand and Rand's[31] series of 64 verified tumors only 13 patients (20.3%) were cured by surgical therapy alone. However, improved methods of radiotherapy[52] and rapidly evolving forms of tumor chemotherapy have brightened the outlook. Moreover, certain problems in childhood, such as neuroblastoma and epidural leukemia, require accurate evaluation to insure cures in the former and judicious palliative therapy in the latter.

Intramedullary Tumors
GLIOMAS

PATHOGENESIS.—These tumors (usually ependymomas or astrocytomas), like those in the cranium, arise as intrinsic masses in the cord substance and expand slowly to compress the normal neural tissue. At times these lesions coexist with developmental disorders such as syringomyelia, neurofibromatosis and meningomyelocele.[11]

CLINICAL AND LABORATORY DIAGNOSIS.—The patient is often seen first because of abnormal posture (scoliosis) (Fig. 17.11,A), gait disturbance or, less commonly, back or abdominal pain or incontinence. Sensory deficit of the posterior column begins just below the lesion and moves down in an irregular fashion. Lower motor neuron signs, including flaccid weakness, areflexia and a superficial dermatome type of sensory loss, also commonly develop. Root pains in the extremities do not often occur and pyramidal tract signs develop late in the course of the disease. The CSF examination may give normal results, and evidence of a subarachnoid block appears late in the course. Bony changes on plain spine x-rays occur commonly with these lesions. They include widening of the interpediculate distances (Fig. 17.11,A and Appendix 10), scalloping of the posterior margins of the vertebral bodies and thinning of the laminae. Myelography typically shows a fusiform swelling of the cord shadow which diverts the column of dye laterally (Fig. 17.11,B), a picture which can usually be distinguished easily from that seen with extramedullary masses.

MANAGEMENT AND PROGNOSIS.—Operative treatment of intrinsic cord tumors presents a major challenge to the surgeon. In attempting tumor removal the operator is faced with the prospect of greatly increasing the existing neurologic deficit. Such possibilities must be reviewed carefully with relatives in advance so that they understand the risks involved. Some workers have advocated removing the tumor in two stages. At the first operation a longitudinal cord incision is made over the mass, a biopsy is taken and the wound is closed without closing the dura. At the second procedure the tumor, which may have extended itself into the wound, is more easily demarcated from normal cord tissue, and not only can the mass be excised, but less damage to normal structures takes place.[18] In general the prognosis is not good. However, in carefully analyzed series not only is clinical improvement noted in most patients, but long-term survival is extended in patients treated by operation and radiation.[2,52]

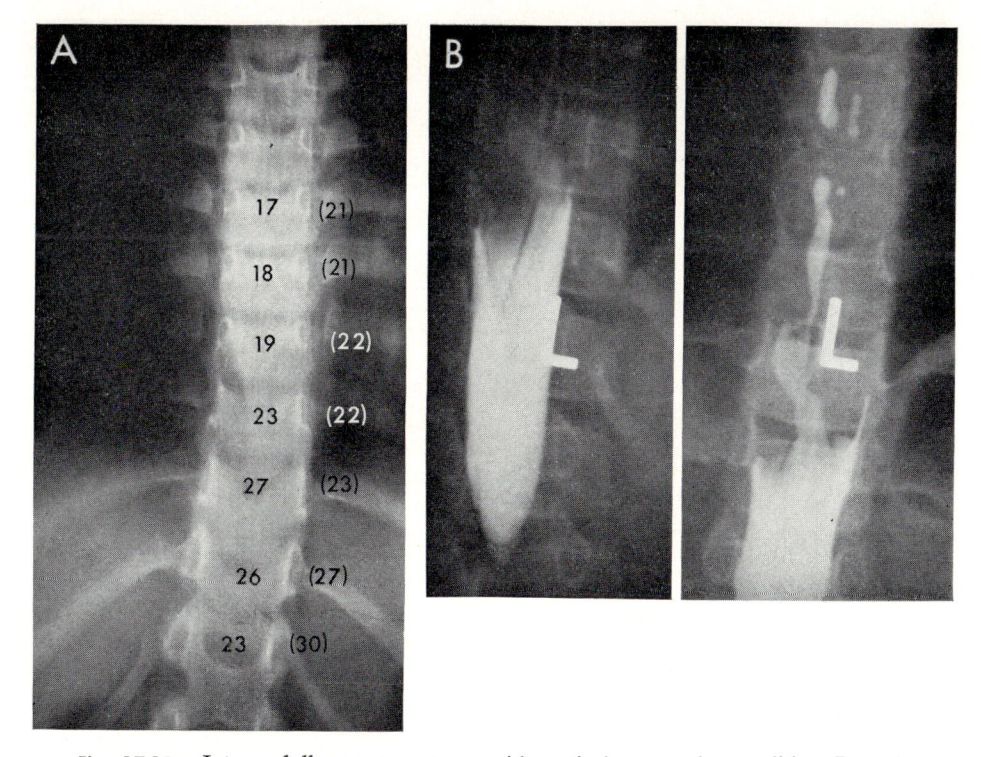

Fig. 17.11.—Intramedullary astrocytoma with typical x-ray abnormalities. Boy, 8, was well until age 3 when abdominal pain and itching of both lower extremities began. An orthopedist found dorsal scoliosis and lumbar lordosis and, after a muscle biopsy revealed normal findings, put him in a back brace. At age 5, a diagnosis of poliomyelitis was made and he was fitted for a plastic jacket and a Milwaukee brace. The latter appliance relieved the abdominal pain for many months. Eventually erosion of the pedicles and widening of the interpediculate distances were noted on plain spine films. In **A**, the actual measurements overlie the vertebrae and the upper normal limits are in parentheses. Neurologic examination revealed only minimal abnormalities: (1) definitely impaired position and vibration sense in both legs, (2) asymmetric tendon reflexes in the legs without pathologic reflexes and (3) mild weakness and diminished bulk of the right quadriceps. **B**, a myelogram revealed fusiform cord swelling maximal at D_{10}, with diversion of the dye column laterally by an intramedullary mass. Attempts at decompression and resection of the intramedullary astrocytoma have been unsuccessful, and the deficit has gradually increased.

Syringomyelia

See Chapter 13.

Extramedullary Intradural Tumors

PATHOGENESIS.—This category of neoplasms is seen least frequently because of the uncommon occurrence of tumors which arise from the nerve and nerve sheath (the controversial nomenclature includes schwannoma, neurilemmoma, neurinoma and neurofibroma) and from the meningeal covers (meningioma). Although these masses may occasionally develop as solitary lesions, they often reflect one manifestation of neurofibromatosis in childhood. One occasionally sees extramedullary seeding from intracranial gliomas, especially medulloblastomas, ependymomas, glioblastomas or brain stem gliomas which have become malignant.

Although "congenital" tumors can arise as extradural masses, more commonly

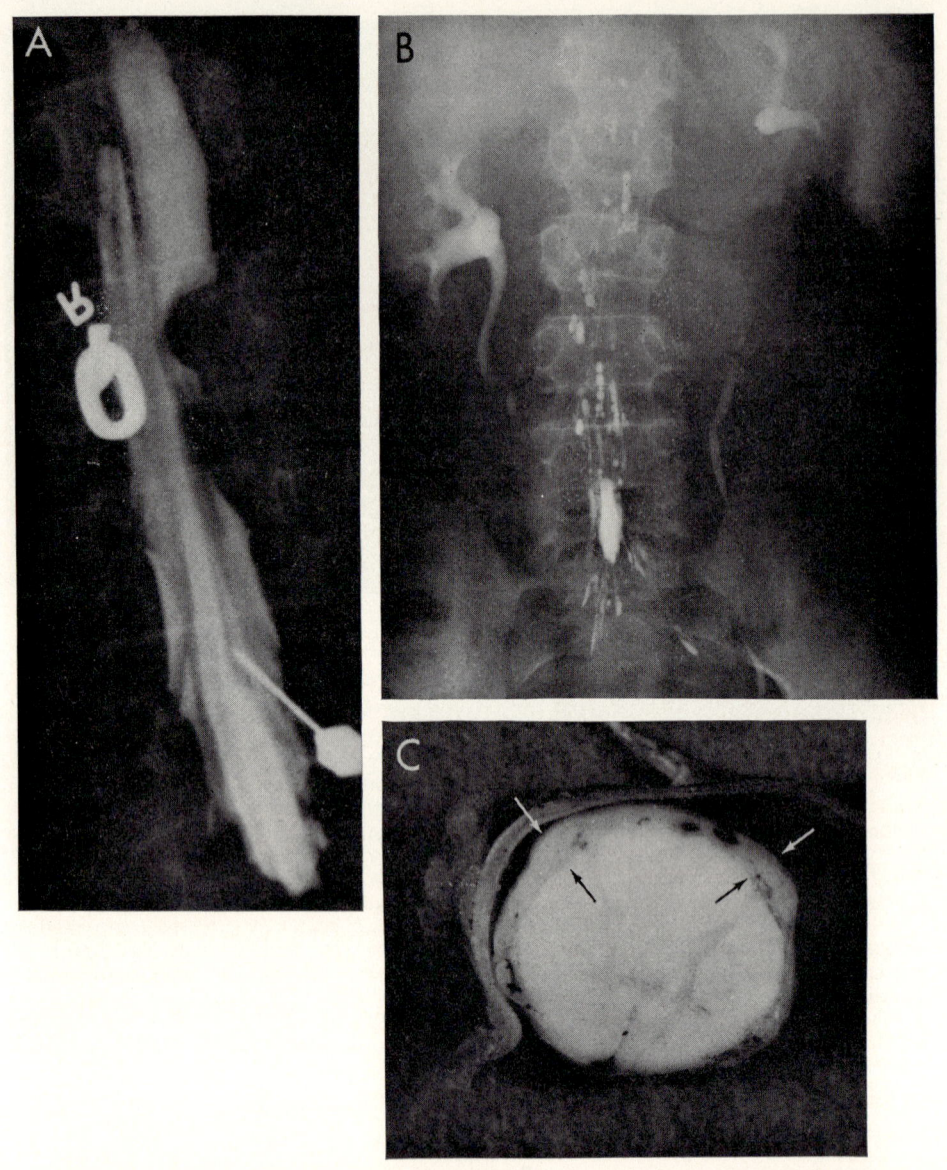

Fig. 17.12.—Extramedullary, intradural spinal tumor—neurofibrosarcoma with neurofibromatosis. Boy, 13, was well until the onset of left thigh pain, a left-sided limp and 15 lb. weight loss over three months. Examination revealed cachexia, mild scoliosis, mild, generalized weakness and increased skin pigmentation and freckling in the skin folds. Focal deficit was restricted to the left lower extremity where signs of L_{3-4} root compression were noted. **A**, lumbar myelogram reveals a large bilobular filling defect at the L_{3-4} level on the left. **B**, intravenous urogram shows the left kidney displaced upward and laterally by a vaguely defined soft-tissue mass at the same level as the intraspinal mass. At laminectomy the intraspinal mass was removed and proved to be a neurofibrosarcoma. Two CSF examinations revealed total *protein values of 121 and 93 mg./100 ml.; glucose values were 0 and 15 mg./100 ml*. Before the posterior abdominal mass could be approached, headache and papilledema developed and the patient died in a short time. At autopsy the large abdominal mass was found along with a cuff of tumor tissue (arrows in **C**) which completely surrounded the spinal cord, causing the hypoglycorrhachia and the terminal hydrocephalus by obstructing the outlets of the fourth ventricle.

they are located in the intradural, extramedullary compartment. Intraspinal teratomas, dermoid cysts and lipomas are located most frequently in the cervical and lumbosacral areas, and they are frequently associated with developmental defects in overlying bone and soft tissue.

CLINICAL AND LABORATORY DIAGNOSIS.—Patients with these lesions often complain of radiating pain in an extremity (Fig. 17.12). On examination there may be evidence of cord compression with unilateral or bilateral pyramidal tract signs and loss of deep sensation. If a sensory level is present, it may be found many segments below the level of the lesion. Patients do not usually exhibit lower motor neuron signs. Patients with congenital tumors often have associated cutaneous lesions (a tuft of hair or a dermal sinus), subcutaneous lesions (palpable lipomas) or occult bony defect in the vertebral column (spina bifida or diastematomyelia).

Lumbar puncture often reveals evidence of a spinal subarachnoid block (Fig. 17.12), and there is usually a markedly elevated CSF protein content. Bony changes in plain spine films may be minimal in the early stages. Later the vertebral canal is enlarged, the posterior aspect of the vertebral body is excavated, and the laminae and pedicles are eroded. In the case of neurinomas which extend into the paraspinal area there is often enlargement of the intervertebral foramen (Fig. 17.12,*B*). On myelography the mass is usually clearly outlined by the Pantopaque (Fig. 17.12,*A*) and the cord is often displaced and compressed. With metastatic gliomas, such as medulloblastoma, the cerebrospinal fluid may contain blood and elevated levels of protein, and myelography may reveal multiple nodular lesions which have become implanted on the surface of the spinal cord. These nodular implants can vary greatly in size.

MANAGEMENT AND PROGNOSIS.—Primary extramedullary intradural tumors should be removed completely if possible. In the case of metastatic gliomas, such as medulloblastoma, the patient should receive a course of fractional radiation over the whole spinal axis. Congenital tumors can usually be excised completely, especially if they are not attached to neural structures in the subdural or extradural space. If the mass is firmly adherent to the cord or nerve, a more conservative approach must be adopted.

The prognosis for primary tumors in this category is very good.

Extradural Tumors

Most extradural spinal tumors in children are malignant (spinal epidural leukemia, neuroblastomas, sarcomas and chordomas).

SPINAL EPIDURAL LEUKEMIA

PATHOGENESIS.—The increasingly common problem of spinal epidural leukemia in children[39,48] deserves special comment and, as a supplement to these paragraphs, the reader is referred to the material on leukemia in the section on Metastatic Intracranial Tumors. Despite the impressive clinical and myelographic evidence of an extradural block in these cases, the tumor tissue is usually diffusely distributed and cannot be recognized as a discrete mass. The epidural infiltrate is often microscopic and may exert some of its ill effects by compromising the vascular supply to the cord. An appreciation of these concepts is essential for proper management.

CLINICAL AND LABORATORY DIAGNOSIS.—These children, who may be in hematologic relapse or remission, often present with root pain in an extremity which, in the early stages, is not accompanied by impressive focal neurologic deficit. Gradually lower motor neuron signs of weakness, atrophy and areflexia develop and, in advanced cases, pyramidal tract signs become prominent as the cord is gradually compressed.

Lumbar puncture should be done with some caution in these patients because sudden signs of cord compromise may develop if fluid is removed and the dynamics are disturbed in a patient with established neurologic deficit. However, since intrathecal therapy is a preferred treatment method, one may be forced to take this risk. A small needle should be used and a small amount of fluid removed. Myelography,

Fig. 17.13.—Extradural spinal tumor—leukemia. Boy, 5½, was treated successfully for acute lymphoblastic leukemia for slightly over two years. Over a one-month period, while still in hematologic remission, he complained of increasing pain in the neck and back as well as pain in the right leg. Examination revealed a partial left peripheral facial palsy, rigidity of the back and lower motor neuron weakness and sensory deficit in the right leg and arm. Pain worsened in the supine position, and urinary incontinence gradually appeared. **A**, on 10/22/63 a complete myelographic block characteristic of a constricting epidural mass was demonstrated with Pantopaque. The contrast material was left in the spinal canal and radiation therapy was started. After 500 r, repeat x-rays (**B**) on 10/29/63 showed partial clearing of the block, but because of worsening paraplegia, pain and incontinence, a laminectomy was done. Some diffusely discolored fatty-looking tissue was found in the epidural space but no discrete obstructing lesion was found. Following a total of 900 r, repeat films (**C**) on 11/2/63 showed further clearing of the epidural block, but without appreciable neurologic change.

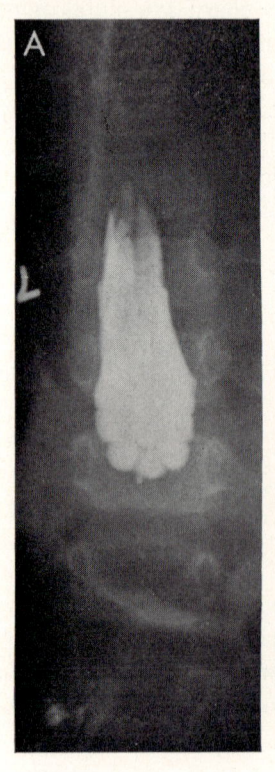

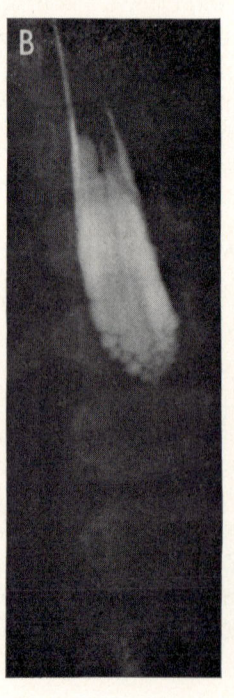

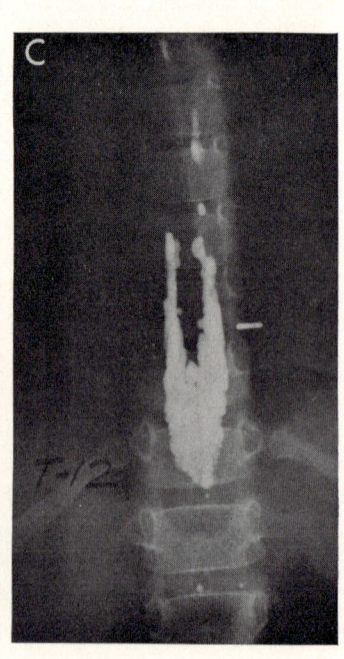

if performed, may show gradual constriction and attenuation of the Pantopaque shadow by the diffuse infiltrative process which surrounds the dura (Fig. 17.13).

MANAGEMENT AND PROGNOSIS.—The principles of treatment are essentially those listed for leukemia in the section on Metastatic Intracranial Tumors. The physician must consider the patient's total welfare in dealing with this problem and must not become too preoccupied with the goals he would set up if he were dealing with a primary extradural cord tumor. More specifically, if the child is entering the terminal stage of acute leukemia, the physician must make the patient comfortable and limit the number of painful diagnostic procedures which he undertakes, especially if the information which he obtains will not affect the treatment plan significantly.

NEUROBLASTOMA (SYMPATHICOBLASTOMA)

The reader should develop thorough familiarity with the behavior of this tumor because of its frequent occurrence in infants and children (second in incidence only to leukemia among 21 childhood malignancies), its remarkably variable clinical picture and the realistic hope for therapeutic cure.[8,14]

PATHOGENESIS.—From a histogenetic point of view, a line of gradation can be drawn between the neuroblastoma, the ganglioneuroblastoma and the ganglioneuroma. The unifying concept can be extended further if one notes the histologic similarity between the ganglioneuroma and the neurofibroma and the clinical coincidence of pheochromocytoma and ganglioneuroma in patients with neurofibromatosis.[35]

One of the commonest malignant tumors in children, the neuroblastoma can be found in the newborn infant[36] (Fig. 17.14) and is seen most commonly in the first two years of life, with two-thirds of the cases occurring under age 5.[14] The tumor can arise from ganglion cells and their precursors (neuroblasts) in the adrenal gland and from the sympathetic nervous system in any part of the body. It is said to arise from the adrenal gland in about half the patients under age 3.[35] In older patients the neoplasm arises most commonly from the sympathetic structures in the retroperitoneal space, the mediastinum and the neck. Spread can occur by direct extension through the extradural spinal space and by blood or lymph channels. Metastatic lesions are seen most frequently in bone, lymph nodes, liver, base of the skull, orbit and leptomeninges. Lesions which metastasize to the head are usually located in the base of the skull or the dural coverings rather than in the brain substance. Such metastatic masses commonly cause increased intracranial pressure.

CLINICAL AND LABORATORY DIAGNOSIS.—Discussion here will be limited largely to the behavior of neuroblastomas which invade the spinal canal from their paravertebral origin. The patient usually presents himself with the complaints of weakness, paresthesias and radiating pain. Examination reveals spastic weakness below the level of the tumor, impairment of deep sensation and light touch, urinary incontinence and extensor plantar responses. These signs will vary greatly depending upon the stage of the disease and the location of the tumor in relation to the cord (i.e., lateral, ventral, etc.). Green and associates[12] have called attention to the fact that occasionally patients with neuroblastoma have a celiac-like syndrome, i.e., chronic diarrhea, abdominal distention and weight loss. They hypothesized that the

274   TUMORS OF THE NERVOUS SYSTEM

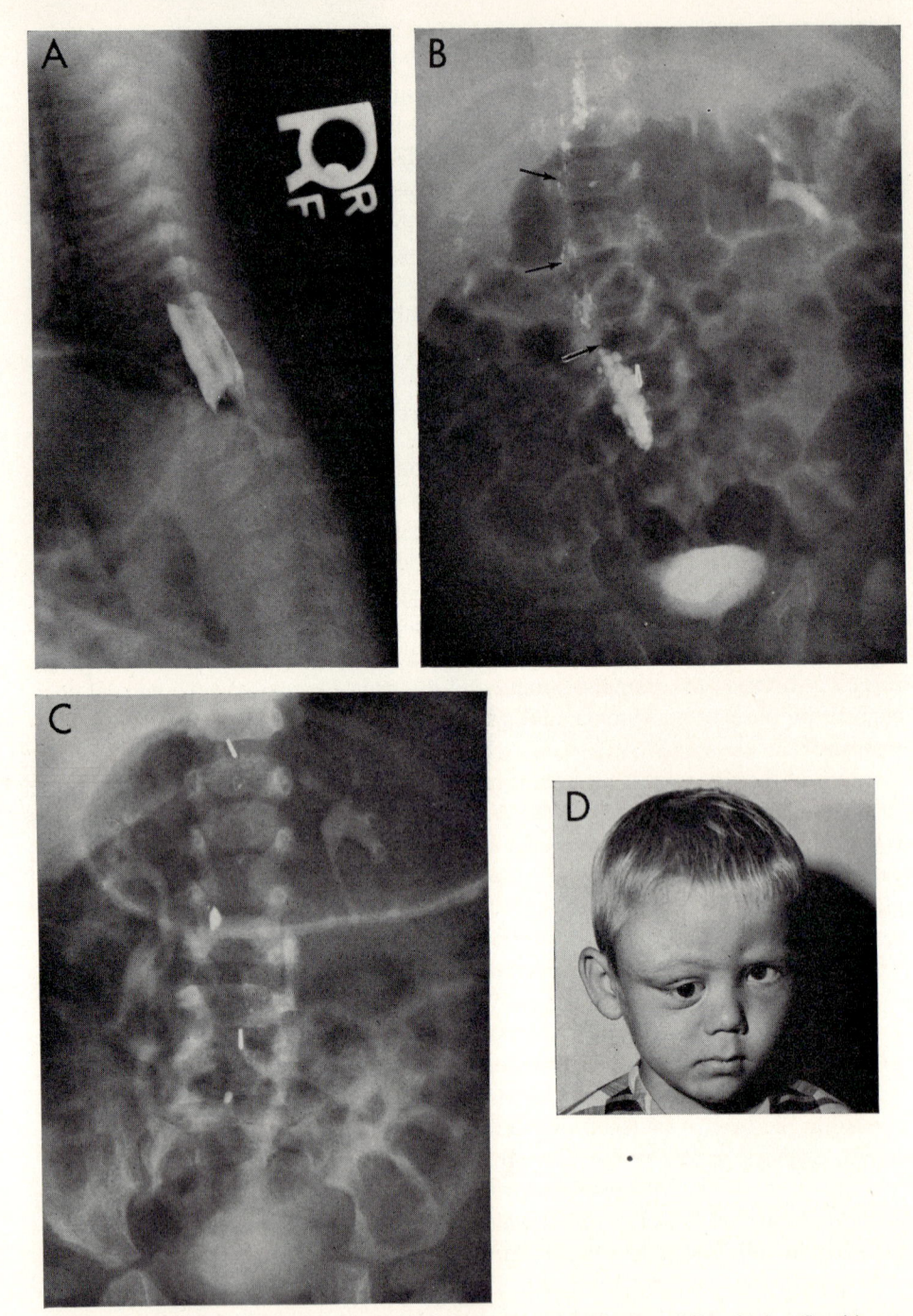

Fig. 17.14.—Congenital extradural spinal tumor neuroblastoma. Boy had a flaccid paraplegia at birth and the mother had noted a paucity of fetal movement during the pregnancy, her seventh. As a newborn, the baby cried when his spine was moved in any direction. Examination at 2 months revealed flaccid weakness of both legs, right more than left, a marked hyporeflexia and partial anesthesia in the legs, and incontinence of urine and feces. Lumbar myelogram revealed no cerebrospinal fluid. A cisternal myelogram was carried out and showed a complete block at D_{11} **(A)**. The extradural mass caused the dye to taper to a point medially in **A**. In **B**, the sweeping arclike indentation of the residual dye (arrows) can be seen when

diarrhea might result from a mechanism similar to that seen in patients with malignant carcinoid, inasmuch as the tumors secrete related chemicals (vanillyl mandelic acid and serotonin).

Except for enlargement of the foramen these masses do not produce striking bony changes on the plain spine x-rays. Myelography usually reveals a sweeping, arclike indentation of the dye column (Fig. 17.14,*B*). If the dural sac is surrounded by tumor tissue, the contrast medium is attenuated or tapered to a point of complete obstruction (Fig. 17.14,*A*). When a mass of this type is detected, especially in a young child, a chest x-ray should be ordered, and an intravenous urogram made promptly. The urogram will often reveal a posterior abdominal mass displacing the kidney laterally (Fig. 17.14,*B*), and a soft-tissue mass may be visualized in the posterior mediastinum on the chest film. In such circumstances one can essentially prove the histologic diagnosis of neuroblastoma by comparing quantitatively the urinary output of 3-methoxy-4-hydroxy mandelic acid (vanillyl mandelic acid or VMA), a product of epinephrine metabolism.[13] Quantities in excess of 12 mg./100 ml. strongly suggest the diagnosis of neuroblastoma. Most normal persons excrete less than 4 mg./100 ml.

MANAGEMENT AND PROGNOSIS.—Over the past 25 years the prognosis for patients with neuroblastoma, especially infants, has improved appreciably. The problem should be managed as a team effort by the surgeon, the medical specialist, the radiologist and the tumor therapist. In patients who have no demonstrable metastases, the mass should be totally excised, if possible, and local radiation therapy then given (Fig. 17.14).[24] The latter approach in a large series reported by Gross *et al.*[14] has led to a cure* ratio of 88%. Partial tumor resection followed by radiation and chemotherapy with vincristine or Cytoxan has produced a cure rate of 64%. In those patients in whom only biopsy has been performed, x-ray irradiation and chemotherapy still produce a cure rate of 38%. Two-thirds of the babies who have had radiation therapy to liver metastases have been cured, but survival following bone metastases is rare (Fig. 17.14,*D*). Currently the overall cure rate in the large series mentioned above is over 36%, whereas in babies under age 1 the cure rate is 56%. Other reports[20,42] support the need for an optimistic outlook although the survival rates in most large series which include older children are not good. Anyone who has dealt with many cases of this tumor recognizes the fact that an occasional spontaneous cure may occur with this unusual neoplasm,

---

*The term "cure" is used in the case of this tumor if the child is well two years after treatment.

---

the complete block had been relieved surgically. A two-stage laminectomy achieved partial removal of a large extradural tumor from D_{11} to S_1. Tissue diagnosis was neuroblastoma, and radiation therapy was given to the left side of the abdomen and spine in a total tumor dose of 3,200 r. The initial intravenous pyelogram **(B)** shows displacement of the left kidney laterally; also note the erosion of the pedicles of L_{1-2-3} (arrows). On follow-up examination at age 2½ the patient was walking, had a normal intravenous pyelogram **(C)** but still had urinary incontinence. The tumor is probably cured.

Metastatic neuroblastoma. This 5½-year-old boy had a retroperitoneal neuroblastoma found at operation when he was 4½. Six months later pain developed in the left arm and head. Tumor cells were found in bone marrow, but no metastatic lesions were demonstrated in an x-ray survey of the skeleton. He was treated vigorously with x-ray, vincristine and Cytoxan. A year after diagnosis a slowly enlarging soft-tissue mass appeared over the right eye **(D)**, together with bone pain, fever and anorexia. At this time metastatic lytic lesions were demonstrable on skull x-rays and he was excreting excessive quantities of VMA in the urine.

especially in young infants. Some workers have advocated serial quantitative urinary catecholamine (VMA) determinations to follow the course of these patients and to aid in more accurate prognosis.[46,50]

Sarcoma

Sarcomas, among the commonest spinal tumors in children, arise from the epidural space, the vertebral bodies or the retroperitoneal or mediastinal space and invade the spinal canal through the invertebral foramen.

Patients with these malignant tumors present with symptoms and signs of cord compression, and the tumor masses produce essentially the same bony and myelographic abnormalities as those described under Neuroblastoma. Definitive diagnosis depends upon surgical biopsy.

The mass is excised as completely as possible and the patient is given a course of local radiation therapy. The prognosis must be guarded with these lesions since the general prognosis is poor, but one can expect an excellent outcome in some cases.[11]

Chordomas

These extremely rare tumors develop at the ends of the notochord. They are seen in the sacrococcygeal spinal canal more often in children and along the clivus in adults. Characterized primarily by destructive bone changes in the vertebrae, these slow-growing masses are associated with typical myelographic signs of an epidural mass.

Tumors of the Skull

Congenital Tumors

PATHOGENESIS.—These rare tumors (dermoid, epidermoid, teratoma) of the scalp and skull may occur as isolated anomalies or they may have direct intracranial extensions. Lesions located near the midline, especially the occipital area, more commonly have intracranial cystic extensions (Chapter 13). Teratomas may reach a huge size and contain a variety of diverse tissue elements.

CLINICAL AND LABORATORY DIAGNOSIS.—These congenital tumors often are seen as a small, firm, rubbery mass beneath the scalp which may communicate with the skin surface.

Radiologically there is a clear area of bone destruction in the skull, the circumference of which is sharply delineated by a line of increased bony density. Laterally located lesions are usually confined to the skin and skull, whereas midline lesions more frequently have intracranial extensions. These roentgen findings must be differentiated from those of metastatic lesions, cavernous hemangiomas of the skull,[43] eosinophilic granuloma, fibrous dysplasia and normal venous lakes.

MANAGEMENT AND PROGNOSIS.—These tumors, including their intracranial extensions, should be removed to prevent infection of the cyst and to prevent the slowly growing intracranial extension from damaging nerve structures by compression.

Primary Neoplasms (Osteomas and Sarcomas)

PATHOGENESIS.—By definition, osteomas are benign tumors and sarcomas are malignant tumors of the skull. Both lesions occur uncommonly.

CLINICAL AND LABORATORY DIAGNOSIS.—Osteomas first appear as hard lumps on the skull which may enlarge greatly. The masses grow outward and are not pulsatile. They are characterized on x-ray by an area of increased density which may be separated (on a tangential view) from the outer table and which rarely extends to involve the diploë or the inner table. Occasional cases may require differentiation from meningiomas.

Sarcomas, in contrast, appear as firm, tender masses over the vault which grow rapidly and may pulsate. On x-ray one sees irregular areas of decreased bone density or destruction. Fortunately rare, these very malignant neoplasms metastasize via the blood stream, often to the lung.

MANAGEMENT AND PROGNOSIS.—Osteomas can be excised completely with an excellent prognosis. Large defects may require cranioplasty.

Malignant sarcomas should be treated by radical excision followed by a course of radiation therapy. Unless the tumor is discovered early, before metastatic spread, the outlook is poor.

BIBLIOGRAPHY

1. Bailey, P., et al.: *Intracranial Tumors of Infancy and Childhood* (Chicago: University of Chicago Press, 1939)
2. Bouchard, J.: *Radiation Therapy of Tumors and Diseases of the Nervous System* (Philadelphia: Lea & Febiger, 1966).
3. Bray, P. F., et al.: Brainstem tumors in children, Neurology 8:1, 1958.
4. Chutorian, A. M., et al.: Optic gliomas in children, Neurology 14:83, 1964.
5. Cummins, F. M., et al.: Treatment of gliomas of the third ventricle and pinealomas, Neurology 10:1031, 1960.
6. Cuneo, H. M., and Rand, C. W.: *Brain Tumors of Childhood* (Springfield, Ill.: Charles C Thomas, Publisher, 1952).
7. D'Angio, G. J., et al.: Roentgen therapy of certain complications of acute leukemia in childhood, Am. J. Roentgenol. 82:541, 1959.
8. Dargeon, H. W.: Neuroblastoma, J. Pediat. 61:456, 1962.
9. Evans, A. E., et al.: Central nervous system complications of children with acute leukemia, J. Pediat. 64:94, 1964.
10. Farber, S.: Chemotherapy in the treatment of leukemia and Wilms' tumor, J.A.M.A. 198:826, 1966.
11. Ford, F. M.: *Diseases of the Nervous System in Infancy, Childhood and Adolescence* (5th ed.; Springfield, Ill.: Charles C Thomas, Publisher, 1966).
12. Green, M., et al.: Occurrence of chronic diarrhea in three patients with ganglioneuromas, Pediatrics 23:951, 1959.
13. Greer, M., et al.: Tumors of neural crest origin, Arch. Neurol. 13:139, 1965.
14. Gross, R. E., et al.: Neuroblastoma sympatheticum—a study and report of 217 cases, Pediatrics 23:1179, 1959.
15. Haft, H., et al.: Spinal cord tumors in children, Pediatrics 23:1152, 1959.
16. Hudson, A. C.: Primary tumors of the optic nerve (a phenomenon of Recklinghausen's disease), Arch. Ophth. 23:735, 1940.
17. Hyman, C. B., et al.: Central nervous system involvement by leukemia in children: I. Relationship to systemic leukemia and description of clinical and laboratory manifestations, Blood 25:1, 1965.
18. Ingraham, F. D., and Matson, D. D.: *Neurosurgery of Infancy and Childhood* (2d ed.; Springfield, Ill.: Charles C Thomas, Publisher, 1961).
19. Jackson, I. J., and Thompson, R. K. (eds.): *Pediatric Neurosurgery* (Springfield, Ill.: Charles C Thomas, Publisher, 1959).
20. James, D. H., et al.: Combination chemotherapy of childhood neuroblastoma, J.A.M.A. 194:123, 1965.

21. Lampkin, B. C., et al.: Response of medulloblastoma to vincristine sulfate: Case report, Pediatrics 39:761, 1967.
22. Lassman, L. P., et al.: Sensitivity of intracranial gliomas to vincristine sulfate, Lancet 1:296, 1965.
23. Leikin, S. L.: Leukemia: current concepts in therapy, Pediat. Clin. North America 9:753, 1962.
24. Lingley, J. F., et al.: Neuroblastoma, New England J. Med. 277:1227, 1967.
25. Low, N. L., et al.: Tumors of the cerebral hemisphere in children, Arch. Neurol. 13:547, 1965.
26. Malamud, N.: Psychiatric disorder with intracranial tumors of the limbic system, Arch. Neurol. 17:113, 1967.
27. Matson, D. D.: Intracranial Tumors, in Farmer, T. W. (ed.): *Pediatric Neurology* (New York City: Paul B. Hoeber, Inc., 1964).
28. Miller, R. W., et al.: Association of Wilms's tumor with aniridia, hemihypertrophy and other congenital malformations, New England J. Med. 270:922, 1964.
29. Moore, E. W., et al.: The central nervous system in acute leukemia, A.M.A. Arch. Int. Med. 105:451, 1960.
30. Odom, G. L., et al.: Brain tumors in children, Pediatrics 18:856, 1956.
31. Rand, R. W., and Rand, C. W.: *Intraspinal Tumors of Childhood* (Springfield, Ill.: Charles C Thomas, Publisher, 1960).
32. Reiquam, C. W., et al.: Wilms' tumors, Rocky Mountain M. J., April, 1965.
33. Rieselbach, R. E., et al.: Intrathecal aminopterin therapy of meningeal leukemia, Arch. Int. Med. 111:620, 1963.
34. Rubin, R. C., et al.: Cerebrospinal fluid perfusion for central nervous system neoplasms, Neurology 16:680, 1966.
35. Russell, D. S., and Rubinstein, L. J.: *Pathology of Tumors of the Nervous System* (2d ed.; Baltimore: Williams & Wilkins Company, 1963).
36. Schneider, K. M., et al.: Neonatal neuroblastoma, Pediatrics 36:359, 1965.
37. Sciarra, D., and Sprofkin, B. E.: Symptoms and signs referable to the basal ganglia in brain tumor, A.M.A. Arch. Neurol. & Psychiat. 69:450, 1953.
38. Selawry, O. S., and Hananian, J.: Vincristine treatment of cancer in children, J.A.M.A. 183:741, 1963.
39. Shaw, R. K., et al.: Meningeal leukemia, Neurology 10:823, 1960.
40. Shuangshoti, S., and Netsky, M. G.: Neuroepithelial (colloid) cysts of the nervous system, Neurology 16:887, 1966.
41. Sullivan, M. P.: Intracranial complications of leukemia in children, Pediatrics 20:757, 1957.
42. Sutow, W. W.: Prognosis in neuroblastoma of childhood, A.M.A. Am. J. Dis. Child. 96:299, 1958.
43. Taveras, J. M., and Wood, E. H.: *Diagnostic Neuroradiology* (Baltimore: Williams & Wilkins Company, 1964).
44. Taveras, J. M., et al.: The value of radiation therapy in the management of glioma of the optic nerves and chiasm, Radiology 66:518, 1956.
45. Vaeth, J. M., and Levitt, S. H.: Five-year results in the treatment of Wilms' tumor of children, J. Urol. 90:247, 1963.
46. Voorhess, M. L., and Gardner, L. I.: The value of serial catecholamine determinations in children with neuroblastoma, Pediatrics 30:241, 1962.
47. Whiteside, J. A., et al.: Intrathecal amethopterin in neurological manifestations of leukemia, A.M.A. Arch. Int. Med. 101:279, 1958.
48. Wilhyde, D. E., et al.: Spinal epidural leukemia, Am. J. Med. 34:281, 1963.
49. Wilkins, L.: *The Diagnosis and Treatment of Endocrine Disorders in Childhood and Adolescence* (Springfield, Ill.: Charles C Thomas, Publisher, 1965).
50. Williams, C. M., and Greer, M.: Homovanillic acid and vanilmandelic acid in diagnosis of neuroblastoma, J.A.M.A. 183:836, 1963.
51. Witcofski, R. L., and Roper, T. J.: A technique for scanning the posterior fossa, J. Nuclear Med. 6:754, 1965.
52. Wood, E. H., et al.: The value of radiation therapy in the management of intrinsic tumors of the spinal cord, Radiology 63:11, 1954.

18

Infections

Meningoencephalitis
    Acute Bacterial Meningitis
        Typical meningitis   Recurrent meningitis
        Meningitis in infancy   Neurologic complications
        Neonatal meningitis
    Acute Viral Encephalomyelitis and Meningitis
    Chronic Meningitis
Abscess Formation
    Brain Abscess   Subdural or Epidural Empyema
Infections with Neurotoxic Organisms
    Tetanus   Botulism (Chapter 20)
    Diphtheritic Polyneuritis
Encephalomyelitis
    Postinfectious
        Measles (rubeola)   Exanthem subitum (roseola)
        Chickenpox (varicella)   Whooping cough (pertussis)
        German measles (rubella)   Smallpox (variola)
        Mumps
    Postvaccinal
        Vaccinia   Pertussis
        Rabies
Disorders of Possible Infectious Etiology
    Acute Cerebellitis (Acute Pontine Encephalitis)
    Acute Labyrinthitis
    Neuritis of the Facial Nerve (Bell's Palsy)
    Infectious Polyneuritis or Neuronitis (Landry-Guillain-Barré)
    Infectious Mononucleosis
    Reticuloendothelioses
    Subacute Inclusion Encephalitis (Subacute Sclerosing Leukoencephalitis)
    Chronic Orbital Cellulitis with Myositis (Orbital Pseudotumor)
    Sarcoidosis
    Cat-Scratch Fever
    "Acute Toxic Encephalopathy" (Chapter 16)

INFECTIONS

UNTIL 10–20 years ago infections of the nervous system—particularly purulent meningitis, poliomyelitis, tuberculous meningitis and postmeasles encephalomyelitis—occupied a position of terrifying pre-eminence, not only as a major cause of death, but also as a group of diseases which handicapped and crippled thousands of patients each year. In no other field of medicine have research advances and their clinical application led to such dramatic reductions in mortality and morbidity rates. The discovery of a potent collection of antibiotic and chemotherapeutic drugs for bacterial infections and the development of selective vaccines for the poliomyelitis and measles viruses have reduced significantly the epidemiologic importance of infections of the nervous system. Despite these therapeutic advances, many problems still exist.

Meningoencephalitis

Many different types of meningitis and encephalitis are clinically indistinguishable, and their differentiation depends upon precise microbiologic laboratory tests.[31,33] For these reasons the disorders will be discussed under the group headings as much as possible, rather than individually.

PATHOGENESIS

ETIOLOGY.—The many different microorganisms which can cause infections of the central nervous system are listed in Table 18.1 according to their basic microbiologic categories.

EPIDEMIOLOGY.—The distinctive epidemiologic characteristics of bacterial meningitis and viral encephalitis deserve special comment because of their diagnostic clinical importance and because of efforts directed to prevention.

Figure 18.1 illustrates graphically the relative frequency of the commonest forms of acute bacterial meningitis in infancy, as well as the common types of prenatal meningoencephalitis. Many reported series have agreed that *Hemophilus influenzae type B* ranks first among the etiologic agents of childhood meningitis. It is rarely seen after age 5 except among the elderly. Like H. influenzae, the *meningococcus* and the *pneumococcus* often cause meningitis in infants under 1 year of age but, unlike H. influenzae, they continue to affect older age groups. Meningoencephalitis during the first two to three months of life is most commonly due to *Escherichia coli* (often associated with obstetric complications), *staphylococci* and the virus of *herpes simplex*. Congenital meningoencephalitis is seen rarely in newborn infants. It is caused by a varied but special group of microorganisms—*cytomegalovirus, rubella virus,* the protozoan *toxoplasma* and the *treponema* of syphilis. All types of meningitis occur sporadically and only meningococcus appears in epidemic proportion. Rarely the dog roundworm, *Toxocara canis,* causes signs and symptoms of encephalitis,[52e] as does *Mycoplasma pneumoniae*.

Viral infections of the central nervous system are contracted in different ways. Arthropod-borne virus infections (*arbovirus*) are transmitted to man and other hosts (birds and mammals) by the bite of arthropods (usually mosquitoes but in some cases ticks or mites). Man-to-man transmission of an arbovirus infection does not occur. *Enteroviruses* which normally inhabit the gastrointestinal tract and

TABLE 18.1.—Etiologic Agents of Meningoencephalitis

Acute
  Bacterial
    Gram-negative bacilli
      Hemophilus influenzae
      Enteric bacteria
    Gram-negative cocci
      Neisseria meningitidis (meningococcus)
    Gram-positive cocci
      Pneumococcus
      Streptococcus
      Staphylococcus
    Gram-positive bacilli
      Listeria
    Gram-negative coccobacilli
      Pasteurella tularensis
      Brucella abortus
  Viral
    Arboviruses
      St. Louis
      Western equine
      Eastern equine
      Japanese B
      Colorado tick fever
    Enteroviruses
      Polio
      Coxsackie
      ECHO
    Mumps virus
    Herpes viruses
      Herpes simplex
      Herpes virus varicella (zoster)
    Rubella virus
    Rabies virus
    Lymphocytic choriomeningitis virus
    Mycoplasma pneumoniae[68b]

Chronic
  Bacterial
  Mycobacterium tuberculosis
  Fungus
  Cryptococcus neoformans
  Coccidioides immitis
  Spirochetal
  Leptospira
  Congenital
  Cytomegalovirus (salivary gland virus) ⎫
  Rubella virus ⎬ Chapter 13
  Protozoal ⎭
  Toxoplasma

nasopharynx of man are transmitted by close human contact, involving contamination with oral secretions or intestinal excreta. Most of the other virus or presumed virus infections, such as mumps, rubella,[52d] herpes and infectious mononucleosis are transmitted by direct contact. Rabies is transmitted by the bite of a rabid animal (usually a dog, but bats, skunks, foxes and other animals also carry the virus), and leptospiral infections are transmitted by the urine of dogs and rats. The rare fungus and yeast forms of meningoencephalitis (cryptococcosis and coccidioidomycosis) are transmitted via the blood stream to the meninges from the respiratory tract after being inhaled. Contamination with pigeon excreta has presumably accounted for an increased incidence of cryptococcosis, whereas coccidioidomycosis is found endemically in arid areas where the spores are readily air-borne.

PATHOLOGY.—In acute *bacterial meningitis* the brain, as well as the basal cisterns and the cord, may be covered with a purulent exudate and the whole cerebrum may appear hyperemic and swollen. Histologically there are collections of pus cells, bacteria and fibrin clumps between the arachnoid and pia mater. Evidence of cerebritis and venous thrombosis is seen at times, especially in fatal cases.

282 INFECTIONS

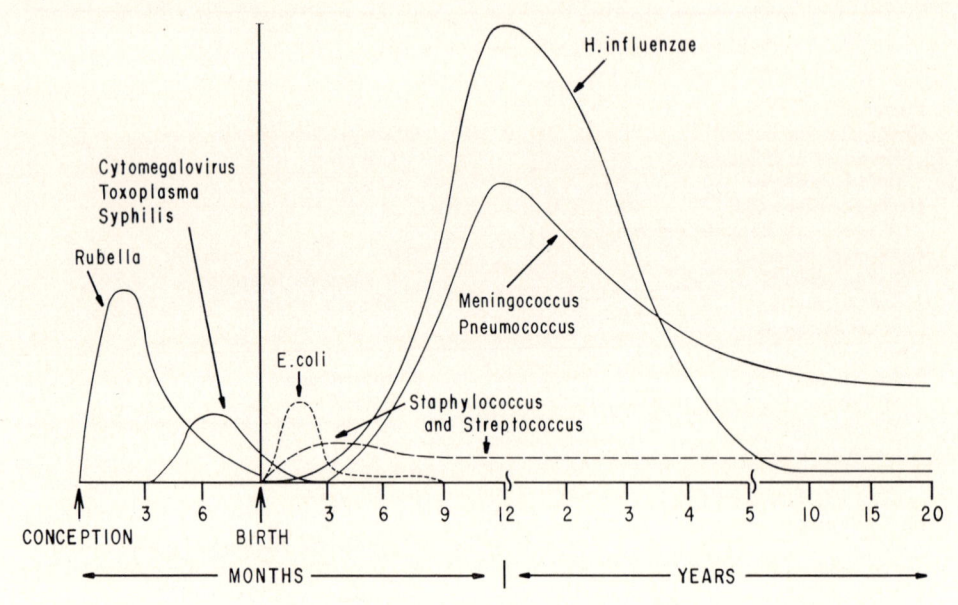

Fig. 18.1.—Age distribution of the common types of childhood meningitis.

The thick pus and inflammatory adhesions at the base can cause noncommunicating hydrocephalus, and the same processes over the surface give rise to communicating hydrocephalus.

In *tuberculous meningitis* the meninges over the convexity have a grayish opacity, and there is a thick, gelatinous exudate around the base of the brain that causes obstructive hydrocephalus in a high percentage of cases. Focal areas of caseation and inflammatory changes in the blood vessels lead, respectively, to small areas of necrosis and ischemic infarction. Other types of *granulomatous meningitis* (cryptococcosis and coccidioidomycosis) produce changes similar to those of tuberculosis.

In general *viral meningoencephalitis,* regardless of specific etiology, causes similar pathologic changes in the nervous system. Grossly the brain and cord appear congested and edematous. Microscopically one sees small hemorrhages, perivascular cuffing or infiltration by neutrophils and mononuclear cells, glial proliferation, varying nerve cell changes and neuronophagia. Inclusion bodies, focal destruction of white matter and arteritis are seen in some cases. With *poliomyelitis* gross changes include petechiae and hemorrhages in the anterior horns of the spinal cord, and microscopically there is varying damage to neurons in the gray matter of the spinal cord, medulla, pons, midbrain and precentral gyrus. Type A intranuclear inclusion bodies are seen in the neurons in *herpes simplex* and *subacute inclusion encephalitis* (Dawson[16] and van Bogaert[58c]). Softening and necrosis of the white matter are seen in herpes simplex, western equine and subacute inclusion encephalitis (or sclerosing leukoencephalitis). A constant arteritis characterizes equine encephalomyelitis. Prenatal infections of the central nervous system are discussed in Chapter 13.

Clinical Diagnosis

Acute Bacterial Meningitis

Typical meningitis.—Fever, vomiting, chills and headache usually occur, with a history of an antecedent upper respiratory infection. Convulsions are common in children, and the patient may show somnolence or marked stupor. Stiffness or rigidity of the neck and back is often present and may be associated with a positive Kernig sign (inability to extend the supine patient's knee completely when the thigh is flexed at the hip), the Brudzinski sign (flexion of the patient's neck elicits flexion of the knee, hip and ankle) or opisthotonos. When petechiae appear on the skin or mucous membranes, one thinks specifically of meningococcemia with or without meningitis. If the hemorrhagic skin eruption evolves rapidly and the patient is in shock, the clinical picture is called the Waterhouse-Friedrichsen syndrome and is associated with bilateral adrenal hemorrhage. Purulent otitis media occurs with both pneumococcal and influenzal infections, and septicemia is the rule with all types of acute bacterial meningitis.

Meningitis in infancy.—These patients have nonspecific signs of acute illness such as vomiting, fever, irritability, a high-pitched cry and convulsions. Meningeal signs (such as nuchal rigidity, the Kernig and Brudzinski signs) may not be prominent, but in many babies a bulging fontanel develops. An essential, general rule for the physician is to do a lumbar puncture whenever the possibility of meningitis enters his mind, especially if a convulsion has occurred and he has not found an adequate alternative explanation for the illness.

Neonatal meningitis.—Subtle and nonspecfiic clinical signs characterize neonatal meningitis.[7] Lethargy, irritability, feeding difficulties, respiratory distress and convulsions are most usual, whereas fever, a tense fontanel and meningeal signs are uncommon. In fact, hypothermia should alert one to the possibility of meningitis in a newborn. Other factors which should heighten suspicion of meningitis in the neonate include perinatal maternal infections and prematurely born infants, especially boys.

Recurrent meningitis.—Recurrent attacks of meningitis usually result when an open path from the intracranial cavity to the outside permits repeated bacterial contamination.[18] This set of circumstances can follow a basilar skull fracture with rhinorrhea and otorrhea (Chapter 15), especially in patients with chronic purulent sinus, mastoid or ear infections. It can be found with a congenital dermal sinus (Chapter 13) or with an intracranial foreign body (shunt tube for hydrocephalus). Recurrent meningitis can also occur in patients with an impaired ability to manufacture antibodies (e.g., agammaglobulinemia).

Management of these patients often poses a difficult clinical problem and requires thorough diagnostic study. The patient's head should be shaved and inspected carefully for a dermal sinus, nasal discharge should be tested for glucose (using Testape), x-rays of the skull, sinuses and mastoids should be taken, and the serum proteins should be fractionated for gamma globulin. If the basic cause or an abnormal port of entry is not demonstrated with these studies, fluorescein or phenolsulfonphthalein may be instilled into the lumbar subarachnoid space. The patient's head is then tilted down so that the exit of the foreign material can be visualized (using Wood's lamp in the case of florescein), especially in the area of the cribriform plate. Some workers have run Lipiodol into the head and looked for evidence of a leak by means of fluoroscopy.

One can expect to see a variety of bacteria as the etiologic agents in recurrent meningitis. Gram-negative organisms in particular, as well as pneumococcus,[60a] H. influenzae and staphylococcus, have been reported.

Neurologic complications of purulent and granulomatous meningitis include (1) subdural effusions (common) and subdural empyema (rare), (2) damage to cranial nerves (II, III, VI, VII, VIII) by basilar adhesions and (3) hydrocephalus (see Pathology), venous sinus thrombosis and brain abscess. The physician should suspect the development of a subdural effusion in any infant who shows persistent fever, a full or bulging fontanel, repeated seizures and focal neurologic deficit. Diagnostic subdural taps should be done if the patient does not improve promptly without persistent signs of infection. Often the cranial nerve deficit proves to be transient, although permanent deafness is not uncommon. Swartz and Dodge[58] have emphasized that papilledema in acute meningitis should make one suspect subdural empyema, venous sinus thrombosis or brain abscess.

Acute Viral Meningoencephalomyelitis

Acute symptoms include fever, headache, vomiting and lethargy, a clinical picture similar to that of acute bacterial meningitis. The patient may have some nuchal rigidity and always manifests varying degrees of an acute mental syndrome—stupor, coma, irritability, delirium and convulsions. Patients with arbovirus infections (Table 18.1) have more cerebral signs, whereas those with enterovirus infections (ECHO, Coxsackie and poliomyelitis) and mumps virus infections exhibit more striking meningeal signs.

Herpes simplex virus infections of the nervous system usually cause a rapidly fulminating clinical picture in which death results from a severe necrotizing inflammation of the brain[62,63] or the patient is left with severe brain damage.[35] Nervous system infections with *varicella-zoster virus* cause radiculitis with pain, a vesicular eruption (Fig. 18.2) and usually mild meningeal signs.

In 1958, laboratory studies consisting of virus isolations and antibody determinations were performed on a series of 511 patients in southern California by Lennette and associates.[36] These workers incriminated viral etiologic agent in almost two-thirds of the patients. Included were infections with 20 different enteroviruses. Among 60 patients with encephalitis, several cases of Coxsackie and ECHO virus infections were encountered. No agent was identified in 55% of these patients. Among 35 patients not vaccinated with polio virus, 26 had paralytic poliomyelitis, in contrast to 3 cases of paralysis among 17 patients who had received three doses of Salk vaccine. Mumps virus infections were seen most commonly in the spring, and enterovirus infections predominated in the summer. The same group of workers[41,42] showed earlier that other enterovirus infections generally cause milder degrees of paralysis than does polio virus. However, severe and even fatal cases of ECHO[57] and Coxsackie infection are occasionally seen.

The *enteroviruses* (polio, Coxsackie and ECHO) cause widespread infection. They can cause neurologic syndromes varying from aseptic meningitis to encephalitis to paralytic illness. At present they fortunately cause a much smaller number of disabling infections of the nervous system than they did previously because of an effective vaccine against poliomyelitis.

Poliomyelitis can be inapparent, abortive, nonparalytic or paralytic. Krugman and Ward[31] report that 90–95% of the population have *inapparent* infections, 4–8% have *abortive* infections and less than 2% develop *nonparalytic* or *paralytic* forms of the disease. In the last two types of poliomyelitis, usually after an initial phase characterized by sore throat, headache, fever and gastrointestinal symptoms, the patient is relatively well for about a week. Then the same symptoms recur, with headache, myalgia, meningeal symptoms and fever followed by weakness or paralysis of almost any of the skeletal muscles. Marked rigidity of the neck, back and hamstrings is seen, with focal weakness, muscle tenderness and hyporeflexia. Paralysis is notoriously asymmetric, often involves the respiratory muscles and, in the case of bulbar poliomyelitis, affects muscles innervated by the lower cranial nerves, especially the facial and the vagus. In severe bulbar disease the vital centers in the brain stem which control pulse, respiration and blood pressure are damaged, causing death in many cases. Patients with poliomyelitis do not have sensory deficit.

Coxsackie and *ECHO virus* infections usually produce a mild, acute febrile illness with signs of meningeal irritation.[31] However, it is important to realize, now that vaccination for poliomyelitis is used widely, that both Coxsackie and ECHO virus infections can cause paralysis occasionally.[23,43] Among 35 unvaccinated patients with acute clinical paralytic illness, 26 (74%) had polio virus infection and 14% had Coxsackie, ECHO or mumps virus infections. Residual paresis was seen only in two patients with Coxsackie infections.[36]

Fig. 18.2.—Herpes zoster radiculitis and meningoencephalitis (complicating Hodgkin's disease). Lumbar puncture revealed clear fluid under normal pressure. The cerebrospinal fluid contained 150 leukocytes (90% mononuclear cells), with a glucose content of 70 mg./100 ml. and protein of 44 mg./100 ml. The culture revealed no growth.

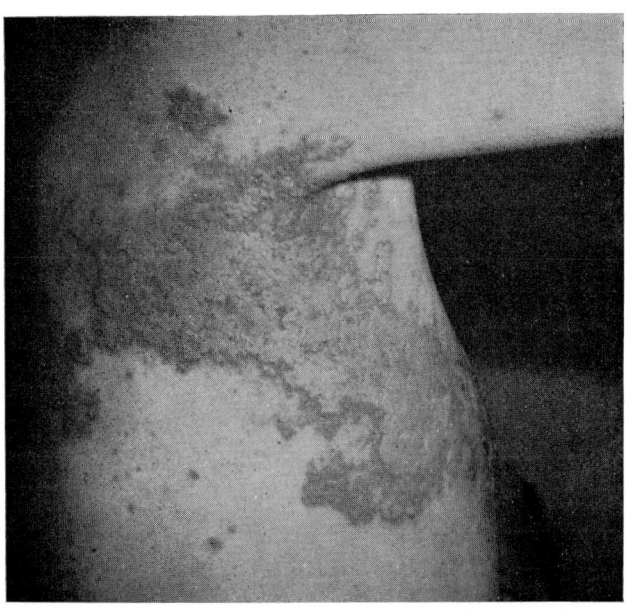

Mumps meningoencephalitis occurs in an estimated 10% of infections, but it usually is a mild type of aseptic meningitis with headache and stiff neck. Rarely, however, a severe, fatal form of the disease occurs. Although mumps meningoencephalitis usually follows the parotitis, it may antedate or occur in the absence of parotitis.

Rabies, an inevitably fatal type of encephalitis, is very uncommon. The disease is characterized by fever, delirium, convulsions, maniacal behavior and painful spasmodic contractions of the muscles of deglutition.

Chronic Granulomatous Meningitis

Tuberculous, cryptococcal[11] and *coccidioidal* meningitis is characterized by the slow but progressive evolution of systemic symptoms (fever, headache, irritability, vomiting) and neurologic manifestations (convulsions, stupor, meningeal signs and evidence of increased intracranial pressure). Not uncommonly at present these patients are studied intensively for brain tumor, brain abscess and subdural hematoma before a definitive diagnosis is made. The presence of papilledema and other signs of increased intracranial pressure usually serves to delay diagnosis because of the common reluctance to do a spinal tap. We think that such patients who have any evidence of infection and who do not have focal neurologic deficit should have a careful diagnostic lumbar puncture with a thorough study of the cerebrospinal fluid. Patients with tuberculosis usually have an abnormal chest x-ray and a positive tuberculin skin test, and patients with coccidioidomycosis may live in an endemic area.

Intracranial tuberculomas now occur only rarely in the United States but are more common in other parts of the world. The symptoms and signs resemble closely those of brain tumor. In the series of Sibley and O'Brien[53] seizures and increased intracranial pressure affected the majority of patients. The lesions can be situated anywhere in the nervous system, and diagnosis is rarely made without operation unless the patient has active tuberculous meningitis.[49] Postoperative meningitis can be prevented by giving antituberculous therapy for two to three months.

Leptospiral meningitis usually produces the typical clinical picture of aseptic meningitis. Distinguishing features such as icterus, oliguria, petechiae, skin rash and formed elements in the urine occur only with Leptospira icterohemorrhagiae infections.

LABORATORY DIAGNOSIS

Acute Bacterial Meningitis

As mentioned before, the physician should do a spinal puncture whenever there is the slightest suspicion of meningitis, knowing that he will do a certain number of "negative" taps but realizing also that almost all practicing physicians who see sick children will overlook the diagnosis of meningitis at some time. The CSF profiles or formulas in different types of meningoencephalitis are shown in Table 18.2. In the average case of acute purulent meningitis, (1) the CSF pressure is over 200 mm. H_2O, and (2) a pleocytosis varying from 10 to 10,000, usually

TABLE 18.2.—CEREBROSPINAL FLUID PROFILES IN MENINGOENCEPHALITIS

Disease	Cell Count Normal = 3 cells/cu. mm.	Glucose Normal = 40 mg./100 ml. or 40% of blood sugar value	Protein Normal = 55 mg./100 ml.
Acute bacterial meningitis	Elevated (polymorphonuclear) 10–10,000	Depressed	Elevated
Viral meningoencephalitis	Elevated (mononuclear) 15–500	Normal	Normal or slightly elevated
Chronic granulomatous meningitis	Elevated (mononuclear) 10–500	Depressed	Elevated

predominantly polymorphonuclear cells, is found. When extremely high CSF leukocyte counts are found one should consider the diagnosis of epidural abscess, subdural empyema or even a brain abscess which has ruptured into the ventricle. (3) The CSF sugar is low, either under 40 mg./100 ml. or less than 40% of a simultaneous blood sugar. (4) The CSF protein is elevated above 55 mg./100 ml. In a small percentage of patients (usually when the tap is done early), the cell count and sugar may be normal in the face of a positive culture later. (5) Gram-stained smear should be done to identify the organism. This can be misleading if the patient has received prior antibiotic therapy and if the technician is not expert. For these reasons, definitive decisions about specific therapy should be based upon (6) the culture report. The result of this laboratory test may also be negative if the patient has received sufficient antibiotic therapy before the spinal puncture is carried out.

Blood culture and *nose and throat culture* often yield the organism which has caused the purulent meningitis. A *leukocytosis* is usually seen, but in severely ill patients, especially young infants, a leukopenia may be found.

Viral Meningoencephalitis

The usual CSF findings in patients with viral infections are shown in Table 18.2. Typically, the fluid is water-clear, but in many cases it will have a ground-glass appearance. The cell count varies from 15 to 500, is predominantly mononuclear in type but may show a slight preponderance of polymorphonuclear cells early in the course. Sugar values are nearly always normal, but a mild elevation of the protein content may occur. In poliomyelitis the CSF protein rises after the first week of illness. Bacterial cultures are sterile. *Enterovirus, mumps* and *herpes virus* infections can be identified by (1) culture of the virus from stool or throat washings or (2) demonstration of a fourfold or greater rise in antibody titer by collecting paired sera in the acute and convalescent phases of the illness. *Lymphocytic choriomeningitis virus* (which causes the clinical picture of aseptic meningitis) can also be identified by the same serologic methods. The specific type of *arbovirus* infection cannot be identified during life by serologic methods, cultures of body fluids or stool. One can only expect to identify the specific agent by culturing the virus from the neural tissue in fatal cases.

Recent studies on the etiologic role of *herpes simplex* virus in infections of the nervous system stress the need for a critical attitude toward serologic and pathologic evidence of infection. In a study of 49 cases of herpes simplex meningoencephalitis, four patients had normal cerebrospinal fluid, indicating that even supposedly dependable clinical laboratory studies do not have complete diagnostic reliability.[49b] Recent reports on the clinical value of thymidine analogues such as idoxuridine in herpes simplex encephalitis,[43a] if confirmed, make it more urgent that diagnosis be made rapidly if one expects to prevent death or permanent neurologic damage.

Chronic Granulomatous Meningitis

The CSF profiles for *tuberculous, cryptococcal* and *coccidioidal* meningitis resemble one another (Table 18.2). Generally, the fluid contains 10–500 leukocytes, with either an even distribution in the differential count or a predominance of lymphocytes. The sugar content is usually abnormally low and the protein is elevated (to the point of pellicle formation in the advanced case). In suspicious cases a number of stains of the CSF sediment should be examined to identify acid-fast bacilli since cultural evidence is usually not obtained for three to four weeks.

An *India ink* preparation of the sediment should be carried out in any patient with a pleocytosis who does not have findings typical of acute purulent meningitis. The India ink stain reveals typical budding yeast cells with their doubly refractile walls in patients who have *cryptococcal* meningitis.[11] The causative organism of the less common infection, *coccidioidal* meningitis, can also be identified on smear by its typical spherule form. Both Cryptococcus neoformans and Coccidioides immitis can be cultured on Sabouraud's medium.

MANAGEMENT, PROGNOSIS AND PREVENTION

Purulent Meningitis

As soon as a tentative diagnosis of purulent meningitis has been made (with lumbar puncture and examination of the fluid), intensive nursing and medical care should be instituted. Therapy should be started *immediately* because any delay raises the mortality and morbidity rate significantly. Vomiting occurs in almost every case, and an intravenous infusion should be started promptly, using a "cutdown" if necessary, to give necessary fluids, electrolytes, whole blood and anticonvulsants.

THERAPY OF PURULENT MENINGITIS
OF UNKNOWN ETIOLOGY

Until a definitive culture report is obtained, therapy should be given as outlined in Table 18.3. If the CSF smear definitely reveals cocci, either gram negative or gram positive, penicillin G intravenously in doses of 10,000,000–40,000,000 units daily and a sulfonamide should be given.

Cephalothin, erythromycin or chloramphenicol can be used in patients who are allergic to penicillin. If one suspects staphylococci, methicillin (Staphcillin) should

TABLE 18.3.—ANTIMICROBIAL THERAPY OF PURULENT MENINGITIS

UNKNOWN ETIOLOGY*	H. INFLUENZAE*	PNEUMOCOCCUS*	MENINGOCOCCUS*	ESCH. COLI*	STAPHYLOCOCCUS*	STREPTOCOCCUS*	PSEUDOMONAS*
Chloramphenicol† Initial dose: 50 mg./kg. I.M. Daily dose: 100 mg./kg. in 4 divided doses	*Chloramphenicol* Same as unknown etiology	*Chloramphenicol* Same as unknown etiology					
Sulfonamide‡ Initial dose: 50 mg./kg. 5% sodium sulfadiazine I.V. or Gantrisin I.M. or I.V. Daily dose: 200 mg./kg. in 4 divided doses for 5 days	*Sulfonamide* Same as unknown etiology		*Sulfonamide* Same as unknown etiology				
Penicillin§ Aqueous crystalline penicillin: 12,000,000 units/day I.M. or I.V.		*Penicillin* Same as unknown etiology	*Penicillin* Same as unknown etiology		*Penicillin* (for sensitive organism) Same as unknown etiology	*Penicillin*§ Aqueous crystalline penicillin G: 12,000,000 units/day I.V. or I.M.	
	Streptomycin 40 mg./kg. I.M. every 12 hr.			*Kanamycin* 25 mg./kg./day I.M. in 4 divided doses (15 mg./kg. in prematures) *Ampicillin* 150 mg./kg./day I.V. or I.M. in 6 divided doses		*Streptomycin* 40 mg./kg./day I.M. in 2 divided doses	
					Methicillin (drug of choice) 150 mg./kg./day in 4 divided doses		*Polymyxin B*‖ 2.5 mg./kg./day I.M. in 2 divided doses 2.5 mg./day intrathecally for 3 days

*Antibiotic therapy is continued arbitrarily for a one-week period after defervescence.
†The use of chloramphenicol in premature and newborn infants requires special caution because of toxic side effects in ordinary therapeutic doses. The daily dose should not exceed 25 mg./kg. Clinical signs of intoxication include vomiting, abdominal distention, diarrhea, cyanosis, shallow respirations, hypothermia and shock.
‡Most workers agree that sulfisoxazole (Gantrisin) causes fewer renal complications (hematuria and anuria) than sulfadiazine and works as effectively.
§In patients who are allergic to penicillin one may substitute cephalothin (Keflin), erythromycin or chloramphenicol. For the treatment of purulent meningitis penicillin should not be given by mouth.
‖Use of polymyxin B should be reserved for the treatment of Pseudomonas meningitis. Polymyxin B can be given intrathecally for this disease but *not* polymyxin E.

be given along with penicillin G. Mathies and co-workers[44] reported a large series in which ampicillin alone was used effectively (rather than the accepted "triple therapy") for the treatment of the common types of meningitis (H. influenzae, pneumococcus and meningococcus). Others have recommended intravenous administration of ampicillin in large doses (150–400 mg./kg./day) in meningitis before the organism is identified.[48a] However, in *infants under 2 months of age,* in whom gram-negative enteric organisms are often encountered, a combination of kanamycin and ampicillin is recommended. Even in older patients an adequate course of ampicillin therapy alone may not suffice to eradicate the meningitis.[64] Therefore, we do not yet recommend this procedure for the treatment of purulent meningitis of unknown etiology because it fails to cover adequately the less common types of meningitis, such as that due to staphylococcus and some gram-negative organisms, and because confirmation of these observations seems desirable.

Antimicrobial agents should be given intravenously (and/or intramuscularly) until vomiting has stopped completely. We agree with those[47] who reserve intrathecal antibiotic therapy for patients who have or are suspected of having Pseudomonas meningitis (p. 291). When the causative organism has been identified by the laboratory, appropriate changes in the treatment program can be made (Table 18.3). Oral penicillin should *not* be used for the treatment of purulent meningitis because of its undependable absorption from the gut. However, chloramphenicol and sulfonamides can be given by mouth when vomiting has ceased.

Glucocorticoids are frequently used in the treatment of acute bacterial meningitis, especially that due to meningococcus, but their precise value has not been demonstrated. The temporary clinical effect may result from their real ability to reduce cerebral edema. Like the corticosteroid drugs, the enzymes such as streptokinase, streptodornase and pancreatic DNA are used empirically to prevent adhesive arachnoiditis, but their value as adjunctive therapy has not been established. Ordinarily, intrathecal enzyme therapy can be considered innocuous, but we have seen a patient in whom the enzyme caused a systemic and meningeal reaction which suggested an incompletely resolved meningitis.[50]

Seizures and coma which are considered secondary to acute brain swelling[61] should be treated immediately with anticonvulsants and agents which reduce cerebral edema, although the value of the latter therapy is still uncertain.[8] Good supportive care requires that severe *dehydration* be corrected promptly, but one must guard against overhydrating these small infants and producing hyponatremia and convulsions due to water intoxication. In our experience over the past 20 years, convulsions secondary to water intoxication are seen much more commonly in large hospitals than death due to dehydration.

In *subdural effusions* (proved by transillumination and diagnostic tap) aspiration is generally recommended, and usually the effusion can be evacuated completely with two or three taps.[5,40,52,55,56] If one suspects membrane formation, surgical excision may be necessary, but this decision should be made only by a neurologist. Inasmuch as evacuation of subdural effusions does not often alter the clinical course dramatically, we urge a cautious and thoughtful approach to the management of this problem. One should not forget that severe purulent meningitis can cause cerebritis, cerebral edema, anoxia from seizures, and venous thrombosis—complications which themselves can cause brain atrophy. In such cases the subdural effusions may result from the cerebral atrophy and not cause it.

SPECIFIC THERAPY OF BACTERIAL MENINGITIS

Meningococcus.—Although the sulfonamides have been considered the drug of choice for years, the recent emergence of sulfonamide-resistant strains of meningococci[34] necessitates the use of at least two therapeutic drugs. Penicillin, ampicillin, chloramphenicol or erythromycin can be employed with a sulfonamide until the organism's sensitivity has been established (Table 18.3).

H. influenzae.—Although chloramphenicol is considered the drug of choice, H. influenzal meningitis can be treated effectively with any of the following regimens: (1) chloramphenicol alone, (2) chloramphenicol and a sulfonamide, (3) chloramphenicol and streptomycin, (4) streptomycin and a sulfonamide, (5) tetracycline and a sulfonamide or (6) ampicillin.

Pneumococcus.—Known cases of pneumococcal meningitis can be treated satisfactorily with high doses of penicillin G. Some authorities[31] recommend combined therapy with chloramphenicol (Table 18.3) or a sulfonamide.

Coli-klebsiella.—Kanamycin and ampicillin, in that order, are considered the drugs of choice for treating coliform meningitis, a common form of the disease in newborn infants.

Staphylococcus.—Methicillin is considered the drug of choice for this type of meningitis unless one is dealing with an organism which is proved to be sensitive to penicillin G.

Pseudomonas.—Parenteral polymyxin B therapy is considered mandatory for this form of meningitis, along with intrathecal use of polymyxin B (2.5 mg./day for three days). One should *not* give polymxin E (colistimethate) intrathecally.[48]

PROGNOSIS.—The mortality and morbidity rates are elevated by the following factors: (1) neonatal meningitis (mortality rate approximately 60%), (2) gram-negative organisms and drug-resistant staphylococci, (3) delay in therapy, (4) the Waterhouse-Friderichsen syndrome, (5) coma and (6) increased intracranial pressure. Chances for cure are enhanced by early diagnosis, the identification of the organism and measurement of antibiotic sensitivity, and thorough immediate treatment.

PREVENTION.—Prophylactic therapy is given to all contacts of patients with meningococcal infection and to sick infant contacts of children with H. influenzal disease. To prevent meningococcal infections, sulfadiazine 0.5–1 Gm. twice a day is given for five days. Penicillin therapy should be added if sulfonamide-resistant strains are found. To prevent H. influenzal infections in sick infant contacts, chloramphenicol 100 mg./kg./day in four divided doses for at least five days is recommended.

Viral Meningoencephalitis

THERAPY.—Excellent nursing care and careful supportive medical care are essential. No specific therapy is available. Anticonvulsant drugs for seizures (Chapter 2) and agents to reduce cerebral swelling (Appendix 2) should be employed when necessary.

Herpes zoster.—Elliott[19] has reported the consistent relief of root pain with high doses of prednisone in patients with herpes zoster radiculitis.

Poliomyelitis.—No attempt will be made here to detail the complexities of the treatment of this disease, which fortunately has become uncommon in most parts of the world. However, some general principles will be mentioned. In symptomatic cases the patient should receive bed rest, sedative drugs if necessary, hot packs for pain relief and careful physiotherapy for tight or paralyzed muscles. In *bulbar* poliomyelitis the patient requires special nursing care, parenteral fluid therapy, mechanical aspiration of secretions and artificial respiration with a mechanical lung. The decisions to use a respirator and to do a tracheostomy should be made only by a physician who has wide experience in the care of such patients.

Herpes simplex.—Marshall[43a] treated a patient with acute necrotizing encephalitis due to this ubiquitous virus with idoxuridine given intravenously and external cerebral decompression. The patient responded well, which led the author to encourage similar trials of therapy in patients in whom early diagnosis could be established.

Measles.—See the section on Encephalomyelitis in this chapter and the text of Krugman and Ward.[31]

PROGNOSIS.—The mortality and morbidity rates for acute viral infections of the nervous system vary with the specific virus, the age of the patient and the epidemic. All of the arbovirus infections represent a major threat to life and threaten residual neurologic disability (mental retardation, seizures, spastic paralysis, organic behavior disturbances, loss of memory and postencephalitic parkinsonism). Most workers believe that the syndrome of parkinsonism complicates encephalitis infrequently compared to the number of cases which fall into the idiopathic or symptomatic categories.[49] Eastern equine and Japanese B encephalitis are considered more malignant than the St. Louis and western equine infections. Serial electroencephalograms are sometimes used to document the progress of acute viral encephalitis (Fig. 18.3).

Poliomyelitis.—The prognosis in abortive and nonparalytic poliomyelitis is very good, but obviously the risk increases with paralytic and bulbar disease. Although the fatality rate is relatively low (5–10%), permanent and disabling weakness often results. In the acute stage of paralytic or bulbar poliomyelitis it is extremely difficult to prognosticate accurately about residual disability. The general statement that patients who survive the bulbar form recover completely is simply not true if a large enough series of patients is followed over a period of years, as emphasized by Bosma.[9]

Other viral infections.—Rabies is almost uniformly fatal, and herpes simplex encephalitis also carries a high fatality rate. Mumps meningoencephalitis is generally (but not always) a benign disease, as are varicella-zoster and lymphocytic choriomeningitis infections of the nervous system.

PREVENTION.—*Viral encephalitis* can be prevented by avoiding a bite from an infected mosquito. Public health measures to destroy mosquito breeding sites are important. Equine encephalomyelitis has been prevented by active immunization of animals, but this measure has not been used extensively in human beings.

Poliomyelitis.—During the past 12 years two vaccines have been developed to prevent this disease—the inactivated, injectable Salk vaccine and the live, attenu-

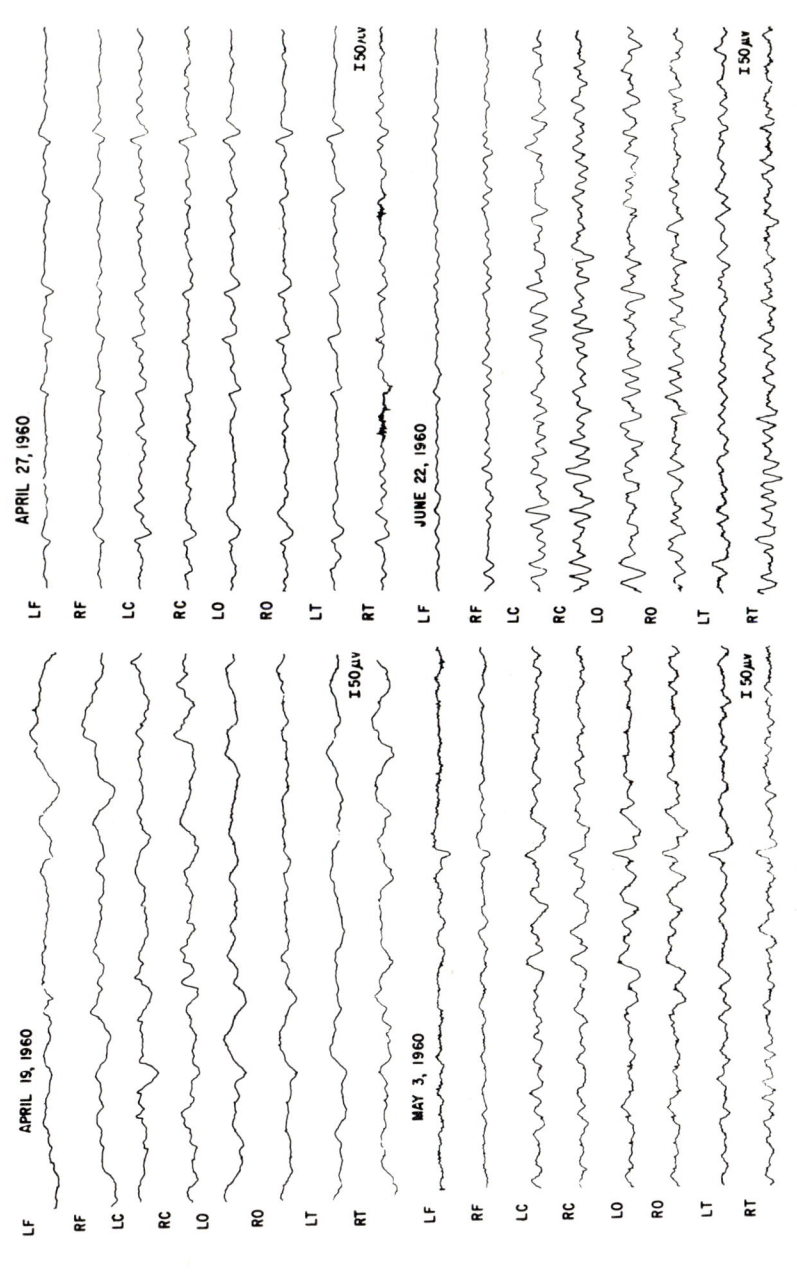

Fig. 18.3.—Postvaricella meningoencephalitis. Serial EEG changes are shown. Note the irregular, low-voltage, slow background frequencies on the initial recording. Subsequent tracings showed gradual and steady improvement with increasingly regular, synchronous frequencies of higher voltage.

TABLE 18.4.—RABIES: GUIDE FOR SPECIFIC POSTEXPOSURE TREATMENT[62a]

NATURE OF EXPOSURE	STATUS OF BITING ANIMAL*		RECOMMENDED TREATMENT (IN ADDITION TO LOCAL TREATMENT)
	At time of exposure	During observation period of 10 days	
No lesion; indirect contact	Rabid		None
Licks			
1. Unabraded skin	1. Rabid		None
2. Abraded skin, scratches and unabraded or abraded mucosa	2. a) Healthy	Clinical signs of rabies or proved rabid (laboratory)	Start vaccine at first signs of rabies in animal
	b) Signs suggestive of rabies	Healthy	Start vaccine immediately; stop treatment if animal is normal on fifth day after exposure
	c) Rabid, escaped, killed, or unknown		Start vaccine immediately
Bites			
1. Mild exposure	1. a) Healthy	Clinical signs of rabies or proved rabid (laboratory)	Start vaccine at first signs of rabies in biting animal
	b) Signs suggestive of rabies	Healthy	Start vaccine immediately; stop treatment if animal is normal on fifth day after exposure
	c) Rabid, escaped, killed, or unknown		Start vaccine immediately
	d) Wild (wolf, jackal, fox, bat, etc.)		Serum immediately, followed by a course of vaccine†
2. Severe exposure (multiple, or face, head, finger or neck bites)	2. a) Healthy	Clinical signs of rabies or proved rabid (laboratory)	Serum immediately; start vaccine† at first sign of rabies in the biting animal
	b) Signs suggestive of rabies	Healthy	Serum immediately, followed by vaccine. Vaccine may be stopped if animal is normal on fifth day after exposure
	c) Rabid, escaped, killed, or unknown		Serum immediately, followed by vaccine†
	d) Wild (wolf, stray dog, jackal, fox, bat, etc.)		

*Schedule applies equally whether or not the biting animal has been previously vaccinated.
†Course of vaccine to be followed by supplemental doses of vaccine, of non-nervous tissue if possible, 10 and 20 days after the last usual dose.

ated, oral Sabin vaccine. The oral Sabin vaccine has emerged as the more effective agent because of its greater immunogenic potency, its protective capacity and its ease of administration.

Monovalent vaccine: Optimal immunization[2] is obtained by giving Types I, III and II, in that order, at six to eight week intervals. The first dose can be given at 2 months of age when DPT immunizations are started. A fourth dose of trivalent vaccine is given to infants at 15–18 months of age. Older children do not need the fourth dose. Older children who have been incompletely immunized should receive the complete series of oral poliovaccine.

Trivalent vaccine: Two doses of oral vaccine are given at six to eight week intervals. Only infants and preschool children need a third dose to insure reliable immunity to Type I.

Rabies.—The use of vaccine in the management of dog bites continues to present one of the most difficult but important decisions the physician has to make because of (1) the inevitably fatal nature of rabies in man, (2) the rarity of the disease in most well-developed countries, (3) the slight risk of encephalomyelitis following vaccination and (4) the 50% incidence of painful local reactions to the vaccine.

The procedures for rabies prevention recommended by the World Health Organization are shown in Table 18.4. It is recommended that the child be immunized with duck embryo vaccine[62a] (the newer duck vaccine carries a lesser risk of postvaccinal encephalomyelitis than does the older rabbit brain vaccine) *if the skin is abraded* and (1) the biting animal is rabid, (2) signs of rabies develop in the biting animal during the 10 day observation period, or (3) the biting animal is unknown, escaped or killed. The patient should be given *hyperimmune rabies serum* immediately (as well as the initial dose of duck vaccine) if (1) bites have been inflicted on or around the head and neck or (2) the animal is wild. Sensitivity tests to horse serum (intradermal or ophthalmic) should be carried out before giving the hyperimmune serum.

DOSAGE

Duck embryo vaccine: 1 ml. subcutaneously every day for 14–21 days depending upon the severity of exposure.

Hyperimmune serum: 0.5 ml./kg. intramuscularly every day for 14 days.

We would like to emphasize that the physician must use his clinical judgment, based upon all the circumstances which surround the possible exposure, including (1) the type and condition of the animal, (2) domesticated or wild animal, (3) extent of the bite or exposure, (4) location on the body and (5) the natural concentration of the virus in the community. Table 18.4 represents a guide to proper judgment.

Rubella.—An effective vaccine for rubella has been developed recently by Meyer and associates.[49a] If its value is confirmed by other workers, it should prevent the crippling congenital anomalies of this intrauterine infection. Babies born with congenital rubella may shed the virus for many months and should be isolated from pregnant women (especially pregnant hospital nurses). Until an effective vaccine is marketed, it is recommended that young girls be exposed to known rubella in order that they acquire a natural infection.

Chronic Granulomatous Meningitis

SPECIFIC THERAPY.—*Tuberculous meningitis.*—These patients are treated with isoniazid (INH) streptomycin and para-aminosalicylic acid (PAS). Isoniazid in a daily dose of 15–30 mg./kg. intramuscularly or orally, streptomycin in a daily dose of 20 mg./kg. intramuscularly and PAS 250 mg./kg./day intravenously or orally is given initially. After two weeks of this therapy the streptomycin is reduced to the point where the patient is given the same dose twice a week for two more weeks and then it is discontinued. Isoniazid and PAS therapy is continued for 18 months. Although definitive controlled studies have not been carried out to prove the worth of glucocorticoid therapy, clinical observations suggest that adrenal steroid therapy has more value in the treatment of tuberculous than in acute purulent meningitis.[58a] All these agents have significant toxic side effects: streptomycin (ataxia, deafness and vertigo), INH (seizures, lethargy, ataxia, psychosis and neuropathy) and PAS (nausea, vomiting, arthralgia, fever, rash and psychosis).

Cryptococcal meningitis.—Patients are given amphotericin B intravenously, 0.25 mg./kg./day in 5% glucose in water over five to six hours. The dose is increased gradually to 1 mg./kg./day and it is given for six weeks.[54]

Coccidioidal meningitis is also treated with amphotericin B (as above).

The management of congenital infections of the nervous system is covered in Chapter 13. No specific therapy for *leptospiral* infections has proved efficacious.

PROGNOSIS.—Before chemotherapeutic agents for tuberculosis were developed, tuberculous meningitis ran an inevitably fatal course in about six weeks. Early detection and therapy have changed the outlook greatly—the mortality rate is now about 20%. However, residual cranial nerve damage, deafness and hydrocephalus from adhesive basilar arachnoiditis still cause permanent residual deficit when the diagnosis is delayed. In general, the same prognostic attitudes prevail in the case of cryptococcal and coccidioidal meningitis, although the outlook may be even graver than with tuberculous meningitis. Leptospiral infections generally carry a good prognosis and will go unrecognized as "aseptic meningitis" unless serologic laboratory studies are carried out.

PREVENTION.—*Tuberculosis.*—Infants and children under age 3 who have a positive response to the tuberculin skin test and children over 3 years who have recently converted to a positive tuberculin reaction or have x-ray evidence of active primary tuberculosis should receive INH prophylactically. The drug is given in the dose of 4–6 mg./kg./day for one year.

Abscess Formation

PATHOGENESIS.—Intracranial abscesses and septic venous thromboses result from (1) direct extension of infection from a purulent otitis media, mastoiditis or sinusitis, (2) bacteremia secondary to chronic lung disease, endocarditis or congenital heart disease with septal defect or (3) direct contamination of the intracranial cavity following a compound skull fracture or craniotomy. Abscesses secondary to otitis and mastoiditis are often located in the temporal lobe or cerebellum, with or without sinus thrombosis. Purulent sinusitis more commonly causes frontal lobe abscesses. Multiple abscesses are often seen in patients with a hematogenous basis for the disease. When an abscess reaches sufficient size, it may rupture and form swollen satellite lesions or it may rupture into the ventricle (Fig. 18.4,*B*). In patients with congenital heart disease, bacteria enter the venous portion of the blood stream, pass through a septal defect and enter the cerebral cir-

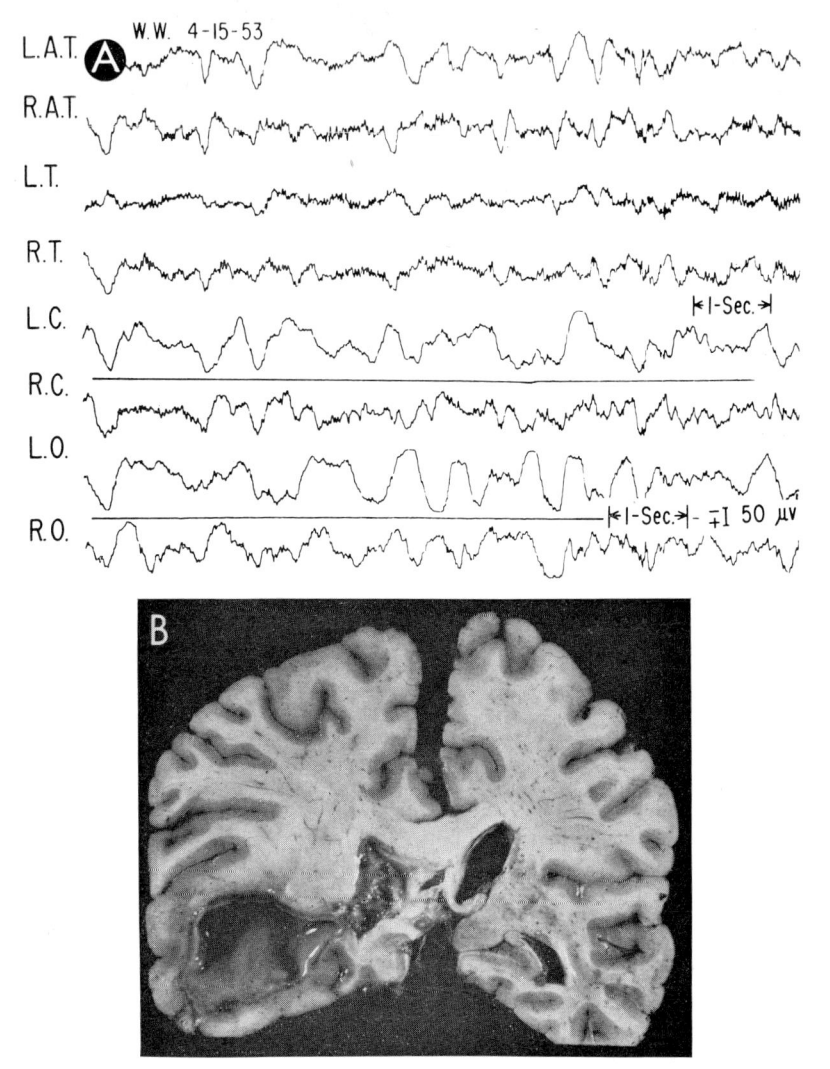

Fig. 18.4.—Brain abscess. A, Delta wave focus on electroencephalogram of a patient with a brain abscess in the left parietal lobe, associated with a ventricular septal defect and a right-to-left shunt. B, Pathologic specimen. Notice how this abscess has ruptured into the body and the temporal horn of the lateral ventricle. (Courtesy of Dr. Abner Wolf.)

culation, bypassing the pulmonary filtration system.[45] Abscesses can form in the subdural or epidural space, and cerebral thrombophlebitis can develop as a result of direct extension from a purulent focus (middle ear, mastoid or sinus) or secondary to a compound fracture of the skull.

The common causative organisms are Staphylococcus aureus or albus and Streptococcus viridans or hemolyticus. Liske and Weikers[37] noted an increase in the incidence of "no growth" cultures since 1950 in a series of 110 cases, presumably because of the increasing use of broad-spectrum antibiotics. The same observation was made by Loeser and Scheinberg[38] in their series of 99 cases.

CLINICAL AND LABORATORY DIAGNOSIS.—In most cases intracranial pyogenic infections complicate focal infections elsewhere in the body, as outlined above. In patients with cardiac septal defects, abscess formation may occur without a history of antecedent infection, usually when an ordinarily innocuous venous bacteremia gains access to the arterial circulation.

The symptoms of any of these septic intracranial conditions resemble one another—fever, headache, vomiting, drowsiness, seizures and neck stiffness. *Brain abscess* often evolves through three stages, although clinical distinctions may be vague: (1) the encephalitic stage, with fever, drowsiness, headache, stiff neck and seizures; (2) the encapsulation stage, in which these symptoms subside or fail to progress for a few days or weeks while the abscess enlarges slowly, and (3) cerebral decompensation, in which signs of increased intracranial pressure, focal deficit and uncal herniation with brain stem compression appear (papilledema, hemiparesis, hemianopia), giving way to progressive stupor, third nerve palsy and change in vital signs (Fig. 8.1, p. 85). Clark[12] believes that percussion tenderness may help to localize the abscess quite accurately.

Skull x-rays in any of these septic intracranial processes may show only signs of increased intracranial pressure. Radioisotopic brain scans or arteriography may help in the process of localization of brain abscesses, and the electroencephalogram is considered especially useful for it often shows a discrete slow wave focus (Fig. 18.4,*A*). If an *empyema* in the extradural or subdural space is suspected, the area is aspirated and the fluid examined and cultured. In the first stage of an abscess the cerebrospinal fluid may show a lymphocytic pleocytosis. Later the pressure becomes elevated but the fluid usually remains sterile, and finally the cell count, pressure and protein content all rise, especially if the abscess ruptures into the ventricle, at which time the pathogenic organism may be identified on culture.

MANAGEMENT AND PROGNOSIS.—*Brain abscess.*—Regardless of the clinical stage of an abscess, broad-spectrum antibiotic therapy similar to that for purulent meningitis of unknown etiology should be instituted immediately. The antimicrobial regimen may need modification, depending upon the identification of the organism and its sensitivities. In the early stages antibiotic therapy may suffice to control the inflammatory process completely. However, with any established abscess, the process should be localized as accurately as possible and the lesion should be aspirated by the neurosurgeon. Thorium dioxide is often instilled to outline the abscess cavity and to follow its progress. At present most workers favor repeated aspirations and antibiotic therapy rather than an attempt to excise the cavity completely. Survivors should receive maintenance anticonvulsant therapy to prevent seizures, a common complication.

Subdural and epidural empyema.—These accumulations of pus should be drained through one or more burr holes if the infected material is liquid. More extensive craniectomy may be required if the pus is loculated by granulation tissue. Intensive chemotherapy and supportive care are required to prevent disability from these serious intracranial infections.

Infections with Neurotoxic Organisms

Tetanus

PATHOGENESIS.—The microorganism which causes tetanus produces an exotoxin which is potentially damaging to nerve tissue. Tetanus bacilli abound in soil and human excreta, and the organisms multiply in contaminated wounds—usually deep puncture wounds, burns, contaminated umbilical cords—or in crushed tissues where conditions promote anaerobic growth. The liberated tetanus exotoxin reaches the central nervous system by direct axonal spread or via the lymphatics. Antitoxin can neutralize toxin which is circulating freely in the bloodstream but not that which is fixed to nerve tissue. The toxin tetanospasmin acts at the myoneural junction and directly upon the motor nerve cells in the spinal cord and cerebrum to produce skeletal muscle spasms and convulsions. No neuropathologic changes have been found in this toxic disease state.

CLINICAL AND LABORATORY DIAGNOSIS.—The disease usually begins with gradually increasing stiffness of the jaw and neck muscles, causing trismus or lockjaw. The physician's attention may not be drawn to the original site of infection and, even when tetanus is considered, often no relationship is found between the benign appearance of the wound and the eventual toxemia. The spasmodic process may be localized or generalized. Gradually the facial muscles go into spasm, causing a sardonic grin, and the muscles of the neck, back and abdomen become involved, causing opisthotonos. Generalized painful muscle spasms which are triggered by mild external stimuli, such as light, sound and touch, represent a major threat to the patient's life, especially if the respiratory muscles and larynx are involved. The paroxysmal muscle spasms can cause asphyxia and eventually coma and death. Except for times when convulsions occur, the patient retains a clear sensorium. In early stages the diagnosis may not be considered, but when the clinical picture is fully developed, no problem in diagnosis is encountered. No diagnostic laboratory procedures are available except for recovery of Clostridium tetani from the wound.

MANAGEMENT AND PROGNOSIS.—Patients with tetanus should have special nursing and supportive care in addition to antitoxin.

1. Hospitalization in a quiet, darkened room with private nursing care is essential.

2. Sedation is given to prevent or lessen the severity of muscle spasms. Barbiturates or paraldehyde may be used in moderate doses.

3. Muscle relaxants are of doubtful value. Curare is sometimes used but its small margin of safety creates hazards. Perlstein and co-workers[51] have reported that meprobamate helps to control muscle spasm.

4. Tetanus antitoxin. After adequate sedation and tests for horse serum sensitivity, 50,000 units of animal antitoxin or 3,000 units of human antitoxin are given intramuscularly.[46] Tetanus antitoxin (horse) is capable of causing serum sickness, serum neuritis and death. The neuritis which complicates antitoxin administration has a peculiar predilection for the brachial plexus, particularly the fifth and sixth cervical roots, with the shoulder girdle, arm and hand being affected in that order.[3]

5. Antibiotics have value in managing secondary complications such as pneumonia and for eradication of the tetanus organism, but they have no effect upon the toxin which has been liberated.

6. Supportive therapy. An adequate airway (oxygen, suction and tracheostomy if necessary), fluids and electrolytes, nasogastric feedings and proper wound care should be provided.

Between one-third and one-half the patients with tetanus die even with optimal care.[28] Neonates who develop the disease rarely survive.

PREVENTION.—Infants should receive tetanus toxoid as part of their routine immunizations in three divided doses, starting at 3 months of age. Booster doses (0.5 ml.) are given at 1 year and every four years thereafter. In older children and adults who suffer perforating injuries or contaminated wounds, a booster dose (0.5 ml.) of tetanus toxoid is given. If one calculates that the patient's level of immunity is poor, if the wound is badly contaminated or if more than 24 hours have elapsed since the time of injury, 1,500 units of animal tetanus antitoxin should be given after testing the patient for horse serum sensitivity. If human antitoxin is available, it should be used in a dose of 250–500 units because it will not cause anaphylactic reactions or serum sickness and it has a longer half-life.[46]

Diphtheritic Polyneuritis

PATHOGENESIS.—Upper respiratory tract or cutaneous infections with the diphtheria organism can cause neuritis. The toxin liberated by the microorganism causes a motor neuropathy after a latent period of three to seven weeks. As a result of widespread immunization this disease is now rarely seen in the United States.

CLINICAL AND LABORATORY DIAGNOSIS.—Primarily a motor neuropathy which clears completely in patients who survive, this complication causes weakness of the palate (nasal voice and nasal regurgitation), ciliary muscles (blurring of vision), facial muscles and diaphragm (dyspnea and tachypnea) and symmetrical weakness and areflexia in the muscles of the extremities. In some patients paresthesias and ataxia develop. The disease may resemble the Guillain-Barré syndrome (p. 305) but it affects cranial nerves more commonly.

The cerebrospinal fluid usually shows an elevated protein content, and the causative organism, Corynebacterium diphtheriae, can often be isolated from the throat or the skin lesions.

MANAGEMENT AND PROGNOSIS.—After the diagnosis is established, the patient should be given diphtheria antitoxin intramuscularly (20,000–60,000 units) in an amount roughly proportional to the extent and severity of the disease. All the usual tests for horse serum sensitivity should be given before the antitoxin is administered. Penicillin or tetracycline should be given in full therapeutic doses until results of *three successive cultures* from the original site of infection are negative.

The prognosis for complete recovery following adequate therapy is excellent in the present day.

As in the case of tetanus, this disease is prevented by routine immunization.

Encephalomyelitis

PATHOGENESIS.—Neurologic syndromes complicate certain common childhood illnesses and vaccinations against microorganisms:

Postinfectious	*Postvaccinal*
Measles (rubeola)	Vaccinia
Chickenpox (varicella)	Rabies
German measles (rubella)	Pertussis
Mumps	
Exanthem subitum (roseola)	
Whooping cough (pertussis)	
Smallpox (variola)	

ENCEPHALOMYELITIS 301

The following three theories concerning the pathogenesis of encephalomyelitis have been proposed, but none has been proved. (1) The pathologic changes are caused by the virus which was involved in the original infection or vaccination. (2) A latent neurotropic virus is activated by the primary viral agent and this causes the disease. (3) The lesions (similar to those seen in experimental allergic encephalomyelitis) are caused by an antigen-antibody reaction—an autoimmune disease.

Perivascular demyelination and perivascular round-cell infiltration characterize the pathologic changes in these disorders. The location of the lesions resembles closely that seen in patients with multiple sclerosis, but the greater inflammatory cell reaction and the destruction of axis cylinders typify the abnormalities in postinfectious and postvaccinal encephalomyelitis.

CLINICAL AND LABORATORY DIAGNOSIS.—Clinical neurologic symptoms and signs of postinfectious or postvaccinal encephalomyelitis can be divided arbitrarily into three general categories: (1) *systemic*—fever, headache and vomiting, (2) *encephalitis*—drowsiness, convulsions and coma, (3) *myelitis*—nuchal rigidity, cranial nerve deficit (optic neuritis—see Chapter 22—facial weakness, deafness), hemiplegia, paraplegia (transverse myelitis—Chapter 22) and ataxia.

The CSF examination usually reveals a mild pleocytosis of 15–250 cells/cu. mm., mostly mononuclear, and an inconstant, mild elevation in the protein content. Electroencephalographic abnormalities are common; usually there is diffuse slow activity in the acute stages, but often residual focal or diffuse epileptiform abnormalities are seen later. Serial electroencephalograms offer a useful method of following the course of the patient severely ill with encephalomyelitis (Fig. 18.3).

Measles causes serious complications more frequently than the other infec-

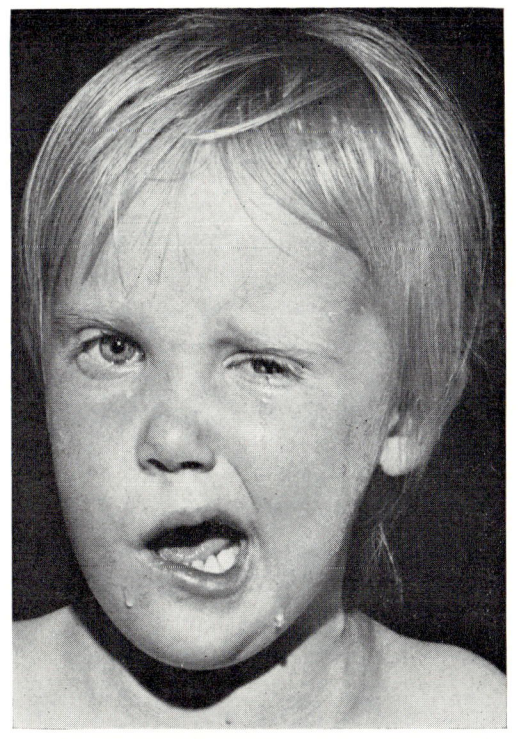

Fig. 18.5.—Bell's palsy due to chickenpox (varicella). This 3-year-old girl was recovering uneventfully from chickenpox until two weeks after the outcropping of the rash. When she awoke in the morning the parents noted weakness of the whole right face. The weakness progressed for about two days and then remained unchanged for one week. No other neurologic deficit was found. Prednisone (1 mg./lb./day) was given for three weeks, and the dose then tapered to nothing over the next two weeks. Coincident with the therapy and the passage of time the patient regained full function of the facial muscles.

tions. It is said that 60% of patients with measles encephalomyelitis recover completely, 15% die and 25% show residual mental retardation, convulsive disorders, severe personality changes and behavior disorders, nerve deafness, hemiplegia or paraplegia.

Chickenpox is associated uncommonly with encephalomyelitis and causes cerebellar ataxia more commonly than the other forms of encephalomyelitis. However, other focal deficits can also appear (Fig. 18.5).

German measles complicated by encephalitis is seen very rarely.[52e] When this complication does occur, the clinical picture resembles other forms of encephalitis. Recovery is usually complete but fatalities have been reported.[31]

Mumps virus usually causes only a benign meningitis (p. 286), but occasionally a severe and even fatal encephalomyelitis is seen. Eighth nerve deafness appears as a common neurologic complication.

Exanthem subitum is frequently ushered in by one or more convulsions associated with fever. As with any severe convulsive episode, occasional postconvulsive deficits such as hemiplegia are noted. Some have considered the incidence of neurologic complications in comparison to the height of the temperature with this disease as inordinately high, and they have suggested an encephalitic component to the disease. This concept is purely conjectural.

A true *pertussis* encephalomyelitis is difficult to distinguish from anoxic cerebral damage secondary to severe coughing paroxysms. The rare convulsions and cerebral damage reported as a consequence of routine DPT immunization have been attributed to the pertussis organisms in the vaccine (Chapter 20).

Smallpox can be complicated by a a demyelinating type of encephalitis as well as a peripheral neuritis. The condition is rarely seen in the United States at present. Vaccination for smallpox produces a rare but serious complication, encephalomyelitis. The clinical picture resembles the general one described above, but the mortality rate has been estimated at 30–40%.

Rabies (see page 295).

MANAGEMENT AND PROGNOSIS.—In general, supportive care represents the most important therapy. Adrenal corticosteroids are widely used for the treatment of the syndrome (prednisone 1 mg./lb./day for 7–10 days) but proof of their effectiveness remains to be demonstrated.[24] Gamma globulin has been given in massive doses to patients with measles encephalitis, but the outcome in treated patients does not differ from a control group given supportive therapy.[1a,31]

The prognosis varies with the etiologic organism, being worse for measles, vaccinia and rabies and better for varicella, rubella, mumps and pertussis. Residual mental retardation, drug-refractory convulsive disorders, motor deficit (hemiplegia or paraplegia) and severe personality changes with behavior disorders occur commonly in the more severe forms of encephalomyelitis.

PREVENTION.—*Measles encephalitis.*—Measles vaccine should be given routinely to all children without a history of measles or measles vaccination.[2] Immunization is especially important for high-risk patients. Among these are patients with asthma, chronic pulmonary disease, heart disease, tuberculosis and cystic fibrosis as well as institutionalized patients. Patients with altered immune responses (leukemic patients and those receiving steroids, antimetabolites, irradiation or alkylating agents) should receive inactivated vaccine. Patients with tuberculosis should be receiving antituberculous therapy before being given measles vaccine.

Specific recommendations can be obtained from the manufacturer's directions or the schedules listed by the American Academy of Pediatrics.[2] In ordinary cases, a single injection of the live, attenuated vaccine is given. This confers lasting immunity. In exceptional cases, one may want to give inactivated vaccine in one or more doses or measles immune globulin with the live vaccine.

The advent of an effective measles vaccine should reduce considerably this major crippling complication of rubeola.

Disorders of Possible Infectious Etiology

Acute Cerebellitis (Acute "Pontine Encephalitis")

PATHOGENESIS.—Several different infectious agents (the varicella virus, poliovirus, ECHO virus type 9, Coxsackie B viruses[6] and to a lesser extent the viruses of measles, mumps and rubella) have been recovered from patients with acute ataxia of unknown etiology. However, the etiology of the majority of such cases remains unknown.[27] It is suspected that other viral agents may cause most cases, but proof is lacking. No pathologic studies on a series of these patients have been reported, primarily because the syndrome is usually not fatal.

CLINICAL AND LABORATORY DIAGNOSIS.—The disorder usually begins abruptly in infants under age 2. The signs often follow an upper respiratory infection, but the patient is usually afebrile before they appear. Sudden ataxia of the gait, trunk and extremities is noted and some patients have coarse horizontal nystagmus. Often the child is unable to stand or sit and seems to prefer to lie flat. In some, movement causes fear and dismay, as though it produced vertigo. Intermittent rapid oscillations of the eyes appear as a prominent feature of the syndrome, suggesting that neural connections in the pons may be affected. A rhythmic tremor of the head, as well as hypotonia and hyporeflexia, is sometimes seen. Vomiting may occur repeatedly, and in a child with profound ataxia this may raise the cogent question of a posterior fossa tumor. However, affected patients do not have signs of increased intracranial pressure.

In other cases the clinical signs of intramedullary brain stem disease predominate. Multiple cranial nerve deficits, corticospinal tract signs, ataxia, nystagmus, headache and vomiting occur. Clinically, such patients are indistinguishable from those with brain stem gliomas. However, pneumoencephalographic studies are normal and the clinical signs usually clear completely under observation.

An attempt should be carried out to demonstrate a viral etiology by culturing throat washings and stools for virus and collecting paired sera for antibody titers. Cerebrospinal fluid examination reveals a mild mononuclear pleocytosis in a small percentage of cases.

MANAGEMENT AND PROGNOSIS.—One can expect complete clearing of the neurologic deficit in about two-thirds of the patients within six months after onset. However, in the series of Weiss and Carter,[60] 33% of the patients showed persistent neurologic deficit in the form of gait and extremity ataxia, truncal tremor, abnormal eye movements (opsoclonus) and poor speech development as well as dysarthria. Evidence of impaired mentality was noted in one-third of these patients, leading the authors to suggest that in many cases the patient may have a "subtle type of cerebral involvement which could not be detected initially." We have had a similar experience and stress the need for caution when discussing the prognosis.

Acute Labyrinthitis

Acute labyrinthitis is uncommon and usually results from a serous or purulent otitis media, mastoiditis or meningitis. At present, the more severe, purulent type of labyrinthitis is rarely seen, but serous collections of fluid in the inner ear can cause symptoms and signs.

The patient usually prefers to lie flat, movement causing vertigo and vomiting. Spontaneous horizontal and rotary nystagmus is seen, with the slow phase toward the side of the inflammation. There is loss of hearing but this may disappear with therapy of a serous process. In purulent labyrinthitis, deafness often ensues and the patient loses all function, including caloric responses (no nystagmus occurs when 5 cc. of ice water is instilled into the ear canal of the affected side).

Intensive, appropriate antibiotic therapy is given, and both medical and surgical measures are taken to insure adequate drainage of fluid from the middle ear. Prognosis for complete recovery of serous labyrinthitis is good, but purulent inflammation (rare at present) causes deafness and a "dead" labyrinth in many cases.

Neuritis of the Facial Nerve (Bell's Palsy)

PATHOGENESIS.—The fact that Bell's palsy sometimes complicates infections of known etiology, such as herpes zoster and varicella (Fig. 18.5), and the fact that many cases follow an acute, nonspecific upper respiratory infection make most workers think that this disorder has an inflammatory etiology, however obscure. Presumably the condition results from inflammation and swelling of the nerve in the fallopian canal of the temporal bone.

CLINICAL AND LABORATORY DIAGNOSIS.—The patient notes the sudden onset of facial weakness, often with a sensation of "stiffness" or even pain in the soft tissues of the face. The sensory symptom of pain may be localized to the ear. All portions of the face are weak so that the patient has difficulty with speech, closing the eye and wrinkling the forehead. Food tends to get caught between the gums and the cheeks, and tears run from the eye because of muscle hypotonia. Taste may be lost over the anterior two-thirds of the tongue if the lesion is proximal to the junction of the chorda tympani with the nerve. When the facial palsy is caused by a herpes zoster infection (usually seen in adults), the inflammation involves the geniculate ganglion and is associated with a vesicular eruption in the ear canal or on the neck (the syndrome of Ramsay-Hunt). The differential diagnosis of a peripheral facial palsy is considered in Chapter 6. About a week or 10 days after the onset, EMG study of the facial muscles may show evidence of denervation.

MANAGEMENT AND PROGNOSIS.—Complete recovery occurs in the vast majority of children with Bell's palsy. Lack of prompt recovery should make one doubt the diagnosis. No specific therapy has proved effective, but adrenal corticosteroids are used widely (prednisone 1 mg./lb./day for 10-14 days). If the eye cannot be closed, an eye patch should be worn and lubricating ointment used to prevent corneal ulceration. Massage and electrical stimulation are often recommended in the early stages, but the value of these measures is probably more psychotherapeutic than physiotherapeutic. If during the course of recovery regenerating fibers are misdirected, movement of one part of the weak side may cause involuntary movement of other parts. Incomplete recovery poses a cosmetic and psychologic problem, especially if it is accompanied by hemifacial spasm. Physical and surgical therapy for incomplete recovery is rarely necessary in children.

Infectious Polyneuritis (Landry-Guillain-Barré Syndrome)

PATHOGENESIS.—As in the case of acute cerebellitis and neuritis of the facial nerve, this clinical syndrome may follow an upper respiratory or gastrointestinal infection, and for this reason it is presumed by many to have an infectious basis. However, no etiologic microorganism has ever been demonstrated, and the pathologic findings in 50 fatal cases described by Haymaker and Kernohan[21] showed very few signs of inflammation. The latent period between the antecedent infection and the symptoms of polyneuritis have led some workers to liken the pathogenesis to that of postinfectious encephalomyelitis and to ascribe an allergic etiology to the condition. Degenerative changes in the nerve fibers with considerable edema and very little cellular response characterize the pathologic findings. The disease affects children less often than adults.

Occasionally lesions in the spinal cord itself are found in patients who have disease of long standing.[52b] Whether these cases have the same etiology as most cases of the Guillain-Barré syndrome is not known.

CLINICAL AND LABORATORY DIAGNOSIS.—The condition has a peak incidence between 4 and 10 years of age. Weakness of the legs frequently ushers in the disease, but paresthesias may appear as the first symptom. Quickly the weakness spreads cephalad (hence the name "Landry's ascending paralysis"), often causing a flaccid quadriplegia with areflexia and facial diplegia. The neurologic involvement usually reaches a peak within one week. Paralysis of the diaphragm and intercostal muscles occurs commonly, and the patient may need to be placed in a mechanical respirator. In addition to the facial nerves, the tenth cranial nerve may be involved and rarely the nerves of the extraocular muscles. Minor degrees of hypesthesia, hypalgesia and impaired deep sensation may be found, along with some dull, aching pain. In the series of Low and associates[39] six of the 30 affected children had transient urinary incontinence and retention as well as constipation. The sensorium is not affected. For reasons which are not entirely clear papilledema is sometimes seen.[22] It has been attributed in some cases to increased intracranial pressure secondary to hypercapnia (secondary to impaired ventilation) and in other cases to impaired reabsorption of cerebrospinal fluid as a result of the high protein content. A CSF examination reveals the so-called "albumino-cytologic dissociation," i.e., high protein content with little or no pleocytosis. No other specific laboratory abnormalities can be expected unless the polyneuritis is a complication of infectious mononucleosis.

Recently Posner and co-workers[52a] pointed out that severe hyponatremia (secondary to the inappropriate secretion of antidiuretic hormone) can cause seizures and mental confusion in patients with this disease.

MANAGEMENT AND PROGNOSIS.—In most cases one can expect the disease to remit starting seven to 10 days after the onset. Complete recovery is seen in most cases, even though the rate of recovery may be slow. Figures for mortality vary, but approximately 20% of patients of all ages die from respiratory failure or intercurrent infections. Although the disease has been considered benign compared to poliomyelitis, in that survivors recover completely, the series of Low and associates[39] showed a significant number of patients with residual weakness and joint contractures.

The acute phase of the illness is managed much the same as poliomyelitis. Special nursing and good supportive medical care are of paramount importance. If bulbar weakness becomes severe, tracheostomy must be performed, and the patient is placed in a tank respirator if the muscles of respiration are badly paralyzed. Adrenal corticosteroid therapy is used in severe cases, but the results defy definitive interpretation. However, the clinical course in some cases of chronic relapsing or recurrent polyneuropathy of obscure etiology is definitely improved by ACTH or corticosteroid therapy. Antibiotics are used to treat specific infections, and careful attention is given to fluid and electrolyte needs. During convalescence, expert physiotherapy should be started to prevent contractures which may require orthopedic correction later. Splints and braces are used when necessary in the patient with residual weakness.

Infectious Mononucleosis (Glandular Fever)

PATHOGENESIS.—Circumstantial clinical and laboratory data suggest that this disorder may be caused by a virus-like microorganism but the actual etiology has never been established. Enlargement of the organs of the reticuloendothelial system (lymph nodes, liver and spleen) regularly occurs. The nervous system is involved only in the exceptional case.

CLINICAL AND LABORATORY DIAGNOSIS.—Neurologic syndromes associated with infectious mononucleosis may be divided into different categories:

    1. Aseptic meningitis. Most often the patient has fever, headache, stiff neck and a lymphocytic pleocytosis.

    2. Encephalitis.[59] The signs of meningitis are associated with convulsions, delirium and coma.

    3. Polyneuritis. The symptoms and signs are identical with those described for the Guillain-Barré snydrome.[17]

    4. Optic neuritis. See Chapter 22 for a fuller discussion of the neurologic findings.

    5. Transverse myelitis.[15] See Chapter 22.

The basic diagnosis is made by finding the atypical lymphocytes on a blood smear or by demonstrating a high titer (1:128) or a rise in titer of heterophil antibodies (sheep cell agglutinins). Central nervous system involvement is associated with a lymphocytic pleocytosis (10–600 cells) with a slightly elevated or normal protein content. The blood serologic test for syphilis may show a false-positive reaction in this disease.

MANAGEMENT AND PROGNOSIS.—Usually a mild, self-limited disease, infectious mononucleosis has no specific therapy, but some neurologic complications require close attention and care. Special nursing and supportive medical care are essential for patients with encephalitis, polyneuritis and transverse myelitis because such complications can be fatal. If respiratory paralysis develops, a mechanical respirator is needed. Adrenal corticosteroids have been used in patients with the serious complications of polyneuritis, transverse myelitis and optic neuritis, and good results have been reported. The natural tendency for this disease to remit completely with good supportive care forces one to treat such reports with skepticism.

Reticuloendothelioses (Histiocytosis X)

PATHOGENESIS.—At present, eosinophilic granuloma, Hand-Schüller-Christian syndrome and Letterer-Siwe disease are classified together in the family of the reticuloendothelioses or histiocytosis X. Although the precise etiology of these disorders is obscure, they are characterized by the accumulation of xanthomatous granulomas in the reticuloendothelial system, skin, membranous bones and portions of the brain.[20] Histologically the granulomas are made up of cholesterol-laden foam cells, eosinophils, giant cells and the fibrous changes of healing, suggesting an infectious or inflammatory etiology. These disorders appear sporadically and do not follow a hereditary pattern.

CLINICAL AND LABORATORY DIAGNOSIS.—Symptoms and signs of these disorders are extremely protean because of their insidious course and disseminated character. The onset of signs and symptoms may occur at age 5 or 6 with exophthalmos, a xanthomatous papular eruption, draining ears, growth retardation, sexual infantilism, diabetes insipidus, seizures, gingivitis and respiratory complaints. The granulomas in the orbit may cause not only exophthalmos but paralytic squint and optic atrophy. The disease process has a predilection for the bones of the skull (Fig. 18.6), and when the granulomas extend from the sella turcica they invade the tuber cinereum and hypothalamus to cause the diabetes insipidus and growth retardation. We have seen a patient whose disease mimicked lateral sinus thrombosis with a draining ear and papilledema, only to have its real nature recognized when skull and mastoid x-rays were taken. Multiple neurologic signs, including bilateral pyramidal tract signs, ataxia and other cranial nerve deficit, have been reported[29] in later stages of the disease, and they have been seen in one of our patients.

Plain films of the skull often reveal sharply defined, "punched-out" osteolytic lesions which vary greatly in size (Fig. 18.6). Similar defects may be found in the pelvis and less commonly in the long bones. Serum lipids are usually normal, as are routine CSF findings. Anemia may develop in advanced cases but no other hematologic abnormalities are seen.

MANAGEMENT AND PROGNOSIS.—The occurrence of spontaneous remissions in these disorders require a critical review of any new form of therapy. However, it is important to view these patients with therapeutic optimism at this time, since Lahey[32] has shown that intensive therapy with x-ray, antibiotics, adrenal steroids and ACTH produces significant benefit by extending longevity. Recent experience of Beier and associates[4] with vinblastine sulfate (Velban) therapy also has been encouraging (Fig. 18.6). The drug is given intravenously at weekly or biweekly

308 INFECTIONS

intervals in the dose of 0.1–0.45 mg./kg. for a total of 8–15 injections, depending on the clinical response and the leukocyte count. Therapy has been effective in about 85% of patients, and better results occur with early therapy. The effectiveness of vinblastine has been noted in patients who are refractory to other therapies and in subsequent courses of therapy in patients who have relapsed after a beneficial prior course of treatment. The drug appears to control the acute proliferative lesions found in the skeleton and skin, but it cannot be expected to abolish the symptom of diabetes insipidus.

Fig. 18.6.—Response to vinblastine therapy of osteolytic skull lesions in patient with histiocytosis. Note the gradual resolution of lytic bone lesions in this patient who has been treated intermittently with vinblastine sulfate (Velban) for nine months. See text for details.

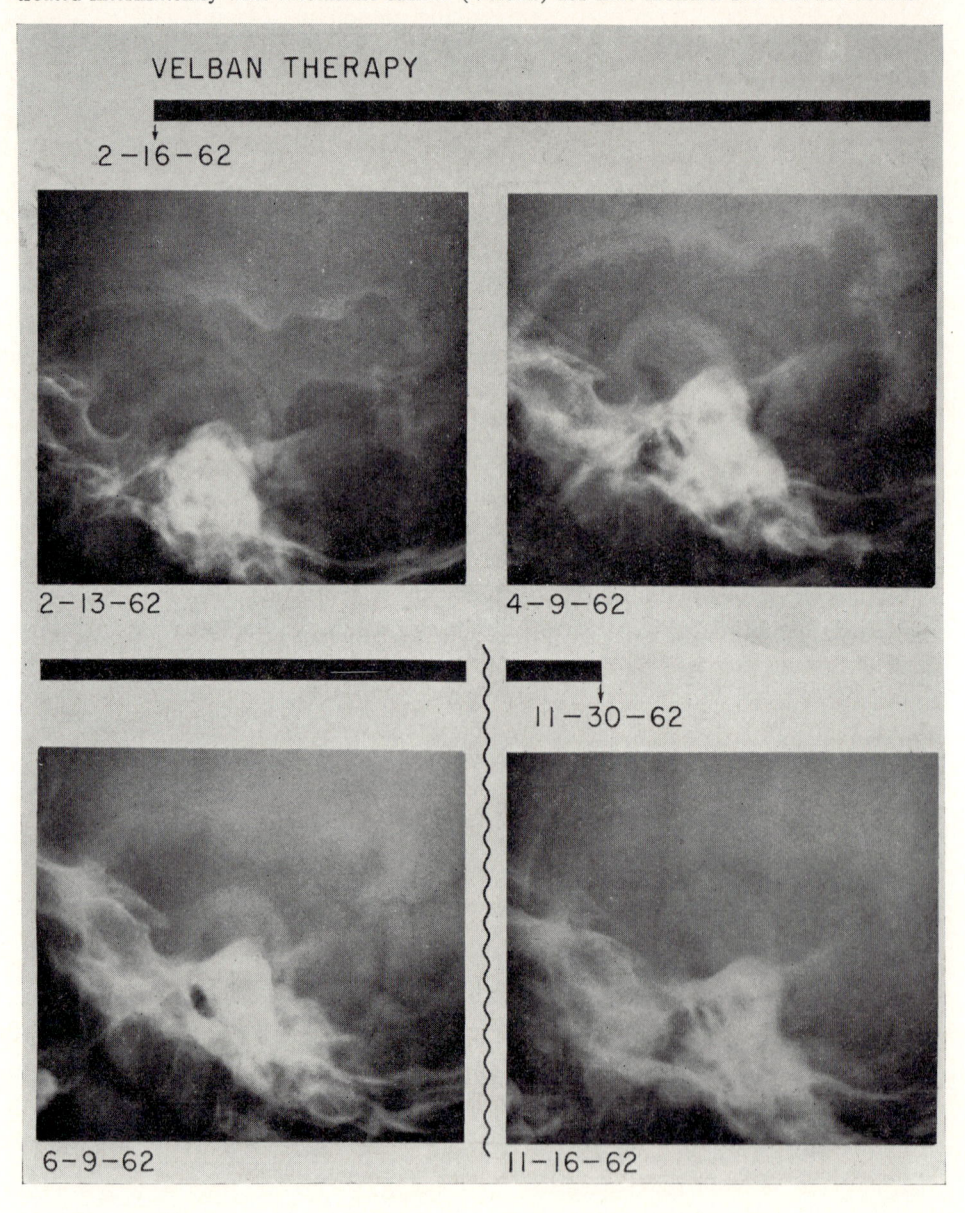

Experience in the treatment of increased intracranial pressure has been limited and results have been inconsistent. Patients with diabetes insipidus can be helped appreciably by the use of pitressin or the new synthetic product, lysyl-8-vasopressin. For details about the treatment of diabetes insipidus, consult Chapter 11. Anticonvulsant therapy is indicated, of course, in patients with seizures.

The prognosis must be guarded since the course of the disorder varies greatly. The young child and those with widely disseminated disease may live only one or two years. However, spontaneous remission, new and beneficial therapies and the observed long-term survival of many patients leave room for considerable hope. Routine examination of the cerebrospinal fluid usually gives normal results.

Subacute Inclusion Encephalitis (Subacute Sclerosing Leukoencephalitis)

PATHOGENESIS.—A subacute type of encephalitis characterized by type A intranuclear inclusion bodies was described by Dawson[16] in 1934. Later (1945) van Bogaert[58e] used the term "subacute sclerosing leukoencephalitis" to describe an electroclinical pathologic entity which is now considered identical with the disease described by Dawson. In cases with a short course, type A inclusion bodies in the nuclei of cortical neurons are prominent, whereas more chronic cases show prominent inflammatory exudate and gliosis in the white matter. Presumably the disease is due to a virus, but the exact agent has not yet been identified. Recently, impressive circumstantial evidence has been collected pointing to the measles virus as the cause of the disease.[52d]

CLINICAL AND LABORATORY DIAGNOSIS.—This rare disease most often affects children between 5 and 10 years and is characterized in the initial stages by subtle personality changes and signs of dementia which progress slowly.[13] Later a variety of involuntary movements, especially myoclonic jerks, appears together with real seizures, ataxia and dysarthria. Eventually there is a generalized "lead-pipe" type of muscular rigidity with severe dementia, leaving the patient in a helpless terminal state. Pyramidal tract signs are not prominent, but cranial nerve palsies and chorioretinitis have been noted in isolated cases.

The most consistent CSF abnormality is a strong, first zone (paretic) colloidal gold curve, indicating a high concentration of gamma globulin, even in an otherwise normal fluid. A highly characteristic but nonspecific EEG abnormality has been described. The background frequencies, which are slow, irregular and of low voltage, are punctuated every 15–30 seconds with brief paroxysmal bursts of generalized, bilaterally synchronous, high voltage, slow (1–3 cycles) and sharp wave discharges.[14,26]

MANAGEMENT AND PROGNOSIS.—Most reports agree that no form of treatment so far employed, including adrenal corticosteroids, has had any significant influence on the course of the disease. Survival time varies from a few months to about five years.

Chronic Orbital Cellulitis with Myositis (Orbital Pseudotumor)

This poorly understood condition presumably results from a subacute or chronic inflammation of the orbital soft tissues and muscles.[1] No etiologic microbial agent

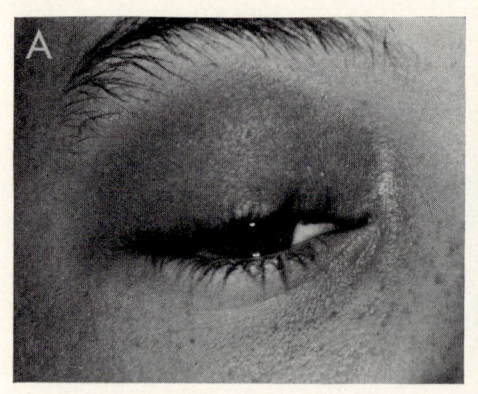

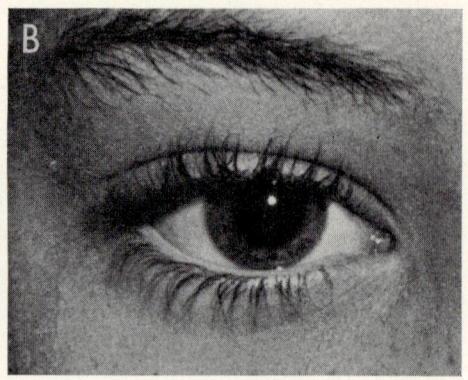

Fig. 18.7.—Chronic orbital cellulitis with myositis (orbital pseudotumor). Boy, 12, had onset of ocular symptoms and signs at age 8½. Intermittent exophthalmos, ptosis and diplopia developed, and he had incapacitating retro-orbital eye pain. Symptom-free intervals would extend as long as three months, and episodes of severe pain lasted from a few hours to two or three days. **A,** examination revealed obvious ptosis, measurable exophthalmos, purplish discoloration of the upper lid and a firm, soft-tissue mass below the upper rim of the right orbit, along with limitation of upward gaze. The patient had normal visual acuity, fields and fundi, and at no time were any laboratory abnormalities detected. Between "attacks" the eye looked relatively normal **(B)**. Because of the continued development of intermittent symptoms an exploration of the orbit was done; thickening of the periorbital soft tissues was found, but no tumor or vascular malformation. Three years later the patient is asymptomatic and free of signs.

has ever been incriminated. Despite our ignorance about the basic etiology and pathogenesis, the physician should be aware of this uncommon and worrisome entity.

Nearly always unilateral, the disorder is characterized by prominent swelling and discoloration of the eyelid and conjunctiva (Fig. 18.7). Proptosis commonly occurs, and the globe may be displaced in other directions. The inflammatory process may cause intermittent ptosis of the involved lid. Pain and diplopia are among the other prominent complaints.

The differential diagnosis of orbital tumors is discussed in Chapter 5.

An awareness of this clinical entity is important in order to guard against unnecessary operation. In some patients enucleation has been performed when the erroneous diagnosis of an orbital tumor has been made. Spontaneous remission can be expected, but the patient may require codeine or other analgesics to relieve severe pain. Kroll and Casten[30] state that systemic prednisone therapy usually brings about prompt improvement in symptoms and signs, and they suggest that a therapeutic trial of this drug provides a useful diagnostic test.

Sarcoidosis

PATHOGENESIS.—This generalized systemic disorder is characterized by a diffuse granulomatous inflammatory process which usually involves the lungs, skin, lymph nodes, eyes, parotid glands and bones. The common coincidence of tuberculosis and sarcoidosis has only heightened the etiologic puzzle of the disease, and its cause remains an enigma. Occasionally the nervous system is involved, most commonly the facial nerve as a result of parotitis. Primary nervous system involvement usually affects (1) the meninges, with secondary cranial nerve involvement (optic and facial) and hydrocephalus and (2) the infundibulum and floor of the third ventricle. In addition to involvement of the uvea, retinal lesions are seen quite commonly. Rarely the brain parenchyma and spinal nerves are affected.

CLINICAL AND LABORATORY DIAGNOSIS.—This disease affects primarily young adults and only occasionally children.[25] In our experience retinal lesions are seen most commonly in children. Unilateral or bilateral facial weakness may occur with parotitis and uveitis (uveoparotid fever), but this too is rare in children. In the more severe forms of the disease in older patients, obstructive hydrocephalus as a result of chronic meningitis and diabetes insipidus or other hypothalamic symptoms secondary to infundibular disease are seen. Seizures and isolated peripheral neuropathies occur rarely, as do corticospinal tract signs, cerebellar deficit and myopathies.[60b]

Diagnosis is based upon systemic signs of the disease, lymph node biopsy, chest x-ray and the Kveim test. Additional laboratory abnormalities include hyperglobulinemia, eosinophilia, leukopenia, and hypercalcemia. In patients with neurologic signs the cerebrospinal fluid may show (1) increased pressure, (2) a lymphocytic pleocytosis (10–200 cells), (3) a moderately decreased sugar content and (4) an elevated protein content.

MANAGEMENT AND PROGNOSIS.—Sarcoidosis runs a chronic course which in many cases is benign and requires no specific therapy. Patients with neurologic symptoms and signs can be benefited by adrenal corticosteroid therapy (prednisone, 1 mg./lb./day). Steroid therapy should be continued up to 8–12 weeks or until a beneficial response is obtained, and then the dose should be tapered gradually. This therapy can be continued for long periods but attempts should be made periodically to withdraw the drug. The disease usually remits after a period of years, the mortality rate being about 5%.

Cat-Scratch Fever

Inasmuch as this disease is benign and self-limited, no knowledge about the underlying lesions has been collected. Presumably due to a filtrable virus, the cause of this acute febrile illness is unknown.

The patient usually first has systemic symptoms of fever, malaise and headache. A papular lesion usually develops at the site of the scratch or bite and is associated with enlargement of the involved regional nodes with redness and tenderness in the area. The nodes may be soft, hard or fluctuant. The central nervous system symptoms have been categorized as those of a mild form of encephalitis, myelitis or radiculitis.[10] The cerebrospinal fluid may show a mild lymphocytic pleocytosis. An intradermal test using cat-scratch antigen has diagnostic value, but it must be interpreted with caution since its specificity is questionable and a positive finding can persist for years.

Patients with this benign illness have a uniformly good prognosis. They usually require only supportive medical care.

BIBLIOGRAPHY

1. Adams, R. D., et al.: *Diseases of Muscle* (New York City: Paul B. Hoeber, Inc., 1954).
1a. Allen, J. E., and Frank, D. J.: The use of gamma globulin in the treatment of measles encephalitis, Pediatrics 17:78, 1956.

2. American Academy of Pediatrics: Report of the Committee on the Control of Infectious Disease, 1966.
3. Bardenwerper, H. W.: Serum neuritis from tetanus antitoxin, J.A.M.A. 179:763, 1962.
4. Beier, F. R., et al.: Treatment of reticuloendotheliosis with vinblastine sulfate, J. Pediat. 63:1087, 1963.
5. Benson, P., et al.: The prognosis of subdural effusions complicating pyogenic meningitis, J. Pediat. 57:670, 1960.
6. Berg, R., and Jelke, H.: Acute cerebellar ataxia in children associated with Coxsackie viruses group B, Acta paediat. scandinav. 54:497, 1965.
7. Berman, P. H., and Banker, B. Q.: Neonatal meningitis, Pediatrics 38:6, 1966.
8. Boe, J., et al.: Corticosteroid treatment for acute meningoencephalitis: a retrospective study of 346 cases, Brit. M. J. 1:1094, 1965.
9. Bosma, J. F.: Residual disability of pharyngeal area resulting from poliomyelitis, J.A.M.A. 165:216, 1957.
10. Brooksaler, F.: Cat scratch disease with encephalopathy, Am. J. Dis. Child. 107:185, 1964.
11. Butler, W. T., et al.: Diagnostic and prognostic value of clinical and laboratory findings in cryptococcal meningitis, New England J. Med. 270:59, 1964.
12. Clark, D. B.: Brain Abscess, in Nelson, W. E. (ed.): *Textbook of Pediatrics* (8th ed.; Philadelphia: W. B. Saunders Company, 1964).
13. Clark, N. S., and Best, P. V.: Subacute sclerosing (inclusion body) encephalitis, Arch. Dis. Childhood 39:356, 1964.
14. Cobb, W.: The periodic events of subacute sclerosing leucoencephalitis, Electroencephalog. & Clin. Neurophysiol. 27:278, 1966.
15. Cotton, P. B., and Webb-Peploe, M. M.: Acute transverse myelitis as a complication of glandular fever, Brit. M. J. 1:654, 1966.
16. Dawson, J. R.: Cellular inclusions in cerebral lesions of epidemic encephalitis, Arch. Neurol. & Psychiat. 31:685, 1934.
17. Eaton, O. M., et al.: Respiratory failure in polyradiculoneuritis associated with infectious mononucleosis, J.A.M.A. 194:609, 1965.
18. Editorial: Recurrent meningitis, Lancet 2:379, 1966.
19. Elliott, F. A.: Treatment of herpes zoster with high doses of prednisone, Lancet 2:610, 1964.
20. Feigin, I.: Xanthomatosis of the nervous system, J. Neuropath. & Exper. Neurol. 15:400, 1956.
21. Haymaker, W., and Kernohan, J. W.: The Landry-Guillain-Barré syndrome: A clinicopathologic report of 50 cases and a critique of the literature, Medicine 28:59, 1949.
22. Janeway, R., and Kelly, D. L.: Papilledema and hydrocephalus associated with recurrent polyneuritis, Arch. Neurol. 15:507, 1966.
23. Jarcho, L. W., et al.: Encephalitis and poliomyelitis in the adult due to Coxsackie virus group B, type 5, New England J. Med. 268:235, 1963.
24. Karelitz, S., and Eisenberg, M.: Measles encephalitis: Evaluation of treatment with adrenocorticotropin and adrenal corticosteroids, Pediatrics 27:811, 1961.
25. Kendig, E. L.: Sarcoidosis among children, J. Pediat. 61:269, 1962.
26. Kiloh, L. G., and Osselton, J. W.: *Clinical Electroencephalography* (2d ed.; London: Butterworth & Co., Ltd., 1966).
27. King, G., et al.: Acute cerebellar ataxia of childhood, Pediatrics 21:731, 1958.
28. Kloetzel, K.: Clinical patterns of severe tetanus, J.A.M.A. 185:559, 1963.
29. Kristensson, K.: Generalized histiocytic reticulo-endotheliosis and leuco-encephalopathy in childhood, Acta paediat. scandinav. 55:321, 1966.
30. Kroll, A. J., and Casten, V. G.: Diseases of the Orbit, in Liebman and Gelles (eds.): *The Pediatrician's Ophthalmology* (St. Louis: The C. V. Mosby Company, 1966).
31. Krugman, S., and Ward, R.: *Infectious Diseases of Children* (3d ed.; St. Louis: The C. V. Mosby Company, 1964).
32. Lahey, M. E.: Prognosis in reticuloendotheliosis in children, J. Pediat. 60:664, 1962.
33. Lawson, D., et al.: Meningitis in childhood, Brit. M. J. 1:557, 1965.
34. Leedom, J. M., et al.: Importance of sulfadiazine resistance in meningococcal disease in civilians, New England J. Med. 273:1395, 1965.
35. Leider, W., et al.: Herpes-simplex-virus encephalitis, New England J. Med. 273:341, 1965.
36. Lennette, E. H., et al.: Viral central nervous system disease, J.A.M.A. 179:687, 1962.
37. Liske, E., and Weikers, N. J.: Changing aspects of brain abscesses, Neurology 14:294, 1964.
38. Loeser, E., and Scheinberg, L.: Brain abscesses: A review of 99 cases, Neurology 7:601, 1957.
39. Low, N. L., et al.: Polyneuritis in children, Pediatrics 22:972, 1958.
40. McKay, R. J., et al.: Collections of subdural fluid complicating meningitis due to H. influenzae (type B), New England J. Med. 242:20, 1950.
41. Magoffin, R. L., and Lennette, E. H.: Nonpolioviruses and paralytic disease, California Med. 97:1, 1962.

42. Magoffin, R. L., et al.: An etiologic study of clinical paralytic poliomyelitis, J.A.M.A. 175:269, 1961.
43. Magoffin, R. L., et al.: Association of Coxsackie viruses with illnesses resembling mild paralytic poliomyelitis, Pediatrics 28:602, 1961.
43a. Marshall, W. J. S.: Herpes simplex encephalitis treated with idoxuridine and external decompression, Lancet 2:579, 1967.
44. Mathies, A. W., et al.: Experience with ampicillin in bacterial meningitis, Antimicrob. Agents & Chemother. 5:610, 1965.
45. Matson, D. D., and Salam, M.: Brain abscess in congenital heart disease, Pediatrics 27: 772, 1961.
46. The Medical Letter 7:13, 1965.
47. The Medical Letter 7:87, 1965.
48. The Medical Letter 8:58, 1966.
48a. The Medical Letter 9:78, 1967.
49. Merritt, H. H.: *Textbook of Neurology* (4th ed.; Philadelphia; Lea & Febiger, 1967).
49a. Meyer, H. M., et al.: Attenuated rubella virus: II. Production of an experimental live-virus vaccine and clinical trial, New England J. Med. 275:575, 1966.
49b. Olson, L. C., et al.: Herpes virus infections of the human central nervous system, New England J. Med. 277:1271, 1967.
50. Parker, R. H., et al.: Toxicity of intrathecally administered pancreatic dornase, J.A.M.A. 192:169, 1965.
51. Perlstein, M. A., et al.: Routine treatment of tetanus, J.A.M.A. 173:1536, 1960.
52. Platou, R. V., et al.: Acute subdural effusions and late sequelae of meningitis, Pediatrics 23:962, 1959.
52a. Posner, J. B., et al.: Hyponatremia in acute polyneuropathy, Arch. Neurol. 17:530, 1967.
52b. Rosenblum, W. I., et al.: Lesions of the spinal cord in polyradiculoneuropathy of unknown etiology and a possible relationship with the Guillain-Barré syndrome, J. Neurol. Neurosurg. & Psychiat. 29:69, 1966.
52c. Schochet, S. S.: Human Toxocara canis encephalopathy in a case of visceral larva migrans, Neurology 17:227, 1967.
52d. Sever, J. L., and Zeman, W. (eds.): Neurology Conference on Measles virus and Subacute Sclerosing Panencephalitis, Neurology, vol. 18, pt. 2, January, 1968.
52e. Sherman, F. E., et al.: Acute encephalopathy (encephalitis) complicating rubella, J.A.M.A. 192:675, 1965.
53. Sibley, W. A., and O'Brien, J. L.: Intracranial tuberculomas, Neurology 6:157, 1956.
54. Siewers, C. M. F., and Cramblett, H. G.: Cryptococcosis (torulosis) in children, Pediatrics 34:393, 1964.
55. Smith, E. S.: Purulent meningitis in infants and children, J. Pediat. 45:425, 1954.
56. Smith, M. H. D., et al.: Subdural effusions complicating bacterial meningitis, Pediatrics 7:34, 1951.
57. Steigman, A. J., and Lipton, M. M.: Fatal bulbospinal paralytic poliomyelitis due to ECHO 11 virus, J.A.M.A. 174:178, 1960.
58. Swartz, M. N., and Dodge, P. R.: Bacterial meningitis: A review of selected aspects, New England J. Med. 272:725, 779, 842, 898, 954, 1003, 1965.
58a. Szabo, G., et al.: Tuberculous meningitis treated with hydrocortisone and cortisone, Pediatrics 19:580, 1957.
58b. Taylor M. J., et al.: Meningoencephalitis associated with pneumonitis due to mycoplasma pneumoniae, J.A.M.A. 199:813, 1967.
58c. van Bogaert, L.: Une leuco-encephalopathie sclérosante subaigue, J. Neurol. Neurosurg. & Psychiat. 8:101, 1945.
59. Walsh, F. C., et al.: Infectious mononucleosis encephalitis, Pediatrics 13:536, 1954.
60. Weiss, S., and Carter, S.: Course and prognosis of acute cerebellar ataxia in children, Neurology 9:711, 1959.
60a. Whitecar, J. P., et al.: Recurrent pneumococcal meningitis, New England J. Med. 274: 1285, 1966.
60b. Wiederholt, W. C., and Siekert, R. G.: Neurological manifestations of sarcoidosis, Neurology 15:1147, 1965.
61. Williams, C. P. S., et al.: Brain swelling with acute purulent meningitis, Pediatrics 34:220, 1964.
62. Wolf, A., and Cowen, D.: Perinatal infections of the central nervous system, J. Neuropath. & Exper. Neurol. 18:191, 1959.
62a. World Health Organization Expert Committee on Rabies: Fifth Report, Technical Report Series No. 321, 1966.
63. Young, G. F., et al.: Necrotizing encephalitis and chorioretinitis in a young infant, Arch. Neurol. 13:15, 1965.
64. Young, L. M., et al.: Relapse following ampicillin treatment of acute Hemophilus influenzae meningitis, Pediatrics 41:516, 1968.

19

Disorders of Muscle

MYOPATHIES

Hereditary Myopathies
    Classic Muscular Dystrophies
        Childhood dystrophy (Duchenne)
        Facioscapulohumeral dystrophy (Landouzy-Déjerine)
        Myotonic dystrophy (Steinert)
        Ocular myopathy (progressive dystrophic ophthalmoplegia)
        Distal myopathy
        Limb-girdle dystrophy (Erb, Leyden-Möbius)
    Hereditary Disorders with Specific Chemical Defects including some Congenital and Limb-Girdle Dystrophies
        Glycogen storage diseases
        Familial myoglobinuria
    Hereditary Disorders with Distinctive Structural Defects
        Central core disease (congenital nonprogressive myopathy)
        Nemaline myopathy
        Abnormal mitochondria
Nonhereditary Myopathies
    Secondary Metabolic Myopathies

NEUROGENIC MUSCULAR ATROPHIES

    Infantile Spinal Muscular Atrophy (Werdnig-Hoffmann)
    Progressive Neural Muscular Atrophy (Charcot-Marie-Tooth)
    Juvenile Proximal Spinal Muscular Atrophy (Kugelberg-Welander)
    Hereditary Spastic Paraplegia (Juvenile Amyotrophic Lateral Sclerosis)
    Enterovirus Infections ⎫
                              ⎬ Chapter 18
    Infectious Polyneuritis ⎭

MYOSITIS

Myositis of Unknown Etiology
    Dermatomyositis
    Acute Polymyositis

Chronic Polymyositis
Other Rare Forms of Myositis
    Collagen vascular diseases with rheumatoid arthritis, rheumatic fever, systemic lupus erythematosus, polyarteritis or scleroderma
    Myositis ossificans

Myositis of Known Etiology
    Bacterial Myositis (Pyogenic, Gas Gangrene Bacillus)
    Viral Myositis (Epidemic Pleurodynia—Coxsackie)
    Parasitic Myositis (Trichinosis)
    Miscellaneous

DISORDERS OF NEUROMUSCULAR TRANSMISSION

Nonhereditary Disorders of Neuromuscular Transmission
    Myasthenia Gravis
    Electrolyte Disorders (Hyper- and Hypopotassemia, Hypernatremia, Hypocalcemia—Chapters 21 and 23)

Hereditary Disorders of Neuromuscular Transmission
    Familial Periodic Paralysis
        Classic hypokalemic type   Normokalemic type
        Hyperkalemic type (adynamia episodica hereditaria)
    Myotonia Congenita   Paramyotonia Congenita

CONGENITAL DEFECTS

Congenital Absence of Muscles
    Abdominals   Diaphragm
    Pectorals   Bulbar

Congenital Contractures
    Clubfoot   Amyoplasia congenita (arthrogryposis)
    Torticollis   Camptodactyly
    Elevation of the shoulder

TUMORS OF MUSCLE

INTOXICATIONS

Tetanus (Chapter 18)
Spider and Insect Bites ⎫
Botulism   ⎬ Chapter 20
Drugs   ⎭

DISORDERS OF MUSCLE

MANY DISEASES manifest themselves clinically by causing muscular symptoms and signs. The term *myopathy* is used here to include any primary disease of muscle, usually (or presumably) metabolic, in which no evidence of an inflammatory or neurogenic etiology is found. It is intended to exclude conditions in which the clinical signs result from primary diseases of the central or peripheral nervous system and of the myoneural junction. Any myopathy which has an hereditary incidence pattern is called a *dystrophy*. The term *neurogenic atrophy* is restricted in the outline given here to conditions in which loss of muscle bulk is a result of lower motor neuron disease, although the reader should realize that the general term *atrophy* is often applied to any condition which is associated with reduction of muscle mass (including the disuse atrophy seen in patients with upper motor neuron lesions or the patient with any advanced myopathy). In this classification system disorders of muscle which have an inflammatory basis (infectious or presumed infectious) are grouped under the term *myositis*. Diseases which produce their clinical effects by blocking or facilitating *neuromuscular transmission* have been placed in a separate category because, by the definition used here, they cannot be placed correctly in the category of myopathies. The classification system devised for this chapter includes the rare categories of congenital defects, tumors of muscle and intoxications.

From the time Duchenne first performed primitive biopsy in patients with muscle disease, techniques have been refined progressively in an effort to reach better understanding of these puzzling processes. At first, histologic criteria were used to distinguish primary myopathies from neurogenic atrophies; later, systemic disorders associated with myositis (such as sarcoidosis and amyloidosis) were diagnosed by the same method. Over the years electromyography has been shown to have definite but limited clinical usefulness. In the past 10 years electron microscopic, histochemical, biochemical, immunologic and tissue culture methods have been developed and have shed new light on these old problems. A myopathy resulting from phosphorylase deficiency has been discovered, and some new and interesting but poorly understood morphologic abnormalities have been uncovered.

The reader is referred to Chapter 3 for a differential diagnostic approach to the common signs and symptoms found in patients with neuromuscular disorders.

Hereditary Myopathies

As in the case of all disorders in which the pathogenesis is poorly understood, many different systems of classification have been suggested. Authorities such as Tyler and Adams[62] have stated that all types of dystrophy probably represent only insignificant variations of a single disease process. In the light of the different patterns of inheritance, the different ages of onset and prognosis, and the new ultrastructural and chemical findings in occasional cases of dystrophy recently described, this point of view is now more difficult to accept. It seems far more likely, despite many clinical, histologic and biochemical features shared in common by patients with dystrophy, that these inherited myopathies (as defined above) comprise different disorders which are well defined clinically and genetically and which have different histologic and biochemical features.

From a practical, clinical standpoint one must separate the different types of dystrophy to provide a sensible basis for (1) prognostication in the child affected and (2) predictions about the recurrence risks in subsequent children. The beginning outline represents a modification of that suggested by Zundel and Tyler[73] and attempts to incorporate the recently described hereditary myopathies with distinctive histologic and chemical features. The reader should realize that the more common types of dystrophy (*Duchenne, facioscapulohumeral* (FSH) and *myotonic*) have a fairly well-defined clinical character, but that so-called *limb-girdle* and *congenital dystrophy* represent wastebasket categories because of their variable clinical and genetic characteristics. Adams and associates[1] use the following classification system:

1. Severe generalized familial muscular dystrophy
    Duchenne's dystrophy (pseudohypertrophic)
2. Mild restricted muscular dystrophy
    Facioscapulohumeral dystrophy (FSH) (Landouzy-Déjerine)
    Scapulohumeral juvenile type (Erb)
    Pelvi-femoral type of limb-girdle dystrophy (Leyden-Möbius)
3. Progressive dystrophic ophthalmoplegia
4. Myotonia dystrophica (Steinert)
5. Late distal muscular dystrophy

For the time being we prefer the outline used at the beginning of the chapter because of (1) the quite dependable inheritance patterns of Duchenne's, FSH and myotonic dystrophy and (2) the undependable genetic characteristics and the new histologic changes being described in families with limb girdle dystrophy.

Classic Muscular Dystrophies

PATHOGENESIS.—In most patients with classic forms of dystrophy the disease is inherited. Presumably the genetic defect causes an abnormality of intracellular muscle metabolism by virtue of either an absent or an altered enzyme system. Abnormal muscle function would then result from this metabolic abnormality.

Excess creatinuria in patients with classic dystrophy was noted years ago, but its exact significance in the pathogenesis remains obscure. It is known that creatine is formed excessively and excreted excessively. Recently it has been shown that creatine phosphokinase (CPK), the enzyme which catalyzes the reversible reaction

$$\text{creatine} + \text{ATP} \underset{}{\overset{\text{CPK}}{\rightleftharpoons}} \text{creatine phosphate} + \text{ADP}$$

and is responsible for energy transfer in muscle cells, is elevated in dystrophic patients[22] and in 80% of the carrier-mothers of dystrophic patients.[61]

Duchenne's dystrophy is inherited in most cases as an X-linked recessive trait (affecting mostly boys). Rarely girls are affected. Whether girls are affected by an autosomal recessive trait or some less common genetic mechanism is uncertain.[73] On the average, half of the boys in a family are affected with the disease and half of the girls are carriers. Patients inherit facioscapulohumeral, myotonic and distal dystrophy via an autosomal dominant trait. Certain cases of limb-girdle dystrophy behave in autosomal recessive fashion but many cases are sporadic. The mode of inheritance of ocular myopathy is poorly defined, but a familial pattern has been seen in many of the reported cases.

318 DISORDERS OF MUSCLE

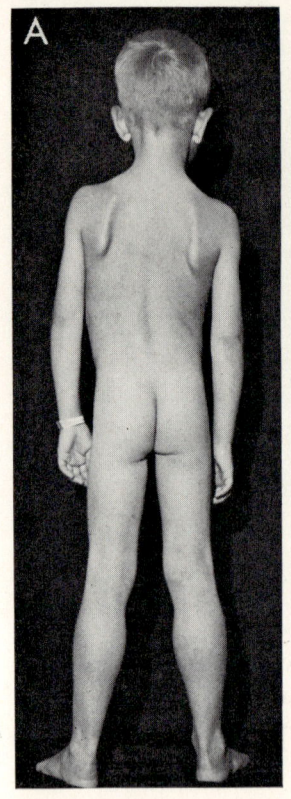

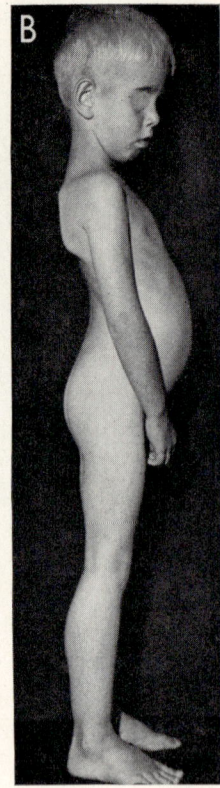

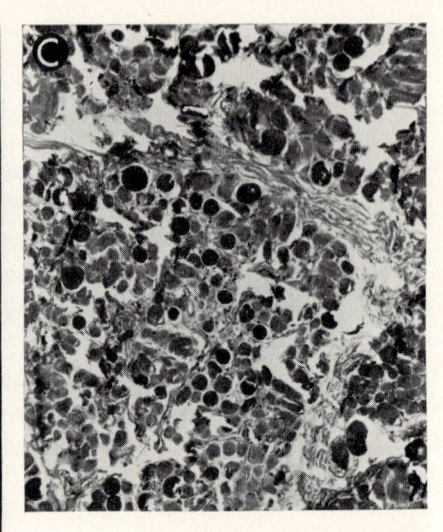

Fig. 19.1.—Childhood or pseudohypertrophic (Duchenne) dystrophy. This 6-year-old boy was asymptomatic during the first year of life but did not walk alone until 18 months. His movements then appeared slower than those of his peers. He could not run well, nor could he climb stairs or raise his hands above his head easily. **A** shows the obvious enlargement of the calves (pseudohypertrophy), shoulder girdle atrophy with scapular winging and a moderate scoliosis. A pronounced lordosis is seen in **B**. He also exhibits the Gower's maneuver on rising to the erect position, a waddling gait and a firm "balsa wood" consistency of calf muscles. Typical light microscopic abnormalities in dystrophic muscle (**C**) include (1) marked variation in size of muscle fibers, (2) fibers in varying stages of degeneration and (3) infiltration with connective tissue and fat.

Childhood Dystrophy (Duchenne)

CLINICAL AND LABORATORY DIAGNOSIS.—This most common and severe form of dystrophy affects boys predominantly. It is not apparent in early infancy, but there is often a history of a delay in walking, frequent falls and clumsiness. The patient exhibits a waddling gait, pronounced lordosis, pseudohypertrophy of the calves (in most cases) and occasionally pseudohypertrophy of the deltoids and triceps (Fig. 19.1). The pseudohypertrophy results from the deposition of fat and fibrous tissue in the weakened muscle, usually the gastrocnemius, and imparts a firmer-than-normal, ropy consistency to the muscle. Often the patient cannot climb stairs or rise normally to the erect position without "climbing" his legs slowly with his arms (Gower's maneuver). The latter sign results from pelvic girdle and trunk weakness, is seen commonly and can appear in other disease conditions that cause pelvic muscle weakness. The weakness and atrophy progress, steadily giving way to contractures, deformities (lordosis and scoliosis) and disability. In the advanced stage of the disease cardiomegaly and electrocardiographic changes (25% of cases) are seen. Studies of intellectual functioning in patients with Duchenne's dystrophy have shown that these patients operate at lower levels than a variety of control groups, but they do not exhibit true dementia.[71]

Recently Mabry and associates[40] described an X-linked form of muscular dystrophy which has a late onset and slow progression. They proposed that four types of X-linked muscular dystrophy can be encountered.

As previously indicated, the serum enzyme, CPK, is elevated in dystrophics and in 80% of the carrier-mothers. The enzyme is remarkably stable in the normal state and is not generally found in liver, lung or erythrocytes. Hence, for practical purposes, CPK levels are elevated only in patients with diseases of skeletal muscle and myocardial infarction. The highest concentrations (50–100 times normal) have been found in infants under 6 months of age who have no clinical signs of the disease.[73] Elevated enzyme levels persist until weakness and atrophy are advanced, at which time normal or only slightly elevated concentrations are found. Patients with neurogenic muscular atrophies generally have normal CPK levels. Many other serum enzymes (such as aldolase, glutamic oxalacetic transaminase, glutamic pyruvic transaminase, lactic dehydrogenase, alpha-glucan phosphorylase and glycerophosphate isomerase) have elevated concentrations in dystrophy, but the levels are also elevated in liver disease and pulmonary and myocardial infarction and so lack specificity.

Muscle biopsy (Fig. 19.1,C) demonstrates (1) striking variation in the size of muscle fibers in a haphazard distribution, (2) fibers in varying stages of degeneration and (3) infiltration of fat and connective tissue. The electromyogram shows action potentials of abnormally low voltage and abnormally brief duration. Urinary creatine output is elevated (see Pathogenesis), and creatinine output, which is quite constant from day to day and is proportional to total muscle mass, is abnormally low. The abnormal creatine/creatinine excretion values are not specific for dystrophy and can be seen in conditions such as polymyositis and chronic thyrotoxicosis. Carriers have been described with muscle weakness in the lower extremities, together with biochemical, histologic and EMG evidence of myopathy.[23]

MANAGEMENT AND PROGNOSIS.—Despite the therapeutic trial of a large group of agents, no effective specific therapy is available for any form of muscle dystrophy. Duchenne's dystrophy runs a relentlessly progressive course, the most rapid progression occurring in patients with disease of early onset. Most patients are confined to a wheelchair by age 10. When patients become inactive because of intercurrent illness or because inactivity is recommended, contractures and skeletal deformities develop quickly. Vignos and associates[67,68] have doubled the duration of ambulation in a small series of patients by carrying out a comprehensive rehabilitation program. Chung and Morton[13] reported a 75% mortality by age 20.

This genetically determined disease is usually inherited as a sex-linked recessive trait and so affects boys almost exclusively. In the exceptional case of autosomal recessive inheritance girls may be afflicted. Using the serum CPK determination, affected asymptomatic male infants can now be identified presumptively and definition of the carrier state in girls may soon be practical. Milhorat and Goldstone[40a] have stated that 79% of definite carrier-mothers have elevation of CPK levels, but they point out the need for caution in genetic counseling. This information should prove useful in both genetic counseling and early diagnosis.

Facioscapulohumeral Dystrophy (Landouzy-Déjerine)

CLINICAL AND LABORATORY DIAGNOSIS.—This milder type of dystrophy is transmitted as an autosomal dominant trait and affects both men and women, usually between age 12 and 20. The disease incidence approaches full penetrance (i.e., 50% of offspring are affected), but the severity of the disorder varies greatly. The mild degree of weakness in many patients leads to many overlooked cases. According to Tyler and Stephens,[63] the muscle weakness appears in approximately the following order: orbicularis oris (inability to purse lips), sternal head of pectoralis, lower fibers of trapezius, brachioradialis and tibialis anticus. Eventually patients cannot elevate the arms, and shoulder weakness develops, followed by lordosis and pronounced winging of the scapulae. In Tyler's experience[61] the serum CPK level is usually normal or slightly elevated. Mild creatinuria may occur. The EMG and muscle biopsy findings cannot be distinguished from those seen in Duchenne dystrophy. Occasionally families with neurogenic atrophy resemble patients with facioscapulohumeral dystrophy quite closely.[27a]

MANAGEMENT AND PROGNOSIS.—Patients with this mild disorder usually can expect a normal life span and remain ambulatory until old age. Parents should be counseled to expect children of either sex to be affected in successive generations, but it is impossible to predict the severity of subsequent cases on the basis of the disease in an affected ancestor.

Myotonic Dystrophy (Steinert)

CLINICAL AND LABORATORY DIAGNOSIS.—This disorder resembles other forms of dystrophy by virtue of the muscle wasting and its hereditary character, but the unique feature lies in the distinctive signs of systemic disease (cataracts, gonadal atrophy, frontal baldness and a high incidence of mental changes). Also, the pattern of muscle wasting has a characteristic distribution, being greater distally than proximally. Weakness of the feet (foot drop) and hands (wrist drop) occurs early, together with pronounced wasting of the neck muscles. Atrophy of the temporalis, masseter and oropharyngeal muscles occurs, as well as ptosis of the eyelids, causing a mournful facial expression (Fig. 19.2,*A*).

The disease generally has its onset in the third decade with myotonia (inability to relax a muscle after strong contraction). This sign may persist alone for several years. The differentiation of myotonic dystrophy from myotonia congenita may be difficult. Some workers have suggested that the two disorders represent two extremes of the same disease, but this concept has not yet been widely accepted. The sign of myotonia may be noted when the patient cannot release his grip on shaking hands. Direct percussion of the muscles, such as the thumb adductors, often evokes visible myotonia. The bilateral lid ptosis leads to marked furrowing of the brow and tilting back of the head to uncover the pupils. Many of these patients have a strikingly nasal voice. Dystrophic heart disease affects this group of patients[29] as frequently as those with the Duchenne type of dystrophy, but its late onset complicates the clinical differentiation from other types of heart disease. Some workers have called attention not only to cardiac muscle involvement but also to clinical symptoms and signs resulting from the effects of the dystrophic process on the involuntary muscles of the gut and respiratory apparatus.[37] A number of workers have emphasized the intellectual and social deterioration of this group of dystrophics.[12] It seems most likely that the dementia is a reflection of degenerative changes in the nervous system because serial air studies in some of these

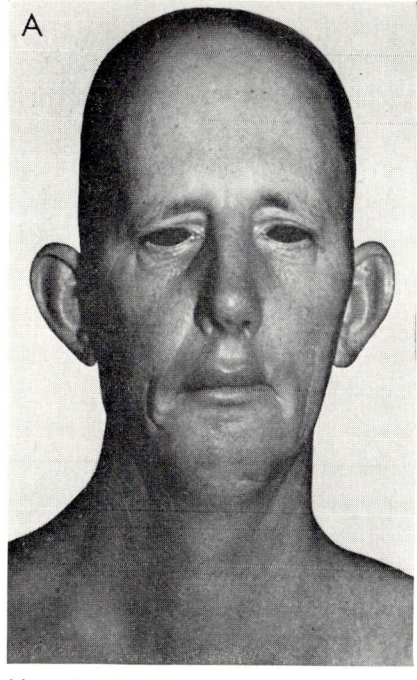

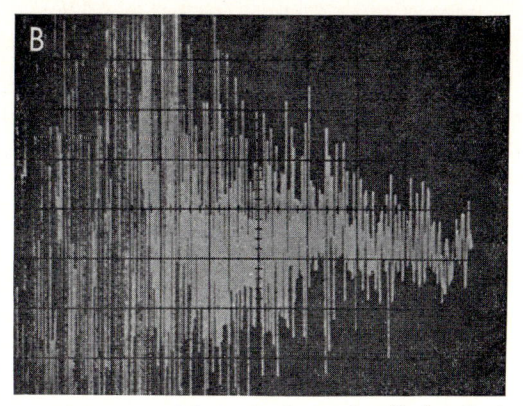

Fig. 19.2.—Myotonic dystrophy (Steinert). **A,** young man with typical myotonic dystrophy exhibits a mournful expression, frontal baldness, weakness, atrophy and "sagging" of facial muscles and bilateral lid ptosis. He also had bilateral foot and wristdrop, mild mental deficiency and testicular atrophy. **B,** the electrical pattern is seen typically in patients with myotonia congenita (Thomsen) and myotonic dystrophy (Steinert) and appears either when a patient relaxes a contracted muscle or when the muscle is stimulated electrically through the EMG needle or by a soft blow. At the beginning one sees a motor unit potential of normal amplitude but, instead of normal electrical silence following, there is a prolonged burst of rapid electrical activity (a mixture of single fiber and motor unit potentials) which subsides very gradually. Audio amplification of this phenomenon suggests the sound of a "dive bomber."

patients show progressive ventricular enlargement[45a] and generalized structural changes.[45b] Myotonic dystrophy is easily confused with Klinefelter's syndrome, but differentiation can be made with a buccal smear. Both myotonia congenita and paramyotonia congenita (p. 344) must also be distinguished from Steinert's disease.

The electromyograms of patients with myotonia, following voluntary contraction or tapping of the muscle or tendon, reveal characteristic, late firing. Instead of the silence which usually follows relaxation in the normal person, one sees and hears a prolonged burst of discharges of gradually diminishing amplitude (Fig. 19.2,*B*), causing the "dive-bomber" effect on audio amplification. The muscle biopsy findings resemble those in other forms of dystrophy, except that central nuclear proliferation is prominent in myotonic dystrophy, and creatinuria is inconstant.

In a penetrating analysis of their own experience and that reported in the literature, Dodge and his group,[18] as well as others,[69] have stressed the unexpected frequency of early symptoms in patients with myotonic dystrophy, contrary to the generally stated impression.[62,73] Dodge and co-workers outlined three clinical syndromes to be expected: (1) onset in infancy of facial diplegia causing feeding difficulty, with hypotonia and retarded motor development, symptoms which usually improve with time rather than getting worse, (2) the solitary symptom of myotonia in early childhood and (3) congenital ptosis. Percussion or grasp myotonia and typical EMG abnormalities helped to establish the diagnosis in all of these early cases.

MANAGEMENT AND PROGNOSIS.—Attempts have been made to relieve the patient's myotonia with quinine, corticosteroids and procaine amide, but the side effects and toxicity of these agents prohibit their regular use. Androgen therapy sometimes helps adults who suffer impotence or loss of libido, but these hormones do not benefit the basic myopathy. Cataracts may require removal if they impair vision seriously or cause glaucoma.

This disease is transmitted as an autosomal dominant trait, with marked variation in the extent and severity of clinical signs.

Ocular Myopathy

This rare disorder can begin at any age and characteristically causes bilateral ptosis of the lids and progressive ophthalmoplegia without pupillary involvement. In some patients weakness of other facial muscles appears, but only rarely are the muscles of the neck, shoulder girdle and trunk affected. This clinical syndrome is generally considered a true myopathy, but in some cases in which neurologic deficit appears a neurogenic basis has been suspected. If muscle biopsy is performed, changes compatible with dystrophy are usually found.

Treatment of this slowly evolving disorder is limited to plastic surgical procedures to correct ptosis of the lids. Familial cases of the disorder have been reported, but a dependable pattern of inheritance has not been delineated.

Distal Myopathy

This rare disorder begins after age 30. It involves the small muscles and extensors of the hands and feet. Typically the myopathic process is entirely distal. The EMG and muscle biopsy findings are compatible with a dystrophic process.

Limb-Girdle Dystrophy (Erb, Leyden-Möbius)

As previously stated, many authorities have considered this group a wastebasket category of dystrophies which do not fit the diagnostic criteria of the other types.[25,46,73] Either sex may be affected, cases may appear sporadically or be inherited in a recessive or dominant fashion and the rate of progression varies. Clinically the signs of muscle involvement are intermediate in location and severity to those of the Duchenne and FSH types. Weakness in either the shoulder or pelvic girdle begins in the first or second decade, and facial involvement rarely occurs. By age 20 both pelvic and shoulder weakness is established. Much variability is seen in the progress of the disease, in the serum enzyme concentrations, the EMG and muscle biopsy findings and in the frequency of cardiac involvement. In some patients with recessively inherited limb-girdle dystrophy, serum enzyme concentrations may be elevated in the preclinical stage of the disease.[35a]

Good supportive care helps the patient with limb-girdle dystrophy to lead a useful, productive life. Patients should be encouraged to continue exercise to tolerance. Contractures can be prevented for a long period by active exercise and passive stretching. When the patient can no longer walk, he should be provided with bracing, training in ambulation and operative procedures when necessary. The rate of progression of this syndrome varies greatly. Inheritance patterns of limb-girdle dystrophy also vary considerably, and this complicates genetic counseling. However, one should expect a familial incidence in many cases.

HEREDITARY DISORDERS WITH SPECIFIC CHEMICAL DEFECTS

True congenital dystrophies rarely occur, and they probably constitute a group of disorders rather than a single entity. Banker and associates[5] and others[35,60] demonstrated myopathic changes in the muscles of patients with the clinical diagnosis of arthrogryposis (p. 348). Gradually, new chemical disorders and morphologic abnormalities are being described in this group of patients. The reader should be reminded that most patients with congenital neuromuscular disorders which are apparent in infancy have progressive spinal muscular atrophy.

Glycogen Storage Diseases

PATHOGENESIS.—It is now known that at least six different forms of glycogen storage disease occur with separate and identifiable enzymatic defects (Table 19.1). Muscular manifestations appear primarily in Cori's Types 2 and 6 and to a lesser extent in Type 3. The nervous system can be damaged indirectly by the attacks of hypoglycemia and acidosis which occur in the hepatic types of glycogenosis, especially Cori's Type 1 or von Gierke's disease (Chapter 2). These rare metabolic disorders are all inherited as autosomal recessive traits and result from absence or deficiency of specific enzymes which are involved in the degradation of glycogen, as indicated in Table 19.1. Disease results from the abnormal deposition of glycogen in skeletal and cardiac muscle. In the cardiomuscular type (Cori's Type 2—glycogenosis), neurons from the cerebral cortex to the basal ganglia and the anterior horn cells may be distended with glycogen.

CLINICAL AND LABORATORY DIAGNOSIS.—The common clinical signs in the muscle glycogenoses are listed in Table 19.1.

Cardiomuscular glycogenosis.—Pompe's disease (Cori's Type 2), a rare disorder, produces symptoms and signs in early infancy which mimic closely more common conditions, such as infantile muscular atrophy, cretinism, mongolism and other causes of hypotonia[14] (Chapter 3). These babies appear retarded, fail to grow and have considerable feeding difficulty because of macroglossia, dysphagia and an absent gag reflex. Muscular hypotonia, drooling, cyanosis and dyspnea are seen commonly and seizures have been reported. Cardiomegaly occurs as a rule, and heart failure may cause death.[72] Hepatosplenomegaly rarely occurs. The diagnosis is established by muscle biopsy findings (and enzymatic assay).

Myophosphorylase deficiency.—The clinical findings in this disorder (McArdle's syndrome—Cori's Type 5), a rare but specific metabolic defect, have been reported in only a small number of patients. Episodes of painful weakness develop after muscular exertion. The symptoms usually begin in childhood.

Muscle biopsy reveals increased glycogen content. The deficiency in muscle phosphorylase can be demonstrated by the failure of venous blood lactate of patients to be elevated following strenuous exercise[28] (normally there is a brisk rise). Patients with this rare disorder also may have myoglobinuria at times.[48]

TABLE 19.1.—The Muscle Glycogenoses*

Cori Type	Enzyme Defect	Organs	Eponymic Name	Suggested Clinical Name	Clinical Manifestations
Muscle glycogen storage diseases					
2	1,4-Glucosidase (acid maltase)	Heart muscle (generalized)	Pompe's disease	Generalized glycogenosis or cardiomuscular glycogen storage disease	Hypotonia and feeding difficulty in infancy with growth failure, macroglossia, drooling, cyanosis and dyspnea, cardiomegaly (rarely hepatosplenomegaly) and heart failure, mental defect and seizures
3	Amylo-transglucosidase (debrancher)	Liver, heart muscle, leukocytes	Forke's disease	Limit dextrinosis	Symptoms similar to those of hepatorenal glycogenosis (Cori Type 1); in addition, muscular hypotonia is seen
5	Myophosphorylase	Skeletal muscle	McArdle's disease	Myophosphorylase deficiency	Periodic muscle pain, weakness and stiffness caused by exertion
	Phosphofructokinase	Muscle	Layzer-Rowland-Ranney	Muscle phosphofructokinase deficiency	Muscle pain and cramps after exertion
Other muscle glycogenoses					
1	Glucose-6-phosphatase	Liver, kidney	von Gierke's disease	Hepatorenal glycogenosis	
4	Amylo-transglucosidase (brancher)	Liver	Andersen's disease	Amylopectinosis	
6	Liver glycogen Phosphorylase	Liver, leukocytes	Hers' disease	Hepatophosphorylase deficiency	

*Modified from Field.[28]

Muscle phosphofructokinase deficiency.—Recently Layzer and associates[38b] described a patient with symptoms which were indistinguishable from those seen in muscle phosphorylase deficiency. In an excellent study they demonstrated an inherited deficiency in muscle phosphofructokinase.

MANAGEMENT AND PROGNOSIS.—No specific therapy has been developed for these rare disorders. In patients with myophosphorylase deficiency strenuous exercise should be avoided. Exercise tolerance is allegedly increased by taking glucose orally.

Since all of these disorders behave as recessive traits, they can be expected to cluster in sibships. Patients with cardiomuscular glycogenosis usually do not live beyond age 2. Nasogastric tube feedings circumvent the common feeding problems.

Familial Myoglobinuria

Nosologic confusion complicates a clear understanding of this disorder. In a detailed review of this rare condition, Rowland and associates[48] emphasize that "idiopathic myoglobinuria" represents a heterogeneous group of disorders. Jarcho and Adams[35b] state clearly that, in any disease which results in the rapid destruction of striated muscle fibers, myoglobin and other muscle proteins may enter the blood stream and appear in the urine. Myoglobinuria has been seen, for example, in a patient with lateralized status epilepticus and ipsilateral rhabdomyolysis,[17] as well as in states of muscle exertion.[33a] The pigment imparts a dark red color to the urine.

PATHOGENESIS.—Familial myoglobinuria has been reported repeatedly. It may or may not be associated with pathologic changes in the skeletal muscles. The histologic findings differ, but they usually show muscle fibers in varying stages of degeneration.

CLINICAL AND LABORATORY DIAGNOSIS.—Attacks of painful muscle weakness, stiffness and tenderness are usually precipitated by strenuous exercise. The excessive myoglobin in the urine may be precipitated in the renal tubules, causing acute renal failure and anuria. Pigmenturia (a dark red or wine-colored urine) follows within 24-48 hours. In general the urinary pigment can be identified as myoglobin by virtue of a positive urine guaiac test in the absence of erythrocytes. The differentiation of myoglobinuria from hemoglobinuria and porphyria and the positive spectroscopic identification of myoglobin have been outlined by Rowland *et al*.[48] Fatalities may occur in the acute stage of the illness.

MANAGEMENT AND PROGNOSIS.—In general, strenuous exercise must be avoided to prevent attacks. Acute episodes are treated by complete rest. Some workers have advocated sodium bicarbonate orally to lessen the risk of renal damage. However, alkalinization of the urine must be carried out carefully, because administration of excessive sodium to the anuric patient may complicate the problem by causing fluid retention. Usually attacks subside spontaneously but recurrent episodes over a lifetime can be expected. The inheritance pattern of this familial disorder has not been clearly defined.

HEREDITARY MYOPATHIES WITH DISTINCTIVE STRUCTURAL DEFECTS

During the past 10 years siblings with clinical evidence of muscle disease and unusual microscopic changes in muscle have been described by Shy and his co-workers and other workers.[34,51,52] Patients with nonprogressive, benign myopathies have exhibited *central core disease* and *nemaline myopathy*.[27] More recently enlarged mitochondria (*megaconial myopathy*) and abnormally numerous mitochondria (*pleoconial myopathy*) have been demonstrated in the electron microscopic study of muscle in siblings with clinical signs of myopathy.[15,45,50,53] Another clinically similar type of slowly progressive myopathy characterized by centrally placed nuclei in most muscle fibers has been described (*familial centronuclear myopathy* or *myotubular myopathy*).[35c,49a]

These provocative findings heighten interest in the puzzling group of children in whom the etiology of hypotonia and weakness has remained obscure. What the ultimate significance of these morphologic changes will be in terms of pathogenesis and disease specificity remains to be demonstrated. As more reports and observations accumulate, it becomes increasingly apparent that these morphologic changes may not have specificity for separate myopathic diseases.[3,15,26,32,54] We would like to re-emphasize that the conditions listed above are not discussed in the usual fashion under Pathogenesis, Diagnosis and Management because their identity as diseases has not yet been proved.

Nonhereditary Myopathies

Myopathies which are secondary to endocrinopathies (such as hypothyroidism, Cushing's disease and prolonged glucocorticoid therapy) are so uncommon in children that the reader is referred to the text of Adams, Denny-Brown and Pearson[1] for a complete discussion.

Neurogenic Muscular Atrophies

Much has been written about the hypotonic, "limp" or "floppy" child. The nomenclature is unnecessarily confusing. The reader is referred to Chapter 3 where an attempt has been made to present the common symptoms, signs and differential diagnosis of this syndrome. In this section, only the muscular atrophies which result from specific diseases of the lower motor neuron are discussed.

Infantile Spinal Muscular Atrophy (Werdnig-Hoffmann)

PATHOGENESIS.—This inherited disorder of early infancy often affects several children in a family because it is transmitted as an autosomal recessive trait.[9] The basic morphologic defect is seen in the degeneration of the anterior horn cells of the spinal cord and brain stem. These cells are reduced in number and the remaining cells show degenerative changes. Distinctive pathologic changes in the muscle are seen, the most outstanding finding being great variation in the size of muscle fibers. Most of the fibers are very small with preservation of both longitudinal and cross striations, whereas others are of normal size or very large, presumably as a result of compensatory hypertrophy. Fat and fibrous connective tissue infiltrate the muscle in moderate amounts (Fig. 19.3,*C*) without any cellular infiltrate. If an underlying biochemical anomaly exists, its nature is not understood.

The nomenclature which has been employed to classify spinal muscular atrophy of infancy has created considerable confusion, not only because of different eponyms (Werdnig-Hoffmann and Oppenheim), but because neurologists have not always agreed whether the syndrome represented different diseases or whether it represented a single disease of differing clinical severity. We support the view, until further basic metabolic evidence is documented, that most cases represent infantile spinal muscular atrophy, and that a small group of weak, atrophic and areflexic

Fig. 19.3.—Infantile spinal muscular atrophy (Werdnig-Hoffmann). **A**, boy, 9, was considered normal until 8 months of age when the family noted slow motor development. At the time of a traumatic leg fracture at age 1 the poorly developed muscles were noted and biopsied. Over the next eight years the child has been increasingly incapacitated by muscle weakness, atrophy and recurrent pneumonia. He has no elicitable deep tendon reflexes. No other neurologic deficit is present. Tracheostomy was required for treatment of a recent episode of pneumonia (**A**).

B, x-rays of extremities of a baby girl whose family noted paucity of leg movements at 4½ months of age. Examination showed a fat but floppy baby who was diffusely weak, hypotonic and areflexic. No other general or neurologic abnormalities were noted. Films show greatly diminished muscle mass with some evidence of fatty infiltration. Note the associated bone atrophy (from inactivity) and the discrepancy between total amount of soft tissue and muscle bulk itself, findings typical of infantile muscular atrophy. **C** shows the typical abnormal histologic features, i.e., bundles of normal-appearing muscle fibers (center of field) and small, atrophic, poorly staining fibers in the upper field (longitudinal section) and lower field (cross-section).

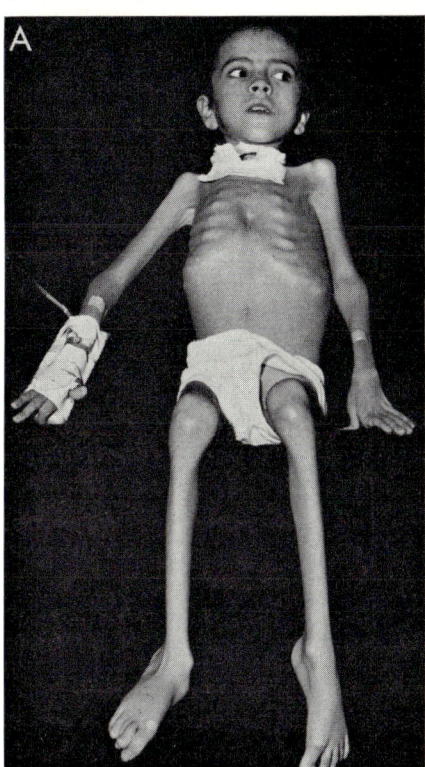

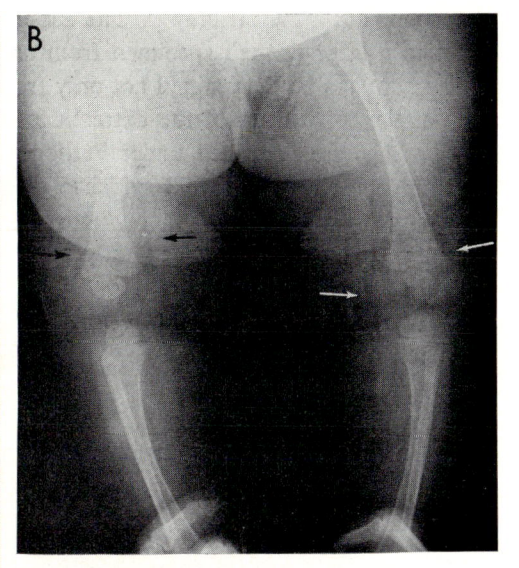

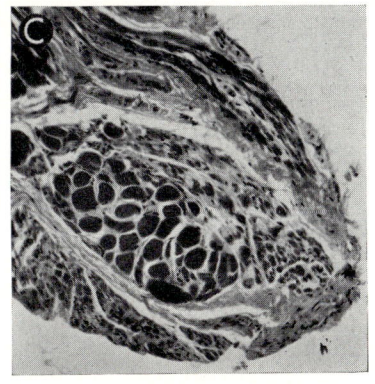

infants may be placed in a clinical group of varied etiology sometimes called "amyotonia congenita"[8] (Chapter 3).

CLINICAL AND LABORATORY DIAGNOSIS.—The most prominent symptoms—hypotonia, weakness and areflexia—are usually obvious in the early weeks or months of life (one-third of Brandt's 112 cases were congenital[10]), but at times they are not noticed until the child fails to achieve the expected motor milestones of sitting, standing and walking. The marked hypotonia gives rise to extreme hyperextensibility of joints. The severe muscle atrophy is often overlooked at first, since the child appears deceptively well nourished because of a large accumulation of subcutaneous fat. All muscle groups in the trunk and extremities are involved initially, whereas the diaphragm and muscles above the neck are spared until the terminal phase of the illness (Fig. 19.3,*A*). The exclusively diaphragmatic breathing causes "seesaw" respiratory movements and a weak cry and cough, the latter leading to frequent bouts of pneumonia. In the late stages of the illness the tongue may show fasciculations and atrophy, fasciculations in the other muscles being hidden by subcutaneous fat. In nearly all patients the deep tendon reflexes are absent. If they are present, one must consider other diagnoses seriously. Few other bulbar muscles are involved, and no sensory or intellectual deficit is found.

The diagnosis of this disorder can be established with the greatest certainty by carrying out a muscle biopsy. One should be sure that the surgeon is instructed to obtain a large enough specimen from an involved muscle. The sites of muscle involvement can be determined not only from the clinical examination but from an x-ray of the soft tissues of the extremities (Fig. 19.3,*B*). The pathognomonic biopsy findings are described under Pathogenesis and are shown in Figure 19.3,*C*. Electromyography may reveal evidence of denervation, and nerve conduction velocity studies reveal delayed conduction times. Cerebrospinal fluid examination gives normal results. One must study each case fully because no single diagnostic method can be considered foolproof. For example, Drachman and associates[21] recently pointed out that typical "myopathic" changes were seen on muscle biopsy in a small number of patients who were afflicted with chronic denervation or neurogenic muscular atrophy.

The differential diagnosis includes all of the disorders which can cause the syndrome of the "limp infant" or the "floppy baby" (Chapter 3). One must remain alert to the possibility of infectious polyneuritis when diffuse flaccid weakness develops in infants who were previously well. A significantly elevated CSF protein level can be expected at some time in the course of polyneuritis but does not appear in patients with spinal muscular atrophy.

MANAGEMENT AND PROGNOSIS.—Therapy for this progressive disorder is directed at the maintenance of good general health and the prevention and treatment of respiratory tract infections. Physical therapy may have some supportive value, and orthopedic appliances may facilitate walking in children whose symptoms have a late onset. The prognosis of this pathetic disorder is poor. In one of the largest reported series[10a] it was noted that 50% of children die within a year of onset and 80% within four years. Rarely patients live to early adult life in a markedly disabled state. In general, the earlier the onset of symptoms the shorter the life span.

Parents must be alerted to the rather high recurrence risk of this *recessive* disorder in any subsequent children.

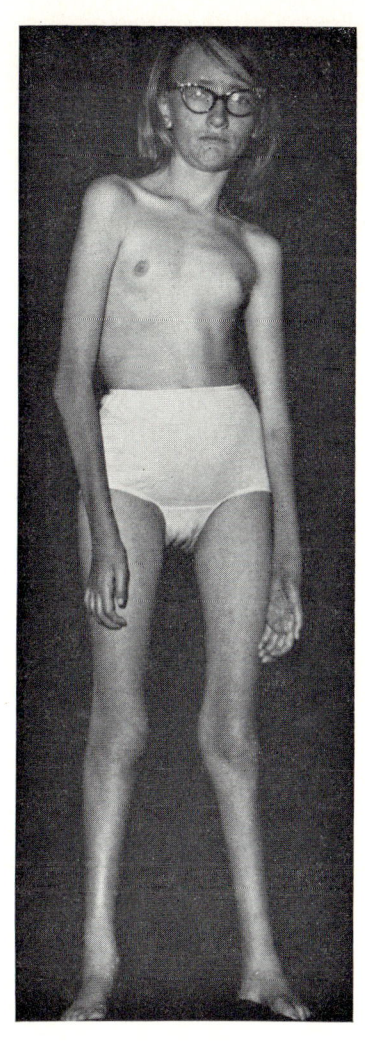

Fig. 19.4.—Progressive neural muscular atrophy (Charcot-Marie-Tooth). Girl, 14, did not walk until age 2½ and had impaired use of her hands since infancy. Examination showed bilateral foot drop, marked limitation of hand use and severe distal atrophy in all four extremities. She has been areflexic and has shown progressive loss of deep sensation over the past six years. Muscle biopsy revealed typical evidence of neural atrophy (see Fig. 19.3,*C*; compare normal fibers below to the atrophic ones above). These findings are diagnostic of Charcot-Marie-Tooth disease. She died at age 15.

Progressive Neural Muscular Atrophy (Charcot-Marie-Tooth)

PATHOGENESIS.—This uncommon familial disorder is characterized by slowly progressive neural muscular atrophy. It is inherited usually as an autosomal dominant trait. Although the basic etiology is totally unknown, it resembles a peripheral neuritis pathologically, except that the changes in the spinal cord resemble those found in some cases of spinocerebellar degeneration. Degenerative axonal changes and demyelination of the distal nerves of the extremities are the most prominent findings, but degeneration of nerve roots, anterior horn cells and posterior columns also occurs. The histopathologic changes in muscle resemble those seen in any type of neural atrophy. One sees both small and large muscle fibers and infiltration of muscle with fat.

CLINICAL AND LABORATORY DIAGNOSIS.—Symptoms and signs usually have their onset between ages 5 and 15 with insidious weakness and wasting of the distal lower extremities (Fig. 19.4). Cramping pains and paresthesias occur commonly, but sensory loss is slight and usually involves deep sensation (vibration and position sense) in late stages of the illness. Muscle atrophy is usually symmetrical and nearly always leads to foot drop and pes cavus deformity. Eventually the muscle atrophy below the knees becomes severe and produces a "stork-leg" deformity, and later the distal third of the thigh atrophies to the point of causing an "inverted champagne bottle" appearance. Despite the common name for the disorder, *peroneal muscular atrophy,* the atrophy is almost never limited to the peroneal muscles, but instead involves the intrinsic muscles of the hands and forearms, producing claw-hand deformities. The face, trunk and proximal limb muscles escape the atrophic process almost completely. The distal deep tendon reflexes, especially the ankle and knee jerks, disappear and the plantar reponses are silent. The mental state, cerebellar function and sphincter control are unaffected except for those variants described below.

Muscle biopsy reveals evidence of neural muscular atrophy (see Pathogenesis and Fig. 19.3,*C*), and conduction velocity studies show slowing of motor nerve conduction rates. Cerebrospinal fluid is normal except for occasional slight elevation of total protein content.

Variants of this disorder which exhibit scoliosis, optic atrophy, retinitis pigmentosa, ataxia and even corticospinal tract signs are impossible to distinguish at times from some of the hereditary cerebellar ataxias (see Friedreich's and Lévy-Roussy ataxias, Chapter 21). Myotonic dystrophy may also resemble peroneal muscular atrophy because of the predominantly distal wasting. However, in myotonic dystrophy weakness of the facial and neck muscles and a myotonic response are distinctive. Hypertrophic interstitial neuritis (Déjerine-Sottas) is differentiated by the palpably thickened peripheral nerves. All other types of peripheral neuropathy must be differentiated in the early stages of this disease, but this is usually not difficult if one remembers the inheritance pattern, the symmetrical distal wasting, the deformities and the mild posterior column sensory loss in progressive neural atrophy. The differential diagnosis of chronic polyneuropathy in childhood has been reviewed by Byers and Taft.[11a]

MANAGEMENT AND PROGNOSIS.—Although no specific therapy is available, orthopedic appliances will keep the patient ambulant for long periods. The decision to carry out operative procedures, especially for the correction of a foot drop, must be made and timed carefully to avoid an actual increase in the patient's functional disability. We have seen arthrodeses performed on several patients with an unstable gait, only to have the patient confined permanently thereafter to a wheelchair. Although these patients would probably have reached this plight eventually regardless of the management, they tend to fix the blame on the operative procedure.

Parents must be warned about the high risk of passing this dominant trait on to one or more children. Fortunately the disease is slow in its progression and may not shorten life or disable the patient seriously.

Juvenile Proximal Spinal Muscular Atrophy (Kugelberg-Welander)[38]

PATHOGENESIS.—This uncommon hereditary neuropathy bears a close clinical resemblance to childhood dystrophy (Duchenne)[24] and a close pathologic and genetic likeness to infantile muscular atrophy (Werdnig-Hoffmann). The disorder behaves usually as an autosomal recessive but occasionally as a dominant trait and consists of anterior horn cell and motor fiber degeneration.[3a,59]

In the absence of more precise etiologic information it is obviously difficult to separate this entity from slowly progressive cases of infantile muscular atrophy. For the present it seems reasonable to consider it separately.

CLINICAL AND LABORATORY DIAGNOSIS.—Weakness of the proximal leg muscles (the large muscles of the buttocks and thighs) with loss of knee jerks is seen first, followed by atrophy and weakness of the upper arm muscles. The face and neck muscles are not affected but the more distal limb muscles are involved later in the course. Signs and symptoms may appear in early childhood (as in dystrophy) or in adolescence.

Muscle biopsy and diagnostic electrical studies (electromyography and conduction velocity) establish the neurogenic basis of the disease and distinguish it from dystrophy and other types of muscular weakness in childhood.

MANAGEMENT AND PROGNOSIS.—The importance of considering this disorder as an entity apart from dystrophy lies in the fact that affected patients have a normal life expectancy.[31] Hence, the prognosis differs greatly from that of dystrophy. Treatment is symptomatic (Chapter 3).

Hereditary Spastic Paraplegia (Juvenile Amyotrophic Lateral Sclerosis)

PATHOGENESIS.—This familial form of spastic paraplegia can be inherited in a variety of patterns, dominant or recessive, sex-linked or autosomal. Byers and Banker[11] consider hereditary spastic paraplegia (with amyotrophy) the same disease as juvenile amyotrophic lateral sclerosis.[33] It seems likely that amyotrophic lateral sclerosis in childhood and in adult life are different disorders. However, one can sometimes elicit a positive family history for motor neuron disease even when symptoms begin in adult life, and Kurland[38a] considers it generally a dominantly inherited disease with incomplete penetrance. The overlap between classical amyotrophic lateral sclerosis and the various forms of spinal muscular atrophy has been reviewed recently by Pearce and Harriman[44] and a new classification proposed based upon the hereditary and nonhereditary nature of the various clinical syndromes. Although the number of reported pathologic studies is limited, one usually sees severe degeneration of (1) the anterior horn cells in the spinal cord, (2) the motor nuclei of the brain stem and (3) the Betz cells in the motor cortex, with secondary degeneration of the corticospinal and corticobulbar tracts. The pathologic changes in the muscle vary according to the stage of the disease at the time of biopsy, but they closely resemble those seen in other types of spinal or neural muscular atrophy. Unless the case represents a variant of another type of spinocerebellar ataxia (Chapter 21), other portions of the cord and brain are normal.

Whatever point of view one adopts about the classification of these disorders, he must do it arbitrarily because the total lack of precise etiologic information in both age groups makes dogmatic statements impossible.

CLINICAL AND LABORATORY DIAGNOSIS.—Signs and symptoms may appear at any age, but most cases are recognized in infancy or early childhood. Limited movement or delayed walking may be noted in infancy. Examination reveals spasticity of the lower extremities with scissoring of the legs, hyperreflexia, ankle clonus and extensor plantar responses (Fig. 19.5). Weakness is obvious and disuse atrophy becomes increasingly severe as the patient grows older. In a review of the literature Byers and Banker[11] found no patients with childhood amyotrophic lateral sclerosis in whom spasticity, hyperreflexia and Babinski signs did not appear as the initial signs. No sensory defect, sphincter difficulty or abnormal laboratory findings are present in this disorder.

Differential diagnosis must include intramedullary spinal cord disease, including multiple sclerosis, and the causes of spinal cord compression, including tumor and spondylitis. The age of onset, the unremitting progressive nature of the signs, normal sensory examination, the family history and the absence of spinal subarachnoid block should serve to exclude other diagnoses.

MANAGEMENT AND PROGNOSIS.—Despite the lack of specific therapy, patients can be helped greatly by orthopedic appliances such as braces and crutches and by corrective surgery, including tendon-lengthening and muscle-releasing procedures similar to those for congenital cerebral palsy (Chapter 3). The course of the disease varies greatly, but continued medical attention often contributes to a useful life with a near-normal life expectancy. A gradually progressive downhill

Fig. 19.5.—Hereditary spastic paraplegia. A, this 19-year-old woman has a history of slow motor development in infancy (she did not walk until 22 months) and a remote past history of seizures treated with phenobarbital. She has always walked with crutches and has had multiple orthopedic procedures to relieve the spasticity and joint deformities in the legs. B shows her 5½-year-old son. He appeared normal until 1 year of age, when slow motor development was linked to marked hyperreflexia and spasticity of the thigh abductors which were causing scissoring of gait.

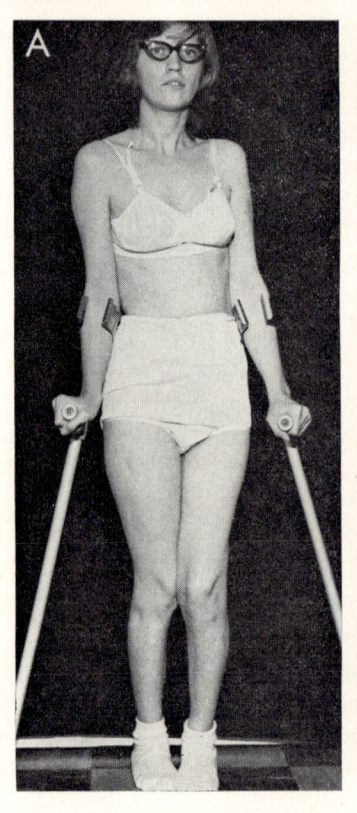

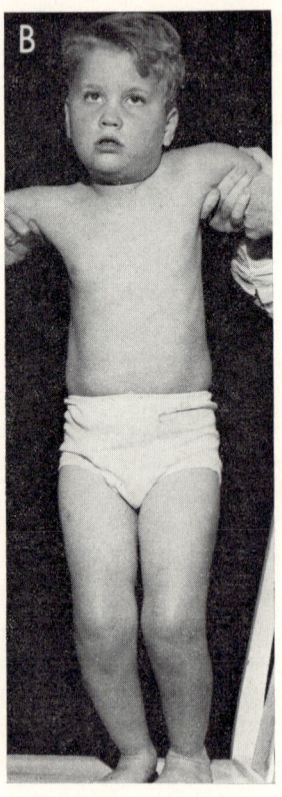

course is seen in some patients, with death resulting from intercurrent infection. However, many individuals appear to have a static deficit.

The risk of recurrence in siblings and descendants is sufficient to warrant careful counseling.

Myositis of Unknown Etiology

These uncommon myositides are poorly understood in terms of etiology and pathogenesis. They are generally grouped according to (1) their cardinal clinical and pathologic manifestations (i.e., dermatomyositis, polymyositis) and (2) the evidence of associated systemic disease (e.g., dermatomyositis or polymyositis secondary to generalized connective tissue diseases such as rheumatoid arthritis and rheumatic fever, systemic lupus erythematosus, polyneuritis, scleroderma). A brief description of myositis ossificans is also given.

Dermatomyositis and Polymyositis

PATHOGENESIS.—These uncommon disorders of unknown etiology must be separated primarily upon the basis of the tissues which are involved. In *dermatomyositis,* the most common of the myositides in childhood, the skeletal muscle and skin reflect the inflammatory process. This clinical-pathologic entity is detailed in the description of eight children with the disorder by Banker and Victor.[4] In *polymyositis* only the skeletal muscles are affected; if other connective tissues are involved, the combined term is used, viz., collagen vascular disease (e.g., rheumatoid arthritis) with dermatomyositis. The etiology of all these conditions is unknown. No infectious agent has been incriminated, nor has a single hypersensitivity or metabolic cause been found. An impressive association between dermatomyositis and malignant disease has been noted in adults but not in children. It seems probable that different basic causes (viral infections, hypersensitivity reactions to infectious illnesses, drugs, neoplastic disease and obscure metabolic disorders) may give rise to similar inflammatory reactions in skin, muscle and connective tissue.

Pathologically one finds *constant degeneration or necrosis of muscle fibers with an inconstant inflammatory cell infiltrate* in the muscle or skin.

CLINICAL AND LABORATORY DIAGNOSIS.—*Dermatomyositis; acute polymyositis.*—This rare disorder is quite evenly distributed from early childhood to old age. It has an insidious onset. Skin lesions may precede or follow the onset of muscle symptoms. A pink, maculopapular eruption is found on or around the eyelids (Fig. 19.6,*A*), the face, the upper trunk and the backs of the hands. The skin may become indurated and darkly pigmented, similar to the changes seen in scleroderma. Periorbital edema occurs commonly.

Muscle symptoms in both dermatomyositis and acute polymyositis usually begin with painful, symmetrical weakness of the proximal limbs and are noted when reaching above the head, combing the hair, climbing stairs or arising from a squatting position. Importantly, about half the patients have dysphagia. Eventually there is weakness of the facial, neck and jaw muscles, but ocular weakness is rarely seen. Muscular pain and tenderness may develop, but this sign is inconstant. The deep tendon reflexes become diminished or absent as the disease progresses. Low-grade fever occurs at times, as do lymphadenopathy and hepatospleno-

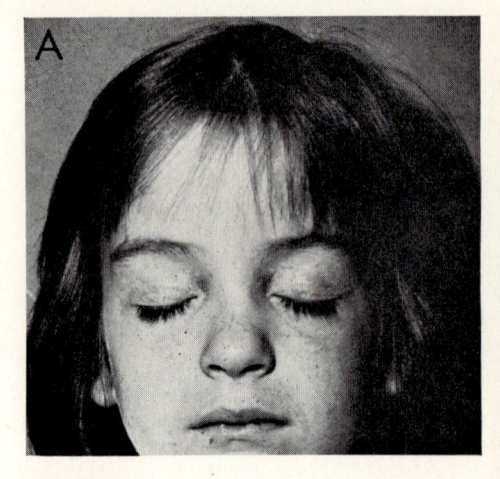

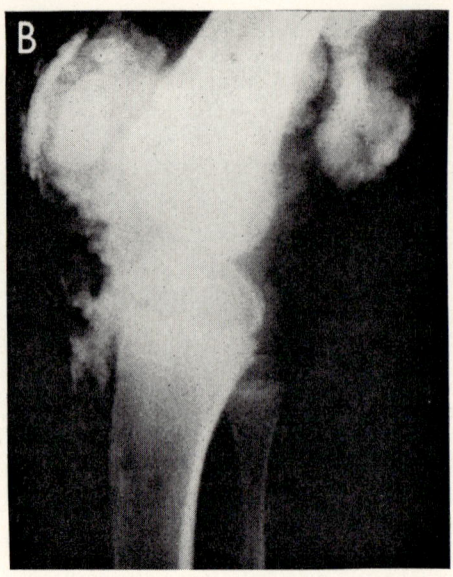

Fig. 19.6.—Dermatomyositis. **A,** this girl exhibits a prominent pink macular rash over the eyelids, a favorite site for the eruption. The extensive subcutaneous calcifications seen in the chronic stages of this disease are shown in **B.**

megaly, but the absence of these systemic signs does not preclude the diagnosis. In severe cases muscle atrophy, areflexia, fibrosis and contractures may develop. Widespread subcutaneous calcinosis occurs in chronic cases (Fig. 19.6,*B*). Involvement of pharyngeal and/or the respiratory muscles carries a grave prognosis.

Widespread gastrointestinal ulceration leads commonly to symptoms of abdominal pain, hematemesis and melena. Death is said to occur almost invariably as a result of a perforated viscus with subsequent peritonitis or mediastinitis.[4] When one suspects the diagnosis, a thorough study should be undertaken to rule out all of the collagen vascular diseases.

Chronic polymyositis.—This disorder has an even more insidious onset and may be difficult to distinguish from polyneuritis and a rapidly advancing dystrophy. Adults are affected more often than children. The patient may complain first of malaise and easy tiring. Later the proximal limb muscles become tender and weak and eventually there is diffuse muscle involvement. As a rule these patients do not have oropharyngeal weakness. Pseudohypertrophy may occur, and the major weakness and atrophy may be located distally. After a protracted course the patient may become incapacitated by the wasting and contractures. Calcification in muscles may be seen. Gradual loss of deep tendon reflexes occurs but no true sensory deficit is expected. In advanced stages a diagnostic differentiation from a chronic polyneuropathy or dystrophy may be difficult.

The diagnosis of polymyositis may present no problem if the clinical features and the biopsy findings are typical. However, in the acute form the muscle biopsy is sometimes nondiagnostic because of the limited extent of the disease, and in the chronic form the biopsy findings may be indistinguishable from those in dystrophy. In the latter situation, if there is no family history of muscle disease, definitive diagnosis may be impossible. In any case, the diagnosis is essentially a clinical one and the laboratory studies, except for muscle biopsy, are nonspecific or unreliable.

MANAGEMENT AND PROGNOSIS.—None of the therapeutic programs produces dependably predictable benefit. However, Tyler and Adams[62] recommend (1) aspirin every four hours during the day (this agent must be used with caution in children to prevent intoxication), (2) prednisone in a dose of 1 mg./lb./day for one month, with very gradual tapering of the dose over weeks or months and (3) physiotherapy consisting of gentle massage, passive movement and resistance exercises as signs of the disease subside. The pathologic changes in the acute form of polymyositis resemble experimentally produced viral infections, vitamin E deficiency and intoxication with the antimalarial plasmocid. This has led to the clinical trial of vitamin E and antibiotics but without appreciable benefit.

In dermatomyositis or the acute form of polymyositis patients often recover after a prolonged stationary period. However, one-third to one-half the patients have died, in many instances as a consequence of pharyngeal and respiratory muscle weakness.[7a,46] A relatively small percentage recover completely, most being left with residual atrophy and contractures. Bitnum and co-workers[7a] reviewed the literature and their experience with 13 cases. They concluded that current therapy has not improved the prognosis significantly but point out that prednisone therapy sometimes offers dramatic benefit in the acute stage. They also conclude that one-third of the patients recover completely, one-third die and one-third survive with contractures and deformities.

Chronic polymyositis runs a more protracted course and has a lower mortality rate.

Other Rare Forms of Myositis

Collagen vascular diseases.—In patients with a variety of connective tissue disorders (rheumatoid arthritis, rheumatic fever, systemic lupus erythematosus, polyarteritis and scleroderma), clinical and pathologic signs of myositis may develop. Adams, Denny-Brown and Pearson[1] have emphasized that all of these disorders cause an interstitial, nodular or miliary inflammatory reaction in skeletal muscle. This finding differs from those seen in dermatomyositis or polymyositis, but the interstitial myositis is not an aid in distinguishing one type of collagen vascular disease from another.

The reader is referred to other reference sources for a discussion of the differential diagnosis and management of the various collagen vascular diseases.[70]

Myositis ossificans.—This rare disorder of childhood is characterized by the progressive deposition of fibrous tissue and calcium in the muscles, tendons and ligaments. In 75% of the patients other congenital anomalies have been found, including microdactyly (especially of the thumbs and great toes), joint contractures, syndactyly, deformed ears and spina bifida. Biopsy material from muscle shows proliferation of connective tissue with degeneration of muscle and transformation into bone. Little or no inflammatory cell reaction is seen. The disorder may be familial.

Symptoms and signs often are noted in early childhood. Firm masses in the soft tissue of the neck, back or shoulders are noted, often after an injury, although trauma is not considered significant in this disorder.[65] The painless lumps eventually ossify, and the overlying soft tissue may ulcerate and discharge chalky material. As the disease progresses, ankylosis of joints occurs and the patient is increasingly incapacitated. This disorder must be distinguished from other syndromes of multiple congenital anomalies and other arthropathies, such as rheumatoid arthritis, rheumatic fever, localized traumatic ossifying myositis and multiple exostoses.

Only supportive therapy has value. Death may supervene from intercurrent pulmonary infection in early adult life. As mentioned above, the disorder may be familial but the mode of inheritance has not been defined.

Myositis of Known Etiology

Bacterial Myositis

Pyogenic infections of skeletal muscle behave clinically like other purulent, soft-tissue infections. They respond to treatment in the same way and hence do not merit any more detailed discussion in this text. *Gas gangrene* infections (infections with Clostridium welchii) develop in contaminated, traumatized, deep puncture wounds where anaerobic growth conditions prevail. The rapidly destructive myositis is associated with swelling, crepitus (gas bubble formation in the soft tissues) and edema.

The incubation period varies from a few days to several weeks. In gas gangrene the rapidly destructive myositis is associated with swelling, discoloration of the skin, crepitus and severe signs of systemic infection.

The organism can usually be recovered from a wound culture. However, the symptoms and signs are usually sufficiently typical to make a presumptive diagnosis on clinical grounds without awaiting a culture report. When the diagnosis of gas gangrene is made clinically, therapy should be started immediately. Prompt and radical surgical intervention should be carried out to provide drainage and wound aeration and to obviate further tissue necrosis. Intravenous penicillin should be given promptly in the daily dose of 10,000,000–20,000,000 units. It is recommended that 100,000 units of polyvalent gas gangrene antitoxin be given intravenously as an initial dose, followed by 50,000 units every four to six hours. Intensive supportive therapy with blood, electrolytes and maintenance fluids should be provided to combat shock, dehydration and anemia.

Viral Myositis

Epidemic pleurodynia or the devil's grip (Bornholm) represents the most common type of viral myositis. Various members of the group B Coxsackie viruses are commonly the agents, although in some cases group A microorganisms are implicated. Presumably an inflammatory process of muscle (diaphragm and intercostals), the basic pathologic process is not understood because the disease is self-limited and no reliable studies have been reported.

Patients may be any age, but children and young adults are most commonly affected and often in epidemics. There may be symptoms of a common cold followed by the sudden onset of severe chest pain. The pain is located at the costal margins, substernally or often in the interscapular area, and is aggravated by breathing, coughing and sneezing. Mild muscle tenderness may occur, and the patient may complain of hyperesthesia of the overlying skin. Systemic symptoms of acute infection are common, and signs of a friction rub may be noted. Aseptic meningitis may accompany the illness.

Coxsackie B viruses can be recovered from body fluids, but definitive diagnosis depends upon the demonstration of a rise in titer of neutralizing or complement-fixing antibodies. When aseptic meningitis occurs concomitantly, a lymphocytic CSF pleocytosis can be found.

Treatment of this self-limited disease is purely symptomatic. Aspirin, codeine and morphine provide relief when pain is disabling. The disease usually runs its course in four to seven days.

Parasitic Myositis: Trichinosis

This disease is caused when pork contaminated with the nematode Trichinella spiralis is ingested. After fertilization, the female burrows into the intestinal wall and later discharges larvae into the blood stream. The larvae become encysted only in skeletal muscle, despite their widespread distribution in the body. The muscles of the diaphragm, the eye, the tongue, the deltoid, pectoral and intercostals are affected most commonly.

Initially a gastroenteritis develops within 24 hours after the ingestion of the contaminated meat. Over the next six weeks symptoms of a myositis appear—fever, edema of the eyelids and conjunctivae, muscle pain and tenderness. The diagnosis is aided by the presence of an eosinophilic leukocytosis (15–50% eosinophils) and positive skin test results to the trichina antigen (a 5 mm. wheal develops within 30 minutes after the intradermal injection of 0.01 ml. of 1:10,000 antigen).

Management includes rest, good nutrition and pain relief. Piperazine citrate therapy (as prescribed for pinworm infestations) is recommended if the patient has symptoms of a gastroenteritis after eating poorly cooked pork.

Generally the prognosis is good, but fatalities can occur in severe, high-dose infestations. The epidemiologic importance of this inflammation in the United States is slight. The disease can be prevented if pork is cooked adequately or if it is frozen to -15 C. for 20 days or to -18 C. for 24 hours.

Miscellaneous

The rarity of other microbial and parasitic myositides of known etiology (actinomycosis, cysticercosis, echinococcosis, sarcosporidiosis, toxoplasmosis and trypanosomiasis) places them beyond the scope of this text. The reader is referred to the excellent monograph by Adams, Denny-Brown and Pearson[1] for detailed information on these other infections and infestations of muscle.

Nonhereditary Disorders of Neuromuscular Transmission

Myasthenia Gravis

This disorder causes weakness and easy fatigability of any skeletal muscle, but ocular and bulbar muscles are affected most prominently. Although the disease is uncommon in children, its early recognition and proper management may be life-saving. In childhood the disease occurs at any time, including the neonatal period.[42,43]

PATHOGENESIS.—For many years study of the disease mechanism was devoted almost exclusively to a search for a biochemical or physiologic defect at the neuromyal junction. This preoccupation resulted from the fact that the symptoms of myasthenia gravis resembled those following administration of the drug curare, and the fact that the weakness was corrected partially by giving the anticholinesterases physostigmine or neostigmine (Prostigmin). Subsequently several etiologic hypotheses were considered: (1) a deficiency or inadequate production of acetylcholine, (2) an excess of cholinesterase which destroys acetylcholine, (3) the existence of some other substance with a curare-like action. However, a variety of factors suggested that an acetylcholine-cholinesterase defect at the motor end-plate did not explain the whole problem: (1) Prostigmin and other anticholinesterase or cholinergic drugs produce only minimal benefit in many patients; (2) the patient may enter remissions spontaneously, and (3) the patient who recovers has no sign of neurogenic muscular atrophy.

More recently a possible pathogenic relationship between the thymus gland and myasthenia gravis has been suggested. This association is supported in Schwab's experience[49] which disclosed an 85% incidence of thymus gland abnormalities in patients with myasthenia gravis. About 18% of the patients had thymomas and the rest showed hyperplasia or immature lymphoid follicles.

Recently a number of workers demonstrated elevated levels of circulating antibodies to normal tissues (muscle, thyroid and thymus), raising the possibility that the disease may be an autoimmune disorder.[2,6,56,66] Conceivably, antibodies which are produced, stimulated or controlled by the thymus may in some way interfere with normal end-plate function.

All of these observations are extremely provocative, but the exact pathogenesis of this disorder remains tantalizingly obscure.

CLINICAL AND LABORATORY DIAGNOSIS.—*Juvenile myasthenia gravis.*—Symptoms have their onset in middle childhood and affect girls more often than boys. Diplopia, bilateral lid ptosis and easy fatigability often develop, and a change is noted in facial expression, smile and quality of voice. The face is relatively immobile, and the smile looks like a snarl because the lips can be elevated but cannot be retracted. Many patients have cyclical variations in the severity of weakness during a 24-hour period, often feeling strong after a night's sleep but having symptoms worsen late in the day. Such regular variations in strength must be considered when recommending the time to administer an anticholinesterase drug. In exacerbations or progression of the disease bulbar and respiratory muscle weakness can be life-threatening. Environmental factors such as emotional stress, respiratory infections, lack of sleep and menstruation can accentuate the symptoms. Pregnancy has a variable effect upon the course of the disease.

Traditionally, patients with myasthenia show no consistent histologic abnormalities in the muscles except for the inconstant collections of lymphocytes ("lymphorrhages"). However, exceptional patients show atrophic changes (from disuse), and a few exhibit muscle abnormalities which resemble those of dystrophy or polymyositis.[47]

Diagnostic signs of easy muscle fatigability can be demonstrated easily by having the patient sustain upward gaze for a minute or two. Generally this will cause ptosis and even diplopia (Fig. 19.7,*A*). The diagnosis can be confirmed by the intramuscular injection of neostigmine (Prostigmin) or the intravenous injection of edrophonium hydrochloride (Tensilon). Tensilon has become the more popular diagnostic agent because its effect reaches a peak within a minute after injection and any cholinergic side effects disappear within a few minutes. A dose of 1 mg. (0.1 cc.) Tensilon is given intravenously to children under 75 lb. and 2 mg. (0.2 cc.) to those above 75 lb. as an initial test dose. If no benefit occurs, the child under 75 lb. should be given an additional 4 mg. (0.4 cc.) and the older child or adult 8 mg. (0.8 cc.). In a patient receiving therapy for myasthenia gravis one should never give more than 2 mg. (0.2 cc.) (see Management). An intramuscular Prostigmin test may be carried out if Tensilon is unavailable. This test is often used in newborns.

An EMG study of myasthenics often reveals the Jolly reaction. A series of high-frequency, repetitive (200–500/sec.) stimuli causes an initial high-amplitude muscular response followed by a series of muscle contractions of rapidly diminishing amplitude (Fig. 19.7,*B* and *C*). All patients should have laminograms of the chest made to evaluate the size of the thymus and to search for a thymic tumor.

Neonatal myasthenia gravis.—This must be considered in any feeble, weak,

Fig. 19.7.—Juvenile myasthenia gravis. In girl, age 11, periodic generalized muscular weakness gradually developed, along with occasional dysphagia, dysarthria and diplopia. Though the weakness was usually a little worse in late afternoon, she had to keep an anticholinesterase drug (Prostigmin or Mestinon) at her bedside so she could take it before getting out of bed in the morning. Symptoms were greatly exacerbated by any respiratory infection and by emotional stress. **A**, sustained upward gaze for about 60 seconds caused ptosis, eye muscle imbalance and diplopia. Intravenous administration of Tensilon brought about abrupt, temporary relief of weakness at the outset of the illness. EMG studies revealed findings pathognomonic of myasthenia gravis. In **B**, the nerve to a muscle is stimulated electrically by a rhythmic series of shocks; a progressive failure in the muscle's response occurs (myasthenic reaction). In **C**, the "Jolly reaction" is demonstrated: a high-frequency, tetanic electrical stimulus causes a strong initial twitch followed by progressively smaller contractions.

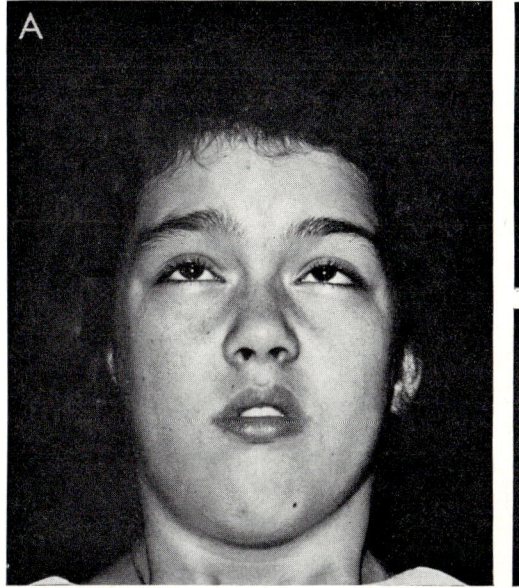

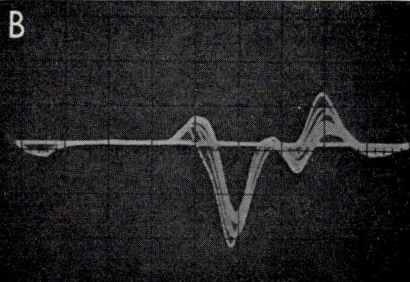

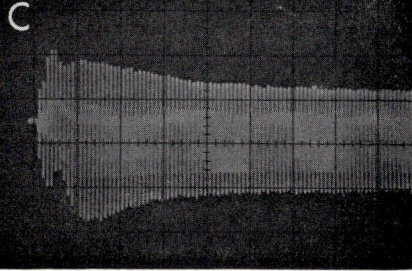

hypotonic infant or in one who is having respiratory or swallowing difficulty. All infants with this disorder are born of myasthenic mothers, and the severity of the infant's symptoms bears no direct relationship to the status of the mother's disease. In almost all cases, however, the weakness is transient and babies do well even though they may require anticholinesterase therapy for a short period.

Occasionally persistent symptoms are seen in babies with neonatal myasthenia and, although they suffer milder symptoms, they may exhibit refractoriness to drug therapy. These patients have been distinguished from the "transient neonatal myasthenia gravis" patients by Millichap and Dodge,[41] who assign the name "persistent neonatal myasthenia gravis" or "congenital myasthenia gravis."

MANAGEMENT.—The average physician often feels ill equipped to handle these patients, not only because the disease is rare, but also because many problematic aspects of medical and surgical therapy arise in young patients with this alarming disorder. It is generally accepted that a spontaneous remission nearly always benefits the patient more than the most expertly administered drug therapy.

Currently Mestinon (pyridostigmine bromide) enjoys the widest usage for maintenance *medical therapy* of juvenile myasthenia gravis. Other anticholinesterase drugs include Prostigmin (neostigmine)—the agent which has been in use for the longest time—and Mytelase (ambenonium chloride), which has been considered by some as preferred therapy in patients with bulbar weakness. As with anticonvulsant drug regimens, the necessary dosage varies among individuals. In general, the patient is given Mestinon 30–60 mg. (1–2 tablets) every four to six hours. In all but the severest cases all medication is given during the day. However, some patients must keep the early morning dose at the bedside because of weakness upon wakening. In patients who need larger doses the long-acting (180 mg. Timespan) tablet of Mestinon may take effect as quickly as the regular tablet, and its effect may have twice the duration. One must be prepared to raise the drug dosage until improvement occurs or until cholinergic, muscarinic side effects develop (abdominal cramps, diarrhea, lacrimation, sweating and salivation). These reactions can be controlled partially or completely by giving atropine sulfate along with the anticholinesterase drug. Although most experienced persons would agree that medical therapy of the disease does not influence the remission rate, resistance to drug therapy may appear, especially in patients receiving Prostigmin. If a patient begins to manifest weakness after having shown improvement with the initial therapy, two possibilities must be considered:

1. Myasthenic crisis. In this situation the patient's symptoms worsen because he is not receiving a large enough dose of drug. This state is recognized if the response to a Tensilon test is an improvement in strength. The maintenance dose of Mestinon is then raised. *Under no circumstances* should more than 2 mg. (0.2 cc.) Tensilon be used in the test lest a dangerous, cholinergic crisis be precipitated.

2. Cholinergic crisis. In some patients on therapy, progressive weakness of the bulbar and respiratory muscles develops because of overmedication with anticholinesterase agents. One may suspect this because of apparent muscarinic side effects, but often one cannot distinguish the cholinergic from the myasthenic crisis clinically. In this situation a Tensilon test (using 2 mg. or 0.2 cc.) fails to benefit the patient and, in fact, may make him worse. Such an observation calls for a smaller maintenance dose of Mestinon.

Some experienced workers like to use ephedrine sulfate as an adjunctive drug because of its alleged smoothing-out effect on the drug requirement, but its worth must be individualized in each case. Similar claims have been made recently for germine diacetate.[29a] Drug therapy in patients with severe myasthenia may be of no benefit, and the patient may require tracheostomy and care in a mechanical respirator.

Among the most difficult decisions to make in managing the severe myasthenic is that of recommending *surgical therapy* (thymectomy). If a tumor is suspected on the basis of the chest laminograms, thymectomy should be carried out to avoid the high risk of thymic malignancy. Theoretically the young woman who has had severe disease for less than five years and who has responded poorly to medical therapy represents the best candidate for thymectomy. One has to balance the operative risk against the chance for spontaneous remission and the probable need to give drug therapy postoperatively. Further, one must plan on doing a tracheostomy in any person whose disease is severe enough to warrant operation in order to lessen the operative risks. In summary, the proper management of the patients with severe disease calls for experienced and dedicated medical, surgical and nursing care.

PROGNOSIS.—The prognosis of myasthenia gravis in any age group must be guarded. In general most babies with neonatal myasthenia survive the illness, but they should be given anticholinesterase drug therapy if they have any bulbar or respiratory weakness. However, in persistent neonatal or congenital myasthenia the children are refractory to therapy and the course is protracted.[41] In juvenile myasthenia the prognosis is less favorable. Patients can enter severe and sudden relapse with what appears to be a mild respiratory infection. Consequently the patient and parents should be educated about the nature of the illness, and close medical supervision should be provided.

Hereditary Disorders of Neuromuscular Transmission

Familial Periodic Paralysis

PATHOGENESIS.—This very rare disorder is characterized by bouts of muscular paralysis and temporary hyporeflexia without neurologic signs in patients who are strong and healthy between attacks.[64] The disorder is inherited as an autosomal dominant trait and is associated with histopathologic changes in the muscle in some cases (Fig. 19.8).[41a] Three types of familial paralysis have been described, their differentiation being based upon the serum potassium level: (1) *hypokalemic type,* the commonest variety, (2) *hyperkalemic type* (adynamia episodica hereditaria) and (3) *normokalemic type*. Patchy fiber loss has been seen in some patients, but no cellular reaction or unique morphologic changes have been noted. In the hypokalemic variety the serum potassium level drops sharply during an attack in some patients. This apparently results from a sudden shift of potassium into the intracellular space, since no rise in urinary potassium is noted. Attacks are precipitated in some of these patients by excess carbohydrate intake and rest after strenuous exercise. For further details the reader is referred to the thorough discussion on periodic paralysis by Streeten.[58]

342   DISORDERS OF MUSCLE

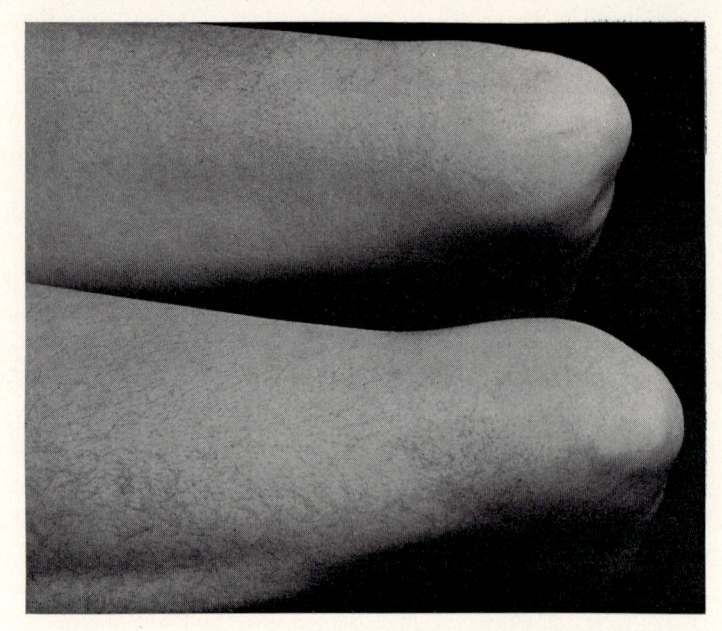

Fig. 19.8.—Familial periodic paralysis. Man, 26, with normokalemic familial periodic paralysis was included in a study reported by Tyler et al.[64] when he was 13. At age 26 he sought help from another doctor because of progressive weakness and disability. Atrophy of the thighs was noted (above). Muscle biopsy showed some loss of cross striations, variation in the staining characteristics of the muscle fibers and their nuclei and an occasional small fiber and histologic muscle abnormalities. This was interpreted erroneously as "muscular dystrophy." Some atrophy occurs in some of these patients. We have had the opportunity to examine two sons of this patient who have periodic paralysis without any objective neuromuscular deficit. The disorder behaves as an autosomal dominant trait.

CLINICAL AND LABORATORY DIAGNOSIS.—*Classic hypokalemic type.*—Periodic attacks of weakness without loss of consciousness usually begin in middle childhood, reach a peak in the third decade and often subside in middle or old age. The disease appears with greater frequency and intensity in males. Except for hyporeflexia during the attack, no neurologic deficit occurs in most cases. Some older patients, in whom attacks continue to occur, may show persistent weakness and atrophy, but this is exceptional (Fig. 19.8). Although the bulbar muscles above the neck are rarely involved, respiratory muscle weakness can occur and deaths have been reported. The attack may last from a few minutes to several days and may be associated with hypokalemia (Table 19.2). The patient often awakens in an episode of weakness. In some cases of classic periodic paralysis, cardiac arrhythmias have been noted.[36] Other conditions which may offer some difficulty in differential diagnosis include adynamia episodica hereditaria, myasthenia gravis, hypokalemia secondary to diarrhea, diabetic acidosis or metabolic alkalosis due to intestinal obstruction, and hyperaldosteronism (potassium-losing nephritis of Conn).

Hyperkalemic type (adynamia episodica hereditaria).[30]—This disorder resembles classic periodic paralysis very closely, but its milder nature and better prognosis justify its differentiation. Adynamia usually has an earlier onset, often in

TABLE 19.2.—DISTINGUISHING FEATURES OF THE THREE TYPES OF PERIODIC PARALYSIS[57,58]

	Hypokalemic Type	Hyperkalemic Type (Adynamia Episodica Hereditaria)	Normokalemic Type
Age of onset	7–21 years	First decade	First decade
Duration of attacks	1 hr. to 4 days (usually several hours)	Less than 1 hr.	2 days to 3 weeks
Serum potassium during attack	Low	High	Normal or slightly low
Factors which induce attacks	Rest after exertion, large high-carbohydrate meals, cold, infections, trauma, mental tension, alcohol	Rest after exertion, cold and damp, hunger	Rest after exertion, sleeping late, alcohol, cold and damp, mental stress
Iatrogenic induction	Glucose and insulin, ACTH, DCA, fluorohydrocortisone, epinephrine	Potassium chloride	Potassium chloride
Severity	Frequently complete paralysis, sparing face and respiratory muscles	Usually mild weakness, often localized	Often complete paralysis, including jaw and cough reflex
Time of onset	Awaken paralyzed	Usually during the day	Awaken paralyzed
Sex differences	More severe in males	More severe in males	Similar in both sexes
Sensory changes	None	May have paresthesias	Peripheral hypesthesia (one patient)
Metabolic changes	Potassium and, usually, sodium retention	No retention of potassium or sodium	Potassium retention
Prophylaxis	Spironolactone, very low-sodium diet, diuretics	Gentle exercise after exertion, carbohydrate feedings, acetazolamide	Gentle exercise after exertion, fluorohydrocortisone and acetazolamide
Treatment of attacks	Potassium salts	Calcium gluconate	Sodium chloride

infancy, and it is inherited as an autosomal dominant trait. The attacks occur in the daytime, are milder and briefer and can be precipitated by giving potassium salts. In normokalemic periodic paralysis no consistent change in serum potassium is found, but clinical attacks can be precipitated by giving potassium.

Normokalemic type.—The pathogenesis of this form of periodic paralysis is not understood. The paralytic episodes may last from two days to three weeks (Table 19.2).

The clinical and laboratory features which distinguish the three types of periodic paralysis as modified from Streeten[57,58] are shown in Table 19.2. A fourth variant of periodic paralysis distinguished by premature ectopic heart beats has been described in one family.[36]

MANAGEMENT AND PROGNOSIS.—*Hypokalemia.*—In patients with hypokalemic periodic paralysis having frequent attacks, the oral administration of 4–8 Gm. of potassium chloride in divided doses may prevent further episodes. Rarely in patients with acute respiratory or pharyngeal paralysis must one use potassium chloride intravenously. The intravenous route must be used with great caution, since overdosage will cause hyperkalemia which by itself can cause flaccid paralysis and cardiac arrhythmias. Some have suggested the use of amphetamine or dextroamphetamine to help these patients "get started" upon arising, since their symptoms may be worse at that time. Inasmuch as this is an autosomal dominant trait with a high penetrance rate, affected parents may have one or more children with the disease.

Hyperkalemia.—In contrast to the hypokalemic form, the attacks in patients with adynamia may be relieved by giving glucose and may be precipitated by giving potassium. Dexedrine (10–15 mg. per day in Spansule) appears to help some patients.[22a]

Normokalemic type.—This type of paralysis is provoked by potassium administration and relieved by sodium infusions without appreciable changes in serum electrolyte concentrations. These patients may unconsciously recognize the beneficial effect of salt ingestion.

Myotonia and Paramyotonia Congenita

PATHOGENESIS.—Myotonia congenita (Thomsen) resembles myotonia dystrophica by virtue of the muscle myotonia and the dominant mode of inheritance. The nosologic controversy is exemplified by the separate disease status assigned to myotonia congenita by Adams and associates,[1] versus the contention by Maas and Paterson[39] that it represents just one manifestation of myotonia dystrophica. Others have lumped myotonia congenita and paramyotonia congenita (von Eulenberg) into the same disease category, conceding that a cold environment accentuates myotonia in the latter form.

Myotonia congenita is inherited as an autosomal dominant trait.

CLINICAL AND LABORATORY DIAGNOSIS.—*Myotonia congenita.*—Symptoms develop insidiously before age 6, usually as a result of increased tone. Infants may walk later than expected, and they appear extremely muscular. Percussion myotonia may not be demonstrable until middle childhood, but the child or parent may report that he must "warm up" before he engages in any athletic activity to "iron out" the increased tone. The slowness of relaxation is best seen in the muscles of the hands, the orbicularis oculi and the tongue. As mentioned, above, Maas and Paterson[39] have noted mild dystrophic changes late in the course of the disease, but this observation is exceptional. Cataracts, frontal baldness and testicular atrophy do not as a rule develop in these patients.

Typical EMG abnormalities similar to those described in myotonia dystrophica (Fig. 19.2,*B*) are noted in patients with myotonia congenita. Muscle biopsy ordinarily reveals only hypertrophy of most muscle fibers.

Paramyotonia congenita.—Patients with this rare disorder have symptoms similar to those of myotonia congenita. Slowness and stiffness of movement are precipitated by environmental cold. This mild myotonia is often restricted to the hands, the eyelids and the tongue. Periodic attacks of weakness are also induced by cold or they may develop spontaneously. Layzer and co-workers[38c] have provided evidence which strongly suggests that paramyotonia congenita and hyperkalemic periodic paralysis are identical conditions.

Congenital Defects

Congenital Absence of Muscles

PATHOGENESIS.—True congenital absence of skeletal muscles is uncommon. The defect may appear as an isolated benign anomaly or may be associated with other malformations, and it may at times interfere with normal function. In approximate order of descending frequency the following muscles are congenitally absent: pectoralis (sternocostal portion), trapezius, quadriceps, serratus anterior, semimembranosus, abdominals, deltoids, sternomastoids.[1,7] Almost any muscle may fail to develop, but those which have the greatest clinical importance include (1) the abdominals (often bilateral), (2) the pectoralis major (unilateral), (3) diaphragm (unilateral), (4) facial muscles (often bilateral), (5) lid elevators and (6) external rectus. Although the etiology is not known, the common familial incidence pattern suggests a basic genetic etiology. No consistent pathologic changes are found in the nervous system of patients with congenitally absent muscles.

CLINICAL AND LABORATORY DIAGNOSIS.—*Abdominal muscles.*—Often a bilateral anomaly in boys, this defect interferes with the acts of breathing, defecating and urinating. Weakening of respiration and impaired coughing often cause pneumonia which may lead to death at an early age. Patients may be constipated, and they often exhibit dilated bladders, ureteral reflux and bilateral hydroureters and hydronephrosis. Superimposed chronic renal disease may cause early death.

Pectoralis major.— If this anomaly occurs alone, no real problem is encountered, but often the nipple on the same side is underdeveloped and the breast is absent, presenting a major cosmetic and psychologic problem in girls. Deformity of the ipsilateral hand with syndactyly as well as bony defects in the thorax and spine may be seen concomitantly. Muscular dystrophy has been reported in a number of patients with congenital absence of the pectoral muscles.[7]

Diaphragm.—Congenital absence of a hemidiaphragm may lead to atelectasis with serious pulmonary insufficiency, often as a result of herniation of the abdominal viscera into the chest.

Defects of bulbar muscles (Duane's syndrome and Möbius' syndrome) are discussed in Chapter 13.

Congenital ptosis.—This disorder often behaves as a dominant familial trait and causes both functional and cosmetic problems. When the defect, which is usually bilateral, is severe, the pupils are covered and vision is impaired. This causes the patient to tilt his head backward and wrinkle his brow in an effort to widen the palpebral fissures. On examination one should look especially for evidence of superior rectus weakness and also for other anomalies (epicanthi, cataracts, syndactyly and polydactyly).

Patients whose congenital muscular anomalies warrant further study (abdominals, pectorals, diaphragm) should have chest x-rays and urinary tract studies, including a voiding cystourethrogram. Surveys of the bony skeleton may disclose anomalies.

MANAGEMENT.—A detailed discussion of the management of these congenital muscular defects lies beyond the scope of this text. Most definitive therapy is surgical, but in the case of secondary pulmonary and genitourinary complications patients benefit from good supportive medical care. Patients with congenital ptosis can be helped functionally and cosmetically with corrective operations.[16] The reader is referred to textbooks of ophthalmology for details of surgical therapy.

Congenital Contractures

For the sake of clinical convenience, common congenital contractures of muscles such as *clubfoot* (talipes), *torticollis* (wryneck), *elevation of the shoulder* (Sprengel's deformity), *amyoplasia congenita* (arthrogryposis) and *camptodactyly* (stiff little finger) are discussed together. In general most workers think that a number of different pathogenic explanations must be invoked to account for these various deformities. The evidence suggests that the etiologies include (1) multiple congenital anomalies, (2) isolated hereditary trait (viz., camptodactyly and some cases of clubfoot[55]), (3) hereditary trait linked to muscular dystrophy (absence of the pectoral muscle), (4) primary anomaly of the nervous system with secondary joint contracture, (5) primary defect in the muscle without evidence of neuronal disease (e.g., clubfoot) and (6) factors operating prenatally which immobilize the fetus at critical periods during embryogenesis.[19] Experimental animal studies by Drachman and Coulombre[20] using fetal immobilization have produced an arthrogryposis-like syndrome. Confirmation of this provocative observation should be sought since it has logical theoretical appeal. A more complete discussion of the pathogenesis of these problems can be found in the text of Adams, Denny-Brown and Pearson.[1]

Clubfoot.—Although clubfoot is one of the most commonly encountered joint deformities, its pathogenesis is poorly understood. Most cases appear sporadically but the hereditary nature of the defect in some cases is adequately documented, since it may behave as a dominant or at other times a recessive trait.[55] Most often clubfoot appears as an isolated anomaly. However, in other instances it is seen as (1) one in a constellation of anomalies (e.g., certain of the chromosomal anomalies), (2) one of the many joint contractures in patients with arthrogryposis, or (3) a manifestation of an hereditary spinocerebellar ataxia (Friedreich's ataxia or peroneal muscular atrophy). In most studied cases no anomalies of the nervous system have been seen, but variation in the fiber size of the agonist and antagonist muscles of the foot have been noted.[1]

The disorder is obvious in early infancy, and it may be unilateral or bilateral. When used in the broadest sense, the term encompasses a variety of foot and ankle joint deformities, but talipes equinovarus (plantar flexion of the ankle with inversion and adduction of the foot) is the commonest type and is said to account for 77% of all cases.[1] Usually the foot cannot be forced into the normal position because of shortened muscles and ligaments. With growth, in untreated cases there may be underdevelopment of certain muscles, such as the peroneal, and shortening of the gastrocnemius.

In order to insure the best functional end result, orthopedic treatment of this common deformity should be initiated promptly. The foot (or feet) is casted in an overcorrected position or the patient is placed in a Denis-Browne splint. Surgical correction should be carried out only in the exceptional case.

Torticollis (wryneck).—The cause of this condition has not been proved. It does not have a hereditary pattern of occurrence. The evidence at present suggests that it may result from ischemic contracture of the sternocleidomastoid muscle (often as a result of a traumatic birth), similar to that seen in Volkmann's ischemic contracture of the hand or foot in adults.

The head is tilted to one side and on the same side one can feel a firm, taut sternocleidomastoid muscle. The head is usually rotated slightly so that the occiput is nearer the side of the shortened muscle and the chin is turned to the opposite side and tilted upward. In many cases of congenital torticollis there is a fusiform swelling in the belly of the sternocleidomastoid muscle. This so-called "sternomastoid tumor of infancy" is usually absorbed in two or three months, but a fibrous contracture may ensue and give rise to torticollis. Secondary deformities of the head, face, spine and shoulder are frequently noted as the child ages. The ipsilateral side of the face is shortened and sometimes broadened and recessed, while the frontal eminence of the skull is flattened and the occipital bone bulges slightly on the side of the shortening. The head on the opposite side shows prominence of the forehead and flattening of the occiput. A dorsal scoliosis may develop and one scapula is often elevated above the other.

Of great importance in dealing with this clinical sign is an accurate differential diagnosis before therapy is started. In young children, associated congenital anomalies of the spine together with birth injuries, such as fractured clavicles, should be excluded. In older children, localized infections in the neck or spine, focal muscle weakness (poliomyelitis), arthritis (acute rheumatic fever and rheumatoid disease), posterior fossa tumors (Chapter 17) which cause head tilt and other causes of scoliosis (Chapter 8) must be considered. In adolescent children the onset of spasmodic torticollis should suggest, in addition to functional disorders, such conditions as chlorpromazine intoxication, dystonia musculorum deformans, kernicterus, Hallervorden-Spatz disease, chronic progressive chorea (Huntington) and hepatolenticular degeneration (Wilson).

In the majority of cases of this disorder the "sternomastoid tumor" is gradually resorbed and the wryneck disappears. Babies with this deformity should be followed carefully and, if the wryneck does not disappear by 5 or 6 months of age, surgical section of the involved muscle may be required. If this plan is not followed, irreversible facial and skull asymmetry may develop. Once the asymmetry has become established surgical correction of the wryneck may serve only to make the facial asymmetry more obvious to the patient.

Elevation of the shoulder.—This malposition and malformation of the scapula may result from defective innervation or development of the trapezius or serratus anterior muscles. At times malformation is associated with cervical spina bifida or Klippel-Feil deformity of the spine.

The affected scapula is usually elevated and rotated so that the lower angle lies closer to the spine, and it is often shorter and broader than the scapula on the normal side. It is usually fixed to the ribs or spine by fibrous or bony attachments so that limitation of active and passive motion is noted. This fixation in turn limits abduction of the ipsilateral arm at the shoulder. Anomalies of the bony spine may be seen on x-ray study.

No regularly satisfactory treatment of this deformity has been developed. Attempts to free the bony or fibrous fixation of the scapula have been carried out. This may permit a wider range of arm abduction, but the scapula tends to assume a more elevated position, thus limiting activities of the arm which require shoulder fixation (e.g., pushing).

Amyoplasia congenita (*arthrogryposis*).—Most workers think that this clinical syndrome does not constitute a discrete pathologic entity. Multiple causes for this syndrome have been found, as indicated previously.

Multiple congenital joint contractures characterize this crippling syndrome. The joint position deformities may vary greatly, but in most cases the arms are partially extended and pronated, the hands are flexed in ulnar deviation and fingers may be held in a position of general flexion. The knees are often flexed and the hips are flexed and externally rotated. Congenital dislocation of the hip, clubfoot and scoliosis may occur secondarily. The range of joint motion is markedly limited, although the joints may appear prominent because of the muscle atrophy. Actually, no pathologic joint changes are seen on x-ray but marked loss of soft-tissue muscle shadow is obvious. Muscles above the neck are usually spared except for rigidity of the temporomandibular joints in some patients. Deep tendon reflexes are usually not elicitable, and electrical studies of muscles show feeble responses without evidence of denervation. In exceptional cases anomalies are found in other organ systems. Patients with this syndrome usually have normal mentality.

The management is best carried out by a team of persons including the orthopedic surgeon, the physiatrist and ancillary medical personnel who work regularly with children who have chronic motor handicaps.

Camptodactyly.—This contracture of the fifth finger at the interphalangeal joints behaves as a dominant trait with variable penetrance[55] and it is apparent in early infancy. Ford[29b] describes a progressive type which appears almost exclusively in girls in later childhood. The etiology of the latter malformation is not defined.

These patients have contractures of both interphalangeal joints but none at the metacarpophalangeal joints. The disorder is not really disabling.

This mild deformity usually requires no therapy and any decision to operate should be made by an experienced orthopedist.

Tumors of Muscle

The rarity of primary muscle tumors in childhood precludes their discussion in this text. The reader is referred to Adams and associates[1] for detailed information.

BIBLIOGRAPHY

1. Adams, R. D., et al.: *Diseases of Muscle* (2d ed.; New York City: Paul B. Hoeber, Inc., 1962).
2. Adner, M. M., et al.: An immunologic survey of forty-eight patients with myasthenia gravis, New England J. Med. 271:1327, 1964.
3. Afifi, A. K., et al.: Congenital nonprogressive myopathy, Neurology 15:371, 1965.
3a. Armstrong, R. M., et al.: Familial proximal spinal muscular atrophy, Arch. Neurol. 14:208, 1966.
4. Banker, B. Q., and Victor, M.: Dermatomyositis (systemic angiopathy) of childhood, Medicine 45:261, 1966.
5. Banker, B. G., et al.: Arthrogryposis multiplex due to congenital muscular dystrophy, Brain 80:319, 1957.

BIBLIOGRAPHY

6. Beutner, E. H., *et al.*: Studies on autoantibodies in myasthenia gravis, J.A.M.A. 182:46, 1962.
7. Bing, R.: Über angeborene Muskel-Defekte, Virchow's Arch. path. Anat. 170:175, 1902.
7a. Bitnum, S., *et al.*: Dermatomyositis, J. Pediat. 64:101, 1964.
8. Brandt, S.: Amyotonia congenita—a symptom and not a separate disorder, J. Child. Psychiat. 1:266, 1948.
9. Brandt, S.: Hereditary factors in infantile progressive muscular atrophy, Am. J. Dis. Child. 78:226, 1949.
10. Brandt, S.: Course and symptoms of progressive infantile muscular atrophy: A followup study of 112 cases in Denmark, Arch. Neurol. & Psychiat. 63:218, 1950.
10a. Brandt, S.: *Werdnig-Hoffmann's Infantile Progressive Muscular Atrophy* (Copenhagen: Ejnar Munksgaard, 1950).
11. Byers, R. K., and Banker, B. Q.: Infantile muscular atrophy, Arch. Neurol. 5:140, 1961.
11a. Byers, R. K., and Taft, L. T.: Chronic multiple peripheral neuropathy in childhood, Pediatrics 20:517, 1957.
12. Caughey, J. E., and Myrianthopoulos, N. C.: *Dystrophia Myotonica and Related Disorders* (Springfield, Ill.: Charles C Thomas, Publisher, 1963).
13. Chung, C. S., and Morton, N. E.: Discrimination of genetic entities in muscular dystrophy, Am. J. Human Genet. 11:339, 1959.
14. Clement, D. H., and Godman, G. C.: Glycogen disease resembling mongolism, cretinism, and amyotonia congenita, J. Pediat. 36:11, 1950.
15. D'Agostino, A. N., *et al.*: Familial myopathy with abnormal muscle mitochondria, Arch. Neurol. 18:388, 1968.
16. Dayal, Y., and Crawford, J. S.: Evaluation of the results of surgery to correct congenital ptosis of the upper eyelid, Canad. M. A. J. 94:1172, 1966.
17. Diamond, I., and Aquino, T. I.: Myoglobinuria following unilateral status epilepticus and ipsilateral rhabdomyolysis, New England J. Med. 272:834, 1965.
18. Dodge, P. R., *et al.*: Myotonic dystrophy in infancy and childhood, Pediatrics 35:3, 1965.
19. Drachman, D. B., and Banker, B. Q.: Arthrogryposis multiplex congenita, Arch. Neurol. 5:77, 1961.
20. Drachman, D. B., and Coulombre, A. J.: Experimental clubfoot and arthrogryposis multiplex congenita, Lancet 2:523, 1962.
21. Drachman, D. B., *et al.*: "Myopathic" changes in chronically denervated muscle, Arch. Neurol. 16:14, 1967.
22. Ebashi, S., *et al.*: High creatine phosphokinase activity of sera of progressive muscular dystrophy, J. Biochem. 46:103, 1959.
22a. Egan, T. J., and Klein, R.: Hyperkalemic familial period paralysis, Pediatrics 24:761, 1959.
23. Emery, A. E. H.: Clinical manifestations in two carriers of Duchenne muscular dystrophy, Lancet 1:1126, 1963.
24. Engel, W. K.: 2. A clinical approach to the myopathies. Symposium Review of Current Concepts of Myopathies. Clinical Orthopaedics and Related Research 39:6, 1965.
25. Engel, W. K., and Hogenhuis, L. A. H.: 4. Genetically determined myopathies. Symposium Review of Current Concepts of Myopathies. Clinical Orthopaedics and Related Research 39:34, 1965.
26. Engel, W. K., and Resnick, J. S.: Late-onset rod myopathy: A newly recognized, acquired and progressive disease. (Abstract) American Academy of Neurology Meeting, April 25-30, 1966, Philadelphia.
27. Engel, W. K., *et al.*: Nemaline myopathy, Arch. Neurol. 11:22, 1964.
27a. Fenichel, G. M., *et al.*: Neurogenic atrophy simulating facioscapulohumeral dystrophy, Arch. Neurol. 17:257, 1967.
28. Field, R. A.: Glycogen Deposition Disease, in Stanbury, J. B., Wyngaarden, J. B., and Fredrickson, D. S. (eds.): *The Metabolic Basis of Inherited Disease* (2d ed.; New York City: McGraw-Hill Book Company, Inc., 1966).
29. Fisch, C., and Evans, P. V.: The heart in dystrophia myotonica, New England J. Med. 251:527, 1954.
29a. Flacke, W., *et al.*: Treatment of myasthenia gravis with germine diacetate, New England J. Med. 275:1207, 1966.
29b. Ford, F. R.: *Diseases of the Nervous System in Infancy, Childhood and Adolescence* (5th ed.; Springfield, Ill.: Charles C Thomas, Publisher, 1966).
30. Gamstorp, I.: Adynamia episodica hereditaria, Acta paediat., upsal. 45 (supp. 108): 1, 1956.
31. Garvie, J. M., and Woolf, A. L.: Kugelberg-Welander syndrome (hereditary proximal spinal muscular atrophy), Brit. M. J. 1:1458, 1966.
32. Gonatas, N. K., *et al.*: Nemaline myopathy: The origin of nemaline structures, New England J. Med. 274:535, 1966.

33. Gordon, R. G., and Delicati, J. L.: The occurrence of amyotrophic lateral sclerosis in children, J. Neurol. & Psychopath. 9:30, 1928.
33a. Greenberg, J., and Arneson, L.: Exertional rhabdomyolysis with myoglobinuria in a large group of military trainees, Neurology 17:216, 1967.
34. Greenfield, J. G., et al.: The prognostic value of the muscle biopsy in the "floppy infant," Brain 81:461, 1958.
35. Gubbay, S. S., et al.: Clinical and pathological study of a case of congenital muscular dystrophy, J. Neurol. Neurosurg. & Psychiat. 29:500, 1966.
35a. Jackson, C. E., and Strehler, D. A.: Limb-girdle muscular dystrophy: Clinical manifestations and detection of preclinical disease, Pediatrics 41:495, 1968.
35b. Jarcho, L. W., and Adams, R. D.: Myoglobinuria, in Harrison, T. R., (ed.): *Principles of Internal Medicine* (5th ed.; New York City: McGraw-Hill Book Company, Inc., 1966).
35c. Kinoshita, M., and Cadman, T. E.: Myotubular myopathy, Arch. Neurol. 18:265, 1968.
36. Klein, R., et al.: Periodic paralysis with cardiac arrhythmia, J. Pediat. 62:371, 1963.
37. Kohn, N. N., et al.: Unusual manifestations due to involvement of involuntary muscle in dystrophia myotonica, New England J. Med. 271:1179, 1964.
38. Kugelberg, E., and Welander, L.: Heredofamilial juvenile muscular atrophy simulating muscular dystrophy, A.M.A. Arch. Neurol. & Psychiat. 75:500, 1956.
38a. Kurland, L. T.: Epidemiologic investigations of amyotrophic lateral sclerosis: III. A genetic interpretation of incidence and geographic distribution, Proc. Staff Meet. Mayo Clin. 32:449, 1957.
38b. Layzer, R. B., et al.: Muscle phosphofructokinase deficiency, Arch. Neurol. 17:512, 1967.
38c. Layzer, R. B., et al.: Hyperkalemic periodic paralysis, Arch. Neurol. 16:455. 1967.
39. Maas, O., and Paterson, A. S.: Myotonia congenita, dystrophia myotonica and paramyotonia: Reaffirmation of their identity, Brain 73:318, 1950.
40. Mabry, C. C., et al.: X-linked pseudohypertrophic muscular dystrophy with a late onset and slow progression, New England J. Med. 273:1062, 1965.
40a. Milhorat, A. T., and Goldstone, L.: The carrier state in muscular dystrophy of the Duchenne type, J.A.M.A. 194:130, 1965.
41. Millichap, J. G., and Dodge, P. R.: Diagnosis and treatment of myasthenia gravis in infancy, childhood, and adolescence, Neurology 10:1007, 1960.
41a. Odor, D. L., et al.: Familial hypokalemic periodic paralysis with permanent myopathy, J. Neuropath. & Exper. Neurol. 26:98, 1967.
42. Osserman, K. E.: Studies in myasthenia gravis, New York J. Med. 56:2512, 2672, 1956.
43. Osserman, K. E.: *Myasthenia Gravis* (New York City: Grune & Stratton, Inc., 1958).
44. Pearce, J., and Harriman, D. G. F.: Chronic spinal muscular atrophy, J. Neurol. Neurosurg. & Psychiat. 29:509, 1966.
45. Price, H. M., et al.: New evidence for excessive accumulation of Z-band material in nemaline myopathy, Proc. Nat. Acad. Sc. (USA) 54:1398, 1965.
45a. Refsum, S., et al.: Dystrophia myotonica, Neurology 17:345, 1967.
45b. Rosman, N. P., and Rebeiz, J. J.: The cerebral defect and myopathy in myotonic dystrophy, Neurology 17:1106, 1967.
46. Rowland, L. P.: Muscular dystrophies, polymyositis and other myopathies, J. Chron. Dis. 8:510, 1958.
47. Rowland, L. P., and Eskenazi, A. N.: Myasthenia gravis with features resembling muscular dystrophy, Neurology 6:667, 1956.
48. Rowland, L. P., et al.: Myoglobinuria, Arch. Neurol. 10:537, 1964.
49. Schwab, R. S.: Management of myasthenia gravis, New England J. Med. 268:596, 1963.
49a. Sher, J. H., et al.: Familial centronuclear myopathy, Neurology 17:727, 1967.
50. Shy, G. M., and Gonatas, N. K.: Human myopathy with giant abnormal mitochondria, Science 145:493, 1964.
51. Shy, G. M., and Magee, K. R.: A new congenital non-progressive myopathy, Brain 79:610, 1956.
52. Shy, G. M., et al.: Nemaline myopathy: A new congenital myopathy, Brain 86:793, 1963.
53. Shy, G. M., et al.: Two childhood myopathies with abnormal mitochondria: I. Megaconial myopathy; II. Pleoconial myopathy, Brain 89:133, 1966.
54. Spiro, A. J., and Kennedy, C.: Hereditary occurrence of nemaline myopathy, Arch. Neurol. 13:155, 1965.
55. Stern, C.: *Principles of Human Genetics* (San Francisco: W. H. Freeman and Co., 1960).
56. Strauss, A. J. L., et al.: Immunofluorescence demonstration of a muscle-binding, complement-fixing serum globulin fraction in myasthenia gravis, Proc. Soc. Exper. Biol. & Med. 105:184, 1960.
57. Streeten, D. H. P. (modified from Poskanzer, D. C., and Kerr, D. N. S.): A third type of periodic paralysis, with normokalemia and favourable response to sodium chloride, Am. J. Med. 31:328, 1961.
58. Streeten, D. H. P.: Periodic Paralysis, in Stanbury, J. B., Wyngaarden, J. G., and Fred-

rickson, D. S. (eds.): *The Metabolic Basis of Inherited Disease* (2d ed.; New York City: McGraw-Hill Book Company, Inc., 1966).
59. Tsukagoshi, H., *et al.:* Kugelberg-Welander syndrome with dominant inheritance, Arch. Neurol. 14:378, 1966.
60. Turner, J. W. A., and Lees, F.: Congenital myopathy—a fifty-year follow-up, Brain 85:733, 1962.
61. Tyler, F. H.: Unpublished data.
62. Tyler, F. H., and Adams, R. D.: Chronic Muscular Wasting and Paralysis, in Harrison, T. R. (ed.): *Principles of Internal Medicine* (5th ed.; New York City: McGraw-Hill Book Company, Inc., 1966).
63. Tyler, F. H., and Stephens, F. E.: Studies in disorders of muscle: II. Clinical manifestations and inheritance of facioscapulohumeral dystrophy in a large family, Ann. Int. Med. 32:640, 1950.
64. Tyler, F. H., *et al.*: Studies in disorders of muscle: VII. Clinical manifestations and inheritance of a type of periodic paralysis without hypopotassemia, J. Clin. Invest. 30:492, 1951.
65. vanCreveld, S., and Soeters, J. M.: Myositis ossificans progressiva, Am. J. Dis. Child. 62:1000, 1941.
66. VanderGeld, H., *et al.*: Multiple antibody production in myasthenia gravis, Lancet 2:373, 1963.
67. Vignos, P. J., and Watkins, M. P.: The effect of exercise in muscular dystrophy, J.A.M.A. 197:843, 1966.
68. Vignos, P. J., *et al.*: Management of progressive muscular dystrophy of childhood, J.A.M.A. 184:89, 1963.
69. Watters, G. V., and Williams, T. W.: Early onset myotonic dystrophy, Arch. Neurol. 17:137, 1967.
70. Wedgwood, R. J.: Diseases of Mesenchymal Tissues, in Nelson, W. E. (ed.): *Textbook of Pediatrics* (8th ed.; Philadelphia: W. B. Saunders Company, 1964).
71. Worden, D. K., and Vignos, P. J.: Intellectual function in childhood progressive muscular dystrophy, Pediatrics 29:968, 1962.
72. Zellweger, H., *et al.*: Glycogen disease of skeletal muscle, Pediatrics 15:715, 1955.
73. Zundel, W. S., and Tyler, F. H.: The muscular dystrophies, New England J. Med. 273:537, 1965.

20

Intoxications and Adverse Reactions to Therapy

Poison Control Centers
General Manifestations and Therapy

Specific Manifestations and Therapy

POISONINGS

Insecticides, Pesticides and Herbicides
    Arsenic
    Chlorinated Phenoxyacetic Acids
        (e.g., 2,4-D)
    Thallium

Fuels, Paints, Solvents and Antifreeze
    Carbon Monoxide
    Lead
    Alcohols
Food Poisoning
    Botulism
    Mushroom
Spider Bites and Snake Bites

Organic Phosphates (Parathion and
    Malathion)
Chlorinated Hydrocarbons (e.g.,
    Lindane, Chlordane)
Strychnine

Ethylene Glycol (Antifreeze)
Kerosene
Solvent Sniffing (Glue, Gasoline)

Coyotillo
Shellfish

ADVERSE REACTIONS TO THERAPY

Sedatives
    Barbiturates
    Narcotics and Potent Analgesics
Stimulants
    Amphetamine Derivatives and Xanthines
Salicylates

Phenothiazine Tranquilizers

INTOXICATIONS AND ADVERSE REACTIONS TO THERAPY

Antimicrobials
- Tetracyclines
- Penicillin
- Isoniazid (INH)
- Nitrofurantoin (Furadantin)
- Streptomycin
- Kanamycin
- Gantrisin
- Chloroquine

Water and Electrolyte Therapy
- Water Intoxication and Hyponatremia
- Hypernatremia

Hormones
- Adrenal Corticosteroids
- Insulin

Anticancer Drugs
- Vincristine and Vinblastine

Immunizations
- DPT
- Rabies } Chapter 18
- Vaccinia

Diets and Supplements
- Cow's Milk
  - Idiopathic hypercalcemia
  - Neonatal tetany (Chapter 2)
- Vitamin K
- Vitamin A

Miscellaneous
- Aminophylline
- Mercury
- Methysergide (Sansert)
- Oxygen
- Antiserum

Anticonvulsants (Chapter 2)

IN THE UNITED STATES poisoning is a leading cause of death, especially among poison-prone toddlers between the ages of 1 and 4. The incidence pattern of poisonings has varied with (1) the more frequent prescriptions for drugs of all types, especially tranquilizers, antibiotics and "pep pills" (amphetamine compounds), (2) the more widespread use of herbicides and insecticides, (3) the increasing awareness of the poisonous nature of certain commercial products (e.g., the virtual elimination of lead-base paints on household furniture and the replacement of lead battery casings with plastic ones), (4) the growing tendency to dispense poisonous products, such as aspirin, with candy flavoring, thereby making them more attractive to children and (5) the changing types of fuel (e.g., gas instead of kerosene).

The scope of this chapter will be limited to (1) an outline for the immediate general treatment of all poisonings, (2) the diagnosis and therapy of the more common specific poisonings and adverse reactions which can cause neurologic signs and (3) a limited discussion of specific antidotal therapy.

Poison Control Centers

It has been estimated that more than 500,000 different household products are commercially available and that 1,500 new substances are marketed each month. For this reason the coverage in this chapter must be limited. Every physician who expects to handle the acute emergency of a poisoned patient should be familiar with the *poison control center* concept. The centers are provided with up-to-date information on the toxic ingredients in nearly all registered commercial products and can provide the pertinent information to the physician. The information service is available over the phone and around the clock, and every practitioner and hospital should keep the phone number readily accessible. Obviously, no one person or reference source can provide specific current information on every product, but the poison control centers provide an important aid to the individual physician.

A list of the commoner poisons is included in the preceding outline and in Table 20.1, which gives the nature of the toxic ingredients and the distinctive clinical features of the intoxication. The reader is referred to other informational sources including those of Done[21] and Lucas and Imrie[44] for greater detail. The latter reference also includes a list of poison control centers in the United States and Canada.

General Manifestations and Therapy
CLINICAL AND LABORATORY DIAGNOSIS

Any general practitioner must consider the possibility of poisoning in a patient in whom another diagnosis is not clearly established. Through long experience pediatricians have established this habit, and they rarely fail to consider at least the possibility of an intoxication. Although the manifestations of poisoning may vary greatly, the commonest *acute* clinical signs are:

1. Acute gastrointestinal symptoms and signs (vomiting, abdominal pain and diarrhea) which may mimic acute gastroenteritis, acute appendicitis, peritonitis and intestinal obstruction
2. Acute mental changes (irritability, personality change, delirium and psychosis) suggesting acute meningoencephalitis or functional personality disorders
3. Signs of acute central nervous system excitation (acute mania, convulsions, tonic or tetanic rigidity), also suggesting acute nervous system infections and other causes of convulsions
4. Signs of central nervous system depression (stupor or coma)

The neurologic manifestations may be confused with meningitis, encephalitis, hypocalcemic tetany or a convulsion attributed to some other cause. Somewhat less often one sees respiratory symptoms and signs such as cough, dyspnea and tachypnea (see Table 20.1).

In the *subacute* or *chronic* stage of poisoning one can expect neurologic signs of:

1. increased intracranial pressure (headache, papilledema, suture separation)
2. cranial nerve deficit
3. peripheral neuropathy (flaccid weakness, hyporeflexia, paresthesias and pain, loss of sensation and ataxia)

TABLE 20.1.—CLINICAL MANIFESTATIONS OF CNS POISONINGS AND ADVERSE DRUG REACTIONS

PART I. CATEGORIES OF NEUROLOGIC SYMPTOMS AND SIGNS

1. Mental symptoms: irritability, personality change, delirium, psychosis
2. CNS excitation: acute mania, seizures, tonic or tetanic rigidity
3. CNS depression: stupor, coma
4. Increased intracranial pressure: headache, drowsiness, papilledema, suture separation
5. Cranial nerve deficit: I-XII
6. Peripheral neuropathy: flaccid weakness, hyporeflexia, paresthesias, sensory loss, ataxia
7. Movement disorders: tremor, ataxia, fasciculations, dystonia, athetosis
8. Corticospinal tract deficit: spastic weakness, hyperreflexia, pathologic toe signs
9. Autonomic signs: sweating, salivation, bronchospasm, lacrimation, bradycardia, miosis, fasciculations

CATEGORIES OF SYSTEMIC SYMPTOMS AND SIGNS

10. Gastrointestinal: vomiting, abdominal pain, diarrhea, melena
11. Respiratory: cough, dyspnea, tachypnea, malodorous breath
12. Hepatic: jaundice, hepatomegaly
13. Renal: oliguria, edema, albuminuria, hematuria, hypertension
14. Cardiovascular: arrhythmia, murmurs, bruits, rubs
15. Skin: rash, redness

PART II. CLINICAL MANIFESTATIONS*

TYPE OF POISON	CNS Acute	CNS Subacute, Chronic	SYSTEMIC Acute	SYSTEMIC Subacute, Chronic
Insecticides, pesticides and herbicides				
Arsenic	2	6	10	14,13
Chlorinated phenoxyacetic acids (e.g., 2, 4-D)	2	6	10	
Thallium		1,2,3,5,6	10	15 (alopecia)
Organic phosphates	9,1,2,3,7 (parasympathomimetic)			
Chlorinated hydrocarbons (chlordane, lindane)	1,2			
Strychnine	2,7			
Fuels, paints, solvents and antifreeze				
Carbon monoxide	1,2,3		10,12,15	
Lead	1,2,3,4			
Alcohols (ethanol, methanol, isopropanol)	1,2,3,4		10(12,13)	
Ethylene glycol	1,2,3		10,13	
Kerosene	1,2,3		11	
Solvent sniffing (glue, gasoline)		(see text)		
Food				
Botulism	5,6,2,3		10	
Mushrooms	9,1,3		10	
Arachnidism				
Black widow spider bites	6		Pain, 10	
Tick paralysis	6		10	
Medications				
Sedatives and narcotics	1,2,3			
Phenothiazine tranquilizers	1,2,3			
Anticonvulsants	(Chapter 2)			
Amphetamines	1,2			
Salicylates	2,3		11	
Tetracycline, penicillin, furadantin, isoniazid	4			
Vitamins	4		15	
Aminophylline	2,3	4	10,11	
Mercury		1,6		10,15

*The numbers in Part II of the table refer to the numbered categories of neurologic and systemic symptoms and signs in Part I. They are used to illustrate (1) the type of neurologic deficit and systemic signs seen with different poisonings and (2) the stage in the poisoning when the signs usually appear.

4. movement disorders (tremor, ataxia and fasciculations)

Signs of peripheral neuropathy develop usually after long-term administration or exposure, and they have become an increasingly important problem with the emergence of more potent antimicrobial and cancer drugs. After the immediate, acute stage of poisoning, systemic signs of *liver insufficiency* (anorexia, nausea, vomiting, jaundice, hepatomegaly) and *renal insufficiency* (edema, hypertension, oliguria, albuminuria and hematuria) are common.

These neurologic and systemic symptoms and signs are listed in Table 20.1. Each category is assigned a number for the purpose of tabulating the clinical signs to be expected with different types of intoxications. The poisons are listed in the approximate order of their neurologic importance.

Laboratory studies are valuable in the diagnosis of selected poisonings and may provide a useful guide for the necessary therapeutic vigor and the prognosis.

Blood.—Most hospital laboratories are now equipped to measure salicylate and barbiturate blood levels. Done[19] devised a nomogram to serve as a therapeutic and prognostic guide in patients with salicylate poisoning. Blood alcohol levels can also be measured, and this determination primarily has medicolegal value. Spectrophotometric determination of carboxyhemoglobin in the blood may provide the only definitive diagnostic information in patients with carbon monoxide poisoning.

Urine.—In patients with suspected heavy metal poisoning, quantitative determinations of lead or arsenic can be carried out on 24-hour urine specimens collected in metal-free containers. Most state or local public health laboratories can provide this service. Also in lead poisoning a rough quantitative test will often show elevated amounts of coproporphyrin in the urine.

Hair.—In questionable cases of arsenic or thallium poisoning, a test for heavy metal content of the hair is helpful in diagnosis.

X-rays.—Patients with suspected *lead* poisoning should have films of the long bones to identify the dense metaphyseal lead line. X-rays of the paint chips may provide proof of the source. Pneumonia is usually demonstrable within four hours of ingesting *volatile petroleum hydrocarbons* such as kerosene. Of special interest to the pediatrician and the neurologist are the skull and long bone abnormalities seen in patients who have been intoxicated with vitamin A or D.

Management and Prognosis

The principles of therapy are directed at (1) prevention of further absorption by (*a*) induction of emesis or (*b*) gastric lavage and (*c*) instillation of a universal or specific antidote into the stomach, and (2) good supportive care. It has been proved experimentally that emesis eliminates the poison more effectively than gastric lavage.

Initially parents often seek advice over the phone in a state of panic. The physician should offer a few simple, calm words of advice and, if the situation warrants, arrange to see the patient immediately in his office or in the hospital emergency room.

Prevention of Further Poison Absorption.—Immediate induction of vomiting is recommended *except in the following situations*: (1) the child who has ingested a caustic or corrosive, (2) the child who has ingested a volative petroleum hydrocarbon, such as kerosene, (3) the child who is severely stuporous or comatose and (4) the child with convulsions. If advice is sought over the phone, the parent should be instructed to have the child drink a glass of salt water (2–3 teaspoons of table salt in a glass of lukewarm water) and follow this by stimulating the gag reflex in the posterior pharynx with the index finger. The child should be brought to the hospital in the meantime and, if vomiting has not occurred, should be given *syrup of ipecac* (*not* fluidextract) in a dose of 20 cc. Another dose of 10 cc. is given in 10 minutes if the patient has not vomited.

If these measures fail to induce emesis within 15 minutes (and failure to vomit under these conditions is seen in only 5% of patients), gastric lavage is carried out. When a very toxic poison has been ingested, lavage should be carried out promptly and an emetic then given to *avoid unnecessary delay*. The child is "mummified" in a sheet restraint, placed in the prone Trendelenburg position and a reasonably large gastric rubber tube is passed through the mouth (*not the nose*) into the stomach. Using a large-bore syringe, one should aspirate as much of the stomach contents as possible without instilling anything. This step also serves to guarantee that the tube is in the stomach and not the tracheobronchial tree. Lavage is then carried out with not more than 1 qt. of water. The initial stomach contents should be saved if the need for laboratory analysis is anticipated.

With rare exceptions, to be mentioned, the best *universal antidote* is *medicinal* or *activated charcoal* (not to be confused with wood charcoal or burnt toast). This is introduced into the stomach either by having the patient drink it or by instilling it through the lavage tube. Five to 6 heaping teaspoonfuls of activated charcoal are mixed with water to form a thin paste. Shortly after it has been ingested or instilled, this charcoal is removed and some fresh charcoal is added and left in the gut.

An attempt is being made in many areas to make "poison prevention kits"

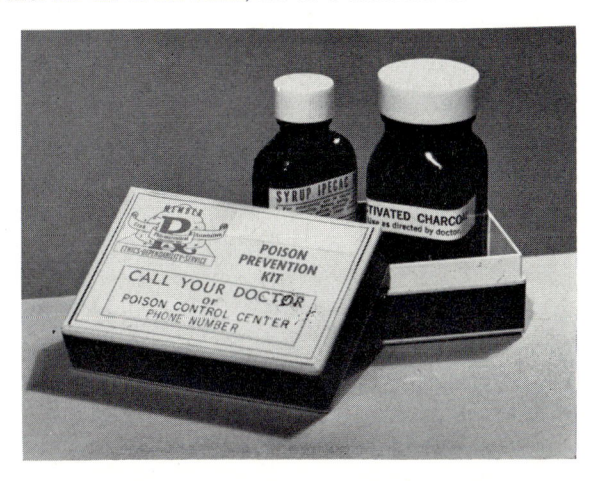

Fig. 20.1.—Poison prevention kit. This kit is marketed under the name Ipechan by Hoyt. It is intended for first-aid use in the home, *not* as a substitute for definitive medical treatment.

available through local pharmacies and to encourage families to keep them in the home for emergencies (Fig. 20.1).

GOOD SUPPORTIVE CARE.—While the preceding measures are being carried out, relatives, police ad public health officials should aid in the identification of the poisonous product if its nature is unknown. This may require only simple common sense, but in some instances it takes detailed detective work. The area where the poisoning took place should be inspected carefully, and relatives should be quizzed about all medications and household products which are within reach of the child. Parents are often extremely naive—sometimes because of a sense of guilt or irresponsibility—about the ability of a 2-year-old to obtain and open bottles of medicine from the top shelf of a cupboard. More difficult usually than identifying the nature of the poison is an accurate estimate of the amount that was ingested. Again ordinary common sense and simple arithmetic help to answer this question. Next, one should assess the patient's physical condition and institute necessary treatment while guarding against overtreatment. In patients with moderate or severe poisoning, serum for sodium, potassium, chloride, CO_2 and pH determinations should be obtained while hydrating solutions are started (Appendix 3).

Maintain oxygenation.—After the general emergency measures have been carried out, an adequate airway should be established, if necessary, with a tracheostomy. Oxygen should be given via a nasal catheter or a BLB mask. Positive-pressure oxygen can be given with a Bird or Bennett respirator (in patients with respiratory depression such as that seen in salicylate or barbiturate intoxication), either letting the patient trip the positive-pressure mechanism with his own inspiratory effort or putting the device on "automatic" and setting an arbitrary mechanical respiratory rate. In severe cases that require oxygen under positive pressure the patient often benefits if he is seen and followed by an anesthesiologist or a member of the hospital inhalation therapy team.

Circulatory collapse.—Shock or circulatory collapse should be treated as outlined in Appendix 4. Blood and plasma should be given along with pressor agents to maintain blood pressure in the hypotensive patient.

Fluid and electrolyte therapy.—Clear fluids should be given orally if the poisoning is not severe and the patient is not vomiting or severely obtunded. In general, more harm is done by overzealous and unwise administration of fluids and electrolytes than follows dehydration and electrolyte loss. A possible exception to this statement may be that of salicylate intoxication, but even here overcorrection of metabolic acidosis with alkali therapy will cause alkalosis with tetany, pulmonary edema and hypernatremia (p. 374).

Anticonvulsant therapy.—Convulsions, a common sign of central nervous system excitation from a variety of poisons (Table 20.1) should be managed as outlined in Appendix 1. If the seizures are related to coexistent cerebral edema, the latter should be managed as outlined in Appendix 2.

Analgesics.—Pain can be relieved with appropriate doses of codeine or meperidine hydrochloride (Demerol), but caution should be employed in order not to aggravate any nervous system depression caused by the poison itself.

Infections.—A chemical type of pneumonia complicates many cases of poisoning with volatile hydrocarbons. Hypostatic pneumonitis may appear in those patients whose ventilation and activity have been impaired by a state of coma. In general, therapy directed at a specific organism (grown in culture) works more effectively than so-called prophylactic treatment.

Dialysis.—In the past five or 10 years more and more patients with severe poisoning by agents such as barbiturates and salicylates have been treated with some form of dialysis. A detailed consideration of the indications and contraindications for this special therapy is beyond the scope of this text. Suffice it to say that hemodialysis using the artificial kidney offers the most efficient technique for ridding the body of poisons, but the technique is more complex than peritoneal dialysis and is associated with higher risks. Peritoneal dialysis, though not as efficient, can be carried out using simpler methods at minimal risk of complication. Exchange transfusion has also been used in selected cases of salicylate and barbiturate intoxication.

Specific Manifestations and Therapy

In addition to the textual descriptions that follow the reader should consult Table 20.2 which outlines the limited number of specific antidotes recommended for poisonings affecting the nervous system, as modified from Done's review.[20] Obviously, we have had to be arbitrary about placing some intoxications under

TABLE 20.2—RECOMMENDED SPECIFIC ANTIDOTES*

POISON	ANTIDOTE AND DOSE
Narcotics (natural and synthetic)	Nalorphine (Nalline) 1–2 mg. I.V. (small children) or
	Levallorphan (Lorfan) 0.25–0.5 mg. I.V. (small children) for *severe poisoning only* (see p. 372)
Phenothiazine (causing dystonia or athetosis)	Benadryl 5 mg./kg./24 hr.
	Biperiden hydrochloride (Akineton) 0.04 mg./kg.
Amphetamines	Chlorpromazine 1–2 mg./kg. I.M.
Thallium	Activated charcoal 0.5 Gm./kg.
	KCl 3–5 Gm./day
	Dithizon 10 mg./kg. orally or by nasogastric tube twice daily for 5 days
Organic phosphate insecticides (parathion, malathion)	1. Atropine sulfate in relatively large doses for 24 hr. Child: 0.5–1 mg. I.M. Adult: 2–3 mg. I.M. Repeated doses every 30 min. if necessary 2. PAM or PAMS 30 mg./kg. I.V. or I.M. over 30 min.
Mushroom poisoning	Atropine sulfate in relatively large doses for 24 hr. Child: 0.5–1 mg. I.M. Adult: 2–3 mg. I.M. Repeated doses every 30 min. if necessary
Heavy metals (lead, arsenic, mercury) chronic poisoning	EDTA 75 mg./kg./day I.M. (see text, Lead poisoning) BAL 2.5–3 mg./kg. every 4 hr. for 2 days, every 6 hr. on the third day and then every 12 hr. for 10 days or until recovery (see text, Arsenic poisoning)
Carbon monoxide	Oxygen

*Other antidotes are used for some poisonings (see text) but either their value is doubtful or they are dangerous. These data were provided through the courtesy of A. K. Done.

the heading of "Poisonings" and others under "Adverse Reactions." The decision was based on the commonest clinical experience with each agent in children.

Poisonings

Insecticides, Pesticides and Herbicides

Poisonings in increasing number are related to the growing list of substances developed by the chemical industry for killing pests and weeds. With the exception of arsenic and organic phosphates, most of the agents used have proved remarkably safe. Accidental poisoning with other substances is rare and in some cases remains unproved. Both precaution in the use of these substances and education about their toxicologic properties are called for.

Arsenic

This substance is used not only in weed killers and rodenticides (rat poison), but in the past enjoyed widespread medical use. In the form of Fowler's solution arsenic was used in the treatment of miscellaneous groups of refractory medical disorders. Arsenic now accounts for 7% of childhood deaths in the United States and ranks as the fourth leading cause of poison deaths.

In the acute stage of intoxication there are intense gastrointestinal symptoms and profound urinary urgency, often followed by collapse and death. Occasionally signs of nervous system excitation (headache, mania and convulsions) appear in the early stage of poisoning, and rare cases of acute hemorrhagic encephalopathy have complicated the intravenous administration of arsenic. Usually, however, neurologic signs in the form of a polyneuropathy indicate chronic poisoning due to prolonged medical use. In cases of chronic arsenic poisoning, one must consider in the differential diagnosis all the other clinical causes of polyneuropathy. A definitive diagnosis depends upon demonstrating elevated levels of arsenic in the urine or the hair. Normally not more than 0.1 mg. elemental arsenic is excreted in 24 hours. Poisoned patients will excrete 0.3 mg. or more in a 24-hour specimen.

In addition to the usual supportive measures, BAL therapy should be instituted. The efficacy of BAL in acute arsenic poisoning is undisputed, but it has little effect upon the established polyneuropathy. The drug is given intramuscularly in a dose of 2.5–3 mg./kg. every four hours for two days, every six hours on the third day and then every 12 hours for 10 days or until recovery. BAL injections are painful and by themselves can cause nausea and vomiting which may be indistinguishable from the usual acute toxic gastrointestinal symptoms. Pretreatment with antihistamines, such as Benadryl, will partially prevent the side effects of BAL. Treatment of arsenic poisoning with penicillamine has been suggested because of its lower toxicity, but it may be a less potent chelating agent than BAL.

Chlorinated Phenoxyacetic Acids (e.g., 2,4-D)

This extensively used group of herbicides or weed killers does not often cause intoxication. The clinical picture is not yet well defined, but it is clear that in the acutely intoxicated person one sees prominent gastrointestinal symptoms. Convulsions constitute the major sign of neurotoxicity, but cases of peripheral neuropathy have been associated with, though not proved to result from, these weed killers.[6]

Treatment at present consists of supportive, symptomatic care.

Thallium

Thallotoxicosis remains a serious cause of childhood poisoning. It results most commonly from the ingestion of rodenticides (rat poison) and insecticides. The incidence of thallium poisoning is augmented in many instances by the addition of thallium to cookies or biscuits to attract the pests. Instead the food attracts children. Poisoning formerly resulted from the use of depilatories for the cosmetic removal of facial hair in women and the treatment of scalp ringworm, but depilatories containing thallium have recently been removed from the market. A thorough study by Reed and co-workers[54] pointed up (1) the seriousness of this public health problem in the southern United States, (2) a 13% mortality rate among 72 children and (3) residual neurologic deficit in over half the surviving patients.

In the acute stage of the illness gastrointestinal symptoms predominate, followed in two to five days by neurologic signs of delirium, convulsions and coma. Smaller doses of poison may cause ataxia, neuropathy, a variety of movement disorders and even retrobulbar neuritis. Prominent among the signs of chronic intoxication are *alopecia* and evidence of neurologic deficit.

As yet no good antidote or chelation therapy for thallium poisoning has been discovered, other than general measures to promote excretion and intensive supportive care. BAL has been abandoned for the treatment of this intoxication, but diphenylthiocarbazone (Dithizon) has been used, albeit without impressive results. Dithizon in a dose of 10 mg./kg., given orally or by nasogastric tube twice a day for five days, has been suggested.[13,54]

Organic Phosphates (Parathion and Malathion)

Patients are usually poisoned with these substances by contact with insecticides—either by ingestion of contaminated food or water or by absorbing the substances through the skin or lungs at the time of crop spraying. These compounds have a "nicotinic" and "muscarinic" cholinergic action, i.e., they inhibit the action of cholinesterase. Their effects are multiple and complex, with symptoms similar to those occurring in overtreatment of myasthenia gravis (Chapter 19). The muscarinic effects (gastrointestinal complaints, sweating and bronchospasm) develop first and are followed by the nicotinic signs (muscle fasciculations, cramps and weakness) and variable neurologic manifestations, both excitatory and depressant. The diagnosis can be confirmed (1) by reduction of erythrocyte cholinesterase, (2) by demonstrating the organic phosphates or their metabolites in the urine or (3) by a therapeutic test with atropine.

Treatment consists of (1) relatively large doses of atropine to combat the muscarinic effects and (2) "cholinesterase regenerators" for the nicotinic effect (see Table 20.2). In patients with severe muscarinic symptoms, the danger of undertreatment with atropine is greater than the risk of atropine poisoning.[21] A small child is given 0.5–1 mg. of atropine sulfate intramuscularly (2–3 mg. for an adult) with repetition of this dose every 15–30 minutes, depending upon the response to the first dose. Careful atropinization (oral) should be maintained for at least 24 hours. The most commonly used cholinesterase regenerators, PAM (2-pyridine aldoxime methiodide) or PAMS (soluble methane sulfonate of PAM), are given intravenously or intramuscularly in doses up to 30 mg./kg., depending upon the severity of the poisoning.[44] The agent is infused over a 30-minute period.

Chlorinated Hydrocarbons (Lindane, Chlordane, etc.)

This most widely used group of insecticides has proved very safe when restricted to its ordinary commercial use. However, accidental ingestion by children causes a serious constellation of neurologic signs as well as some systemic manifestations. No common basis of toxicity has been defined for these compounds, possibly because of the different solvents used for the different compounds. Patients develop signs of nervous system excitation followed by parasympathomimetic signs and nervous system depression. A predominantly motor neuropathy has been seen following prolonged exposure to these chemicals.[37] Gastrointestinal symptoms as well as hepatotoxic and nephrotoxic effects have been reported.

Only supportive and symptomatic treatment is available for this type of poisoning (see General Manifestations and Therapy).

Strychnine

This potent neurointoxicant is still widely used as a rat poison and continues to be consumed accidentally by children. Its former popularity as a medicinal tonic, laxative and aphrodisiac has waned. When taken in large quantities it causes death in about half an hour. The direct, global stimulant effect upon the nervous system causes excitement, muscle fasciculations and tetanic rigidity, as well as convulsions which usually have a spinal basis. Death results from damage to the medullary respiratory center. In the absence of a clear history of strychnine ingestion, the clinical picture must be differentiated from tetanus, tetany, phenothiazine intoxication, cerebral seizures and other types of poisonings.

Treatment must be directed immediately toward intensive supportive care and adequate sedation. Rapid-acting intravenous barbiturates—amobarbital (Amytal) or pentobarbital (Nembutal)—are given even before gastric lavage because the latter procedure may precipitate more spinal seizures. The barbiturate is infused slowly until the patient is quiet and free from convulsions. Mephenesin, the centrally acting skeletal muscle relaxant, has been recommended in a dose of 20 mg./kg. by slow intravenous infusion as an adjunct to sedation.[21] Obviously, close attention must be devoted to an adequate airway and proper oxygenation in this dire medical emergency. When the reflex hyperexcitability has been controlled with sedatives and mephenesin, gastric lavage with a 1:10,000 solution of potassium permanganate is carried out, followed by instillation of activated charcoal into the stomach.

Fuels, Paints, Solvents and Antifreeze

Carbon Monoxide

This type of poisoning results either from the accidental (more common in children) or intentional (more common in adults) inhalation of fuels which are incompletely burned. In the United States the fumes from automobile exhausts or a defective stove or furnace which burns coal, oil, gasoline or wood can cause intoxication. Carbon monoxide, a colorless, tasteless and essentially odorless compound, forms a normal constituent of illuminating or coal gas but is not a component of natural gas. It forms carboxyhemoglobin with a much greater affinity than oxygen, and its affinity for hemoglobin eventually leads to tissue hypoxia. This occurs more readily in children than in adults because of the child's faster metabolic rate and greater respiratory minute volume.

Mild intoxication causes headache, drowsiness, mental confusion and vomiting (sometimes hematemesis), whereas severe poisoning leads to convulsions, coma, fecal and urinary incontinence and respiratory arrest. In addition, the patient may exhibit so-called "cherry red cyanosis," but this may disappear in a short time after he is removed from the poisonous atmosphere. The diagnosis depends upon a compatible history, "cherry red cyanosis" or the demonstration of carboxyhemoglobin in the blood. Carboxyhemoglobinemia may not be evident if the blood sample is not obtained until after the patient has been treated and all of the CO has been excreted. In many patients skin erythema and even bullae are seen. If a definitive diagnosis is not made with these measures, the carbon monoxide content of the air at the site of the poisoning should be measured.

The poisoned patient should be given 100% oxygen immediately, using a hyperbaric chamber if one is available. Blood transfusions and other supportive therapy should be provided. Patients usually die within 48–72 hours or recover completely. However, in a small percentage of patients organic mental changes, spasticity, choreoathetosis, cortical blindness and polyneuropathy appear as residual deficits.

Lead

Fortunately, lead is losing its position of pre-eminence as one of the commonest fatal intoxicants in the United States. Nonetheless, cases of lead poisoning continue to appear in infants and young children, mostly as a result of gnawing on articles painted with lead-containing paints. Many other causes are known, including insecticides, ointments, powders, liquids ingested from lead pipes and lead-containing fumes from storage batteries that are burned for fuel. Many of these agents are being eliminated from general use.

CLINICAL AND LABORATORY DIAGNOSIS.—Acute lead poisoning occurs rarely and then produces primarily gastrointestinal symptoms. *Chronic lead poisoning* causes a variety of neurologic and systemic signs, the major difference in adults and children being that polyneuropathy afflicts adults and encephalopathy afflicts children almost exclusively. Fundamental to an understanding of both the clinical signs and the management is the knowledge that severe cerebral edema occurs in most cases. Irritability and listlessness, followed by convulsions, hemiparesis or decerebrate rigidity commonly occur. Papilledema, bulging fontanel and suture separation reflect the increased intracranial pressure.

Careful routine laboratory studies often provide sufficient evidence for a diagnosis. Glycosuria, albuminuria and basophilic stippling of the erythrocytes on a blood smear are seen almost routinely. There is elevated pressure of the cerebro-

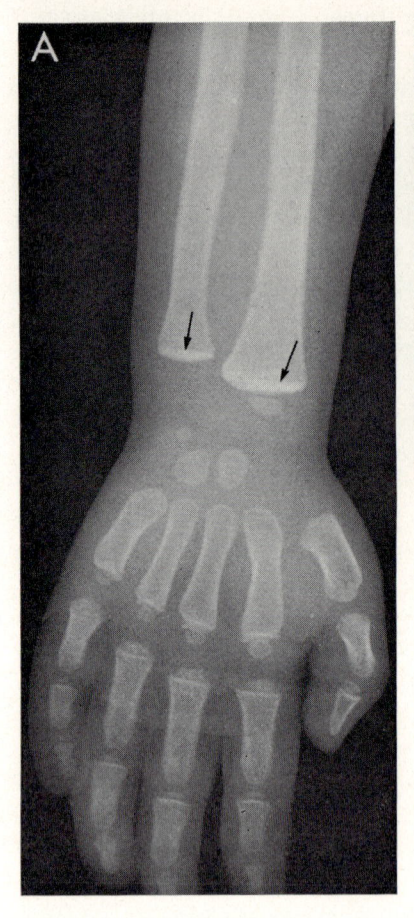

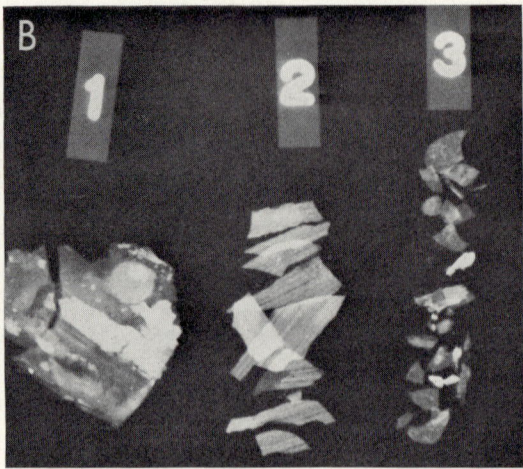

364 INTOXICATIONS AND ADVERSE REACTIONS TO THERAPY

Fig. 20.2.—Lead poisoning. Girl, 2, was admitted because of the sudden onset of an ocular squint. The parents reported that vomiting had occurred intermittently the past three months and had become more intense recently. Laboratory studies initially showed only persistent glycosuria without acetonuria, hyperglycemia or signs of dehydration. Shortly after admission she had her first seizure and then continued to have left-sided focal seizures. Examination revealed a comatose child with a flaccid left hemiparesis and a right sixth nerve palsy. The fundi appeared normal and there was moderate hepatomegaly. Lumbar puncture revealed clear, colorless fluid under 350 mm. H$_2$O with a protein content of 100 mg./100 ml. Wrist x-rays **(A)** revealed lines of increased density at the ends of the radii, and skull films showed suture separation. Diagnosis of lead poisoning was confirmed by x-rays of paint chips from the suspected source **(B)**. Despite extensive efforts to arrest the epileptic status and to reduce the cerebral edema medically the child died without recovering consciousness.

spinal fluid as well as an elevated protein content. X-rays show a line of increased density at the ends of the long bones (Fig. 20.2,*A*). Flecks of radiopaque lead can often be seen on a flat plate of the abdomen or in the paint chips from the suspected source (Fig. 20.2,*B*). Coproporphyrinuria can be demonstrated early in the course of lead poisoning with a qualitative or quantitative urine test (24-hour excretion of coproporphyrin over 250 μg.). Quantitative urinary lead determinations show elevated levels with this protean clinical picture. The differential diagnosis must include subdural hematoma, meningitis or encephalitis, brain tumor, other types of poisonings and the many other causes of seizures and acute neurologic deficit (Chapter 9). The physician should suspect lead poisoning in *any young child with a convulsion who has glycosuria, albuminuria, anemia or stippled red blood cells.*

MANAGEMENT AND PROGNOSIS.—If the patient has only mild symptoms, removal of the lead source constitutes sufficient therapy. In severe poisoning with encephalopathy, treatment is directed at (1) reducing cerebral edema (Appendix 2), (2) controlling convulsions (Appendix 1) and later (3) promoting lead excretion with chelating agents. Saline cathartics and enemas should be given before starting chelating therapy if lead flecks are seen on x-rays of the abdomen. The best current method of "deleading" the patient consists of giving EDTA (ethylenediaminetetracetic acid) or its analogue DTPA (diethylenetriaminepentacetic acid).

After much experience, Byers[9] recommends that EDTA, 75 mg./kg./day be given intramuscularly as 20% normal saline solution with 0.5% procaine. This treatment is continued for five days, then omitted for five days and then repeated for five days if the patient's symptoms persist or if the urinary coproporphyrin values remain high (250 μg./24 hours). Chisolm[14] has reported more rapid excretion of toxic metabolites with combined BAL (p. 360) and EDTA therapy than with EDTA alone. This therapy will remove most of the soft-tissue lead, but the metal fixed in bone is excreted slowly over a period of many months.

If the medical management of cerebral edema (Appendix 2) does not suffice, extensive surgical decompression has been advocated by Ingraham and Matson[36] and others.[32,48] Whether such heroic therapy reduces the mortality and morbidity rates is conjectural. Two-thirds of affected children die of lead encephalopathy, and many of the survivors have residual deficits, such as mental retardation, seizures and spastic weakness. The grave nature of this toxic syndrome calls for a total therapeutic effort by all of the specialists who might have something valuable to contribute to saving the patient's life.

Alcohols

ETHANOL.—Ethanol, the usual alcohol in beverages intended for consumption, is also found in varying concentrations in a variety of shaving lotions, perfumes, colognes, hair tonics, mouth washes and in some varnishes and shellacs. Children show a variable tolerance to ethanol, as do many adults, and some may be intoxicated by apparently small amounts. Clinical signs include lethargy, stupor, convulsions, coma and vomiting. These signs are very nonspecific when one considers all the other neurointoxicants that have similar manifestations. Unless what was ingested is known or an alcoholic odor to the breath is recognized, diagnosis may be difficult. The physician must learn to consider this diagnostic possibility, so that a blood alcohol determination may be made to provide definitive proof. Hypoglycemia, a common result of high ethanol intake, should alert one to the possibility of ethanol poisoning.

Only supportive treatment can be recommended, but this should include intravenous administration of 50% glucose for patients with hypoglycemia.

METHANOL.—Methyl alcohol (or wood alcohol) poisoning results from the ingestion of solvents for paints, shellacs, varnishes, canned fuels and nonpermanent antifreeze. The clinical signs resemble those of ethanol poisoning, but in addition most patients exhibit two other distinctive clinical features: *impairment of vision* and *metabolic acidosis*. (The latter results from the accumulation of formaldehyde and formic acid, oxidative products of methanol.) Diagnosis depends on the history of ingestion, the odor of methanol on the breath, severe acidosis and rapid loss of vision. Examination may reveal dilated, poorly reactive pupils, impaired acuity, papillitis and visual field constriction.

Treatment consists of good supportive care, including hydration (see Appendix

3), the administration of ethyl alcohol and treatment of acidosis (p. 374). Dialysis is now considered an effective way to rid the system of methanol.

ISOPROPANOL.—Isopropyl alcohol is most accessible to children in the form of rubbing alcohol and certain shaving or skin lotions. Intoxication with isopropanol produces the same clinical signs as poisoning with ethanol, but isopropanol possesses twice the toxicity. Hence, with the same dose patients may exhibit more severe nervous system depression. Acetonuria commonly results, inasmuch as the body converts isopropanol to acetone. However, acidosis is not usually found.

Good supportive care and proper hydration represent the only therapies.

Ethylene Glycol

Permanent antifreeze provides the commonest source of this intoxicant, though it is also widely used as an industrial solvent. Presumably the oxalic acid which is formed from ethylene glycol determines the toxicity. The clinical signs are essentially the same as those in severe ethanol poisoning. Renal insufficiency develops in the advanced stages of severe poisoning.

General supportive care is most important to insure recovery. Intravenous administration of ethanol is now recommended, and intravenous calcium gluconate is used to precipitate the toxic intermediary metabolite, oxalic acid.

Higher Alcohols, Glycols, Aldehydes, Ketones, Esters

The reader is referred to Done's[21] review of the toxicology and management of these various substances which form constituents of many solvents, fusel-oil, hydraulic brake fluid, some antifreezes, dry cleaning solvents, "meta fuel," "buzz bomb" fuel and "Jamaica ginger."

Kerosene

A large variety of petroleum distillates are used as fuels, solvents and lubricants, but kerosene will be discussed as the common prototype of these toxic substances.[21] Kerosene causes "chemical pneumonia" (both by its direct inhalation and by its pulmonary excretion) and has a narcotizing effect on the nervous system. The diagnosis is usually obvious because of the characteristic odor and x-ray evidence of a hilar and basilar bronchopneumonia.

The advisability or inadvisability of gastric lavage has been debated for years. Done[21] recommends lavage when (1) a large amount of material has been ingested or (2) the petroleum product has a potent narcotizing effect (benzine, gasoline). This would mean that patients who have ingested small amounts of kerosene should not have lavage. Vomiting should never be induced in these patients. Other forms of therapy are strictly supportive. Although antibiotics are commonly used in cases of chemical pneumonia, it seems likely that they do not affect the course of recovery.

Solvent Sniffing

The sniffing of glue or other volatile hydrocarbons has been practiced by young thrill-seekers for years and is for the most part innocuous. In the past few years "glue sniffers" have attained much notoriety with this habit, a sign of social maladjustment and not a major challenge to conventional medical therapy.[53]

Food Poisoning

Botulism

This rare but highly fatal type of poisoning results from eating improperly canned foods, particularly vegetables such as string beans and beets. The toxin of the organism Clostridium botulinum causes paralysis of both skeletal and smooth muscle. At first the patient may or may not have nausea, vomiting and either constipation or diarrhea, which are followed later by signs of bulbar palsy. Paralysis of both intrinsic and extrinsic ocular muscles is seen (loss of accommodation and convergence, diplopia and ptosis), together with dysphagia, dysarthria and chewing difficulty. Eventually weakness in the extremities appears, followed in severe cases by convulsions and coma. Neurologic symptoms and signs usually appear after a latent period of 12–15 hours. A definitive diagnosis is difficult to establish, but the ingestion of home-canned food followed by the typical clinical picture is most suggestive. The differential diagnosis must include bulbar poliomyelitis, myasthenia gravis and pontine encephalitis.

If the diagnosis is suspected strongly, the patient should be given polyvalent botulinus antitoxin after testing for horse-serum sensitivity. An immediate intravenous dose of 50,000 units of both type A and type B antitoxin is given, followed by daily doses of 10,000–20,000 units. As in the case of tetanus, the administered antitoxin can be expected to neutralize only the toxin which has *not* been fixed in nerve tissue. If the patient is seen early, which seldom happens, gastric lavage is carried out. Intensive supportive care is essential, much as in patients with bulbar poliomyelitis. The disease carries a fatality rate of 50–65%, death resulting from respiratory failure or pneumonia. Survivors recover completely.

Mushroom Poisoning

Many different species of mushrooms are intoxicating. Only some of these produce neurologic deficit. The reader is referred to another source for detailed information on different mushroom species.[21]

In most poisoned patients prominent gastrointestinal symptoms develop early, followed by muscarinic neurologic signs (sweating, salivation, bronchospasm, bradycardia, miosis, lacrimation) and sometimes convulsions and coma. Later diffuse liver, renal and cardiac insufficiency may develop.

Good supportive treatment is essential, and in most cases atropinization is beneficial. Atropine, 0.02 mg./kg., is given intravenously and the dose repeated at intervals, depending upon the patient's course.

Coyotillo

Karwinskia humboltiana is a poisonous shrub of the buckthorn family which grows in the southwestern United States and in central and northern Mexico. Ingestion of the berries from this plant causes a progressive, symmetrical polyneuropathy which starts in the lower limbs and ends with respiratory and bulbar paralysis. The clinical picture closely resembles the Guillain-Barré syndrome (Chapter 18), but the cerebrospinal fluid is normal. Surviving patients recover slowly and usually completely.[10a]

Shellfish

The reader is referred to Done's[21] review for a discussion of the rare neurointoxications which occasionally result from eating *shellfish* and certain *tropical fish*.

Spider Bites and Snake Bites

Arachnidism

Black widow spider bites cause 99% of cases of arachnidism, i.e., disease caused by spider bites.[35] In the United States this black insect has a "red hourglass" mark on the abdomen. Its venom causes severe local burning pain, followed by dizziness, weakness, abdominal cramping and boardlike rigidity of the abdominal muscles. The disorder must be differentiated from an acute abdominal catastrophe, tetanus, strychnine poisoning, lead colic and porphyria.

When the diagnosis is established, gradual but steady relief follows the intramuscular injection of an ampule (2.5 ml.) of antivenin (Lyovac Antivenin—Merck Sharp & Dohme). Bennett[5] states that among 1,300 cases the mortality rate varied from 2.4 to 6%. Other supportive therapy should be given, including adequate analgesia, hot baths, intravenous calcium gluconate, corticosteroids and opiates if necessary.

Tick Paralysis

The gravid female wood tick, Dermacentor andersoni, and the dog tick, Dermacentor variabilis, on rare occasions can cause poisoning. While the tick is embedded in the skin it injects its toxin and, when it is removed, the symptoms and signs clear rapidly. Prodromal symptoms of irritability and diarrhea develop 24 hours before a diffuse, slowly progressive, flaccid paralysis occurs. The weakness may be severe, spread to the bulbar musculature and abolish the deep tendon reflexes. The disorder closely resembles polyneuritis, epidural masses, bulbar poliomyelitis and other intoxications.

Removal of the tick is followed by prompt improvement. A drop of gasoline, kerosene or ether on the tick facilitates removal of the intact parasite. Good supportive care must be provided, especially if the bulbar or respiratory muscles are involved.

Snake Bites

PATHOGENESIS.—Most snakes are not venomous, and fatality rates from the bites of poisonous reptiles vary greatly around the world. In the United States and Europe less than 1% of persons bitten by venomous snakes die, whereas in places such as Brazil and Burma the fatality rate is much higher because of the greater number and potency of poisonous reptiles.

Most snake venoms contain a mixture of proteins and enzymes which poison the patient by virtue of their *necrotizing, neurotoxic* and *hemolyzing* properties.

The natural habitat of poisonous snakes determines the geographic incidence and type of venomous bites. In the United States most poisonings result from bites by the pit vipers (rattlesnakes, water moccasins and copperheads). Occasionally coral snake bites are encountered in the southern tier of states.

CLINICAL DIAGNOSIS.—*Pit viper* venom has strong necrotizing and hemolyzing properties and may cause circulatory collapse. The patient usually suffers immediate and severe local pain, swelling with necrosis appearing later. Hematemesis, bloody diarrhea, convulsions and circulatory collapse constitute the systemic reactions.

Coral snake bites occur less commonly and cause little local pain or swelling. The systemic reactions are primarily neurotoxic. Within 10–15 minutes diffuse numbness and weakness develop, followed by ataxia, ptosis, nonreacting pupils, dysarthria and dysphagia. In severe cases coma, convulsions and respiratory arrest ensue, with death occurring within eight to 72 hours.

The severity of any poisonous bite is greater in the case of (1) children, (2) a bite on the trunk or face, (3) a large snake whose venom glands are full (spring more than fall), (4) associated clostridium wound infections and (5) excess exercise after the bite.

MANAGEMENT AND PROGNOSIS.—As indicated above, most snake bites fortunately are not poisonous, and the fatality rate is low even with poisonous types. *If progressive, local pain and edema or systemic numbness and weakness do not develop within 20 minutes, one can almost assume that the bite is probably not poisonous.* The most important therapy for poisonous snake bites consists of (1) immobilization of the patient (with splinting if the bite is on an extremity), (2) administration of antivenin and (3) proper supportive care, including analgesics (aspirin, Demerol), sedatives (barbiturates but not morphine), treatment of shock, anticonvulsants, artificial respiration if necessary, tetanus toxoid or antiserum and antibiotics. Use of adrenal corticosteroids will help to prevent reactions to horse serum in sensitive patients, but their specific value for snake bites has never been demonstrated.

The value of tourniquets, incision and suction, and local cooling of the bite area is a matter of controversy among experts. Opinions abound but data are lacking. Despite the lack of a consensus, we would recommend that a tourniquet be used intermittently in the field, but not after the patient gets to the hospital. Incision and suction are probably useful if the incision is made carefully only through the skin and if suction is applied along with gentle finger massage. Local cooling (not extreme cold or freezing) may have value if a delay as long as eight hours in giving antivenin is anticipated.[62]

Pit viper antivenin is available as Antivenin Crotalidae Polyvalent (Wyeth)—North and South American antisnakebite serum.

Coral snake antivenin is now commercially available as Antivenin, Micrurus fulvius, Monovalent (Wyeth). It can be obtained through state departments of health in areas where coral snake bites occur, from the nearest zookeeper or from the manufacturer in Marietta, Pennsylvania.

The patient is given 3–5 ampules of antivenin intramuscularly or intravenously, depending upon the severity of the bite. Repeated doses are given according to the progression of toxic signs. Some workers advocate local infiltration of 10 ml. of antiserum around the wound if it can be given within two hours after the bite.

Adverse Reactions to Therapy

Today's practicing physician has at his fingertips a vast number of drugs, diets, hormones, antibiotics and assorted chemicals. The range of toxicity and adverse reactions to these substances is not well understood in many cases, despite the

TABLE 20.3.—Neurologic Complications of Systemic Therapy

Therapy	Clinical Symptoms and Signs	Mechanism
Antimicrobials		
Gantrisin (prematures)	Kernicterus	Hyperbilirubinemia
Streptomycin	Deafness and ataxia	Eighth nerve toxicity
PAS	Psychosis	Direct neurotoxicity
Tetracyclines	Increased intracranial pressure	Cerebral edema
INH	Seizures, psychosis, neuropathy, ataxia	Direct neurotoxicity
Water and Electrolytes		
Too much H$_2$O, too little sodium	Seizures (A.T.E.*)	Hypervolemia and hyponatremia, cerebral edema
Too much sodium	Muscular twitching, convulsions	Hypernatremia, intracranial hemorrhage, severe vascular congestion
Hormones		
Adrenal corticosteroids: prolonged, high-dose therapy	Seizures (A.T.E.*) Weakness	Hypertension and cerebral edema "Cortisone myopathy"
Insulin treatment of diabetes mellitus	Seizures, mental retardation	Hypoglycemia
Anticancer Drugs		
Vincristine, vinblastine	Peripheral neuropathy†	Direct neurotoxicity
6-Mercaptopurine	Encephalomalacia	Cerebrovascular accident
Diets and Supplements		
Cow's milk formula	Tetany or seizures Hypocalcemia	High phosphorus content Transient hypoparathyroidism
?Cow's milk formula	Mental retardation	High calcium content ?Vitamin D hypersensitivity
Vitamin K (prematures)	Kernicterus (athetosis, rigidity)	Hyperbilirubinemia
Miscellaneous		
Mercury: metallic mercury in powders, ointments, disinfectants	Irritability, personality changes, neuropathy	Direct neurotoxicity
Antimigraine therapy: methysergide (Sansert)	Urinary and cardiac complaints, insomnia, confusion	Arteritis and regional fibrosis
Oxygen		
Excessive O$_2$ in prematures	Blindness	Retrolental fibroplasia
Vigorous mechanical ventilation in chronic pulmonary disease	Seizures, coma, chorea	Induction of alkalosis
Horse antiserum	Brachial plexus neuritis	?Horse serum sensitivity

*A.T.E. = Acute toxic encephalopathy (Chapter 8)
†Pain, weakness, hyporeflexia, atrophy

extravagant claims by some manufacturers. For this reason we would like to recommend strongly that the reader become aware of "disease of treatment," a concept well formulated by Lasagna[40] and others, and that he follow the ancient hippocratic warning, ". . . as to diseases, make a habit of two things—to help, or *at least to do no harm.*"

The material which follows covers the neurologic complications of systemic therapy. The textual data are summarized in Table 20.3 (p. 370). Complications which result from the treatment of various neurologic diseases are covered in their respective chapters.

Sedatives

All the widely used agents—the barbiturates, narcotics, tranquilizers and anticonvulsants—have a primary depressant effect upon the central nervous system. The action of barbiturates will be discussed in general terms as the prototype. The manifestations and treatment of sedatives which have specific neurologic effects will be outlined briefly.

Barbiturates

CLINICAL AND LABORATORY DIAGNOSIS.—Patients exhibit varying degrees of somnolence, stupor and coma, depending upon the type of barbiturate, the amount ingested and time elapsed since ingestion. A number of workers have recommended the categorization of poisonings into mild, moderate and severe to sharpen the diagnostic focus and to aid in treatment and prognosis. Mildly intoxicated patients are drowsy and slightly disoriented and show poor judgment, slurred speech, a drunken gait and nystagmus. Moderately intoxicated patients can be aroused only with vigorous stimulation. They lose the deep tendon reflexes but retain the corneal reflexes and exhibit shallow respirations. The severely poisoned patient is deeply comatose, unresponsive, sometimes cyanotic, has slow, shallow respirations and no corneal or gag reflexes. The pupils are small and react to light, but in asphyxiated patients the pupils become dilated and unreactive, an ominous sign.

Clinically, barbiturate poisoning cannot be differentiated from other causes of central nervous system depression, and for this reason blood barbiturate levels have importance in therapy. The correlation of coma with the blood barbiturate level varies with the specific agent involved: coma occurs at about 2 mg./100 ml. with secobarbital (Seconal) or pentobarbital (Nembutal), 3 mg./100 ml. with amobarbital (Amytal) and 6 mg./100 ml. with phenobarbital. The electroencephalogram has no appreciable diagnostic value since the superimposed 20–25 cycles/second fast activity may result from a variety of other sedative drugs. However, Hockaday and associates[34] have suggested that in the comatose patient with fixed, dilated pupils, whose vital signs are being maintained with artificial respiration and pressor drugs, the "flat" electroencephalogram with loss of distinguishable wave forms may provide one of the most reliable signs of irreversible brain damage. These patients, who also have markedly elevated CSF protein values, have suffered severe asphyxia and do not recover. (See Chapter 12, p. 120.)

MANAGEMENT AND PROGNOSIS.—All of the general measures previously outlined, including (1) maintenance of oxygenation, (2) prevention of further drug absorption and (3) treatment of circulatory collapse, are essential for survival of these patients. Specific therapy of barbiturate poisoning in selected cases is directed at (1) the administration of central nervous system stimulants or analeptics, a treatment over which there is considerable controversy and (2) dialysis and urea-induced diuresis to hasten elimination of the drug. In general, analeptic therapy, e.g., with bemegride (Megimide), pictrotoxin or Metrazol, is contraindicated in patients with mild or moderate degrees of intoxication because of the risk of convulsions from these powerful stimulants of the cerebral cortex. Megimide may be given to severely poisoned patients in amounts sufficient to improve ventilation, but its ability to alter the mortality rate remains doubtful.[18] In no case should analeptic drugs be allowed to reduce the intensity of supportive care.

Dialysis, using either the peritoneal method or the artificial kidney, may hasten the elimination of barbiturate in badly intoxicated patients who are not responding to the above measures. The administration of urea and alkalization of the urine (with lactate) causes an osmotic diuresis in the case of phenobarbital (but not with most other barbiturates used in the United States) and this in turn hastens excretion. Myschetzky and Lassen[50] have outlined the details of the latter treatment, which can be used in conjunction with both general measures and dialysis.

Barbiturate-induced coma has a mortality rate of at least 5%, and death usually occurs in three to four days. Patients who recover from this type of poisoning usually have no residual neurologic deficit. Isolated patients who die of complications of barbiturate poisoning have shown laminar cortical necrosis and degeneration—classic neuropathologic signs of anoxia.[58]

Narcotics and Potent Analgesics

Narcotics and potent analgesics in widespread use, such as codeine, meperidine (Demerol) and dextropropoxyphene (Darvon), have primarily depressant action but occasionally cause excitation of the central nervous system (fasciculations and convulsions). Consequently the clinical manifestations of narcotic poisoning closely resemble those of the barbiturates.

In the mildly or moderately intoxicated patient only good supportive care is given. In the severely poisoned patient, and *only in those with signs of severe poisoning,* the narcotic antagonists, nalorphine (Nalline) and levallorphan (Lorfan), counteract the signs of central nervous system depression effectively. An intravenous dose of Nalline (0.1 mg./kg.) or Lorfan (0.02 mg./kg.) is given and can be repeated in 15 minutes if no improvement is seen. Repeated doses every two to three hours may be required. The reader should understand that the narcotic antagonists may aggravate the depressant effect of the poisonous narcotic if the patient is only mildly or moderately intoxicated or if the patient is depressed for other reasons. These agents should be used only in the severely narcotized patient.

Phenothiazine Tranquilizers

All of these agents in sufficient dose cause central nervous system depression resembling that described for barbiturates. They also have the capacity to increase the frequency of seizures in known epileptics and to initiate seizures in a patient without a prior history of convulsions.[11,39,57a] Some of the phenothiazines also cause a peculiar type of dystonia or athetosis which may be confused diagnostically with meningitis, encephalitis, seizure, spasmodic torticollis, bulbar poliomyelitis, tetanus, hysteria or poisoning with strychnine. Ayd[3] has reviewed this complication among 3,775 patients treated with phenothiazines, 1,472 of whom developed extrapyramidal signs: 21.5% had akathisia (inability to sit still), 15.4% had parkinsonism and 2.3% dyskinesia. Agents which have caused this dystonic syndrome include: prochlorperazine (Compazine), chlorpromazine (Thorazine), perphenazine (Trilafon), triflupromazine (Vesprin), mepazine (Pacatal), thiopropazate (Dartal), fluphenazine (Permitil, Prolixin) and trifluoperazine (Stelazine). This reaction has been seen most frequently in young children as a result of Compazine therapy to prevent vomiting. It should be clearly understood that the extrapyramidal signs which complicate long-term phenothiazine administration may persist permanently.[3,26,33,56]

Recognition of the true nature of the drug-induced dystonia is most important since the problem is usually self-limiting and clears spontaneously. A urinary ferric chloride test in the presence of phenothiazines produces a peach or lavender color, but care must be taken to distinguish this positive reaction from other "positive ferric chloride" tests caused by aspirin, acetone and phenylpyruvic acid (PKU). The toxic extrapyramidal syndrome is often alleviated dramatically by giving an intravenous dose of diphenhydramine (Benadryl)[61] (Table 20.2, p. 359).

The long-term, high-dose administration of chlorpromazine (Thorazine) has been associated with the occurrence of convulsions, often in known epileptics, but also in patients who have not had seizures previously. This toxic effect should be borne in mind when Thorazine is given to patients with epilepsy or chronic mental illness.

Stimulants

Amphetamine Derivatives and Xanthines

Widely used as "pep pills," "mood elevators" and appetite suppressants, these stimulants have accounted for an increasing number of poisonings. The agents most commonly incriminated are amphetamine sulfate (Benzedrine), dextroamphetamine sulfate (Dexedrine), dextroamphetamine combined with amobarbital (Dexamyl) and phenmetrazine (Preludin), but a number of other related compounds have been marketed. Toxic signs include those of central nervous system stimulation—hyperactivity, delirium and in severe cases convulsions—along with evidence of sympathetic nervous system stimulation—tachycardia, hypertension, sweating and arrhythmias.

In the mildly or moderately poisoned patient no specific therapy is usually required, except that the child should be prevented from injurying or mutilating himself. Barbiturates have been used to quiet these patients, but one must guard against overtreatment and a resulting delayed depressant reaction. More recently, intramuscular administration of chlorpromazine (Thorazine), 1–2 mg./kg., has produced striking reversal of the behavioral disturbances with a less noticeable effect upon the sympathomimetic signs.[25a] This dose may be repeated several times if necessary.

If one is treating a combined intoxication due to amphetamine-barbiturate (e.g., Dexamyl) with chlorpromazine, special caution must be used to avoid overtreatment because it is well known that chlorpromazine potentiates the action of barbiturates. As a result, serious hypotension and apnea may be encountered. In such cases, half the above dose is recommended.

Salicylates

Aspirin and oil of wintergreen are the common causes of salicylism. Convulsions and CNS respiratory depression, along with vomiting and hyperventilation, occur quite often in children with severe salicylism.[20] Practically speaking, most children (in contrast to adults) have reached a state of metabolic acidosis by the time the blood pH and CO_2 are measured. Although at first one finds evidence of respiratory alkalosis, it can be assumed that any young child with severe symptoms six to eight hours after ingestion of the drug and a *serum CO_2 content less than 10 mEq./L.* is suffering from significant acidosis.[22] In addition to the acid-base disturbances, severe poisoning in children is accompanied by dehydration, loss of potassium and, in some cases, by hyponatremia. A urine ferric chloride test in which the purple color does *not* disappear from a previously boiled urine specimen (as it does in a test for acetone) indicates the presence of salicylates. However, one must depend upon (1) a quantitative serum level of salicylates and (2) the time elapsed since ingestion to evaluate the severity of the poisoning.[19]

Therapy after instituting the necessary supportive measures: (1) treat shock if necessary (Appendix 4), (2) establish urine flow (Appendix 3), (3) start maintenance fluid therapy (Appendix 3), (4) treat severe acidosis if present by adding 7.5 mEq. of sodium bicarbonate (8.5 ml. of 7.5% solution) to 500 ml. of "electrolyte 75" solution (Appendix 3). These measures usually suffice to correct the acidosis and dehydration, but their efficacy should be checked by repeating the blood chemistries. In cases of extreme acidosis in which limited amounts of sodium must be given (cardiac and renal insufficiency), one may give the alkalinizing agent tromethamine (THAM) in an intravenous dose of 5 ml./kg. of 0.3 molar solution. *Convulsions* are managed as outlined in Appendix 1. If *tetany* complicates alkali therapy, one should stop the alkalinizing agents, give a dose of calcium gluconate intravenously and try CO_2 inhalation. Severe *CNS respiratory depression* must be managed as outlined under General Manifestations and Therapy.

Antimicrobials

Tetracyclines

The antibiotics of this group, including oxytetracycline (Terramycin) and tetracycline (Achromycin), are employed much less widely than they were 10 years ago, but still enjoy wide enough usage for physicians to be aware of their toxicity. We shall consider only the sign of neurologic toxicity—"bulging fontanel." A number of articles in the literature report this reaction to the tetracyclines.[27] Presumably this sign results from transient increased pressure or "pseudotumor cerebri," although the evidence for actual increased intracranial pressure is poorly documented and its pathogenesis is not understood. Nonetheless the problem must be recognized and differentiated from other acute causes of intracranial hypertension, such as meningitis, subdural hematoma, tumor, etc. (Chapter 8). The problem subsides quickly when the drug is stopped, and no other treatment is required.

Penicillin

Rarely patients who receive penicillin in extremely high doses (usually intravenously) will show neurotoxic signs. Most often they have generalized seizures[7,52] associated with transient EEG abnormalities. In some, psychotic mental states and stupor have been reported.[59] Most observers think that such reactions have a toxic basis because the convulsant effect of experimental penicillin lesions in an animal's brain is well known.

Less often anaphylactic reactions to penicillin have led to acute and chronic organic mental syndromes.[15]

Isoniazid (INH)

Isoniazid enjoys widespread use because of its effectiveness in the treatment of tuberculosis. However, a wide variety of neurotoxic signs have been attributed to this drug and have been well documented. These neurotoxic manifestations include (1) peripheral neuropathy,[17] (2) psychosis, (3) convulsions,[42,55] (4) diffuse encephalopathy[1,2] and (5) the syndrome of neuromyelitis optica.[17] The physician must be aware that the drug can cause various central and peripheral neurologic signs. The CSF findings are usually normal, and the electroencephalogram shows nonspecific abnormalities.

Chronic neurologic toxicity is treated by prompt withdrawal of the drug. Acute poisoning with INH is managed with good general supportive care and measures to lessen chances for absorption (emesis or gastric lavage) and to hasten excretion (dialysis and exchange transfusion[38]).

Patients who survive acute or mild chronic intoxications usually recover completely. However, severe permanent damage to the nervous system has been reported in many patients with chronic poisoning.

Nitrofurantoin (Furadantin)

This drug has enjoyed widespread use for the treatment of genitourinary infections because it causes relatively few systemic toxic effects and because resistant strains do not commonly result. However, prolonged usage, especially in patients with impaired renal function, readily produces peripheral neuropathy.[16,25,40a,43] Painful extremities, paresthesias, weakness, hyporeflexia and atrophy are seen. Discontinuation usually eliminates the sensory complaints, but the motor deficit may be irreversible.

Streptomycin

No problems are seen when streptomycin is given for periods up to 10-14 days. Prolonged use (four to six weeks) of full doses for diseases such as tuberculosis carries the risk of eighth nerve damage. Tinnitus, vertigo, progressive nerve deafness, nystagmus and ataxia develop. Once the neurologic signs are established, one can expect little or no functional recovery. Most of the neurologic deficit is irreversible, as reflected by persistent deafness and ataxia with an absent labyrinthine response (nystagmus) when the ear is irrigated with ice water.

Kanamycin

Although this drug has been used for a relatively short time, it is apparent that it has neurotoxic properties that resemble those of streptomycin. It can cause eighth nerve damage with symptoms and signs of vertigo, tinnitus and deafness. Kanamycin in full therapeutic doses for 10–12 days in infancy apparently does not cause eighth nerve deficit which is apparent after a follow-up of five years.[24] An unusual case of kanamycin-induced peripheral neuropathy following the instillation of the drug into the epidural space after a lumbar disk operation has been reported.[29]

Gantrisin

Like other substances, such as synthetic vitamin K analogs, Gantrisin potentiates the development of hyperbilirubinemia in the premature (Chapter 23). It does not apparently have neurotoxic properties in older infants and children.

Chloroquine

This agent is one of the more effective antimalarial drugs now in use and is also employed in the treatment of amebiasis, rheumatoid arthritis and some skin disorders. Myopathy (potentially reversible) and peripheral neuropathy (weakness, EMG abnormalities and typical muscle biopsy changes) have been attributed to prolonged use of the drug.[23]

Water and Electrolyte Therapy

Water Intoxication and Hyponatremia

Children are easily overloaded with water and depleted of salt (sodium) when parenteral fluids are given to correct losses from dehydration, operation or any severe prolonged illness. The resulting hypervolemia and hyponatremia may cause cerebral edema with clinical symptoms.

The same end result has been reported repeatedly in patients with a variety of central nervous system infections (meningitis, severe anomaly and metastatic malignancy) and certain pulmonary diseases (bronchogenic carcinoma and tuberculosis).[12,46,47,51,57] In most of the latter cases the hyponatremia and concentrated urine have been attributed to an "inappropriate secretion of ADH" (antidiuretic hormone), but the mechanisms of simple water intoxication or "cerebral salt wasting" have been implicated in some patients.

Clinical signs in patients with water intoxication and hyponatremia include mental confusion, stupor or coma, and convulsions. One must be careful not to attribute the signs and symptoms of the central nervous system disease (usually meningitis in children) to the disturbance of salt and water metabolism, because the treatment is obviously different. There are abnormally low serum sodium and chloride values and hypertonic urine (measured roughly by a high specific gravity or more accurately by osmolality).

These patients usually respond promptly and well to a sharp limitation of water intake and administration of a 3% sodium chloride solution. A safe rule-of-thumb dosage for 3% sodium chloride would be 0.6 × weight in kilograms × 7.5. The sodium chloride is given in a small volume of water over a period of not more than an hour. Serial electrolyte determinations should be obtained during the course of therapy. Although patients usually recover completely from water intoxication, permanent brain damage can occur.[41]

Hypernatremia

Hypernatremia which is severe enough to cause brain changes is seen with accidental salt poisoning and hypertonic dehydration. One finds widespread vascular dilatation and congestion, subarachnoid and intracerebral hemorrhage and dural sinus thrombosis. These findings have been well documented by Finberg and associates,[28,45] and the clinical conclusions are supported by experimental observations.[45a]

Widespread muscular twitching, especially of the eyelids and face, and convulsions constitute the usual neurologic signs. Vomiting, severe thirst and respiratory distress in infants also occur. By definition, an elevated serum sodium level is diagnostic of the disorder. In the series of Finberg and associates[28] results of serum sodium determinations among the symptomatic and fatal cases varied from 164 to 244 mEq./L.

Hypernatremia with neurologic signs which results from an overload of salt constitutes an urgent medical problem. Experience suggests that peritoneal dialysis with 5-8% glucose-water solution reduces serum sodium levels quite effectively, provided proper technique is used.[28] Affected infants should be given low-electrolyte solutions (oral or parenteral), since they are often dehydrated by the time treatment is started. The physician should not use such intensive therapy for the more commonly seen hypernatremia—that of hypertonic dehydration.

Hormones

Adrenal Corticosteroids

These agents can cause both cerebral edema and myopathy when given in large doses for prolonged periods. The recognition and treatment of cerebral edema is covered in Chapter 8.

Cortisone myopathy, an adverse reaction which is not well understood, causes scattered degeneration and regeneration of muscle fibers without signs of inflammation—changes which resemble those in chloroquine myopathy. The patient's symptoms and signs disappear within a few weeks after the steroid therapy is stopped, and no other therapy is needed.

Insulin

Insulin therapy can cause hypoglycemia in any diabetic. In "brittle" childhood diabetes one may encounter the difficult problem of hypoglycemia, which, in turn, causes the seizures and signs of permanent brain damage (behavior disorders or mental retardation). This complication of insulin treatment usually reflects the severity of the disease rather than therapeutic indiscretion.

Anticancer Drugs

With the advent of a growing number of potent chemicals for the treatment of neuroblastoma, Wilms' tumor, leukemia and some brain tumors in children, it has become apparent that some of these agents have a destructive, toxic effect upon nerve tissue. Peripheral neuropathy (painful weakness, hyporeflexia and atrophy) has resulted from the use of vincristine and vinblastine.[49] For reasons that are not clear, sensory symptoms apparently affect adults more often than children. Greenhouse et al.[32a] reported widespread encephalomalacia following the heroic attempt to treat a glioblastoma with intracarotid methotrexate. Only time will tell whether some of the other new potent oncolytic agents will exhibit neurotoxic properties.

Whenever these powerful chemicals are used the patient should be watched closely and therapy discontinued if significant signs of neurotoxicity develop. Obviously, the risk of inducing neuropathy in patients with cancer is worth taking because the tumors being treated are usually lethal.

Immunizations

Convulsions which occur within hours of routine immunization with DPT (diphtheria-pertussis-tetanus) vaccine have been noted infrequently. It is generally accepted that pertussis is the offending agent in the triple vaccine. The universal use of the vaccine and the rarity of this neurologic complication make one wonder, of course, whether a cause and effect relationship exists. However, the persistent seizures and permanent neurologic deficit which have been seen by careful observers in children who were apparently previously well must be regarded seriously.[10] When convulsions complicate DPT immunizations, no further pertussis immunization should be carried out and diphtheria and tetanus toxoids should be given alone.

Diets and Supplements

Cow's Milk

PATHOGENESIS.—Hypercalcemia, which is sometimes associated with mental retardation, has been reported frequently in the United Kingdom but rarely in the United States. The basic cause for this disease is unknown, but several hypotheses have been suggested. One is the excessive dietary ingestion of calcium; nearly all reported patients have been drinking cow's milk, which contains four to five times more calcium than human milk. Another is a hypersensitivity to vitamin D. Whether and how this disorder is related to the hypercalcemia in children with structural anomalies of the cardiovascular system (Chapter 13) is conjectural. See Chapter 2 for a discussion of neonatal tetany.

CLINICAL AND LABORATORY DIAGNOSIS.—This disease manifests itself in early infancy with nonspecific signs and symptoms, including anorexia, vomiting, growth failure, hypotonia, constipation and irritability. Some authors have suggested that affected babies have a characteristic "elfin" facies with prominent upper lip and epicanthic folds, drooping lower lid and nostrils pointing forward. Mental retardation occurs in most affected infants.

All patients have hypercalcemia (serum calcium 12–18 mg./100 ml.) and some show bands of increased density in the metaphyses of long bones. Some exhibit osteosclerotic changes at the base of the skull around the orbits. As an associated complication a few patients have "base-losing nephritis" or renal acidosis with alkaline urine, hyperchloremia, low serum pH and low serum carbonate (Lightwood syndrome).

MANAGEMENT AND PROGNOSIS.—Therapy is directed primarily at lowering the serum calcium levels. This is effected by placing infants on a special low-calcium formula, such as Locasol.* Vitamin D supplements are withheld. Oral administration of sodium sulfate may be helpful in diminishing the intestinal absorption of calcium. Adrenal corticosteroid therapy has value in lowering serum calcium levels, but one must weigh carefully the benefit it brings against the side effects of continued use. The vigor of therapy can be relaxed if and when the metabolic derangements are corrected.

Parents must be made aware of the likelihood of mental retardation in most of these babies.

Vitamin K

Vitamin K, used to prevent hemolytic disease of the newborn, potentiates the development of hyperbilirubinemia in the premature by causing hemolysis. The hyperbilirubinemia can cause kernicterus.

The diagnosis and management of hyperbilirubinemia with kernicterus are discussed in Chapter 23 (p. 474).

Vitamin A

Intoxications with vitamin A usually occur when infants are mistakenly given teaspoonful quantities of dropper vitamin preparations or when adolescents (usually girls) receive inordinately large amounts of the vitamin for the treatment of acne.[49a] The neurologic syndrome of pseudotumor (increased intracranial pressure without localizing signs) results. The patient often appears surprisingly well despite the increased pressure, in contrast to many other conditions which elevate intracranial pressure. Headache, diplopia, papilledema, sixth nerve palsy, separated sutures and, in infants, a bulging fontanel are commonly seen. Cracking and peeling of the skin provides ancillary evidence of vitamin A intoxication (Fig. 20.3). An awareness of this drug-induced form of pseudotumor cerebri is the physician's greatest responsibility, since the diagnostic and therapeutic management should be restricted to discontinuation of the vitamin preparation.

Miscellaneous

Aminophylline

Among the stimulants classified as xanthines (caffeine, theophylline and theobromine), aminophylline causes more intoxications among children than all the

---

*Locasol is manufactured by Trufood Ltd., Wrenbury, Nantwich, Cheshire, England.

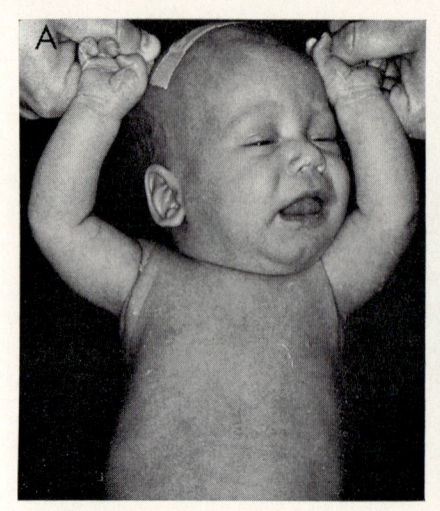

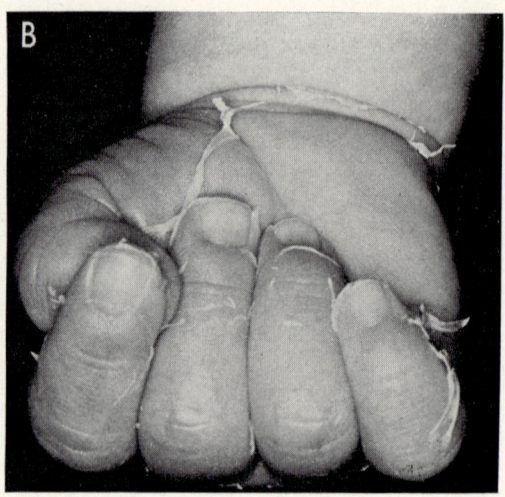

Fig. 20.3.—Vitamin A intoxication. This 9-week-old boy had been completely well until six days before this photograph was taken, when he became increasingly irritable and anorectic. At the same time the parents noted that the skin was peeling and the urine was dark yellow. Examination showed an irritable baby with a bulging fontanel (A) and peeling skin (B). In addition, the head transilluminated excessively. Further history-taking revealed he had been receiving 12,000 units of vitamin A daily (normal requirement, 1,500). Serum carotene level was 140 gammas/100 ml. (normal, 40–150). The baby's general behavior returned to normal completely in about two weeks.

others. Aminophylline is a combination of the stimulant theophylline and the solvent ethylenediamine, and it is widely used in children with bronchial asthma, asthmatic bronchitis and acute bronchiolitis. Toxic levels are reached because it is often administered in a rectal suppository form to patients who are vomiting, and therefore many cases of aminophylline intoxication must be classed as iatrogenic. Further, the toxic effects of the compound resemble closely the signs of the diseases which it is intended to alleviate—asthma and bronchitis—thereby causing dangerous clinical confusion. Restlessness, delirium and convulsions, together with vomiting (occasionally blood or "coffee-ground"), dyspnea and fever occur. The patients may have clinical signs of cerebral edema, with elevated CSF pressure, diffuse, slow wave EEG abnormalities, central respiratory failure and circulatory collapse. The clinical differentiation from other causes of acute increased intracranial pressure and convulsions may be difficult if the physician is not familiar with the syndrome of aminophylline or theophylline poisoning.

CASE EXAMPLE

A 5½-month-old boy was hospitalized because of crouplike symptoms. Three days previously dyspnea, wheezing and cough had developed. Despite intensive therapy with steam and antibiotics the baby had not improved. In the hospital he was given aspirin, Tedral and potassium iodide solution. The Tedral was given in a dose of one-half teaspoon (theophylline 32 mg.) every four hours. About 24 hours later vomiting of "coffee-ground" material which contained blood occurred, temperature was 106 F., and the baby became stuporous. After another 24 hours, right focal motor seizures began. He had become comatose with persistent dyspnea during this time. Spinal and subdural taps gave negative findings. Intravenous administration of calcium gluconate, phenobarbital and urea brought about an equivocal response. Then the Tedral therapy was stopped.

During the next 24 hours the baby became more alert and less dyspneic. He had no more seizures.

Most important in therapy are discontinuation of the drug and good supportive care. Small doses of anticonvulsants (phenobarbital and paraldehyde) may be given to control seizures.

Mercury

Chronic mercury poisoning in children has been seen with diminishing frequency in the United States because of the greatly reduced medicinal use of mercury. Exposure usually results from mercury-containing powders, ammoniated mercury ointment, merthiolate applications in the mouth and use of calomel (HgCl) as a laxative.

In milder poisonings only gastrointestinal symptoms, such as anorexia, abdominal pain, vomiting, gingivitis and stomatitis are seen. In more severe intoxications neurologic signs become prominent. Personality changes, irritability and psychotic behavior occur commonly. The saying "mad as a hatter" probably results from the regular industrial use of metallic mercury in the manufacture of felt hats. We have seen one psychotic "hatter" who was suffering from mercury poisoning. Ataxia, signs of peripheral neuropathy and coarse tremors are characteristic of this intoxication.

The etiology of the syndrome *acrodynia* (pink disease) was cloaked in mystery for many years until Warkany and Hubbard[60] showed that most cases result from chronic exposure to mercury. Acrodynia is characterized by pinkish discoloration and peeling of the skin, perspiration, painful extremities, paresis and areflexia, and marked irritability. Some workers have suggested that this syndrome results from a peculiar sensitivity to mercury rather than an overt intoxication.

Patients with chronic mercury poisoning usually improve when the source of exposure is removed. In patients with severe symptoms, treatment with BAL (p. 360) or EDTA (p. 365) may hasten improvement.

Methysergide (Sansert)

The use of this drug for the treatment of migraine headaches cannot be recommended despite its effectiveness in some patients when given prophylactically. Graham and co-workers[31] have pointed out that its capacity to cause retroperitoneal fibrosis, a serious complication, is a contraindication to its use unless the patient's symptoms are incapacitating enough to warrant the risk. Fibrotic lesions accompanied by a marked arteritis have also been noted.[8] Speculation suggests that the vasoconstrictive properties of the drug cause vascular spasm, arteritis and regional fibrosis, but this theory has not been proved. However, it is known that with discontinuation of Sansert the symptoms clear and many of the signs regress. If this drug is used, the patient should be examined every three to four months for heart murmurs, friction rubs, symptoms of renal disease and bruits over major vessels. Friedman and Elkind[30] also report psychologic side effects, such as insomnia, feelings of unreality, confusion and nervousness.

Oxygen

The prolonged administration of oxygen to small premature infants for respiratory distress or as a prophylactic measure may cause retrolental fibroplasia. For many years this problem grew in importance at the same time that a greater number of prematures were surviving with partial or complete blindness. All premature nurseries now carefully restrict oxygen therapy to prevent this tragic disease. However, Silverman[57b] observed several cases of retrolental fibroplasia in very small infants who received only brief exposure to oxygen, suggesting that all cases may not result from excessive oxygen therapy.

The too-rapid correction of hypercapnia in patients with chronic pulmonary disease is discussed in Chapter 23.

Antiserum

Antitoxin made with horse serum is commonly used for the treatment of tetanus. This therapy often causes "serum sickness" and, much less commonly, anaphylactic deaths. The reader is reminded here that on rare occasions a *neuritis* complicates antiserum therapy. This neuritis has a peculiar predilection for the brachial plexis, particularly the fifth and sixth cervical roots, with the shoulder girdle, arm and hand being affected in that order of frequency.[4] No specific therapy alters the clinical course of recovery.

BIBLIOGRAPHY

1. Adams, B. G., and Davies, B. M.: Neurological changes associated with P.A.S. and I.N.A.H. therapy, J. Ment. Sc. 107:943, 1961.
2. Adams, P., and White, C.: Isoniazid-induced encephalopathy, Lancet 1:680, 1965.
3. Ayd, F. J.: A survey of drug-induced extrapyramidal reactions, J.A.M.A. 175:1054, 1961.
4. Bardenwerper, H. W.: Serum neuritis from tetanus antitoxin, J.A.M.A. 179:763, 1962.
5. Bennett, I. L.: Spiders, scorpions, insects and other arthropods, in Harrison, T. R. (ed.): *Principles of Internal Medicine* (5th ed.; New York City: McGraw-Hill Book Company, Inc., 1966).
6. Berkley, M. C., and Magee, K. R.: Neuropathy following exposure to dimethylamine salt of 2,4-D, Arch. Int. Med. 111:351, 1963.
7. Bloomer, H. A., et al.: Penicillin-induced encephalopathy in uremic patients, J.A.M.A. 200:121, 1967.
8. Buenger, R. E., and Hunter, J. A.: Reversible mesenteric artery stenoses due to methysergide maleate, J.A.M.A. 198:558, 1966.
9. Byers, R. K.: Lead poisoning, Pediatrics 23:585, 1959.
10. Byers, R. K., and Moll, F. C.: Encephalopathies following prophylactic pertussis vaccine, Pediatrics 1:437, 1948.
10a. Calderon-Gonzalez, R., and Rizzi-Hernandez, H.: Buckthorn polyneuropathy, New England J. Med. 277:69, 1967.
11. Cares, R. M., et al.: Therapeutic and toxic effects of chlorpromazine among 3,014 hospitalized cases, Am. J. Psychiat. 114:318, 1957.
12. Carter, N. W., et al.: Hyponatremia in cerebral disease resulting from the inappropriate secretion of antidiuretic hormone, New England J. Med. 264:67, 1961.
13. Chamberlain, P. H., et al.: Thallium poisoning, Pediatrics 22:1170, 1958.
14. Chisolm, J. J., and Harrison, H. E.: The treatment of acute lead encephalopathy in children, Pediatrics 19:2, 1957.
15. Cohen, S. B.: Brain damage due to penicillin, J.A.M.A. 186:889, 1963.
16. Collings, H.: Polyneuropathy associated with nitrofuran therapy, A.M.A. Arch. Neurol. 3:656, 1960.
17. Dixon, G. J., et al.: The relationship of neuropathy to the treatment of tuberculosis with isoniazid, Scot. M. J. 1:350, 1956.
18. Dobos, J. K., et al.: Acute barbiturate intoxication, J.A.M.A. 176:268, 1961.

19. Done, A. K.: Salicylate intoxication: Significance of measurements of salicylate in blood in cases of acute ingestion, Pediatrics 26:800, 1960.
20. Done, A. K.: Clinical pharmacology of systemic antidotes, Clin. Pharmacol. Ther. 2:750, 1961.
21. Done, A. K.: Intoxications of the Nervous System, in Brennemann-Kelley: *Practice of Pediatrics* (Hagerstown, Md.: W. F. Prior Company, Inc., 1965), vol. IV, ch. 11.
22. Done, A. K.: Salicylate Intoxication, in Gellis, S. S., and Kagan, B. M. (eds.): *Current Pediatric Therapy* (Philadelphia: W. B. Saunders Company, 1966).
23. Eadie, M. J., and Ferrier, T. M.: Chloroquine myopathy, J. Neurol. Neurosurg. & Psychiat. 29:331, 1966.
24. Eichenwald, H. F., and Shinefield, H. R.: Antimicrobial Therapy, in Shirkey, H. C. (ed.): *Pediatric Therapy* (St. Louis: The C. V. Mosby Company, 1966).
25. Ellis, F. G.: Acute polyneuritis after nitrofurantoin therapy, Lancet 2:1136, 1962.
25a. Espelin, D. E., and Done, A. K.: Amphetamine poisoning, New England J. Med. 278:1361, 1968.
26. Evans, J. H.: Persistent oral dyskinesia in treatment with phenothiazine derivatives, Lancet 1:458, 1965.
27. Fields, J. P.: Bulging fontanel: Complication of tetracycline therapy in infants, J. Pediat. 58:74, 1961.
28. Finberg, L., *et al.*: Mass accidental salt poisoning in infancy, J.A.M.A. 184:187, 1963.
29. Freemon, F. R., *et al.*: Unusual neurotoxicity of kanamycin, J.A.M.A. 200:410, 1967.
30. Friedman, A. P., and Elkind, A. H.: Appraisal of methysergide in treatment of vascular headaches of migraine type, J.A.M.A. 184:125, 1963.
31. Graham, J. R., *et al.*: Fibrotic disorders associated with methysergide therapy for headache, New England J. Med. 274:359, 1966.
32. Greengard, J., *et al.*: The surgical therapy of acute lead encephalopathy, J.A.M.A. 180:660, 1962.
32a. Greenhouse, A. H., *et al.*: Brain damage after intracarotid infusion of methotrexate, Arch. Neurol. 11:618, 1964.
33. Hall, R. A., *et al.*: Neurotoxic reactions resulting from chlorpromazine administration, J.A.M.A. 161:214, 1956.
34. Hockaday, J. M., *et al.*: Electroencephalographic changes in acute cerebral anoxia from cardiac or respiratory arrest, Electroencephalog. & Clin. Neurophysiol. 18:575, 1965.
35. Horen, W. P.: Arachnidism in the United States, J.A.M.A. 185:839, 1963.
36. Ingraham, F. D., and Matson, D. D.: *Neurosurgery of Infancy and Childhood* (2d ed.; Springfield, Ill.: Charles C Thomas, Publisher, 1961).
37. Jenkins, R. B.: Nutritional, Endocrine and Toxic Disorders, in Farmer, T. W. (ed.): *Pediatric Neurology* (New York City: Paul B. Hoeber, Inc., 1964), ch. 6.
38. Katz, B. E., and Carver, M. W.: Acute poisoning with isoniazid treated by exchange transfusion, Pediatrics 18:72, 1956.
39. Kurtzke, J. F.: Seizures with promazine, J. Nerv. & Ment. Dis. 125:119, 1957.
40. Lasagna, L.: The diseases drugs cause, Perspect. Biol. Med. 7:457, 1964.
40a. Lindholm, T.: Electromyographic changes after nitrofurantoin (Furadantin) therapy in nonuremic patients, Neurology 17:1017, 1967.
41. Lipsmeyer, E., and Ackerman, G. L.: Irreversible brain damage after water intoxication, J.A.M.A. 196:286, 1966.
42. Livingston, S., *et al.*: Convulsive reaction in a two-year-old child following the accidental ingestion of an overdosage of isoniazid, Pediatrics 18:77, 1956.
43. Loughridge, L. W.: Peripheral neuropathy due to nitrofurantoin, Lancet 2:1133, 1962.
44. Lucas, G. H. W., and Imrie, R. J.: Acute Poisoning, in Gellis, S. S., and Kagan, B. M. (eds.): *Current Pediatric Therapy* (Philadelphia: W. B. Saunders Company, 1966).
45. Luttrell, C. N., and Finberg, L.: Hemorrhagic encephalopathy induced by hypernatremia: I. Clinical, laboratory and pathological observations, A.M.A. Arch. Neurol. & Psychiat. 81:424, 1959.
45a. Luttrell, C. N., *et al.*: Hemorrhagic encephalopathy induced by hypernatremia. II. Experimental observations on hyperosmolarity in cats, A.M.A Arch. Neurol. &. Psychiat. 1:153, 1959.
46. Mangos, J. A., and Lobeck, C. C.: Studies of sustained hyponatremia due to central nervous system infection, Pediatrics 34:503, 1964.
47. McCrory, W. W., and Macaulay, D.: Idiopathic hyponatremia in an infant with diffuse cerebral damage, Pediatrics 20:23, 1957.
48. McLaurin, R. L., and Nichols, J. B.: Extensive cranial decompression in the treatment of severe lead encephalopathy, Pediatrics 20:653, 1957.
49. Moress, G. R., *et al.*: Neuropathy in lymphoblastic leukemia treated with vincristine, Arch. Neurol. 16:377, 1967.

49a. Morrice, G., et al.: Vitamin A intoxication as a cause of pseudotumor cerebri, J.A.M.A. 173:1802, 1960.
50. Myschetzky, A., and Lassen, N. A.: Urea-induced osmotic diuresis and alkalization of urine in acute barbiturate intoxication, J.A.M.A. 185:936, 1963.
51. Nyhan, W. L., and Cooke, R. E.: Symptomatic hyponatremia in acute infections of the central nervous system, Pediatrics 18:604, 1956.
52. Oldstone, M. B. A., and Nelson, E.: Central nervous system manifestations of penicillin toxicity in man, Neurology 16:693, 1966.
53. Press, E., and Done, A. K.: Solvent sniffing: Physiologic effects and community control measures for intoxication from the intentional inhalation of organic solvents. I and II, Pediatrics 39:451, 611, 1967.
54. Reed, D., et al.: Thallotoxicosis: Acute manifestations and sequelae, J.A.M.A. 183:516, 1963.
55. Reilly, R. H., et al.: Convulsant effects of isoniazid, J.A.M.A. 152:1317, 1953.
56. Schmidt, W. R., and Jarcho, L. W.: Persistent dyskinesias following phenothiazine therapy, Arch. Neurol. 14:369, 1966.
57. Schwartz, W. B., et al.: Further observations on hyponatremia and renal sodium loss probably resulting from inappropriate secretion of antidiuretic hormone, New England J. Med. 262:743, 1960.
57a. Shaw, E. B., et al.: Phenothiazine tranquilizers as a cause of severe seizures, Pediatrics 23:485, 1959.
57b. Silverman, W. A.: Retrolental Fibroplasia, in Dunham's *Premature Infants* (3d ed.; New York City: Paul B. Hoeber, Inc., 1961), ch. 16.
58. Slager, U. T., et al.: The neuropathology of barbiturate intoxication, J. Neuropath. & Exper. Neurol. 25:237, 1966.
59. Utley, P. M., et al.: Acute psychotic reactions to aqueous procaine penicillin, South. M. J. 59:1271, 1966.
60. Warkany, J., and Hubbard, D. M.: Mercury in urine of children with acrodynia, Lancet 1:829, 1948.
61. Waugh, W. H., and Metts, J. C.: Severe extrapyramidal motor activity induced by prochlorperazine: Its relief by the intravenous injection of diphenhydramine, New England J. Med. 262:353, 1960.
62. Ya, P. M., and Perry, J. F.: Experimental evaluation of methods for the early treatment of snake bite, Surgery 47:975, 1960.

21

Hereditary Metabolic and Degenerative Diseases

DEMENTIA ± SEIZURES ± SPASTICITY ± BLINDNESS

Hereditary Metabolic Defects

    Primary Aminoacidurias: Generalized Enzymatic Defects (Overflow Type)

        Phenylketonuria
        Maple syrup urine disease
        Histidinemia
        Hyperglycinemia (+ uria)
        Disorders of urea synthesis
            Argininosuccinicaciduria
                (no threshold)
            Citrullinemia (+ uria)
            Hyperammonemia
        Congenital lysine intolerance (hyperlysinemia) with periodic ammonia intoxication
        Cystathioninuria (no threshold)
        Homocystinuria (no threshold)
        Tyrosinemia and Tyrosinosis
        Isovaleric acidemia
        Hypophosphatasia

No textual description of the disorders listed below has been included because of the limited number of reported cases. See references.

        Hydroxyprolinemia and hyperprolinemia[45,46,122,128]
        Sarcosinemia[56]
        Hypervalinemia[139]
        Hydroxykynureninuria[80a]
        Tryptophanuria[138]
        Indolylacroyl glycine excretion[95]
        Hyperserotoninemia[132]
        Joseph's syndrome[73]
        Carnosinemia[112a]

    Primary Aminoacidurias: Disorders of Amino Acid Transport (Renal or Intestinal Absorption Defects)

        Hartnup disease
        Methionine malabsorption
        Renal tubular acidosis (including oculocerebrorenal syndrome of Lowe)

    Secondary Aminoacidurias

        These secondary disorders are not all discussed in the text but are included here to demonstrate the need for a broad overview in the critical interpretation of any laboratory measurements. See references.

Other hereditary enzymatic defects
    Galactosemia (see below)   Vitamin-D–resistant rickets[148a]
    Wilson's disease (see below)
Intoxications
    Heavy metals (lead, etc., Chapter 20)
    Out-dated tetracycline[52]
Deficiency diseases[44]
    Rickets
    Scurvy
Congenital anomalies of the genitourinary tract[44]
Chronic liver or renal disease[44]

Carbohydrates
    Hypoglycemia   Glycogen storage disease of muscle (Chapter 19)
    Galactosemia   Fructosuria with hypoglucosemia (hereditary fructose intolerance)

Polysaccharidoses
    MPS   I. Autosomal recessive gargoylism (Hurler)
    MPS II. X-linked recessive gargoylism (Hunter)
    MPS III. Heparitinuria (Sanfilippo)
    MPS IV. Keratosulfaturia (Morquio)
    MPS V. Adult type (Scheie)

Lipids (Cerebral Lipidoses)
    Brain and reticuloendothelial system (reticuloendothelioses)
        Niemann-Pick disease
        Gaucher's disease
    Nervous system and retina
        Infantile amaurotic familial idiocy (Tay-Sachs)
        Juvenile amaurotic familial idiocy (Bielschowsky, Batten, Spielmeyer-Vogt, and Kufs types)
    Leukodystrophies (diffuse scleroses)
        Globoid cell leukodystrophy   Metachromatic leukodystrophy
            (Krabbe)   Sudanophilic leukodystrophy
        Pelizaeus-Merzbacher disease   (Schilder)

Hormones
    Hypothyroidism   Pseudohypoparathyroidism
    Hypoparathyroidism

Vitamins
    Pyridoxine dependency and deficiency

Hereditary Neoplastic Degenerative Disorders
    Tuberous Sclerosis or Epiloia (Bourneville)
    Neurofibromatosis (von Recklinghausen)

HEREDITARY METABOLIC AND DEGENERATIVE DISEASES

Dementias of Unknown Etiology
    Spongy Degeneration of White Matter (Canavan)
    Necrotizing Encephalomyelopathy of Childhood (Leigh)
    Degeneration of Cerebral Gray Matter (Alpers)

ATAXIA AND OTHER MOVEMENT DISORDERS

Hereditary Metabolic Defects
    Amino Acids and Proteins
        Hartnup syndrome (see above)
        Ataxia-telangiectasia
        Acanthocytosis (Bassen-Kornzweig)
        X-linked primary hyperuricemia
    Disease of Mineral Metabolism
        Hepatolenticular degeneration (Wilson)
Degenerative Diseases of Unknown Etiology
    Spinocerebellar Ataxia (Friedreich)
    Chronic Progressive Hereditary Chorea (Huntington)
    Progressive Myoclonus Epilepsy (Unverricht)
    Hallervorden-Spatz Disease
    Dystonia Musculorum Deformans
    Paramyoclonus Multiplex

WEAKNESS, ATROPHY, AREFLEXIA AND SENSORY DEFICIT

Degenerative Diseases of Unknown Etiology
    Infantile Spinal Muscular Atrophy (Werdnig-Hoffmann, Chapter 19)
    Progressive Neural Atrophy or Peroneal Muscular Atrophy (Charcot-Marie-Tooth, Chapter 19)
    Familial Periodic Paralysis (Chapter 19)
    Syringomyelia and Syringobulbia (Chapter 13)
    Hereditary Sensory Radicular Neuropathy
    Progressive Bulbar Palsy

WEAKNESS AND SPASTICITY

Hereditary Spastic Paraplegia (Chapter 19)

LOSS OF VISION

Hereditary Optic Atrophy (Leber)
Pigmentary Degeneration of the Retina
    Laurence-Moon-Biedl Syndrome
    Hallervorden-Spatz Syndrome (see above)
    Retinitis Pigmentosa (Familial Night Blindness)
    Refsum's Syndrome
    Acanthocytosis (see above)
Amaurotic Familial Idiocy (see above)

FAMILIAL DYSAUTONOMIA

388 HEREDITARY METABOLIC AND DEGENERATIVE DISEASES

IN THIS CHAPTER we define hereditary metabolic disorders as those rare conditions which are inherited in a predictable manner and in most of which a biochemical anomaly has been demonstrated. In the past two decades we have seen a rapid growth in the number of "new" disease conditions, the biochemical pathology of which is at least partially understood. All of these conditions result from the absence of one or more enzymes—due usually to a single defective gene. Most are inherited in an autosomal recessive fashion, i.e., they affect both boys and girls, often more than one sibling, and no ancestors are affected. Until recently most patients with autosomal recessive diseases could not produce and the disease was not passed on to succeeding generations. However, this situation can be expected to change with development and refinement of treatment regimens. Many of these "inborn errors of metabolism" manifest themselves in early life, and damage from the disease may develop rapidly. The damage to the nervous system may take place over a short time, after which the body compensates by developing alternate metabolic pathways or by becoming resistant to further damage in its more mature state (e.g., phenylketonuria). When these rare diseases begin later in life, they follow a less rapid course.

Hereditary "degenerative" diseases are transmitted in a predictable mendelian fashion, most of them being autosomal dominant traits. Often one or more ancestors is affected, and the disease is transmitted to children of affected patients. Marked variation in the severity of the disease ("expressivity") is seen frequently, and the percentage of affected patients ("penetrance") may be low. In 1902 Gowers coined the term "abiotrophy" to describe the degenerative diseases, implying that they resulted from "defective vital endurance" of certain portions of the nervous system. Inasmuch as they are inherited and progress slowly but relentlessly, most workers think that these conditions also have a metabolic basis. However, in almost all cases the biochemical basis is still obscure. Degenerative diseases of the nervous system tend to affect selected groups of neurons, long fiber tracts or "systems" (e.g., spinocerebellar degenerations), and a classification with a pathologic-clinical basis is used most commonly.

In this clinical text the classification is based primarily upon the cardinal clinical manifestation and secondarily upon the pathologic abnormality. This method seems more practical than a strictly neuropathologic classification because biopsy of the nervous system is rarely performed. Also, autopsy information is obtained infrequently and always retrospectively.

Dementia ± Seizures ± Spasticity ± Blindness

Primary Aminoacidurias

Most of the well-documented aminoacidurias are included in the textual description. If only a few cases of a disease have been reported, the disease is included in the outline, a bibliographic reference is given but no discussion is now offered. An attempt has been made to include those disorders which meet one or more of the following criteria: (1) the diagnosis can be made in most hospital laboratories (Table 21.1), (2) the disease has one or more distinctive clinical features

TABLE 21.1.—AMINOACIDURIAS

Disease	Pathogenesis	Clinical Diagnosis	Blood	Laboratory Diagnosis Urine	X-ray	Other	Pattern of Inheritance	Treatment
Phenylketonuria	↓ Phenylalanine hydroxylase	Sz, MR, eczema, blond hair	↑ Phenylalanine	Pos. FeCl$_3$ test ↑ o-OH phenylacetic ↑ p-OH phenyllactic	—	Epileptiform EEG	Autosomal recessive	Low-phenylalanine diet
Maple syrup disease	Impaired decarboxylation of branched-chain amino acids Val, Leu, Ileu	First wk. of life: feeding difficulty Spasticity, sz, maple syrup odor	↑ Val ↑ Leu ↑ Ileu (↓ Blood glucose)	Pos. DNPH test Pos. FeCl$_3$ test ↑ Val ↑ Leu ↑ Ileu	—		Autosomal recessive	Diet low in branched-chain amino acids
Histidinemia	↓ Histidase	MR	↑ Histidine	Pos. FeCl$_3$ test ↑ Imidazolepyruvic acid ↑ Histidine No FIGLU (formiminoglutamic acid)	—	Skin biopsy for histidase activity ↓ Sweat urocanic acid	?	?Value Low-histidine diet
Hyperglycinemia	See text	(1) Vomiting, ketonuria, coma, MR, sz (2) MR, sz	↑ Glycine	↑ Glycine	—	(1) Neutropenia, thrombopenia (2) Epileptiform EEG	Autosomal recessive	?Value Low-protein diet, added Na benzoate; avoid "toxic" amino acids
Argininosuccinicaciduria	↓ Argininosuccinicinase	MR, sz, ataxia, abnormal hair (white, brittle), periods of unconsciousness	±↑ Blood ammonia	↑↑ Argininosuccinic acid	—	↑ Argininosuccinic acid in CSF	?	?Low-protein diet (?Citric acid or glutamic acid supplements)

↑ = increased
↓ = decreased
sz = seizures

MR = mental retardation
Val = valine
Leu = leucine
Ileu = isoleucine
DPNH = 2-4-dinitrophenylhydrazine

TABLE 21.1.—AMINOACIDURIAS—CONTINUED

Disease	Pathogenesis	Clinical Diagnosis	Blood	Laboratory Diagnosis Urine	X-ray	Other	Pattern of Inheritance	Treatment
Citrullinemia		MR	↑Citrulline	↑Citrulline	—	↑Citrulline in CSF	?	Low-protein diet (citric acid supplements)
Hyperammonemia		Lethargy, vomiting, coma; MR later	↑Blood ammonia	—	—	—	?	Low-protein diet (supplemental organic acids or phosphoric acid) Same as hyperammonemia
Congenital lysine intolerance (hyperlysinemia)		MR, sz, growth failure, hypotonia, *periods of stupor or coma*	↑Lysine ±↑Arginine and ammonia	↑Lysine ↑Ornithine, ↑γ-Aminobutyric acid, Ethanolamine	—	↑Lysine in CSF	Autosomal recessive	
Cystathioninuria	↓Cystathionase	MR, psychosis, congenital anomalies	—	↑Cystathionine	—	—	?	Vitamin B₆
Homocystinuria	↓Cystathionine synthetase	MR, sz, fine sparse hair, ectopia lentis, thromboembolism, long arms and legs (Marfan's syndrome)	↑Methionine ↑Homocystine	Pos. cyanide-nitroprusside test ↑Homocystine (homocysteine)	Osteoporosis, narrow joint spaces	Absent liver cystathionine	Autosomal recessive	?Dietary supplements of cystathionine and L-serine, restriction of methionine
Tyrosinosis	↓p-OH phenylpyruvic acid oxidase	Slight MR, vitamin-D-resistant rickets, hepatosplenomegaly, growth failure	↑Tyrosine	?Pos. FeCl₃ test ↑Tyrosine	Rickets		?	?Low phenylalanine diet
Isovaleric acidemia	Defect in catabolism of leucine	MR, coma and acidosis precipitated by high-protein intake	↑Isovaleric acid	↑Isovaleric acid			Autosomal recessive	Avoid high milk and protein intake

Disease	Defect	Clinical	Lab	Other lab	Inheritance	Treatment
Hypophosphatasia	Defective calcification of bone matrix	Rickets, long bone deformities, scoliosis, microcrania with craniostenosis	↓ Alkaline phosphatase (↑ Calcium)	↑ Phosphoethanolamine	Rickets	Autosomal recessive	?Vitamin D ?Cortisone
Oculocerebrorenal dystrophy (Lowe)	Defective renal production of ammonia	MR, hypotonia, areflexia, glaucoma, cataracts, rickets. *Males only*	Metabolic acidosis	Generalized aminoaciduria, organic aciduria ↓ NH$_3$	Rickets	X-linked dominant	Vitamin D, Na and K citrate
Hartnup disease	Autosomal recessive defect in (1) intestinal absorption of tryptophan and (2) renal tubular reabsorption of mono-NH$_2$, mono-COOH amino acids	Ataxia, mental disorders, pellagra rash	—	↑ Urinary indoles Distinctive patterned aminoaciduria Ala, Ser, Thr, Asp, NH$_2$, Glu, NH$_2$, Val, Leu, Ileu, Phala, Tyr, Try, His, Cit	—	Autosomal recessive	Nicotinamide 40–200 mg./day High protein diet?
Methionine malabsorption		MR, sz, white hair, abnormal odor ("dried celery")		↑ α-hydroxybutyric acid		?	Low-methionine diet
Galactosemia	↓ Galactose-1-phosphate uridyl transferase	Failure to thrive, hepatosplenomegaly, cataracts, MR	↑ Galactose ↓ Transferase in RBC ±↓ Glucose	Pos. Benedict's test Generalized aminoaciduria (renal tubular disorder secondary to galactose ingestion)		Autosomal recessive	Lactose-free formula (see text) Diet free of milk products
Hepatolenticular degeneration (Wilson's)	Defect in copper metabolism	Hepatomegaly, K-F ring, movement disorder	↓ Copper ↓ Ceruloplasmin	Generalized aminoaciduria ↑ Copper		Autosomal recessive	Penicillamine, Carbo-Resin

(Table 21.2); (3) the disease can be treated with reasonable expectation of benefit. New information is evolving rapidly in our understanding of the pathogenesis, the establishment of the diagnosis and the specific therapy of this group of diseases.

Generalized Enzymatic Defects (Overflow Type)

Phenylketonuria

PATHOGENESIS.—This clinical disorder (PKU) is inherited as an autosomal recessive trait and results from a deficiency in the enzyme phenylalanine hydroxylase (Fig. 21.1) which is necessary to convert the essential amino acid phenylalanine to tyrosine. The defect leads to an excessively high plasma level of phenylalanine, which in some way leads to damage to the developing nervous system and the excessive urinary output of o-OH phenylacetic and phenylpyruvic acids as well as other abnormal metabolites. Some interference with myelin formation does occur, and several other chemical mechanisms, including oxygen consumption, glucose utilization and tyrosine uptake, seem critically impaired.[90a]

CLINICAL AND LABORATORY DIAGNOSIS.—Phenylketonuric newborn infants usually appear normal, but vomiting, lethargy and irritability occur early. Slow motor development, with or without seizures, often ensues and most untreated older infants and children have mental retardation. Intellectual functioning varies from severe retardation (IQ below 50 in the average case) to normal mentality in occasional patients. This variation in the level of mental functioning is sometimes strikingly evident in untreated affected siblings. Other common clinical manifestations include: (1) dilute body pigment, i.e., blond, blue-eyed children are seen more commonly, (2) microcephaly, (3) eczema and (4) a pungent, "musty" odor to the urine and sweat. Electroencephalograms are often grossly disorganized and may show diffuse epileptiform discharges, a pattern described by some as "hypsarhythmia" (Fig. 2.2, page 29).

Before the advent of effective dietary therapy, diagnostic efforts were limited

Fig. 21.1.—Metabolic pathway block in phenylketonuria.

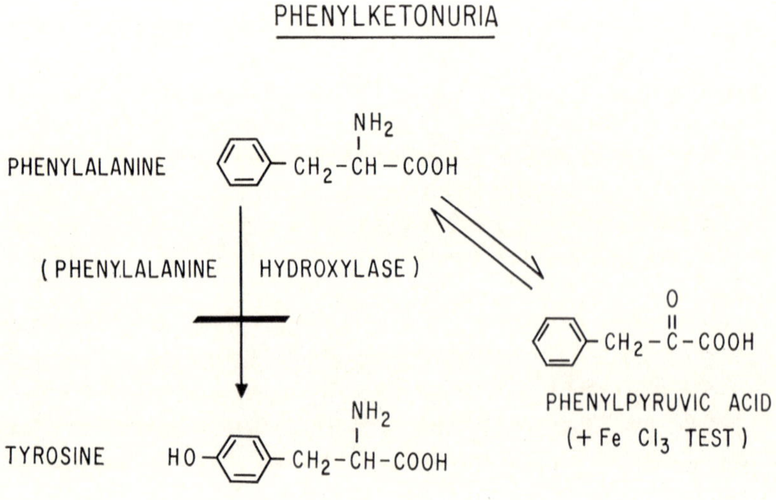

PHENYLKETONURIA

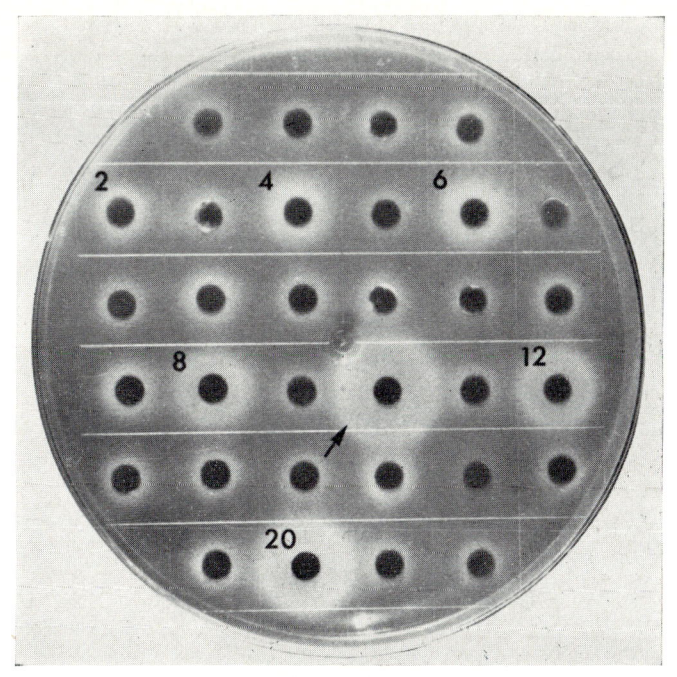

Fig. 21.2.—Guthrie test—routine screening test for PKU. Blood from the newborn infant's heel is absorbed on filter paper. An agar plate containing the phenylalanine antagonist β-2-thienylalanine is seeded with Bacillus subtilis, an organism which needs phenylalanine for growth. Standard-sized disks of blood-impregnated filter paper are punched out and placed on the agar plate in rows, along with standards of known phenylalanine concentration (2, 4, 6, 8, 12, 20 mg./100 ml.). The clear zone around the disk of the patient with known PKU (arrow) reflects bacterial growth and indicates the approximate concentration of phenylalanine (in this case, over 20 mg./100 ml.).

largely to the urinary drop test (when 3–5 drops of 10% ferric chloride are added to 1 ml. of urine an emerald green color develops promptly). False-positive results may be seen in maple syrup urine disease, tyrosinosis, alcaptonuria and methionine malabsorption, in patients taking aspirin or chlorpromazine and in children with histidinemia. A simple stick test (Phenistix) is also used.

The need to establish an early diagnosis and to institute treatment has led now to the mass screening of newborn infants for this disorder. The Guthrie test, a semiquantitative microbiologic inhibition assay procedure, estimates the level of phenylalanine in capillary blood from the infant's heel (Fig. 21.2). One must remain alert to the fairly high incidence of false-positive results (Fig. 21.3) resulting from delayed induction of the enzyme phenylalanine hydroxylase in normal and premature neonates. If the infant is tested before or too soon after milk feedings have been started, false-negative results may occur (Fig. 21.3). If one hopes to detect all affected babies at the earliest possible date, the Guthrie test must be performed just before discharge from the hospital and again at 3 to 4 weeks of age. The urinary ferric chloride test has fallen into disuse as an early detection device because some patients with serum levels over 20 mg./100 ml. have had persistently negative findings with this test. If the quantitative results of the Guthrie test are equivocal, one should (1) send a serum sample to a laboratory that is equipped to perform

LABORATORY CONSIDERATIONS IN THE EARLY DIAGNOSIS OF PKU

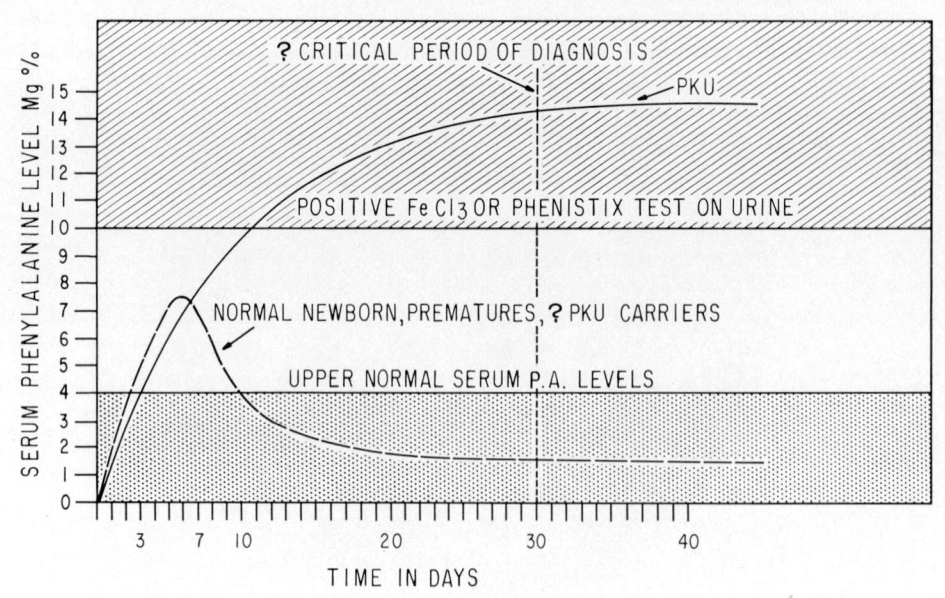

Fig. 21.3.—This diagram indicates the reasons for false-positive results of Guthrie tests (lower left arrow) and false-negative results of ferric chloride tests (upper right arrow) in the neonate.

a more accurate photofluorometric measurement of phenylalanine, (2) carry out phenolic acid chromatography and (3) obtain serum for quantitative phenylalanine and tyrosine determinations. Phenolic acid chromatography will, in practically all cases, demonstrate increased amounts of abnormal metabolites (o-OH phenylacetic and p-OH phenyllactic acids).

Berry and associates[12] have pointed out that nonphenylketonuric neonates may exhibit high levels of phenylalanine as a result of the delayed induction of enzymes which catabolize tyrosine. These workers have discovered that the elevated levels of serum phenylalanine and tyrosine will return to normal 24 hours after the child is given 100 mg. of ascorbic acid.

When an abnormal Guthrie test is reported (serum phenylalanine over 4 mg./100 ml.), the physician should:

1. Continue regular milk feedings until the diagnosis is established in 24–48 hours.
2. Repeat the serum phenylalanine (and tyrosine) determination using a quantitative method.
3. Obtain a urine specimen as soon as possible for a ferric chloride test and phenolic acid chromatography.
4. Give the patient 100 mg. of ascorbic acid and repeat the serum phenylalanine and tyrosine determinations in 24 hours.

MANAGEMENT AND PROGNOSIS.—Affected infants should be placed on a low-phenylalanine diet (Lofenalac or Ketonil) as early as possible, preferably during the first month of life.[14] Careful dietary control of the phenylalanine level at about 4–12 mg./100 ml. will help to prevent hypoproteinemia, edema and hypoglycemia-induced convulsions, all of which have complicated overzealous treatment.

Berry and associates[13] have outlined in detail the biochemical control of the disease by careful dietary manipulation. They maintain rigid control observations by having parents obtain the blood specimens and by having urine specimens collected every day for eight days. Such careful management is certainly laudable, but it will be impractical in many situations at present. The basic treatment aims at providing enough phenylalanine for growth (serum level not below 3 mg./100 ml.) but not an amount which would permit the appearance of o-OH phenylacetic acid in the urine (serum phenylalanine level about 8 mg./100 ml.). The special formula is prepared by mixing 1 packed level measure of Lofenalac with 2 oz. water. One-half cup of the powder supplies 50 calories/lb. body weight and the amount used is adjusted to provide 11 mg. phenylalanine/lb. body weight. The infant is initially regulated on the low-phenylalanine diet and natural foods, including carbohydrates, fats, fruits and vegetables, are gradually added to assure optimal growth. A careful watch on the caloric and fluid needs should be maintained. Progress in regulation is monitored initially with *serum phenylalanine levels;* these are determined using micromethods, so that specimens can be collected in capillary tubes from a heel or finger puncture. Also, *urinary chromatography for o-OH phenylacetic acid* is carried out. These tests should be run every one to two days for the first seven to 10 days, then every week or two for about eight weeks. From the third to the twelfth months serum phenylalanine levels should be obtained about every two weeks.

At about 1 year of age the child usually needs a variety of solid foods in order to meet his protein requirements, and the mother should obtain a list which gives the phenylalanine content of various foods.* During acute illnesses and fever, when the phenylalanine food intake drops, a biochemical paradox is noted in severely affected patients. The serum phenylalanine level rises and o-OH phenylacetic acid appears in the urine presumably as a result of tissue protein catabolism. For this reason Berry *et al.*[13] recommend that the phenylalanine intake be raised about 50% during acute illnesses by offering such foods as broths, soups, gelatin and eggnog. From this outline it is obvious that the management of phenylketonuria requires a great deal of physician time, an intelligent, cooperative mother and special laboratory facilities.

If symptoms have developed before treatment is instituted, the irritability, lethargy and vomiting will usually disappear on the special diet, the seizures and EEG abnormalities may show striking improvement, the child's motor and mental progress may accelerate and the hair color may darken. How long treatment should be carried on and after what age treatment is useless are controversial questions. Most workers are advocating the resumption of a normal diet at age 4[71] and are not recommending institution of the special diet after that age. Precise recommendations about therapy may be altered when more experience is accumulated. Also, the exact value of therapy in a given patient depends upon longitudinal observations on larger series of cases.

The question of how to manage newborn infants with high levels of blood phenylalanine but without other evidence of phenylketonuria is still unsettled.[110]

Phenylalanine Contents of Foods. Handbook available from Barbara Umbarger, Children's Hospital Research Foundation, Cincinnati, Ohio 45229.

Maternal phenylketonuria.—The successful therapy of phenylketonuria in infants solves one problem but creates another, i.e., the threat to the unborn fetus of high circulating blood levels of phenylalanine in pregnant phenylketonuric women. It has been suggested by Mabry et al.[90] and others[48d] that heterozygous babies without the disease may suffer permanent neurologic deficit from this circumstance. Although little experience has been documented on the management of this problem, the obstetrician or any physician managing the pregnant phenylketonuric woman must be prepared to use a low-phenylalanine diet and monitor the blood levels of phenylalanine during gestation.

By a similar line of reasoning it has been suggested that the mother of any mentally retarded child should have a urinary ferric chloride test even though the retarded child has a negative test result.

Maple Syrup Disease

PATHOGENESIS.—This complicated metabolic defect first described by Menkes[97] is probably inherited as an autosomal recessive trait and results from the enzymatically defective decarboxylation of four branched-chain keto acids. In addition to elevated levels of these keto acids in the serum, urine and cerebrospinal fluid, the branched-chain amino acid precursors—leucine, isoleucine and valine—have elevated levels in all of the body fluids. Many of these patients have hypoglycemia, and, although the cause is not clear, it may be the hypoglycemic effect of high blood levels of leucine.[42] The characteristic maple syrup odor of the urine and sweat results from the derivative of alpha-hydroxybutyric acid. Myelin formation in the brains of these infants is defective, and one may see marked astrocytosis.

CLINICAL AND LABORATORY DIAGNOSIS.—Whereas these infants appear normal at birth, symptoms of feeding difficulty, irregular respirations with apnea and cyanosis, opisthotonos, increased muscle tone, an absent Moro reflex and seizures usually appear early in the neonatal period. Rapid deterioration often follows and many patients will die within a month if no therapy is instituted. It is apparent, however, that the disease is not inevitably fatal and is occasionally seen in older infants, but they are usually severely defective and spastic. Isolated cases have been reported by Dancis et al.[37] and others[102] in patients with periodic symptoms of lethargy and ataxia, in whom the typical odor and biochemical abnormalities occur periodically. Permanent neurologic damage does not appear in every case.

The definitive diagnosis is based upon the characteristic maple syrup odor of the patient's urine and a urine test using DNPH (2-4-dinitrophenylhydrazine). When 2 ml. of urine is added to an equal quantity of freshly prepared DNPH, a deep, opaque yellow color develops within one minute. Chromatography of serum and urine should be carried out in all cases because a DNPH test may also give a positive finding in phenylketonuric urine.

MANAGEMENT AND PROGNOSIS.—Special diets, largely synthetic, have been used in the treatment of this rare disorder. Their complex and expensive character make it mandatory that they be supervised carefully by experts who can carry out frequent quantitative measurements of the serum amino acids. If early therapy is instituted, published results[2,131,147,147a] suggest that neurologic deficit can be prevented or limited.

Histidinemia

This disorder in the metabolism of histidine is caused by a deficiency of the enzyme histidase.[3] This defect leads to elevated levels of histidine in both blood and urine and the excretion of imidazolepyruvic acid in large amounts.

The paucity of reported cases and the variable clinical correlates make it difficult at this time to assess the clinical importance of this condition. Retarded speech development, mild progressive ataxia, convulsions, recurrent infections and anomalies in other organ systems have been reported in isolated cases.[58,81,143] A low-histidine diet has been used in a few reported cases but further observations will be necessary before commenting seriously on treatment, prognosis and recurrence risk.

Hyperglycinemia

PATHOGENESIS.—It now appears that at least two defects in the intermediary metabolism of glycine can occur and in both disorders one finds elevated levels of plasma and urinary glycine.

In the original cases of Childs and co-workers[26] available evidence suggests that the defect results from deficient conversion of glycine to serine. Gerritsen et al.[57] have pointed out that another hereditary defect in glycine metabolism is associated with hypooxaluria and results from a deficiency in the enzyme glycine oxidase. To simplify discussion we shall refer to the first as the *ketotic type* and to the second as the *nonketotic type*.

CLINICAL AND LABORATORY DIAGNOSIS.—*Ketotic type.*—This disorder is characterized by the appearance of vomiting, drowsiness and coma, usually in the *first days or weeks of life*. One can screen for the disorder most easily by looking for ketonuria (and ruling out glycogen storage and maple syrup diseases). Amino acid chromatography of the urine and blood reveals hyperglycinuria and hyperglycinemia, but the results must be interpreted carefully because both false-positive and false-negative findings have been reported.[108] Neutropenia and thrombocytopenia, occasionally with purpura, have been noted in most of the patients. Many of these babies die early in life from severe ketoacidosis and mental retardation, and seizures afflict many of the survivors. Affected babies show no distinctive physical abnormalities.

Nonketotic type.—Other children with hyperglycinuria and hyperglycinemia (but without ketoacidosis, neutropenia or thrombocytopenia) usually present with retarded development and refractory seizures.[151] These patients may exhibit striking epileptiform EEG abnormalities. Gerritsen and co-workers[57] demonstrated an abnormally low output of urinary oxalic acid. Without the threat of severe ketoacidosis one could expect to find this disorder more often in older retarded children.

These disorders are distinct from familial glycinuria, a condition with normal serum glycine levels and no neurologic deficit.

MANAGEMENT AND PROGNOSIS.—Experience with these disorders has been limited and still experimental. However, Nyhan[108] appears to have altered the course of the disease successfully in a few patients by preventing or treating the ketoacidosis vigorously. He recommends a diet containing 0.5 Gm./kg. of protein, with or without a diet containing "nontoxic" amino acids—leucine, isoleucine, valine, threonine and methionine. The administration of sodium benzoate helps to maintain low levels of serum glycine.

Argininosuccinicaciduria

This rare disorder results from a block in the synthesis of urea (Fig. 21.4). In a small number of cases argininosuccinase has been absent in the patient's erythrocytes, whereas it is present in normal red blood cells.

Affected infants exhibit severe mental and physical retardation, seizures and anomalies of the hair (trichorrhexis nodosa or monilethrix[62]). Amino acid analysis reveals large quantities of argininosuccinic acid in the cerebrospinal fluid, the plasma and the urine.[88] Intermittent elevation of blood ammonia, especially after a protein meal, has been demonstrated.[86,104] The exact effect of hyperammonemia on the brain development of the young child is not settled.

A similar clinical picture, i.e., a degenerative neurologic condition in infants, especially boys, associated with sparse white hair, has been reported[20,98] in which there is no evidence of argininosuccinicaciduria.

A low-protein diet will reduce the excess output of argininosuccinic acid, and Levin[86] has shown that administration of citric acid, glutamic acid and phosphoric acid will lessen the rise in blood ammonia after a protein meal. However, the diet can be used for only a limited period and no beneficial therapeutic results have been reported as yet. The prognosis for these children is poor.

Citrullinemia

This rare disorder presumably results from a deficiency in an enzyme which converts citrulline to argininosuccinic acid (Fig. 21.4). The actual enzymatic defect has not yet been demonstrated.

A few isolated cases have been reported.[94,103] In one patient, after quite normal development for nine months, vomiting was followed by convulsions and developmental regression. Hepatomegaly, Parkinson-like tremor and hyperreflexia were noted. Elevated levels of citrulline were found in the blood, urine and cerebrospinal fluid and hyperammonemia in the postabsorptive state was noted.

Until more cases are reported, statements regarding treatment, recurrence risk and long-term prognosis must be deferred. Attempts to reduce blood ammonia with neomycin therapy have been made but the results are not impressive.[101]

Hyperammonemia

Whereas various specific aminoacidopathies intoxicate the patient by excessive ammonia production (argininosuccinicaciduria, citrullinemia and congenital intolerance to lysine), several reports have indicated that additional and apparently separate defects in the cycle of urea synthesis cause hyperammonemia (Fig. 21.4). In one report[120] two cousins were found to have a deficiency of transcarbamylase (the enzyme which converts ornithine to citrulline) and chronic ammonia intoxi-

DISORDERS OF THE UREA CYCLE

HYPERAMMONEMIA

1. $NH_3 + HCO_3 + ATP \longrightarrow$ Carbamyl PO_4 + ADP + Pi

2. Carbamyl PO_4 + Ornithine $\xrightarrow{\text{Ornithine Transcarbamylase}}\!\!\!\!/\!\!\!\!\longrightarrow$ Citrulline + Pi

CITRULLINEMIA

3. Citrulline + Asparate + ATP $\xrightarrow{\text{Argininosuccinic acid (ASA) synthetase}}\!\!\!\!/\!\!\!\!\longrightarrow$ ASA + AMP + PP

ARGININOSUCCINICACIDURIA

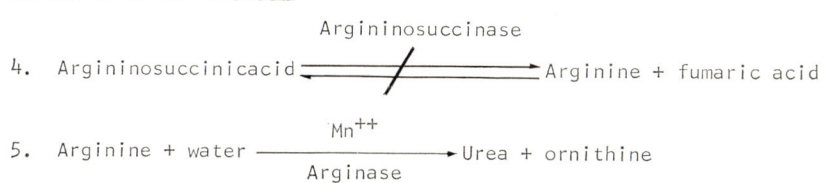

4. Argininosuccinicacid $\xrightarrow{\text{Argininosuccinase}}\!\!\!\!/\!\!\!\!\longrightarrow$ Arginine + fumaric acid

5. Arginine + water $\xrightarrow[\text{Arginase}]{Mn^{++}}$ Urea + ornithine

Fig. 21.4.—Hereditary metabolic defects in the cycle of urea synthesis.

cation without elevation of blood amino acids. Another report[50] describes a similar defect in urea synthesis with ammonia intoxication which suggested a carbamyl phosphate synthetase deficiency.

The clinical picture of lethargy, vomiting, coma and flaccidity should suggest this diagnosis clinically. Differential diagnosis includes seizures, acidosis secondary to diabetes or dehydration and hypoglycemic coma. Most reported patients have been mentally retarded.

The diagnosis can be made by finding elevated fasting or postprandial levels of blood ammonia. The fasting level in normal persons is usually under 60 μg./100 ml. Postprandial levels in these patients may rise to 400–1,000μg./100 ml.

The acute episodes of ammonia intoxication are eliminated impressively by low-protein diets. The protein intake should be reduced to the lowest level compatible with growth, and supplemental organic acids (citric or aspartic) or phosphoric acid can be given.[87] Experience is too limited and too brief to predict whether the mental retardation can be prevented if this condition is detected early in life.

Congenital Lysine Intolerance (Hyperlysinemia) with Periodic Ammonia Intoxication

Occasionally young children with neurologic deficit are found to have extremely high levels of lysine in blood and urine.[59,149] No enzymatic defect to account for this disorder has been demonstrated as yet, and it has been suggested that the biochemical disturbances may result from an inability to incorporate lysine into protein. It has also been suggested that hyperlysinemia may produce some of its clinical signs by causing ammonia intoxication. Some authors have considered hyperlysinemia and congenital lysine intolerance as different disorders, largely on the basis of the different clinical appearances in isolated cases, but it seems probable that they may be one disease. It has not really been proved yet that the abnormality in lysine metabolism is causally related to the neurologic deficit in all patients.[2a]

Symptoms and signs include convulsions, mental retardation, growth failure and hyperextensibility of joints—the last finding producing the syndrome of the "floppy infant." Some patients have episodes of vomiting and coma, at which time the blood ammonia levels are greatly elevated.[31]

Markedly elevated levels of lysine are found in the blood, cerebrospinal fluid and urine of patients. Urine levels of ornithine, gamma aminobutyric acid and ethanolamine are also significantly high.

No proved therapy has been established, but low-protein diets may be useful, especially if ammonia intoxication is present.[32] The regular appearance of mental retardation and the poorly controlled seizures signify a serious outlook in any infant with this biochemical defect.

Cystathioninuria

Presumably due to a defect in the enzyme cystathioninase, this disorder is characterized by the output of very large amounts of cystathionine in the urine (Fig. 21.5).[51,67] Only a few patients have been described with this chemical anomaly,

Fig. 21.5.—Different metabolic pathway blocks in the breakdown of methionine.

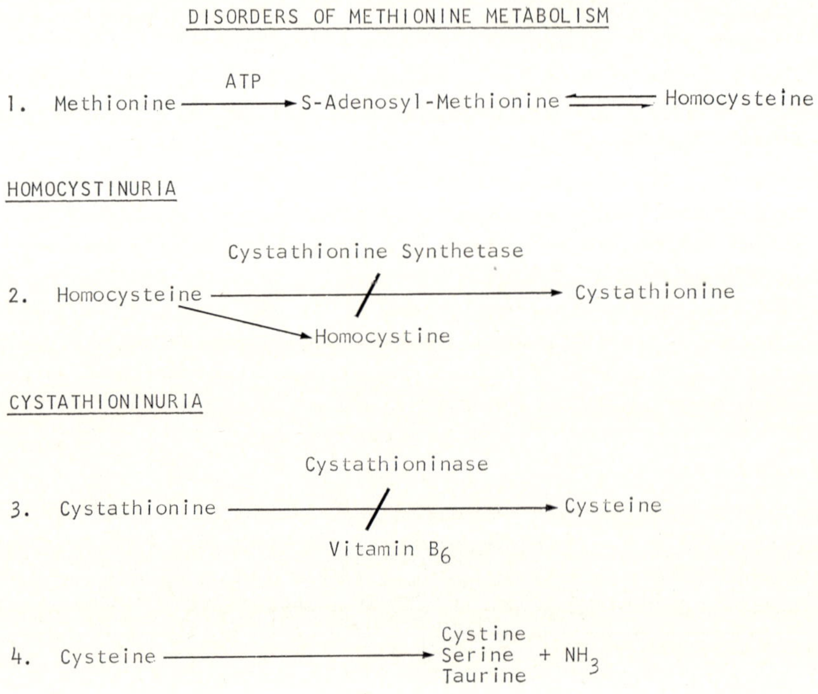

DISORDERS OF METHIONINE METABOLISM

1. Methionine $\xrightarrow{ATP}$ S-Adenosyl-Methionine $\rightleftharpoons$ Homocysteine

HOMOCYSTINURIA

2. Homocysteine $\xrightarrow{\text{Cystathionine Synthetase} \;/\;}$ Cystathionine
   $\searrow$ Homocystine

CYSTATHIONINURIA

3. Cystathionine $\xrightarrow{\text{Cystathioninase} \;/\; \text{Vitamin B}_6}$ Cysteine

4. Cysteine $\longrightarrow$ Cystine / Serine + NH_3 / Taurine

some with mental retardation or psychosis and multiple congenital anomalies and some without any clinical abnormalities.[112b] Further data must be collected before firm conclusions can be reached about the clinical picture. Urine chromatography reveals a large excess of cystathionine.

Several workers have reported beneficial results from large doses of vitamin B_6, the benefit presumably resulting from the fact that this vitamin acts as a coenzyme for the deficient enzyme cystathioninase.[10,53]

Homocystinuria

This unusual hereditary metabolic defect, first reported by Carson and Neill,[22] results from a deficiency or absence of the enzyme cystathionine synthetase which catalyzes the formation of cystathionine and cysteine from homocysteine, serine and methionine (Fig. 21.5). Compared to normal brains which have high levels of cystathionine, biopsy specimens of the brain[55] and the liver[105] from patients with this disorder have no measurable cystathionine. No pathologic morphologic studies have been reported.

Among the small number of reported cases, a consistent constellation of clinical signs have included mental retardation, fine sparse hair, seizures, dislocated lenses and thromboembolic phenomena.[43,124,148] Several reports have emphasized the clinical similarity of this disease and Marfan's syndrome.[141] In isolated cases osteoporosis and narrowing of the joint spaces have been noted.[77]

Amino acid analysis of the blood reveals high levels of homocystine and methionine, whereas the urine has elevated levels of homocystine only.[19] In addition, a cyanide-nitroprusside drop test is diagnostic in some cases. For this test, add 2 ml. of a 5% sodium cyanide solution to 5 ml. of urine. To this mixture add 5 drops of a 5% sodium nitroprusside solution. A stable magenta color develops in the urine of patients with homocystinuria[22,23] (as well as in cases of cystinuria, a neurologically benign condition).

Inasmuch as the brain of one patient contained no measurable cystathionine, compared to high levels in controls, and since these patients have serious neurologic deficit, dietary supplements of cystathionine, L-serine (with restriction of dietary methionine) and cystine have been suggested.[80] However, the value of this theoretical approach has not been established. Also, the limited clinical experience with these patients makes prognosis and intelligent counseling difficult at this time.

Heterozygous parents of children with homocystinuria have been reported to have a striking incidence of psychosis.[22] This provocative observation requires further investigation.

Tyrosinemia and Tyrosinosis

Disorders which cause elevated blood and urine tyrosine levels vary considerably in clinical features, and the terminology employed in their description has increased the confusion. All the facts on the matter have not yet been set down, but it is probable that tyrosinemia and tyrosyluria have a heterogeneous etiology. We shall deal briefly with *tyrosinemia* (a fairly common, transient elevation in blood levels of tyrosine seen in premature and term newborn infants) and *tyrosinosis* (a rare hereditary enzymatic defect associated with hepatic cirrhosis and rickets).

Neonatal tyrosinemia.—Transient, neonatal elevation in blood tyrosine level is probably a benign disorder resulting from a maturational delay in enzyme induction. It has come to attention recently because a Guthrie test for the detection of phenylketonuria will often give a positive result in neonates with transient tyrosinemia. The condition is seen more frequently when the infant has been receiving a high-protein milk and when dietary supplementation with vitamin C is low.[5a] (See discussion of phenylketonuria.) No consistent clinical findings have been noted in this presumably innocuous disorder, and the chemical findings can usually be abolished in 24 hours by giving 100 mg. of ascorbic acid by mouth to the infant.

Tyrosinosis.—This rare hereditary metabolic defect is characterized by cirrhosis, severe hypophosphatemic rickets and renal tubular defects. In addition to elevated serum tyrosine levels, one finds an excess output of various metabolites in the urine resulting from a deficiency in the enzyme pHPPA-oxidase (para-hydroxyphenyl-pyruvic acid oxidase). Preliminary attempts at treatment of this disease by limiting the dietary intake of tyrosine and phenylalanine have been encouraging.[54,66,79,129]

Isovaleric Acidemia

Recently a new hereditary aminoacidopathy was discovered,[140] which results from a genetic (presumably autosomal recessive) defect in leucine metabolism. This disorder causes periodic elevations of serum isovaleric acid, which is a normal breakdown product of leucine.[20a] The two siblings described showed early delayed motor and mental development, recurrent episodes of coma and acidosis and a peculiar odor resembling "sweaty feet" from the skin, breath and urine. They also exhibited an early natural aversion to dietary proteins such as meat and milk, and attacks of coma and acidosis were always precipitated by the ingestion of such dietary proteins.

Analysis of sweat and serum by mass spectrometry and short-chain fatty acid gas chromatography is said to have shown that the odor is due to isovaleric acid, which rises markedly in the serum during bouts of coma and acidosis. A leucine load causes an increase in both the lethargy and the odor.

Limited experience in management of the disorder suggests that excessive dietary meats and milk should be avoided. Whether this dietary restriction will prevent mental retardation must await further reports. Patients who go into coma and acidosis promptly recover their active, alert state in two to five days if they are given 5% glucose in water (2,500 cc./M.^{2}) intravenously.

Hypophosphatasia

This familial disorder is inherited as an autosomal recessive trait and is characterized by a defect in osteoid bone formation and epiphyseal ossification. The disease results in defective growth and skeletal deformities. Signs may appear in early infancy or adult life. Commonly one encounters premature craniostenosis, long bone deformities similar to those seen in ordinary rickets and scoliosis. Patients not only have deformed, small heads, but they also show signs of increased intracranial pressure (bulging fontanel and prominent convolutional markings on x-ray). The eyes may appear prominent, and neurologic signs such as convulsions and mental retardation develop in some cases.

Characteristically, serum alkaline phosphatase concentration is abnormally low for the patient's age and excessive phosphoethanolamine is excreted in the urine (detected by amino acid chromatography). No proved explanation has been established for the association of these two biochemical defects. Hypercalcemia and radiologic evidence of rickets are demonstrable in some patients.

No acceptable therapy has been established for this disorder. Bartler[7] reported results of vitamin D and cortisone therapy in a small number of selected patients, but the outcome has been equivocal or unimpressive. The age of onset of the disease determines its severity and its prognosis to some extent. When the diagnosis is made in early infancy, children rarely live beyond 1 year of age. In adults the disease may remit completely.

Disorders of Amino Acid Transport (Renal or Intestinal Absorption Defects)

Several aminoacidopathies result from defects in amino acid transport (1) across the renal tubular epithelium (cystinuria and Hartnup disease), (2) across the jejunal mucosa (Hartnup disease and methionine malabsorption) or (3) across cell membranes (Lowe's syndrome).[100]

Hartnup Disease

PATHOGENESIS.—This rare familial condition is characterized by a complex and extensive disturbance in amino acid transport, resulting primarily in renal *aminoaciduria of a patterned type*.[6] A defect in the absorption of tryptophan in the intestine (jejunum) (1) allows the formation of decomposition products which can be absorbed and which are in some way toxic to the central nervous system and (2) reduces the amount of nicotinamide synthesized from tryptophan—resulting in a pellagra-like skin rash.[127] The associated severe aminoaciduria involving only the monoamino-monocarboxylic acids (which share a common renal reabsorption mechanism) is critical for the laboratory diagnosis[72] even though it may not be responsible for any of the clinical signs.

CLINICAL AND LABORATORY DIAGNOSIS.—The clinical manifestations are intermittent and variable. Characteristically there is a red, roughened skin on the exposed surfaces—a photosensitivity dermatitis which resembles pellagra. Intermittent cerebellar ataxia occurs as the usual neurologic sign, but personality changes and mental retardation are seen in older children. Both the dermatitis and ataxia tend to improve with age.

The diagnosis of Hartnup disease should be considered in patients with intermittent neurologic signs, whether or not they have dermatitis. Urinary chromatography reveals a severe aminoaciduria which, though not generalized, is multiple and patterned and is not associated with other evidence of renal dysfunction. One also usually finds an excess of indolic substances in the urine.

MANAGEMENT AND PROGNOSIS.—Treatment with nicotinamide has been employed because of (1) the clinical resemblance of the rash in Hartnup disease to that in pellagra and (2) the consistent disturbance in the gut absorption and transport of tryptophan, a metabolic precursor of nicotinic acid. However, the value of this therapy is difficult to assess, especially when one considers the natural tendency of the disease to remit.

Methionine Malabsorption

This disorder is not completely understood and may be related to or the same as "oasthouse urine" disease. Patients with the disorder come to attention clinically because of their peculiar odor, which is likened to dried celery. This odor has been ascribed to alpha-hydroxybutyric acid, which is formed when the poorly absorbed methionine is degraded by intestinal bacteria. The alpha-hydroxybutyric acid is then absorbed and excreted in the urine in excess amounts.

Patients with this rare disorder exhibit mental retardation, convulsions, white hair and an abnormal odor (dried celery). The urine and stool contain abnormally large quantities of alpha-hydroxybutyric acid.

Marked clinical improvement and disappearance of the peculiar odor have been reported with the use of a low-methionine diet.[70] Experience is too limited to generalize about the prognosis in this unusual disease.

Oculocerebrorenal Syndrome of Lowe

This inherited disorder results from a deficiency in the renal production of ammonia, which in turn causes a generalized aminoaciduria and a systemic acidosis. The affected children, usually boys, are born with congenital eye defects (glaucoma, buphthalmos, hydrophthalmos or cataracts) (Fig. 21.6,*A*) and manifest mental retardation and osteomalacia secondary to chronic acidosis (renal rickets). Urine chromatography reveals a generalized aminoaciduria (Fig. 21.6,*B*), and blood studies reflect the state of acidosis. Considerable day-to-day variation in the degree of aminoaciduria should be expected.[27]

Administration of calcium lactate and sodium citrate alleviates the rickets by correcting the chronic acidosis, but no therapy benefits the neurologic and ocular signs.

Carbohydrates

Idiopathic Hypoglycemia

No pathologic lesion can be demonstrated in most cases of childhood hypoglycemia, and most cases which fall into the category of primary hypoglycemia are called idiopathic and may have a familial pattern. Recent work has shown that high-protein meals (specifically casein or leucine[28,29]) will precipitate hypoglycemia, possibly by stimulating the production of insulin.[41,63] Autopsy of a patient with leucine-sensitive hypoglycemia has shown marked islet-cell hyperplasia of the pancreas.[64] Induction of ketosis also lowers the blood sugar significantly in some of these patients, and a tendency for spontaneous improvement with age is seen.

Diagnosis and management of hypoglycemia are discussed in Chapter 2.

Although spontaneous improvement tends to occur in the neonatal and idio-

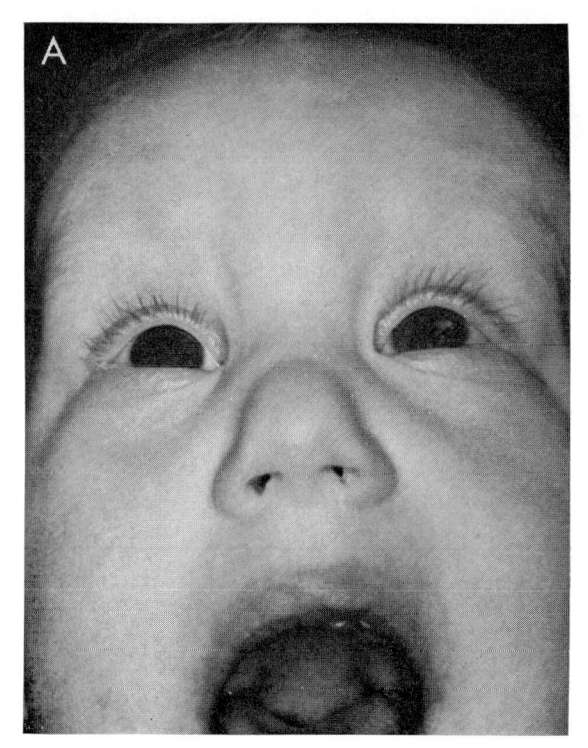

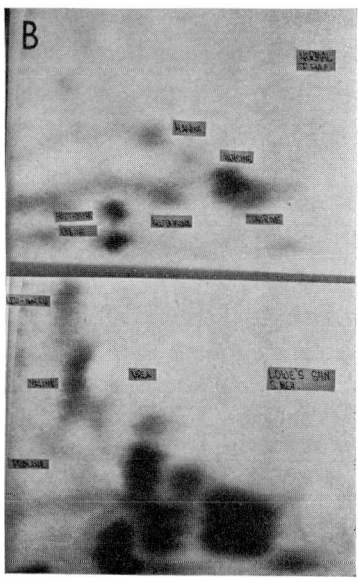

Fig. 21.6.—Oculocerebrorenal syndrome (Lowe) in 9-month-old boy. Bilateral cataracts were noted at 3 days of age. Glaucoma was noted at 5 months and has led to three operations. At age 9 months he exhibits marked hypotonia with hyporeflexia, bilateral dense cataracts, slight buphthalmos, an abnormal appearance of pupils and irides **(A)**, and retardation in both growth and development. Laboratory studies revealed 4+ proteinuria, 1+ acetonuria, generalized aminoaciduria and acidosis, with blood pH 7.29 (normal 7.3–7.45). Note in **B** the generalized aminoaciduria (patient's urine pattern is in the lower half of the figure compared to normal pattern in upper half). Although all patients with this disorder do not have an identical pattern, chromatograms usually show a generalized increase in excretion of amino acids in the urine.

Fig. 21.7.—Neonatal hypoglycemia. This 3-month-old girl was born of a toxemic mother at term. At 14½ hours of age apnea and generalized twitching developed. Blood glucose of 0 mg./100 ml. was noted at 23 hours. Glucose intravenously and ACTH intramuscularly effected normoglycemia. Microcephaly **(A)**, ventricular dilatation **(B)**, mental retardation, refractory seizures and spastic quadriparesis are apparent at 3 months.

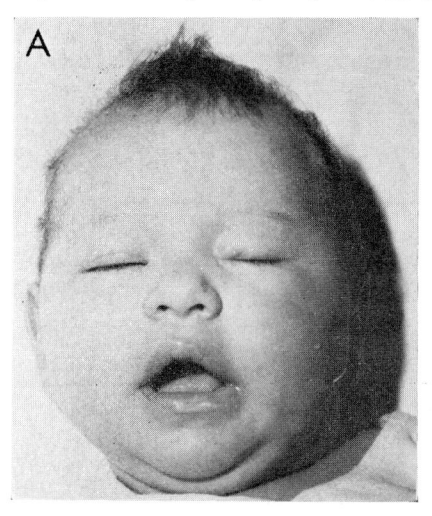

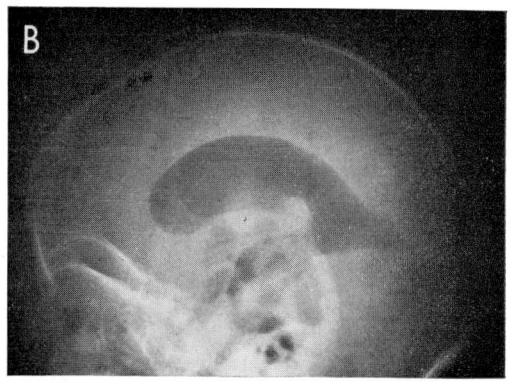

pathic infantile forms of the disease, many of these infants suffer severe damage to the brain, with residual mental defect (Fig. 21.7), refractory seizures, behavior disorders and even focal neurologic deficit.

Galactosemia

PATHOGENESIS.—This disorder is inherited as an autosomal recessive trait and results from an inability to metabolize galactose, the monosaccharide derived from the milk sugar, lactose. It is caused by an inherited deficiency of the enzyme *galactose-1-phosphate uridyl transferase* (Fig. 21.8). This enzymatic block leads to markedly elevated levels of blood galactose-1-phosphate which causes fatty degeneration of the liver followed by cirrhosis, lenticular cataracts and brain damage in the form of neuronal loss and gliosis.

CLINICAL AND LABORATORY DIAGNOSIS.—Galactosemic infants appear normal at birth, but symptoms of vomiting, failure to gain weight and listlessness appear early. Hepatomegaly and jaundice are seen, followed later by lenticular cataracts, splenomegaly and other signs of portal hypertension. The infants show retarded mental and physical development and may have seizures as a result of a secondary hypoglycemia.

A positive result of Benedict's test for urinary reducing substance will be found in *most* patients, and this is the diagnostic test of choice—*not a clini-stix* test, since the latter will give a positive result only if the urinary reducing substance is glucose. The identification of the sugar in the urine as galactose can be confirmed by paper chromatography. Proteinuria and generalized aminoaciduria, the latter presumably due to the "toxic" effect on the renal tubules of marked galactosemia,[35] also occur regularly.

By assay of the transferase activity in red blood cells one can identify the affected individuals (homozygotes have 50% of normal activity) and carriers (heterozygotes have 75% of normal activity) as shown by Kalckar et al.[74] This highly specific test for galactosemia can and should be performed on cord blood of siblings of patients with the disease. Previously the galactose tolerance test was

Fig. 21.8.—Outline of metabolic pathway block in galactosemia (see text).

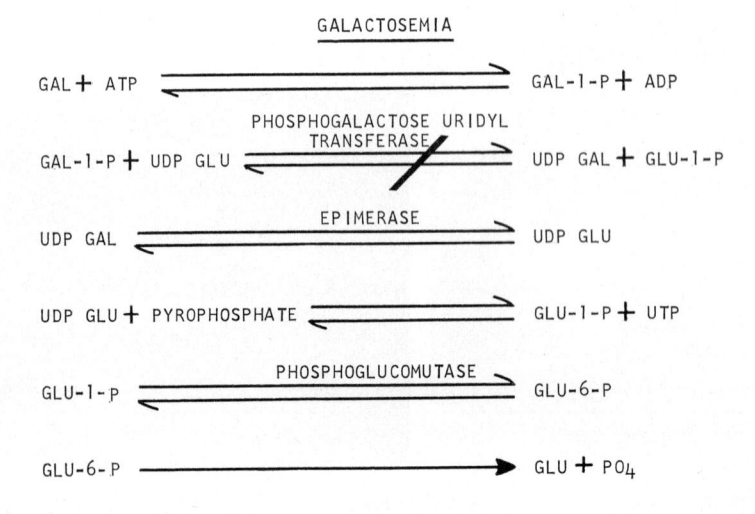

GALACTOSEMIA

GAL + ATP ⇌ GAL-1-P + ADP

PHOSPHOGALACTOSE URIDYL TRANSFERASE
GAL-1-P + UDP GLU ⇌̸ UDP GAL + GLU-1-P

EPIMERASE
UDP GAL ⇌ UDP GLU

UDP GLU + PYROPHOSPHATE ⇌ GLU-1-P + UTP

PHOSPHOGLUCOMUTASE
GLU-1-P ⇌ GLU-6-P

GLU-6-P ⟶ GLU + PO$_4$

used to identify affected patients and heterozygotes, but the development of the more reliable enzymatic assay and the danger of inducing hypoglycemic episodes with a load of galactose have restricted the use of the tolerance test.

MANAGEMENT AND PROGNOSIS.—Affected infants should be placed on a diet free of milk and dairy products. Use of commercially available lactose-free formulas, such as Nutramigen and Mull-soy, reverse the acute symptoms effectively but have little or no effect on established cataracts and mental retardation. Milk and milk products should be avoided until after puberty in all patients, and some patients are maintained on dietary restrictions indefinitely.

Early dietary restriction of milk, even in questionable cases, is important to prevent irreversible damage to the brain, the eyes and the liver. As in other metabolic defects in which the untreated disease varies in severity, it is difficult at this time to define with certainty the age after which dietary therapy is hopeless. Some untreated cases are discovered in mildly affected adults, but patients with more severe disease will die in early infancy if untreated. In undiagnosed cases the majority of surviving patients will exhibit permanent residual damage to the brain, eyes and liver.

Fructosuria with Hypoglucosemia (Hereditary Fructose Intolerance)

PATHOGENESIS.—Although fructosuria usually causes no clinical symptoms, isolated cases in which fructose ingestion causes hypoglucosemia have been reported.[33] Certain hypothetical mechanisms have been proposed to explain the biochemical lesion:

1. The defect in fructose utilization results from a deficiency of fructose-1-phosphate aldolase with an accumulation of fructose-1-phosphate in the tissues, causing damage to the liver and kidneys.
2. The hypoglucosemia may result from insulin overproduction.

CLINICAL AND LABORATORY DIAGNOSIS.—This rare disorder is characterized by small stature, mild mental retardation, attacks of hypoglycemia (vomiting, sweating, somnolence, tremor and seizures) and hepatomegaly with transient icterus. Differential diagnosis must consider idiopathic hypoglycemia of infancy, galactosemia, leucine-induced hypoglycemia, glycogen storage disease, celiac disease and pancreatic insulinoma.

A hypoglycemic response to a fructose tolerance test (50 Gm. fructose/M.^{2} body surface), fructosuria, aminoaciduria (pattern is unclear) and albuminuria are found.

MANAGEMENT AND PROGNOSIS.—Treatment consists in avoiding fruits and cane or beet sugar, since the latter is split into fructose and glucose. This regimen will prevent symptoms and signs of the disease. However, long-term results in patients who receive prompt diagnosis and treatment have not been reported.

Since the disorder is inherited as an autosomal recessive trait, parents should be advised of the high recurrence risk.

Polysaccharidoses

Classification of these inherited metabolic disorders presents the nosologic problem of deciding whether one is dealing with a lipid or a carbohydrate storage disease. This dilemma results from the fact that the ganglioside (lipid) content of the cerebral cortex is increased and the fact that the abnormal storage material in the reticuloendothelial system is a polysaccharide.

PATHOGENESIS.—Although the basic chemical anomaly is not fully understood, it has been known for many years that the urine of patients with classic gargoylism contains abnormally large amounts of four sulfated mucopolysaccharides—chondroitin sulfate A, chondroitin sulfate B (CSB), heparitin sulfate and keratosulfate. As more patients with inherited undiagnosed disease have been studied, the disease definition has been extended on the basis of urinary excretion patterns of acid mucopolysaccharides (AMPS) to the point where five different forms of the disease have now been distinguished.[119,140a] The five types and their distinguishing clinical and chemical characteristics are shown in Table 21.2.

Experience with detailed pathologic studies has been limited largely to examination of tissue from patients with the classic autosomal recessive form of the syndrome. A recent comprehensive case report on the morphologic, histochemical and biochemical studies of the type III disorder (Sanfilippo) has been given by Wallace et al.[145] Grossly the brain may appear enlarged and this is usually due to internal hydrocephalus. The latter results from obstruction to the normal reabsorption of cerebrospinal fluid over the surface by leptomeninges which are thickened by lipid deposits and secondary fibrotic changes. Histologically distention of the neurons with ganglioside-like material is seen primarily in the cerebral cortex and in some of the cells in the basal nuclei and brain stem. Peculiar cavitation is seen in the perivascular spaces. Controversy surrounds the exact nature of the storage

TABLE 21.2.—FIVE MUCOPOLYSACCHARIDE DISORDERS*

	NAME	CLINICAL PICTURE	TOTAL AMPS	OTHER CHEMICAL CHARACTERISTICS
MPS I	Classic autosomal recessive (CSB excreters) (Hurler)	Abnormal facies, skeletal deformities, hepatosplenomegaly, dwarfism, cloudy cornea	↑	CSB:HS = 80:20
MPS II	Classic sex-linked recessive (Hunter)	Late onset, mild skeletal and no corneal abnormalities, no hepatosplenomegaly	↑	CSB:HS = 55:45
MPS III	Neurodegenerative autosomal recessive (HS excreters) (Sanfilippo)	Severe dementia, hepatosplenomegaly	↑ (slight)	Heparitin sulfate (only)
MPS IV	Autosomal recessive musculoskeletal deformity (Morquio or Morquio-Ullrich)	Symmetrical dwarfism, genu valgum, pigeon breast, spine deformities	↑	Keratosulfate (only)
MPS V	Adult type (Scheie)	Corneal opacities	↑	—

*Modified from McKusick et al.[93]
AMPS = acid mucopolysaccharides
CSB = chondroitin sulfate B
HS = heparitin sulfate

DEMENTIA ± SEIZURES ± SPASTICITY ± BLINDNESS   **409**

material found in the liver, heart, cartilage, bone marrow and other viscera, but most believe that it represents acid or sulfated mucopolysaccharides.

CLINICAL AND LABORATORY DIAGNOSIS.—Five types of mucopolysaccharidosis are listed in Table 21.2.[93]

MPS I (Hurler).—One can easily recognize clinically only the classic autosomal recessive type (both sexes are affected) in which the grotesque gargoyle-like facies (large head, flat nose bridge, large lips and tongue with open mouth, bushy eyebrows, low-set ears), the dwarfed stature, noisy stertorous breathing, kyphosis,

Fig. 21.9.—Gargoylism (MPS I). Boy, 14, had onset of symptoms with a generalized seizure at 5 days of age. He has had recurrent infections and noisy breathing all his life. The family noted a hearing loss when he was 3½, and developmental retardation has been evident since age 2. During early and middle childhood the peculiar facial appearance and joint contractures became increasingly obvious. Two siblings are normal. Examination at age 14 reveals a short, partially deaf boy with a slightly large head, a prominent abdomen and continuously noisy respirations. The nose bridge is flat, the tongue prominent and the mouth is held open (**A**). He has joint contractures at elbows, wrists, knees and ankles and a marked hepatosplenomegaly. Typical bony abnormalities are illustrated in **B** and **C**.

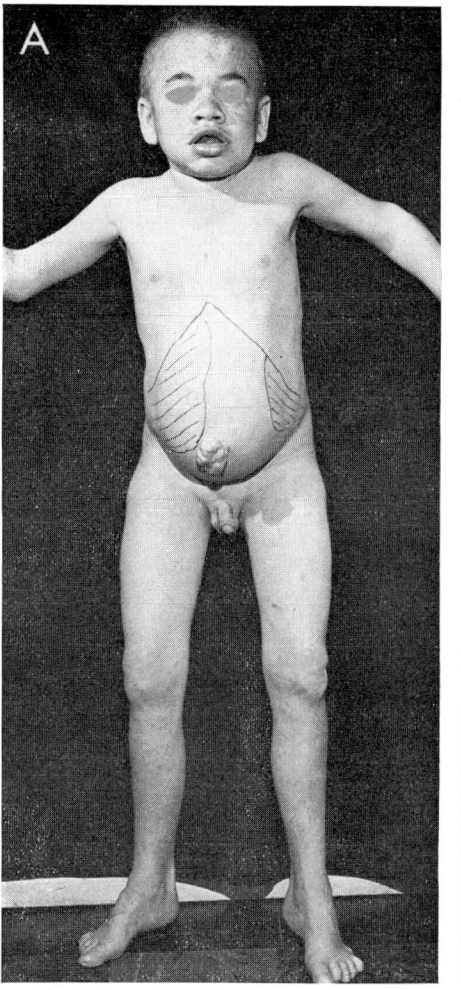

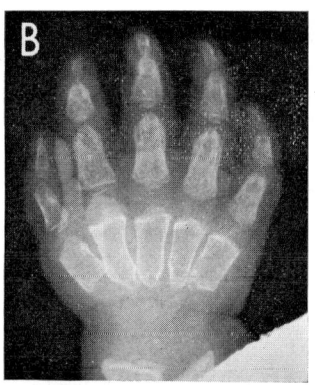

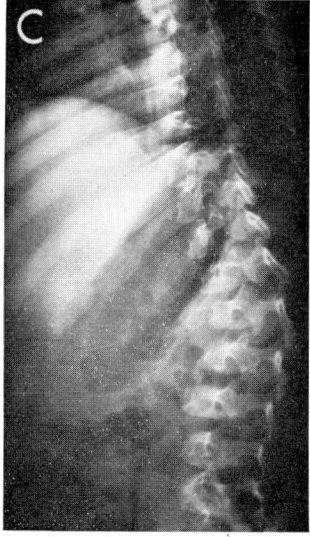

short, tapering, in-curved fingers, joint contractures, umbilical hernia, hepatosplenomegaly, deafness and corneal opacities are evident (Fig. 21.9,*A*). Needless to say, all of these physical signs are not present in every patient, especially in the early months and years of life. Diagnostic x-ray changes are best seen in the upper extremities, the most characteristic alteration being swelling of the midportion of the shaft of the humerus along with undertubulation, shortness and irregular widening of the ulna, radius and metacarpals (Fig. 21.9,*B*). The "hooking" of the first or second lumbar vertebra in the area of the gibbus may be helpful in diagnosis (Fig. 21.9,*C*), but great care must be taken to differentiate this finding from the normal developmental changes.

Chromatograms of the urinary AMPS (Table 21.2) produce the most definitive diagnostic data. The total AMPS are excreted in large excess with the ratio of CSB:HS in the range of 80:20; in other words, the classic autosomal recessive cases are primarily "CSB excreters."

A filter paper "spot test" has been devised for crude screening purposes. Place 5, 10 and 25 μl. of urine on a piece of Whatman #1 filter paper and allow to dry. Using a micropipet, add 5 μl. of urine at a time, letting each application dry thoroughly before the next is made. The paper is then dipped in a 50% ethanol solution of 0.1% toluidine blue and placed in a buffer solution (1% acetic acid in 50% ethanol) for 45–60 seconds. The paper is then washed in 95% ethanol and allowed to dry. Urine from patients with gargoylism produces a purple spot on a blue background. Use 5 μl. of a chondroitin sulfate solution containing 0.10 mg./ml. as a control positive for comparison. This test must be interpreted cautiously because false-positive results may occur, especially in normal infants under age 2.[11]

MPS II (Hunter).—The classic sex-linked recessive form of the disease is not easily recognized clinically. Symptom onset occurs later than in type I, with only mild mental defect, minor skeletal abnormalities and without cloudy corneae. The total urinary AMPS excretion is elevated and the pattern is characterized by a CSB:HS ratio of approximately 55:45, consistently lower than that of patients with the classic autosomal recessive type of disease.

MPS III (Sanfilippo).—Patients with the neurodegenerative autosomal recessive form of the disease show progressive mental and motor deterioration but little else. Hepatosplenomegaly occurs inconsistently and no obvious bone, joint, facial or corneal abnormalities are present. The diagnosis must be made chemically by urine chromatography. The total AMPS excretion is elevated and these patients excrete HS in excess.

MPS IV (Morquio or Morquio-Ullrich).—The classic features of Morquio's disease include dwarfism, normal skull and intellect, short trunk and extremities, pigeon breast and spine deformities, knock-knees, flat feet, muscle weakness and a waddling gait. Roentgen examinations reveal flattening of the vertebral bodies and a central "tongue" formation, metacarpals which point proximally rather than distally, and hypoplasia and irregularity of the carpals. X-rays of the knees show metaphyseal flattening and epiphyseal fragmentation.

Included in the differential diagnosis are cretinism, rickets and syphilis. In cretinism one finds a low protein-bound iodine, high serum cholesterol and different x-ray changes. In Morquio's disease the skeletal changes and stature resemble those seen in gargoylism, but the condition is not progressive, there is no mental defect or hepatosplenomegaly, and an excessive amount of keratosulfate is found in the urine.[119]

In pseudo-Hurler's disease,[84] a familial lipid storage disorder of infants, one finds mental defect, hepatosplenomegaly and changes like those in Hurler's disease, foam cells in the marrow as in Niemann-Pick disease and cerebral and retinal changes like those in Tay-Sachs disease. Hurler's disease may be confused clinically with both rickets and syphilis, but chemical and serologic blood tests are diagnostic of the latter conditions.

MPS V (Scheie).—A fifth and rare form of the disease occurs in adults. It produces mild clinical symptoms, the most prominent being corneal abnormalities. These patients excrete an excess of both CSB and HS, but the distinctive chemical feature rests upon the fact that, unlike the other forms, the excess CSB is not precipitated as the calcium salt with 10% or 20% alcohol.

MANAGEMENT AND PROGNOSIS.—No specific therapy is yet available for this disorder. All the common forms of this condition are inherited as a recessive trait and hence more than one sibling is commonly affected.

In general, patients with the autosomal recessive disorder die between 10 and 20 years of age, whereas those with the sex-linked recessive trait may survive to middle life. The longevity of patients with the atypical, neurodegenerative autosomal recessive disease is quite similar to that of patients with the classic autosomal recessive type.

Cerebral Lipidoses

All of these conditions are characterized by the abnormal accumulation of lipids in the cells of the nervous system and sometimes in other tissues (Table 21.3). Inasmuch as many of these disorders exhibit a hereditary incidence pattern, it is presumed that the disease conditions result from an enzymatic defect in intracellular lipid metabolism. Much progress has been made in identifying the stored lipids but less is known about the exact molecular defect.[18] These diseases have been subdivided according to the other body systems and structures which are involved clinically.

BRAIN AND RETICULOENDOTHELIAL SYSTEM

Niemann-Pick Disease

This lipid storage disorder is inherited as an autosomal recessive trait and is characterized by the accumulation of sphingomyelin in the reticuloendothelial system. It occurs more frequently, but not exclusively, in Jews. Involvement of the brain is frequent but not invariable.

The age of onset is quite variable, and although neurologic symptoms may usher in the disease, more commonly visceral enlargement with failure to thrive and even jaundice appear early. Brownish pigmentation of the skin and pallor secondary to anemia may be present. The motor and mental development is retarded in most but not all patients. A cherry-red macula, indistinguishable from that seen in Tay-Sachs disease, is seen in 25–50% of cases. Seizures occur commonly, and dementia, blindness and spasticity develop in the terminal stage of the disease.

TABLE 21.3.—DIFFERENTIAL DIAGNOSIS OF THE DIFFUSE CEREBRAL SCLEROSES
(LEUKODYSTROPHIES) AND THE NEURAL LIPIDOSES

	AGE OF ONSET, COURSE	FAMILIAL OCCURRENCE	GENERAL EXAMINATION	NEUROLOGIC EXAMINATION	LABORATORY ABNORMALITIES
Leukodystrophies					
Globoid cell (Krabbe)	Infancy Rapid course	+	0	Dementia, spasticity	CSF protein
Pelizaeus-Merzbacher	Early childhood Chronic course	+	0	Dementia, spasticity, movement disorders	
Metachromatic sudanophilic (Schilder) Spongy degeneration	Early infancy Rapid course	+	0	Spasticity, dementia, head enlargement, blindness	0 → 1
Neural lipidoses					
Amaurotic familial idiocy					
Tay-Sachs	Infancy	+	Cherry-red macula	Hyperacusis	
Bielschowsky	3–4 years	+	Optic atrophy, pigmentary degeneration of retina	Blindness, dementia, ataxia, spasticity	0 → 1
Spielmeyer-Vogt	3–10 years	+			
Kufs	15–25 years	+			
Reticuloendothelioses					
Niemann-Pick	2–5 years	+	Hepatosplenomegaly, cherry-red macula in 25–50%	Dementia, blindness, spasticity	Foam cells in marrow (Fig. 21.10)
Gaucher	Infancy	+	Splenomegaly	Spasticity, dementia	Foam cells in marrow (Fig. 21.10)

Bone marrow aspiration or biopsy of the liver or spleen is usually diagnostic because the huge fat-filled "foam cells" are easily seen on microscopic study (Fig. 21.10,*A*). The circulating lymphocytes are vacuolated in most patients with this disease, but this can only be considered supportive, not diagnostic, evidence.

Gaucher's Disease

PATHOGENESIS.—This rare storage disease is characterized by its autosomal recessive incidence pattern and by the accumulation of the cerebroside kerasin in the reticuloendothelial cells of the spleen and liver. Jews are not affected predominantly as in some of the other lipidoses. The material causes a granular, lacy appearance of the cytoplasm and must be distinguished from the foam cells of Niemann-Pick disease. When the nervous system is involved, and this occurs irregularly, one finds primarily neuronal degeneration with neuronal lipidosis appearing only to a moderate degree in the minority of cases.

CLINICAL AND LABORATORY DIAGNOSIS.—Neurologic symptoms and signs are seen inconsistently in this disorder but occur more frequently in the acute infantile form of the disease. Developmental lag may occur at about 6 months of age, followed by ocular squint, opisthotonus, pyramidal tract signs, pseudobulbar palsy (dysphagia, facial immobility and respiratory stridor) and splenomegaly with anemia or pancytopenia and a bleeding tendency. No typical retinal lesions are seen and seizures rarely occur. The patients usually become decerebrate and wasted rather quickly and die of aspiration pneumonia.

Bone marrow aspiration and splenic biopsy often reveal the so-called fat-laden "Gaucher cells." The accumulated kerasin causes a lacy or fibrillar appearance of the cytoplasm (Fig. 21.10,*B*), and such cells are generally distinguishable from the foam cells of Niemann-Pick disease. In practice, however, the morphologic differentiation of the abnormal cells is often difficult and may hinge upon the histochemical staining qualities.

Kampine and associates[75] recently suggested that the low enzymatic activity (enzymes which hydrolyze glucocerebroside and sphingomyelin) of leukocytes from

Fig. 21.10.—Bone marrow "foam cells" in lipidoses. Photomicrographs of foam cells from patients with Niemann-Pick disease (A) and Gaucher's disease (B).

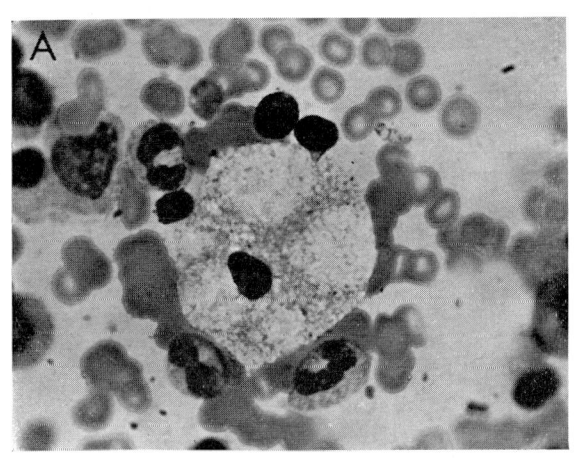

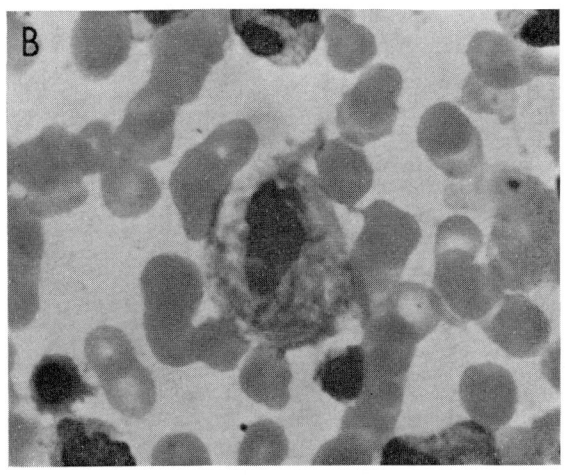

the venous blood of patients with Gaucher's and Niemann-Pick diseases may prove to have diagnostic value. The chronic (adult) form of Gaucher's disease affects the nervous system only rarely.

MANAGEMENT AND PROGNOSIS.—Symptomatic treatment, such as nasogastric tube feeding, antibiotics and transfusion for severe anemia, represents the only form of available therapy. Splenectomy is ineffective in altering the course of the disease. Death usually occurs at about age 1. Parents must be made aware that subsequent siblings have a rather high risk of being similarly affected.

NERVOUS SYSTEM AND RETINA

Infantile Amaurotic Familial Idiocy (Tay-Sachs Disease)

PATHOGENESIS.—Striking distention of the neurons with a material called ganglioside, together with reactive gliosis and moderate demyelination is seen in these patients. The excess lipid material is widely distributed from the neurons of the cerebral cortex to those in the cerebellum, spinal cord and even the myenteric plexus of the rectum. The ganglion cells of the retina are reduced in number and they are also distended with lipid. Tay-Sachs disease is more common in Eastern Europen Jews and is inherited as an autosomal recessive disease.

CLINICAL AND LABORATORY DIAGNOSIS.—These infants may appear normal at birth but usually are retarded in achieving their motor milestones. Hyperacusis (abnormal sensitivity to noise) is seen early in many patients; although this response looks like an exaggerated Moro reflex, it cannot be distinguished readily from a convulsive myoclonic jerk (Fig. 21.11,A). The cherry-red spot of macular degeneration surrounded by a large white halo—the distinctive clinical sign—can be seen on routine funduscopic examination. Early in the disease these patients are hypotonic, but later spasticity and dysphagia supervene, with blindness, generalized seizures and a decerebrate state. Hepatosplenomegaly does not occur, but head enlargement often appears as the result of macrocephaly.

Biopsy of the rectal wall is the most definitive diagnostic procedure if the removed tissue includes neurons of the myenteric plexus. An appropriate fat or hematoxylin-eosin stain reveals the lipid-laden cells[90b] (Fig. 21.11,B). The cerebrospinal fluid may show slight elevation of total protein, but other routine studies give normal findings. The electroencephalogram often shows diffuse but nonspecific slow waves and epileptiform spike discharges. Slight vacuolation of the circulating lymphocytes may be found, but this is not specific for Tay-Sachs disease.

MANAGEMENT AND PROGNOSIS.—Unfortunately, no specific therapy is available for this condition. Anticonvulsant drugs may be used to control seizures and nasogastric tube feeding is usually necessary in the terminal stages. Children with this fatal disorder usually die in the second or third year of life. Consequently, although more than one sibling may be affected, the disease itself usually disappears in a family because subsequent generations are not affected.

Juvenile Amaurotic Familial Idiocy

These disorders, which are inherited as autosomal recessive traits, have been distinguished eponymically (Bielschowsky, Batten, Spielmeyer-Vogt and Kufs

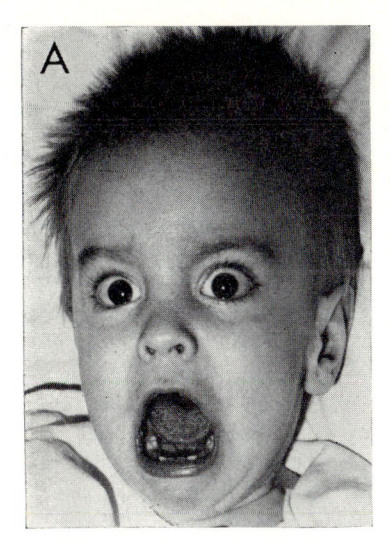

Fig. 21.11.—Tay-Sachs disease. This 19-month-old boy appeared normal until slow motor development was noted at 7 months. Subsequently, retardation in social, language and adaptive spheres became obvious. Examination revealed an exaggerated Moro response **(A)**, bilateral cherry-red spots in the macular areas and bilateral optic nerve pallor. Biopsy of the rectal mucosa revealed lipid-laden ganglion cells in the myenteric plexus **(B)**, confirming the clinical diagnosis of Tay-Sachs disease. The child became increasingly spastic and helpless and died in a cachectic state when he was 22 months old.

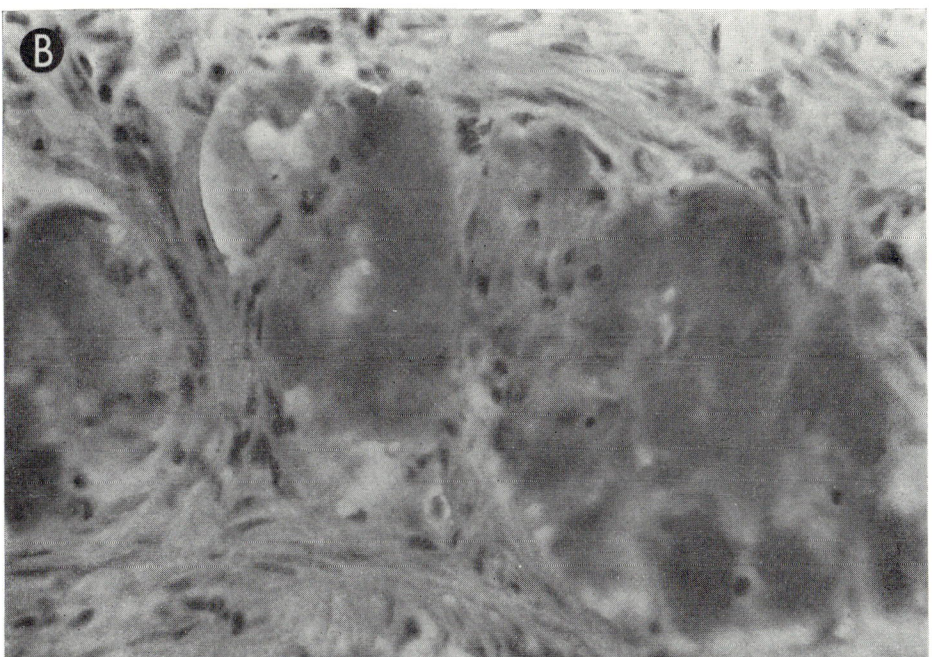

types) according to the age at onset of symptoms. Otherwise their genetic, pathologic, biochemical and clinical characteristics are largely indistinguishable. In general, the earlier the onset of clinical symptoms, the more severe the disease and the more rapid the fatal outcome.

PATHOGENESIS.—The fat-filled neurons characteristic of Tay-Sachs disease are seen also in the other forms of amaurotic familial idiocy, but the degree of cytoplasmic distention is usually less marked. A familial incidence is the rule, but these diseases have no predilection for Jews. Multiple siblings may be affected. The retinal rods and cones may degenerate in the juvenile types, whereas only the ganglion cells of the retina are involved in the infantile form.

CLINICAL AND LABORATORY DIAGNOSIS.—Patients show normal development in early childhood, and the first symptoms are often those of failing vision, seizures, speech and behavior disturbances. Later dementia, movement disorders and gait disturbances appear. The ocular findings vary from optic atrophy to pigmentary degeneration of the retina and macula, but eventually most patients are partially or totally blind. Variable motor system involvement is also seen, with some patients showing parkinsonian rigidity and paucity of movement, others showing athetosis and many eventually having obvious bilateral corticospinal tract signs. The psychotic behavior which some patients manifest may suggest a functional disorder. Ford[49] has collected evidence to suggest that some cases of so-called Heller's infantile dementia may result from cerebral lipidosis (Chapter 1).

No reliable laboratory tests are available for these diseases, the definitive diagnosis depending upon tissue examination. However, recently Bessman et al.[15] described an excessive excretion of imidazole amino acids in the urine of five patients from three different kindreds with late-onset cerebromacular degeneration. Some workers have stressed the diagnostic EEG value of bilaterally synchronous, high-voltage, triphasic sharp waves on a slow background pattern ("burst-suppression"), but this abnormality is found in other diseases.[27a]

MANAGEMENT AND PROGNOSIS.—Anticonvulsant and psychotropic drug therapy may offer temporary symptomatic relief. However, no specific therapy is available for children with this slowly progressive disease. The disorder often terminates with status epilepticus or a fatal infection.

LEUKODYSTROPHIES (DIFFUSE SCLEROSES)

This group includes (1) globoid cell leukodystrophy (Krabbe), (2) Pelizaeus-Merzbacher leukoencephalopathy, (3) metachromatic leukoencephalopathy, (4) sudanophilic leukodystrophy (Schilder) and (5) spongy degeneration of the white matter (Canavan). Brief reference is also made to degeneration of the cerebral gray matter (Alpers).

At present these conditions are distinguished almost exclusively by their histopathology, although a few distinctive clinical features can be used to separate them from one another. This rare group of disorders is characterized by the familial aggregation of cases and by the diffuse dissolution of white matter with the relative sparing of the nerve cell bodies in the cortex. Also, the histochemical qualities of the lipid breakdown products differ distinctly from those which result from almost every other disorder in which myelin destruction is extensive, including the demyelinating lesions of multiple sclerosis, Schilder's disease, cerebral infarction and fiber tract degeneration. Although the exact etiology of the leukodystrophies is unknown, the accumulated histopathologic and histochemical evidence suggests that they result from a metabolic defect in the lipids of the myelin sheath.

Globoid Cell Leukodystrophy (Krabbe)

This familial disorder retards the normal development of young infants and is associated with generalized spasticity or hypotonia in the advanced stages (Fig.

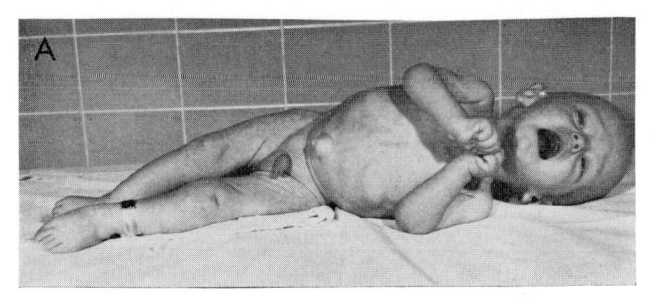

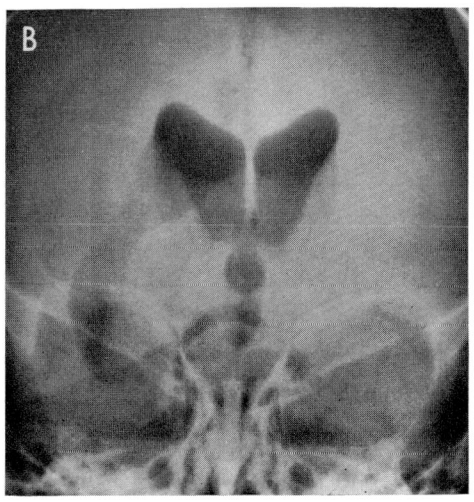

Fig. 21.12.—Krabbe's disease. Patient B.B. was born prematurely but uneventfully, weighing 4 lb. 5 oz., and developed normally until 5 months of age, when gradually increasing developmental retardation and spasticity appeared. At 8 months he was a helpless, irritable, poorly nourished infant with generalized spasticity (A), spontaneous clonus in all four extremities, Babinski signs and impaired swallow. A pneumoencephalogram revealed moderate, diffuse ventricular dilatation (B). Repeated CSF examinations showed markedly elevated total protein (Fig. 21.13). Other laboratory findings were normal. The patient died at 22 months, and autopsy revealed typical gross and microscopic evidence of Krabbe's disease.

21.12,*A*), pyramidal tract signs, dysphagia, opisthotonos and terminal respiratory infection. Pneumoencephalography may show signs of cerebral atrophy (Fig. 21.12,*B*) and the cerebrospinal fluid protein value is often markedly elevated (Fig. 21.13), but no other specific laboratory abnormalities are found.

Examination of nerve tissue in this unique leukoencephalopathy discloses packets of multinucleated cells of spherical shape which resemble foreign body giant cells and which contain lipid breakdown products. Analysis of affected brains has not shown a consistently abnormal chemical pattern, but in most cases there are low concentrations of total glycolipids, cerebrosides and sulfatides. The fact that abnormal storage material is not found in nerve cells or in peripheral nerves means that biopsy procedures are not diagnostic.

Treatment is entirely symptomatic in this rapidly downhill disorder. Multiple siblings may well be affected, but predictions about the likelihood of recurrence cannot be made without autopsy evidence in an affected sibling.

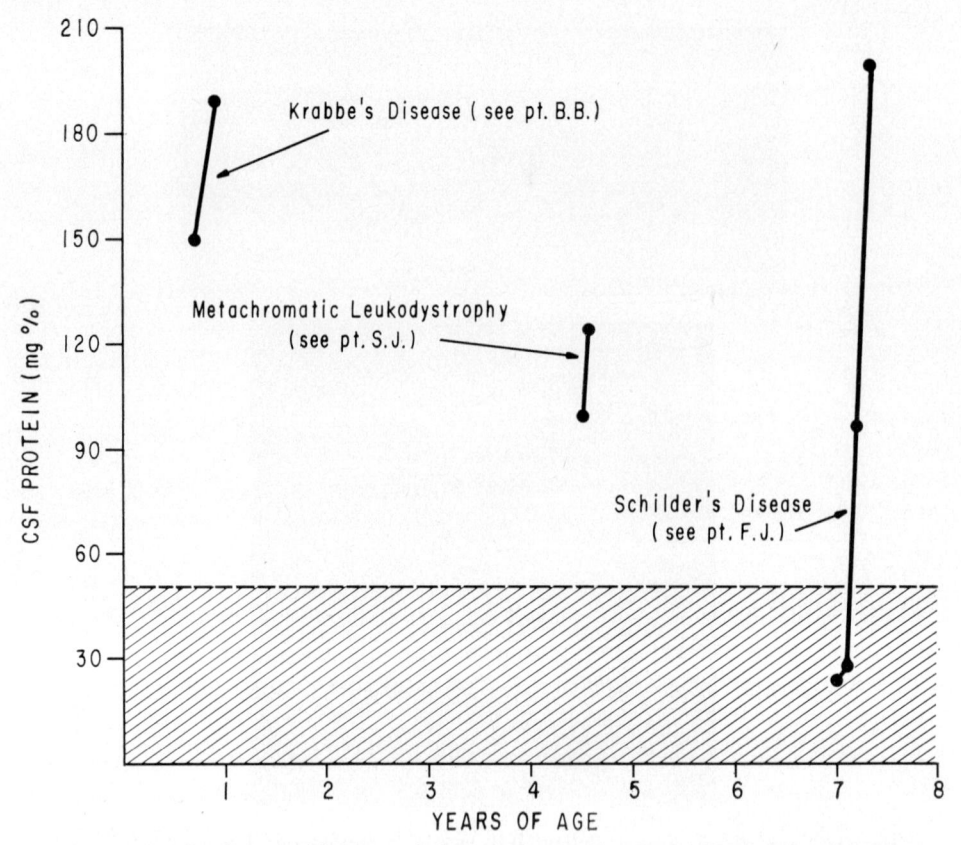

Fig. 21.13.—Cerebrospinal fluid protein in leukodystrophies. Graph illustrates serial CSF protein values from patients with proved leukodystrophies. See legend for Figure 21.12 (Krabbe's disease), Figure 21.14 (metachromatic leukodystrophy) and Figure 21.15 (Schilder's disease).

Pelizaeus-Merzbacher Leukodystrophy

This type of diffuse cerebral sclerosis is characterized by a strong familial tendency and a chronic, slowly progressive course. The disease usually begins in infancy or early childhood, but the patients may live to the third decade. The gradual development of spasticity, dementia, ataxia, choreoathetotic movement disorders and seizures late in the course is characteristic. Widespread but patchy demyelination occurs with relative sparing of axons. Myelin breakdown products, although sparse because of the chronic nature of the disorder, stain as neutral fats (as in sudanophilic leukodystrophy of Schilder) rather than complex lipids (as in metachromatic leukodystrophy). Histochemical and quantitative chemical studies to date have shed no significant light on the pathogenesis of this disorder.[107]

Metachromatic Leukodystrophy (Sulfatide Lipidosis)

PATHOGENESIS.—This disorder is typified pathologically by diffuse metachromasia when tissues are stained with appropriate dyes, such as toluidine blue or cresyl violet. The normal color produced by these dyes is blue or violet whereas the metachromatic color is red or brown. Since the sulfatide (sulfuric acid ester of a cerebroside) content is 5–10 times higher than it is in normal brain tissue and 20 times higher than in normal kidney tissue, and since sulfatide lipids normally show metachromasia, it is assumed that sulfatides are responsible for the characteristic staining reaction in the disease. The fact that metachromatic lipids accumulate in organs outside the brain, including the kidneys, peripheral nerves, liver, pancreas and gall bladder, has both theoretical and practical implications.

CLINICAL AND LABORATORY DIAGNOSIS.—This degenerative neurologic disorder usually begins during the second year of life and terminates between 3 and 6 years of age. It often affects more than one sibling and is thought to behave as a recessive trait. Gait disability commonly appears as the first symptom and may be associated with musculoskeletal deformities such as valgus deformities of the knees and feet[65] as well as genu recurvatum.[40] Whereas initially hypotonia, areflexia and joint deformities predominate, later a spastic quadriparesis, dysphagia, dementia and ataxia gradually develop (Fig. 21.14). This disease should be considered carefully in any hypotonic young child with progressive lower motor neuron disease. If seizures develop, they usually appear late in the course, as do cortical blindness and deafness.

So far no rapid, definitive laboratory diagnostic method has been devised for this disorder although both Austin[4] and Lake[83] have described a "rapid screening test" on the urine of these patients. Cerebrospinal fluid examination may reveal an abnormally high concentration of total protein (Fig. 21.13). The laboratory diagnosis can be made by either a careful stain or a chemical analysis of the urinary sediment. Pink metachromatic granules can be demonstrated in the urinary sediment by staining the sediment with toluidine blue and examining it microscopically. Although this technique is reliable, great care and experience are needed to insure correct interpretation.

A chemical test has also been developed by Austin[5] to demonstrate the excess amounts of metachromatic urinary lipid found in this disorder. For this test, 20 volumes of 2:1 chloroform-methanol is added to the urinary sediment, mixed thoroughly and filtered, and the filtrate is equilibrated against a large volume of water. A white fluff develops at the interface between these solvents. A portion of

Fig. 21.14.—Metachromatic leukodystrophy. Patient S.J. developed normally until 18 months of age when slowly progressive gait disability and incoordination appeared. At age 2 years 9 months she had a spastic quadriparesis with bilateral Babinski signs but was able to walk with a spastic, unsteady gait. Pneumoencephalography at that time was normal. She was hospitalized in a state of decerebrate rigidity (photograph) at age 4 years 5 months. The CSF protein values are shown in Figure 21.13. A toluidine blue stain of the urinary sediment revealed many metachromatic granules. The patient died one month later. Autopsy revealed typical pathologic evidence of metachromatic leukodystrophy.

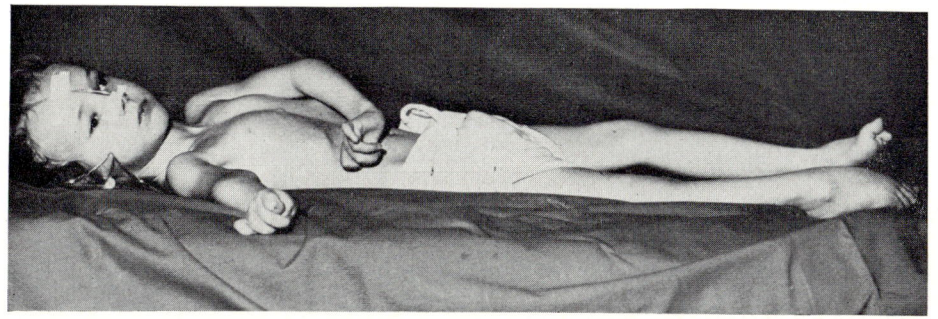

the fluff is applied to filter paper, allowed to dry and then dipped into 0.01% toluidine blue solution in 2% acetic acid. A persistent pink metachromasia represents a positive result, whereas normal samples show either no stain or a blue stain. Inasmuch as false-negative and false-positive reactions are encountered in the tests of urinary sediment, one should confirm the diagnosis by biopsy of a peripheral nerve, e.g., the sural nerve.[150]

MANAGEMENT AND PROGNOSIS.—Although this is a fatal disease with no specific treatment, early diagnosis should be attempted. A prompt and correct diagnosis is important for family planning since the disorder commonly affects more than one child in a sibship.

Sudanophilic Leukodystrophy (Schilder)

PATHOGENESIS.—The morphologic changes which accompany sudanophilic leukodystrophy are well recognized even though the cause or causes of this clinicopathologic syndrome are completely unknown. Most pathologists prefer to classify Schilder's sudanophilic dystrophy as a particular form of multiple sclerosis. Even though familial examples have been reported, most cases occur sporadically. The brain is usually shrunken, with marked, diffuse loss and cavitation of the white matter. The relative sparing of the subcortical arcuate fibers resembles the change seen in multiple sclerosis. Histologically one sees severe demyelination and myelin breakdown products of the sudanophilic type.

CLINICAL AND LABORATORY DIAGNOSIS.—This disorder can only be suspected on the basis of clinical findings, final proof depending upon tissue examination. The disease may develop at any age but is commoner in early childhood. It may occur sporadically or in a familial pattern. The earliest clinical manifestations vary greatly, but disorders of movement commonly herald the onset. Papilledema as a reflection of increased intracranial pressure may occur when massive areas of white matter softening are associated with swelling of the hemispheres. In some cases the papilledema may be a sign of optic neuritis without intracranial hypertension. Later in the course focal or generalized seizures, loss of vision, mental deterioration, aphasia, apraxia and cortical deafness occur. Dementia, generalized spasticity and blindness are seen in the terminal stages (Fig. 21.15,A).

No good specific diagnostic laboratory procedures for this condition are known. When the disease is suspected, the physician must differentiate metachromatic leukodystrophy (by examination of the urinary sediment) and the other neural lipidoses (by the family history and examination of the fundi). The CSF protein is usually elevated (Fig. 21.13). Schilder's disease in adults may be confused with brain tumors, presenile and arteriosclerotic dementias. Subacute inclusion encephalitis (Chapter 18) may resemble Schilder's disease closely, but the former condition is often characterized by paroxysmal, bilaterally synchronous, high-voltage slow and sharp wave EEG abnormalities superimposed upon low-voltage slow background frequencies.[78] Patients with Schilder's disease also have marked slowing and diffusely distributed epileptiform EEG abnormalities of nonspecific type (Fig. 21.15,B).

An interesting but obscure association between this disorder and Addison's disease has been documented by a number of workers.[15a,69a]

MANAGEMENT AND PROGNOSIS.—No specific therapy will influence the course

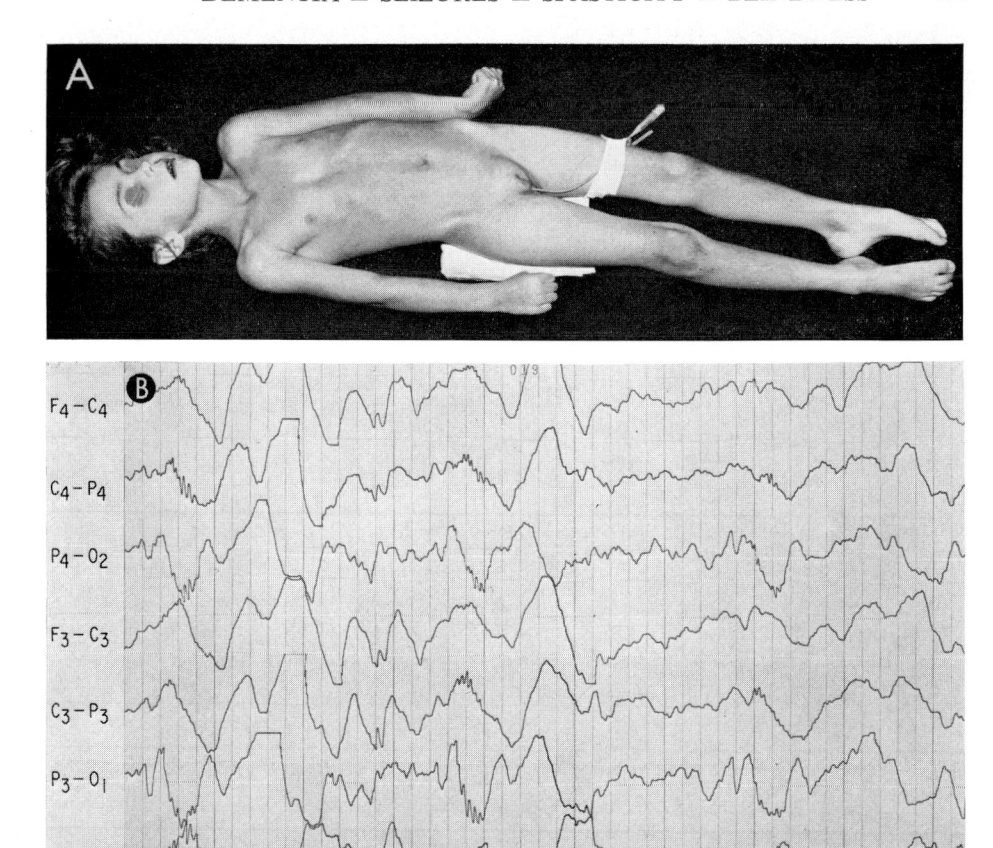

Fig. 21.15.—Schilder's disease. Patient F.J. was well until age 4½ years when she had a generalized seizure. Gradually a progressive change in personality and behavior developed. At age 6 years 10 months the parents reported a progressive deterioration in school work, inattention, dysarthria, unprovoked crying and immature behavior, and a tendency to sit and stare or to stumble into objects. The family history was not remarkable. Initial examination showed a fearful little girl who stared and seemed out of contact much of the time. She cried without provocation and spoke in incoherent, meaningless sentences. Repeated electroencephalograms **(B)** were grossly abnormal with diffuse, paroxysmal, high voltage spikes and slow waves followed by widespread electrical suppression. A trial of cortisone therapy produced some moderate but temporary improvement in behavior. The patient showed increasing lethargy, stupor, dementia, apparent blindness, vomiting and a right hemiparesis. Eventually she reached a decerebrate state **(A)**. The CSF protein rose steadily (see Fig. 21.13). Pneumonia developed and she died six weeks later at age 7 years 2 months.

of this disease. However, vigorous anticonvulsant treatment may be necessary to control seizures if they develop.

Hormones

Congenital Hypothyroidism (Cretinism)

PATHOGENESIS.—Although hypothyroidism may have its onset at almost any age, the forms which impose a threat to the nervous system in the form of mental retardation have their clinical and pathologic onset early in life. The types of hypothyroidism seen in early life may be classified as follows:

Congenital Hypothyroidism	Pathogenesis
1. Sporadic athyrotic cretinism	? Congenital anomaly
2. Familial goitrous cretinism	Inborn metabolic defect (four types[133])
3. Endemic cretinism	Deficient dietary intake of iodine

Approximately two-thirds of patients with congenital hypothyroidism have sporadic athyrotic cretinism and one-third have familial goitrous cretinism.[21] One should realize that not only can athyrotic cretinism occur occasionally in families, but that cretins with thyroid glands have been found in the same sibship with athyrotic cretins. In patients with familial goitrous cretinism, the thyroid glands can accumulate iodine normally, but, because of an inborn metabolic defect (four types have been described[21]), the gland cannot convert iodine into thyroxin. This situation leads to an excess output of pituitary thyroid-stimulating hormone which eventually causes the development of a goiter. Endemic cretinism is almost nonexistent in the United States especially since iodized salt has entered general use. Description of neuropathologic changes in this disorder are limited, but it is said that some brains are small in size, with cortical neurons showing both reduction in number and degenerative changes.

CLINICAL AND LABORATORY DIAGNOSIS.—Regardless of the type of cretinism, signs are usually absent at birth because the baby's needs in utero are supplied by the mother's thyroid function, assuming that the mother has normal thyroid function. Physiologic icterus may be prolonged in these babies, but the typical signs of cretinism do not usually appear for several months. Growth and motor retardation may appear early, together with peculiar changes in the face and body. The puffy eyelids, the open mouth with a thick, protruding tongue, the wrinkled forehead with a low hair line, the broad nose, pale mucous membranes, persistent open fontanel, coarse, scanty hair and dry skin constitute the classic picture (Fig. 21.16,*A*). Umbilical hernias are common, as are excess fat pads in the axillae and above the clavicles, low body temperature and slow heart rate. The infants cry little, sleep much, are constipated and have poor appetites. Carotenemia gives the skin a yellow color but the sclerae remain white. Mental retardation is present in almost all of these infants and this threat makes diagnosis and treatment urgent.

X-rays of the skeleton reveal marked retardation in bone age, even early in life, and when epiphyseal centers do appear they may show multiple foci of ossification (epiphyseal dysgenesis). Levels of serum protein-bound iodine (PBI) or butanol-extractable iodine (BEI) are low, usually under 2 μg./100 ml. (normal values 4–8 μg./100 ml.). Radioactive iodine uptake is low, usually under 10%, and serum cholesterol levels may be high. Goitrous cretinism differs from sporadic athyrotic cretinism only in that the I^{131} value is normal or high and the PBI may not be as low.

The differential diagnosis includes mongolism (present at birth with normal thyroid function), gargoylism (normal thyroid function, hepatosplenomegaly and excess urinary polysaccharides), chondrodystrophy (similarly dwarfed stature but different in all other ways) and pituitary dwarfism (alike only in small stature).

MANAGEMENT AND PROGNOSIS.—Unless the diagnosis of cretinism is made in early infancy and treatment started promptly, the risk of permanent mental retardation and dwarfism is great. In other words, although the early treatment of the cretin does not assure optimal mental development, most authorities agree that the prognosis for satisfactory intellect declines as the period of untreated hypothyroidism is prolonged (Fig. 21.16,B).[130] Even when this warning is heeded, irreversible damage may have occurred during intrauterine life. On the other hand, once the fully developed clinical picture of cretinism is established, replacement thyroid therapy may produce little benefit. Starting with 15 mg. of U.S.P. dessiccated thyroid/day, the dose (given once daily) should be raised by 15–30 mg. increments every one to two weeks until toxic signs appear (diarrhea, tachycardia and hyperactivity); then the dose should be reduced slightly. In infants under age 1 year 45–90 mg./day and in older children 120–200 mg./day will usually be satisfactory. Special attention to early diagnosis and treatment should be paid to newborn infants in families with other goitrous or cretinous children. As a way of measuring therapeutic adequacy, one can aim at PBI levels of 6–8 μg./100 ml.

As indicated, the prognosis for normal or near-normal mental and physical growth depends partly upon early diagnosis and treatment, but the prediction to

Fig. 21.16.—Cretinism. This 4-week-old baby was delivered uneventfully after a pregnancy which was uncomplicated except for a maternal flulike illness in the first trimester. The baby was sleepy, limp, inactive and exhibited a large tongue (A) and a weak cry. No other physical abnormalities were noted. Estimation of bone age revealed no definite retardation. The PBI was 3.7 mg./100 ml. (normal, 4–8 mg.) and I[131] uptake was 23% (normal, 15–45%). Diagnosis was cretinism and the baby was placed on desiccated thyroid therapy (50 mg./day). At age 3½ months the baby was much improved, with good motor development, weight gain and an alert appearance with a less prominent tongue (B).

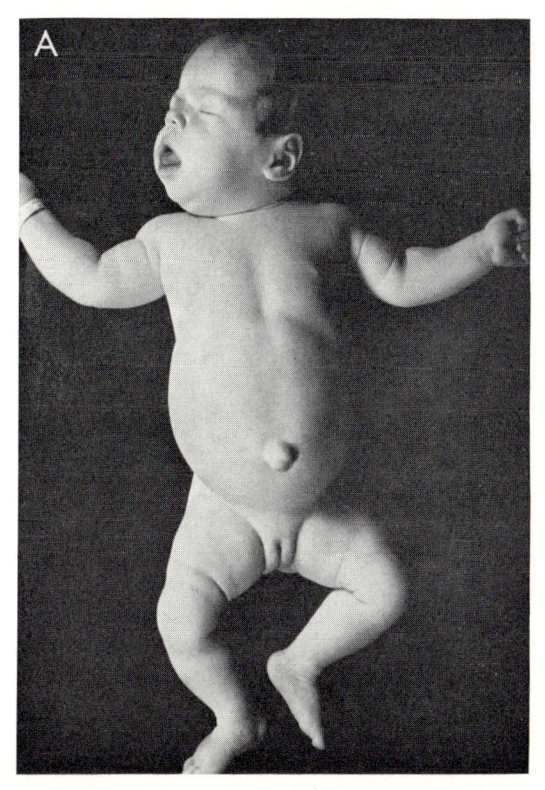

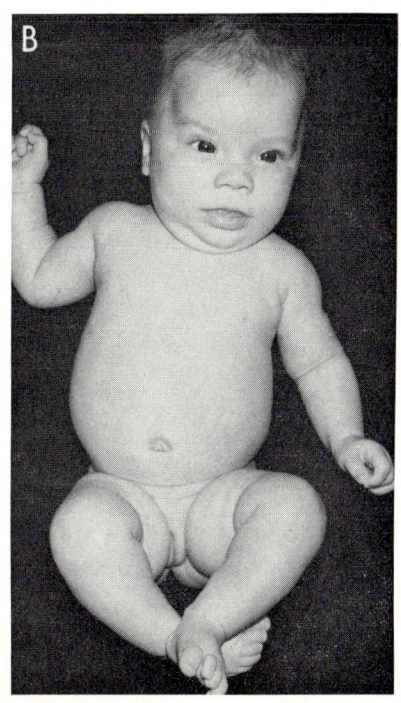

424 HEREDITARY METABOLIC AND DEGENERATIVE DISEASES

parents must be guarded. The recurrence risk is high in familial goitrous cretinism which behaves as an autosomal recessive trait. Athyrotic cretinism usually occurs sporadically, but on rare occasions more than one sibling is affected.

Idiopathic (Chronic) Hypoparathyroidism

PATHOGENESIS.—This disease which occurs uncommonly results from the defective secretion of parathormone and may be associated with adrenal insufficiency.

CLINICAL AND LABORATORY DIAGNOSIS.—The diagnosis of the rare disorder, idiopathic hypoparathyroidism, is often delayed considerably. Average interval between onset of symptoms and diagnosis is 6.3 years.[82] Inasmuch as the commonest presenting symptoms are neurologic (tetany and convulsions), the patient is often managed for years with the diagnosis of "idiopathic epilepsy." Cataracts also occur in almost half of the patients with chronic parathyroid insufficiency. Papilledema is frequently noted, often in association with seizures, and may be associated with suture separation and abnormal prominence of digital markings (Fig. 21.17). Slow wave patterns characterize the EEG abnormality but these findings are highly nonspecific. Mental retardation is common in children with this disorder, whereas psychotic behavior is found more frequently in older patients. Calcifications occur in over 25% of patients and are seen in the region of the basal ganglia on plain x-ray

Fig. 21.17.—Idiopathic hypoparathyroidism. Boy, 21 months, had a massive gastrointestinal hemorrhage wtih hypoprothrombinemia at 3 months. On therapy for the malabsorption syndrome he continued to have diarrhea and bleeding, and development was retarded. Recurrent generalized seizures began at 20 months. Examination at this time showed an obese, retarded baby with blurring of one optic disc and no other abnormalities. Findings of abnormally prominent convolutional skull markings (shown here) and a diffusely slow electroencephalogram suggested increased intracranial pressure. A localized subdural hematoma was suspected but not confirmed by bilateral burr holes. Only then was attention directed to the first serum calcium (8.3 mg./100 ml.) and phosphorus (7.8 mg./100 ml.) determinations. Repeated determinations showed a consistent hyperphosphatemia and a moderate hypocalcemia. Normal levels followed parathyroid hormone administration, and a diagnosis of idiopathic hypoparathyroidism was made. Immediate and long-term response to vitamin D and A.T. 10 therapy was gratifying. All acute signs and symptoms disappeared and he has done well. The IQ at 5 years 9 months was 61.

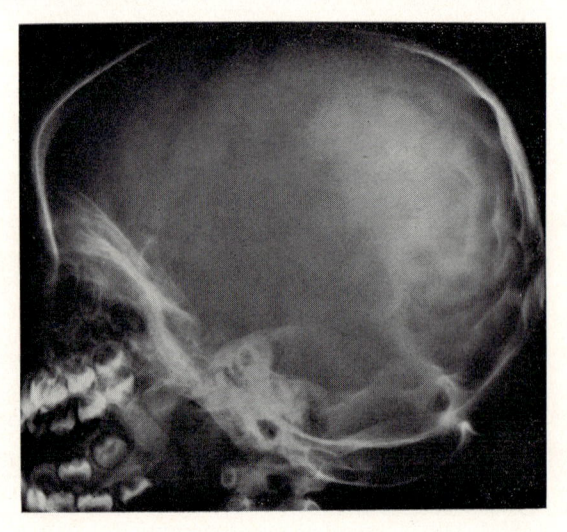

films of the skull. The peculiar association of intermittent diarrhea and steatorrhea with idiopathic hypoparathyroidism may result from coincident malabsorption of fats and calcium. The patient described in Figure 21.17 also had extensive gastrointestinal bleeding, presumably due to vitamin K malabsorption and resultant hypoprothrombinemia. The well-established association of moniliasis and hypoadrenocorticism with hypoparathyroidism also presents a perplexing problem in pathogenesis. The differential diagnosis of tetany is outlined in Table 2.4 (p. 43).

MANAGEMENT AND PROGNOSIS.—The hypocalcemia and phosphorus retention can usually be managed quite easily with the following oral medications: (1) vitamin D_2 (calciferol), 50,000–200,000 units a day, and (2) A.T.10 (dihydrotachysterol), 1–4 ml. daily. Both of these substances promote calcium absorption from the gut, but A.T.10 enhances renal phosphate excretion more effectively. Foods with a high phosphorus content, such as milk products, molasses and cauliflower, should be eliminated from the diet.

During the initial management frequent serum calcium determinations must be carried out. In the long-term management, the urine Sulkowitch test (which measures calcium excretion on a 0, 1+, 2+, 3+ and 4+ scale) should be carried out on bedtime urine to prevent the development of hypercalcemia and serious renal damage. A negative result suggests hypocalcemia, a 3–4+ result suggests hypercalcemia and a 1–2+ finding represents optimal diet and optimal therapy with vitamin D or A.T.10.

Permanent mental retardation of moderate degree affects over 20% of patients with hypoparathyroidism, and its occurrence is probably related to the age of onset, the interval between onset of symptoms and time of diagnosis and the severity of the associated seizures. These factors must be considered in predicting the long-term outcome to parents. These disorders do not generally occur in any predictable hereditary pattern but familial cases are reported.

Pseudohypoparathyroidism

PATHOGENESIS.—This inherited metabolic defect is characterized by blood serum abnormalities which are identical to those in hypoparathyroidism, but here one sees in addition skeletal abnormalities, ectopic calcifications and mental retardation. The disorder behaves as a recessive trait (often affecting more than one sibling), in which the parathyroid glands are normal or hyperplastic but the endocrine organs, kidneys and bone fail to respond to parathyroid hormone with a phosphate diuresis and elevation of serum calcium, respectively.

CLINICAL AND LABORATORY DIAGNOSIS.—The rather typical clinical picture is one of short stature, round face, mild mental retardation, cataracts, brachydactyly and seizures. Patients may be carried with the diagnosis of idiopathic epilepsy. The blood serum shows hypocalcemia and hyperphosphatemia. X-rays show not only the short, thickened bones with exostoses but ectopic calcium deposits in the region of the basal ganglia (Fig. 21.18,*A*) and in the subcutaneous tissue (Fig. 21.18,*C*). Brachydactyly results from characteristically short fourth and fifth metacarpals (Fig. 21.18,*B*). These can be seen best clinically when the patient's fist is closed.

MANAGEMENT AND PROGNOSIS.—This disorder is treated in the same manner

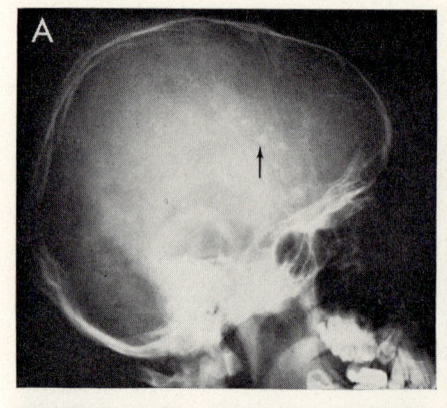

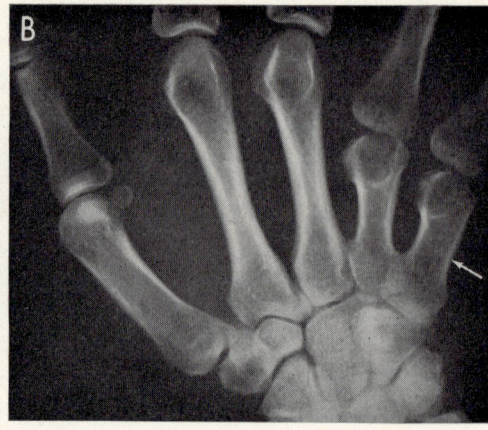

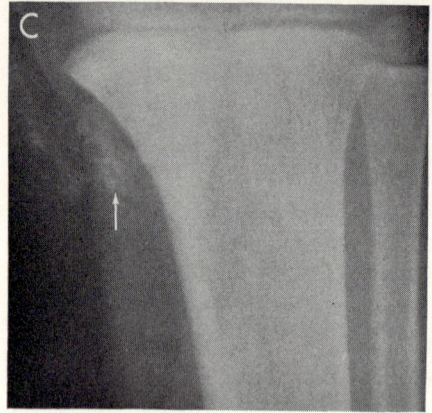

Fig. 21.18.—Pseudohypoparathyroidism. Boy, 13, had neonatal cyanotic episodes and a diagnosis of congenital heart disease was considered but not proved. At age 1 the mother noted "hard lumps" under the skin on his abdomen, similar to lesions which she had. After surgical removal, microscopic examination of this material revealed it was "subcuticular bone." The patient was then well until onset of "fainting spells" at age 13. Precipitated by strenuous exercise, these were brief, generalized tonic episodes. Examination revealed a dull, round-faced boy who had several small, hard deposits near the belt line. Serum calcium was 6.7 mg./100 ml. and serum phosphorus was 9.8 mg./100 ml. Intracranial calcifications were seen in the area of the basal ganglia (**A**), and an Ellsworth-Howard test was diagnostic of pseudohypoparathyroidism (no drop in serum phosphorus level after giving 100–200 units parathormone every six hours for three days). He has done well on vitamin D, 50,000 units every other day. No further seizures have occurred.

Films of another patient with this disorder show the short fourth and fifth metacarpals (**B**) and ectopic calcification (arrow in **C**).

as idiopathic hypoparathyroidism, except that one must remember that patients are less responsive to A.T.10 and parathyroid hormones. Vitamin D and supplementary oral calcium should be used to control symptoms. At the same time guard against signs of overdosage, especially severe hypertension.

Vitamins

Pyridoxine Deficiency and Dependency

PATHOGENESIS.—For the sake of brevity and at a risk of some nosologic inconsistency, we shall discuss both vitamin B_6 deficiency and dependency here. Vitamin B_6 deficiency results from inadequate dietary intake of pyridoxine and from the administration of isonicotinylhydrazide (INH). This vitamin is essential for the normal enzymatic conversion in the brain of tryptophan to nicotinic acid and for the enzymatic activity which converts glutamic acid to gamma-aminobutyric acid (GABA), a naturally occurring anticonvulsive metabolite.

Pyridoxine dependency may affect more than one newborn infant in a sibship and hence this inherited disorder behaves as a recessive trait. The exact biochemical defect is not understood completely, but presumably it is caused by the need for an inordinate amount of pyridoxine to promote satisfactorily the enzymatic processes described for pyridoxine deficiency.

CLINICAL AND LABORATORY DIAGNOSIS.—Vitamin B_6 deficiency is seen rarely, but several rather large series of cases have been reported in infants between 2 and 4 months of age who were receiving SMA formula. In these infants irritability, hyperacusis and generalized seizures developed as a result of the autoclave destruction of the vitamin during preparation of the commercial formula. The seizures in these babies responded to an intake of ordinary amounts of vitamin B_6 and no permanent neurologic deficit or EEG abnormalities resulted. An oral load of L-tryptophan (100 mg./kg.) to vitamin B_6-deficient patients will lead to a consistently increased urinary output of xanthurenic acid.

Pyridoxine dependency may behave as a catastrophic neurologic illness in the newborn and one which may affect a series of siblings. At birth these babies are often meconium-stained and may exhibit respiratory distress as their first problem. Convulsions, generalized clonic seizures or massive myoclonic jerks occur between three and seven hours after birth, and the babies show hyperirritability, hyperacusis, periods of apnea, a high-pitched cry and apparent respiratory distress. A notoriously poor response to standard anticonvulsant drugs has been noted. No biochemical test has been developed for this disease, so that diagnosis depends upon the therapeutic trial of pyridoxine (see below).

MANAGEMENT AND PROGNOSIS.—Both pyridoxine deficiency and dependency are treated by the administration of vitamin B_6, physiologic amounts being effective in the former condition (0.2–0.3 mg./day) and pharmacologic amounts being needed in the latter (10–100 mg./day). Although the clinical syndrome of vitamin B_6 deficiency has essentially disappeared in the United States, vitamin B_6 dependency is being recognized and reported with increasing frequency. In the dependency disorder—often a medical emergency—seizures, EEG abnormalities and other neurologic signs disappear within seconds or minutes after 25 mg. pyridoxine is given intravenously or intramuscularly. A daily maintenance dose of 10 mg. is recommended although this may vary.[126] Experience with long-term management is limited, but daily supplemental B_6 may be required indefinitely.

A lesson can be learned by inspecting the sequence of events in the reported families.[118,144] The first affected patient usually dies with convulsions and respiratory distress and the diagnosis remains obscure. If the second and third children are born with the same clinical picture, the physician becomes increasingly sensitized and vigilant so that a trial of pyridoxine therapy is employed. The immediate and gratifying response to pyridoxine and the almost total failure of other therapeutic measures call for widespread awareness of this syndrome among physicians caring for newborn and young infants.

Hereditary Neoplastic Degenerative Disorders

Tuberous Sclerosis (Bourneville)

PATHOGENESIS.—This distinctive disease is inherited as an autosomal dominant trait with highly variable expressivity. Its precise pathogenic classification (like neurofibromatosis) presents a problem, because it possesses characteristics of both a congenital malformation and a neoplastic process. It has been pointed out that the anomalies belong in the category of hamartomas, in that they are congenital malformations with a potentiality for growth which does not exceed that of the normal tissue in which they arise.[61]

This sublethal trait is characterized by tumorous malformations of the brain, skin, heart, kidneys and lungs. In the cerebral cortex one finds widened, pale, hardened areas ("tubers") which are composed microscopically of large, bizarre nerve cells and dense glial tissue. Similar nodular masses are found in the white matter and basal nuclei, especially projecting into the lumen of the lateral ventricle from the borders of the thalamus like "candle drippings." These masses may calcify and become radiopaque or they may behave as an infiltrating glioma. Brain tumors are quite common in these patients,[75a] and similar tumor-like growths may develop in the retina, kidneys, heart, lungs and other viscera.

CLINICAL AND LABORATORY DIAGNOSIS.—Like many other inherited disorders this one varies greatly in its clinical severity. The fully developed case presents no diagnostic difficulty. The patient exhibits (1) "adenoma sebaceum" (crops of pink papules and flat plaques) in a butterfly distribution on the face (Fig. 21.19,*A* and *B*), (2) seizures, (3) mental deficiency or behavioral disturbances and (4) intracranial calcifications. The greater diagnostic problem, however, is presented by the child who exhibits only seizures and mental disturbances (including typically psychotic behavior) which have no differential specificity. The clue to the diagnosis in such patients may appear later in the form of less typical cutaneous lesions (depigmented spots, café-au-lait spots and raised, rough plaques or "shagreen patches" commonly seen over the lower spine) or the retinal masses which are mushroom-like, yellowish white extrusions called phakomas (Fig. 21.19,*C*). Some patients have minor congenital anomalies, growth retardation, sexual precocity or evidence of tumors involving the kidneys, the heart, the lungs or other viscera. Focal neurologic deficit is uncommon, but hemipareses are seen along with papilledema secondary to associated tumor masses in the brain.

Skull x-rays often show small punctate areas of calcification, especially near the lateral ventricles, and one can demonstrate on pneumoencephalography filling defects in the air shadows where the "candle drippings" project from the floor or roof of the ventricles. Radiographs of the skull and the small bones of the extremities may show small cystic areas and thickening of the periosteum. In some cases sclerotic areas in the bones of the skull cannot be distinguished clinically from intracerebral calcifications. Epileptiform EEG abnormalities are seen in many patients.

In the differential diagnosis one must consider (1) many of the other neurodegenerative diseases discussed in this chapter, (2) true congenital malformations of the nervous system, (3) other "neurocutaneous" disorders such as neurofibromatosis, (4) vascular malformations of the brain, (5) chronic granulomatous infections, such as toxoplasmosis and cytomegalovirus infection, that cause intracranial calcifications, (6) primary and isolated brain tumors, (7) subdural hematoma and (8) idiopathic epilepsy.

MANAGEMENT AND PROGNOSIS.—This progressive degeneration of the nervous system has no specific therapy. Anticonvulsant therapy is used but its effect may

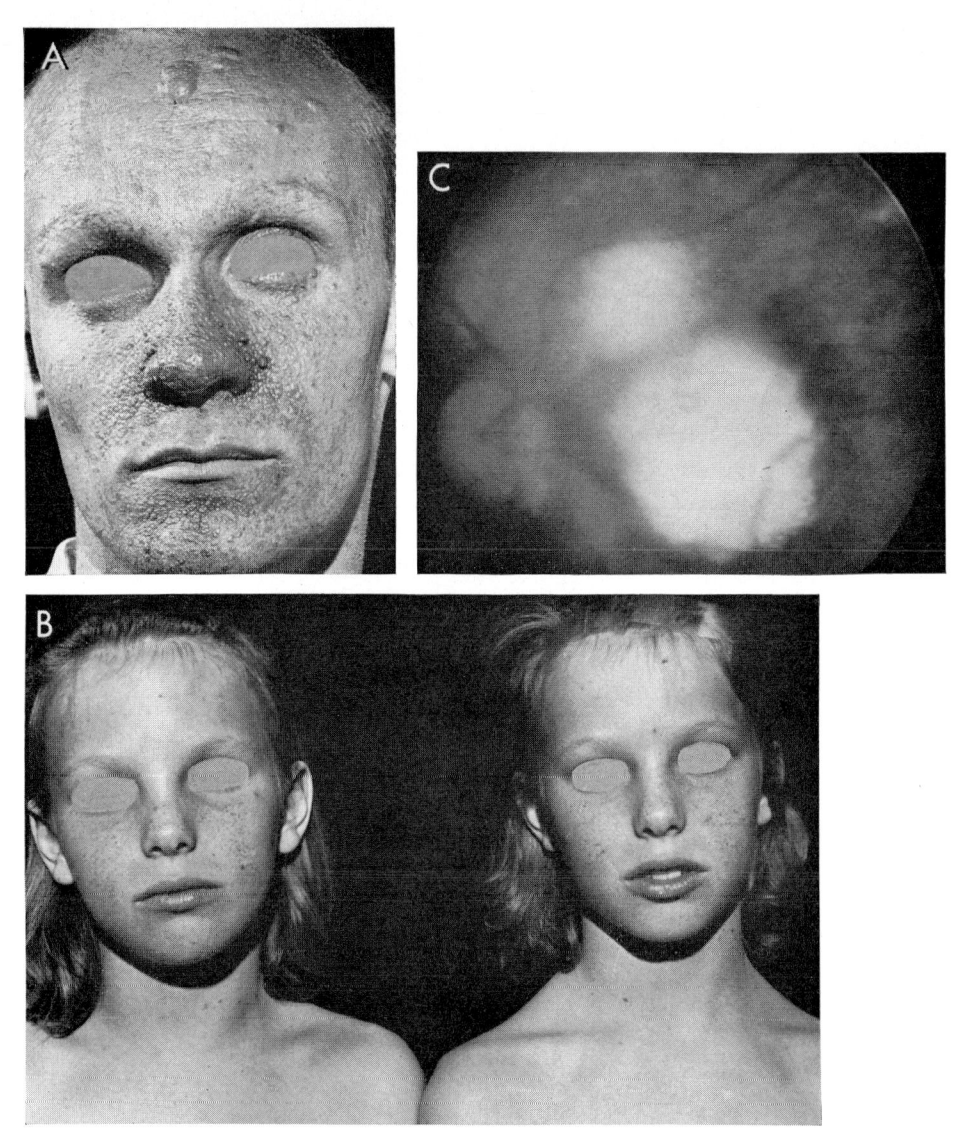

Fig. 21.19.—Tuberous sclerosis. A, patient has advanced form of adenoma sebaceum. B shows identical twins with tuberous sclerosis. Enucleation of the left eye of the patient on the reader's left was done because of glaucoma secondary to a retinal phakoma. The father of the twins had seizures and an organic psychosis in adult life. C, in another patient, note the large piled-up whitish exudates in the retina.

often be limited, many patients succumbing eventually in status epilepticus. Surgical intervention may be necessary if the tumor masses in the brain or other viscera cause obstruction to normal function. Most patients die in early adult life but in exceptional cases there may be near-normal longevity. Because of the sublethal nature of the disease the demand for genetic counseling is uncommon. When the question does arise, however, mildly affected parents should be advised about the dominant inheritance and highly variable clinical expressivity of this serious disorder.

Neurofibromatosis (von Recklinghausen)

PATHOGENESIS.—This complex and variable disorder occurs quite commonly in childhood and behaves as a strongly autosomal dominant trait. Variable expressivity in succeeding generations is almost the rule, but it must be remembered that this trait which has the highest known mutation rate in man, appears commonly in a family without any known affected ancestors.[134] In general, hyperplastic and neoplastic changes in the supporting tissues occur throughout the entire nervous system. The tendency for benign tumors to become malignant, especially near adolescence, has been stressed. One can consider arbitrarily two basic types of neurofibromatosis: (1) *peripheral* disease, in which the tumors arise from the sheaths of the cranial, peripheral and spinal nerves, and (2) *central* disease, in which tumors arise not only from nerve sheaths but also from glia and meninges. If the peripheral manifestations of the disease are striking, few central lesions are usually found, and vice versa.[17] However, this rule has many exceptions. In some cases angiomatous lesions, developmental anomalies (such as meningocele and spina bifida, aqueductal stenosis, syringomyelia and glial heterotopias), pheochromocytomas and ganglioneuromas are seen concomitantly.

Frequently it is taught that a close pathologic alliance exists between neurofibromatosis, tuberous sclerosis and vascular malformation syndromes such as those of Sturge-Weber (Chapter 13) and Lindau. However, proof for this theory is lacking. Admittedly neurofibromatosis and tuberous sclerosis are both inherited as autosomal dominant traits, and pathologic lesions may be found which are common to both diseases. However, the aggregation of all the "neurocutaneous" diseases or "phakomatoses" may represent more a matter of clinical convenience than of pathogenic proof. A close relationship between neurofibromatosis and fibrous dysplasia is also well documented.[119b]

CLINICAL AND LABORATORY DIAGNOSIS.—The cutaneous manifestations of the disease commonly appear. These include café-au-lait spots, heavy freckling (especially in the axillae and other skin creases) and a complexion which is darker than would be expected from the patient's race and family. A detailed survey by Crowe and associates[34] disclosed that 78% of 203 patients had six or more café-au-lait spots, whereas no normal adult had this number. These skin lesions may be inapparent in early life and are commoner in the predominantly peripheral form of the disease. In the latter type of disorder one frequently finds (1) subcutaneous nodules and masses of varied size and consistency along the course of peripheral nerves, and (2) plexiform neuromas which often cause localized enlargement, deformity and asymmetry of the involved tissues, especially the face (Fig. 21.20) and extremities. Sometimes they give rise to the clinical picture of elephantiasis in the affected extremities. The subcutaneous nodules cause neurologic deficit in exceptional cases and the plexiform neuromas may produce rather severe cosmetic problems. In the central form of the disease serious neurologic deficit can result from neurofibromas of the cranial and spinal nerves. These tumors may present with typical signs of pain and root or spinal cord compression, whereas the latter may behave as any other brain tumor, depending upon its location and its pressure effects. Gliomas of the optic nerve develop commonly and may cause exophthalmos and blindness. If the chiasm is involved primarily, there may be a bitemporal hemianopia and signs of pituitary-hypothalamic compression (including growth failure, sexual precocity, diabetes insipidus and pathologic sleep states). One must always remember that sarcomatous malignant changes may develop in patients with long-standing neurofibromatosis[49] and may occur more often in the older patient (Fig. 17.12, p. 270). Mental retardation and seizures occur in many patients with this disorder independent of the direct effects of the neoplastic lesions.

Neurofibromatosis should always be considered in the differential diagnosis of scoliosis because the latter deformity occurs commonly (Fig. 17.12). Other skeletal lesions, such as localized areas of rarefaction or overgrowth, are also seen. In patients with orbital signs or visual symptoms, acuity and field studies should be carried out. Special x-ray views may reveal enlargement of one or both optic foramina as a result of an optic nerve glioma. Similarly, Stenver's views of the internal auditory foramina may show enlargement and erosion in patients who have hearing loss with this disorder. Pneumoencephalography may help in the diagnosis of tumors in the cerebellopontine angle (eighth nerve tumor) and the parasellar region. Angiography and pneumoencephalography may localize tumorous masses as in the case of any other brain tumor. Similarly, lumbar puncture, CSF protein estimation, manometric studies and myelography are valuable in the diagnosis and localization of intraspinal tumors (Fig. 17.12). Chest films and intravenous urog-

Fig. 21.20.—Neurofibromatosis. A, patient has had an obvious, nonprogressive hemihypertrophy of the left side of the head and face since birth. The skin of the left side of the face and neck has increased brownish pigmentation and on the neck a rough, pigskin-like character. There are no skin lesions elsewhere and no subcutaneous nodules or focal neurologic deficits. Recurrent generalized seizures since infancy are associated with a constantly abnormal electroencephalogram. The epileptiform discharges have always been more prominent over the left hemisphere, especially in the posterior quadrants. This boy has made a quite satisfactory social adjustment; IQ is 60 and he receives special education.

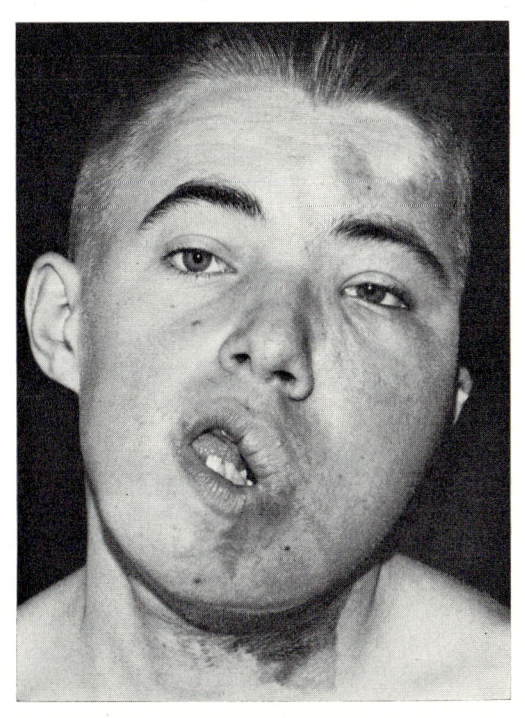

raphy should be performed routinely before operation in patients with intraspinal masses in order to define the extent of the lesions. At times biopsy of peripheral tumors will lead to histologic identification of an obscure mass.

In the peripheral form of the disease the diagnosis is usually obvious. However, the differential diagnosis of intracranial and intraspinal tumors as a whole must be considered in patients with the central type of neurofibromatosis.

MANAGEMENT AND PROGNOSIS.—Surgical removal of lesions which are causing symptoms and signs is indicated. Many patients with one or a few lesions involving the eighth cranial nerve, the optic nerve or spinal roots or cord are given long-lasting clinical relief by judicious operations. However, the patient should be studied fully before operative procedures are undertaken because the decision of when and where to operate is influenced strongly by the number of lesions and their surgical accessibility. Radiation therapy is indicated in this disorder only if the histopathologic changes in the tumor suggest that it is radiosensitive or if it represents a threat to critical functions, such as vision, in which case no other treatment is available. It has been suggested that surgical manipulation of masses in this disorder may lead to malignant changes, but there is little evidence to support this notion. In some young patients with deforming areas of localized tissue overgrowth, plastic cosmetic procedures are carried out, but decisions of this nature should also be carried out only after careful, conservative consideration of the patient's total condition by a team of specialists.

The prognosis varies from a life with few incapacitating symptoms and normal longevity to early fatality in patients with tumors in critical locations or tumors which have undergone malignant changes. The dominant nature of inheritance and the variable expressivity in succeeding generations should be understood fully by the physician who is counseling parents about the recurrence risks in subsequent children or in the marriage plans of an affected adolescent.

Dementias of Unknown Etiology

Many workers doubt the wisdom of separate categories for the entities discussed here. One can only say that characteristic pathologic changes are seen in the nervous systems of some patients who deteriorate and die in infancy or childhood. It seems likely that more than one disease can lead to the changes that are found at autopsy in some or all of these conditions.

Spongy Degeneration of White Matter (Canavan)

The condition nearly always becomes apparent during the first six months of life. Motor deficit is noted first with the appearance of spasticity of the extremities, often associated with hypotonia of the neck and back muscles. Pyramidal tract signs are commonly seen, as are blindness, severe dementia and abnormal enlargement of the head. Death usually occurs by 18 months of age. No useful laboratory studies are known for diagnosis during life. Autopsy examination reveals a heavy, wet, "mucoid" brain which exhibits generalized spongy vacuolation with numerous fluid spaces. The gray matter and the subcortical, white U-fibers are more affected by sudanophilic myelin breakdown products than in most other types of leukodystrophy. The disease is seen more commonly, but not exclusively, in Jews.[69b] Although the familial incidence suggests an inherited enzymatic defect, the basic pathogenesis of the disorder is unknown. Recently Feigin and co-workers[48b] suggested that the spongy state "may not be a valid basis for delineating a nosological entity, spongy degeneration."

Necrotizing Encephalomyelopathy of Childhood (Leigh)

This clinicopathologic entity starts in early childhood and follows a progressive course to death in a variable period. The diagnosis depends upon autopsy evidence of symmetrical necrotizing lesions in the basal ganglia, brain stem, cerebellum and spinal cord. The cause of the disorder is obscure and because of the anatomic resemblance to Wernicke's encephalopathy a metabolic basis is suspected.[48a]

Clinically the course is characterized by progressive motor weakness, ataxia, ophthalmoplegia, disturbances in consciousness and coma leading to death.[119a] The disorder must be distinguished from tumors of the brain stem.

Degeneration of Cerebral Gray Matter (Alpers)

The clinicopathologic syndrome is associated with the onset of minor motor seizures of the myoclonic or akinetic type, convulsions, choreoathetotic disorders of movement, ataxia and progressive spasticity. Progressive dementia and apparent cortical blindness and deafness usually supervene in the advanced stages of the disease, and the patient may die in status epilepticus. The tendency for this disorder to affect several members of a sibship has been noted, but the actual cause is not known.

Pathologic study usually reveals widespread necrosis of the deep layers of the cerebral cortex—the so-called laminar type of necrosis. In addition to neuronal destruction, microglial phagocytosis and astrocytic scarring are evident. These findings are quite nonspecific and are actually indistinguishable from those seen in many patients who have recurrent seizures and anoxia. Some workers believe that this pathologic entity may result from many different obscure hereditary metabolic disorders. They are not convinced that it represents a disease *sui generis*.

Ataxia and Other Movement Disorders

Hereditary Metabolic Defects (Amino Acids and Proteins)

Ataxia-Telangiectasia (Louis-Bar)

PATHOGENESIS.—This rare form of ataxia is inherited as an autosomal recessive trait and is associated with telangiectases of the bulbar conjunctiva and skin, recurrent infections of the respiratory tract and at times choreoathetosis.[16,25] Recent morphologic and serologic data suggesting that the disease may represent a "thymic syndrome" in man[113] include (1) hypogammaglobulinemia, (2) absent or decreased gamma$_1$A globulin, (3) lymphopenia and a paucity of lymph node and tonsillar tissue and (4) an inordinately high incidence of malignancy.[114] Neuropathologic findings have been limited but they have consistently included cerebellar atrophy and degeneration of the posterior column fibers of the spinal cord.[136] A loss of Purkinje and granular cells has been found, together with atrophy of the vermis. Some authors have reported dilatation and engorgement of the cerebellar and meningeal veins, similar to the telangiectases in the skin. Pathologic examination of the lungs has shown only signs of chronic infection.

CLINICAL AND LABORATORY DIAGNOSIS.—After a normal early infancy these babies may not walk until 16–20 months and then manifest difficulties with gait and coordinated movements of the extremities. Athetosis may appear later, with nystagmus, disorders of eye movement, dysarthria and a lack of facial expression. The telangiectases do not usually appear until about age 3. They are seen first on the exposed portion of the bulbar conjunctiva (Fig. 21.21,*A*), the butterfly area of the face, the external ears (Fig. 21.21,*B*), the exposed portion of the neck and upper chest and in the antecubital and popliteal creases.[116] Hypotonia and hyporeflexia are seen later in the disease, but intelligence, sensation and muscle strength are usually normal. Recurrent infections of all portions of the respiratory tract (sinusitis, otitis media, bronchitis and pneumonia) typify this disorder. As a striking correlative finding, these patients have few palpable lymph nodes and little tonsillar and adenoid tissue.[47]

The diagnostic laboratory findings include (1) absent or decreased gamma$_1$A or IgA globulin (immunoelectrophoresis),[9,47,48,76,91] (2) hypogammaglobulinemia

Fig. 21.21.—Ataxia-telangiectasia. Boy, 9, seemed normal until he failed to walk until 19 months, and then gait ataxia was noticed. Recurrent bouts of bronchitis and pneumonia required IPPB and postural drainage. Mental slowness was apparent, but it was difficult to decide whether true dementia existed because of the ataxic speech and movement disorder. Examination revealed (1) moderate choreoathetosis, (2) slow, scanning speech, (3) telangiectasis of conjunctivae **(A)** and pinnae **(B)**, (4) apparent apraxia of eye movements, (5) ataxia of gait and extremities and (6) diffuse pulmonary wheezes and rhonchi. Total serum gamma globulin was at the lower limits of normal. A sister died of the same disorder when she was 12.

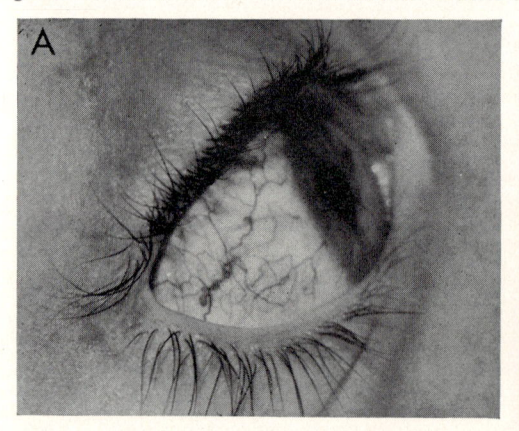

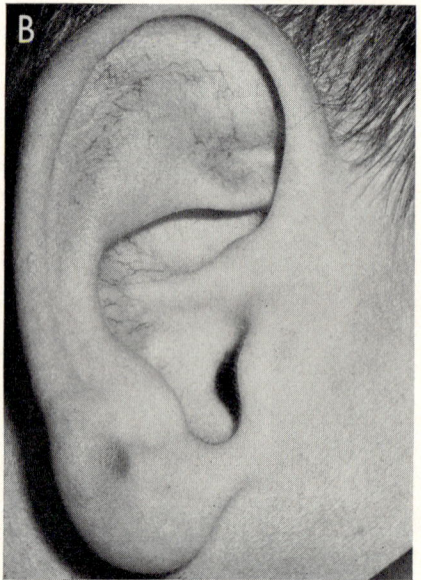

in some cases, (3) lymphopenia and neutropenia at times and (4) an elevated erythrocyte sedimentation rate. Some workers have also shown a sluggish circulating-antibody response to tetanus and diphtheria toxoid as well as to poliomyelitis vaccine, delayed homograft rejection, and almost complete absence of delayed hypersensitivity. Pneumoencephalography has shown evidence of cerebellar atrophy in a few patients, and x-rays of both the sinuses and chest reflect chronic infection in these areas. Of note is that these children recover normally from viral infections.

All other causes of progressive ataxia must be differentiated (Table 9.1, p. 95). However, ataxia-telangiectasia is the only progressive ataxia with onset in infancy.

MANAGEMENT AND PROGNOSIS.—Antibiotic and chemotherapy are of some value in treating specific infections of the respiratory tract. Gamma globulin administration has not produced significant clinical benefit despite the theoretical indications for its use.

The affected child is usually confined to a wheelchair by adolescence because of the severe ataxia and the movement disorder. The slowly progressive nature of the disease usually leads to death in the third decade of life. Parents must be made aware of the recurrence risk in subsequent siblings.

Acanthocytosis (Bassen-Kornzweig)

PATHOGENESIS.—This rare and peculiar autosomal recessive trait causes neurologic deficit, steatorrhea, retinal degeneration and a characteristic deformity of the circulating red blood cells. Reported cases have been noted most frequently in Jewish children of consanguineous marriages. No pathologic studies of the nervous system have been reported, but biopsies of peripheral nerve have shown demyelination. Biopsy of the small intestinal mucosa has shown vacuolation and pallor of the mucosal epithelial cells. The strongest clue to the basic etiology of the disease rests upon the absence of serum beta-lipoprotein.

CLINICAL AND LABORATORY DIAGNOSIS.—Symptoms suggestive of the celiac syndrome (loose, frequent stools with steatorrhea) may occur in infancy, followed in middle or late childhood by unsteady gait, slowly progressive weakness and loss of vision. In the advanced case a variety of deformities may be present, including low hair line, high-arched palate, webbing of the neck, small external ears, thoracic scoliosis, epicanthic folds, thin arms and legs and pes cavus. Neurologic signs include ataxia of both gait and extremities, loss of deep sensation and light touch, areflexia and in some cases Babinski signs. Dysarthria may occur as well as fasciculations of the tongue and ocular squint. Degenerative changes in the retina with pigmentation are associated with loss of visual acuity, constricted visual fields and ring scotomata. The syndrome is reviewed well by Schwartz et al.[125]

The blood smear reveals the characteristic "spiny" projections from the surfaces of the erythrocytes (acanthocytes). Immunoelectrophoresis of the serum discloses absence or marked diminution in the beta-lipoprotein fraction. One can demonstrate malabsorption of fat using Lipiodol and of starches using xylose. The cerebrospinal fluid and skull x-rays give normal findings.

The differential diagnosis must include all other causes of ataxia (Chapter 9), other multiple congenital anomaly syndromes (especially gonadal agenesis or Turner's syndrome), all other causes of scoliosis (Chapter 10) and other progressive degenerative disorders of movement. However, the morphologic and serologic findings in the blood are diagnostic.

MANAGEMENT AND PROGNOSIS.—Although no specific medical therapy is available, these patients should receive long-term physical therapy and orthopedic assistance if necessary. The disease gradually leads to great motor disability and deformity in adult life, along with loss of vision. Dependable data on longevity are not available. Parents must be warned adequately about the high recurrence risk in other siblings.

X-Linked Primary Hyperuricemia

Recently Lesch and Nyhan[85] described an unusual inherited defect in uric acid metabolism with clinical signs of severe central nervous system involvement. The disorder usually behaves as an X-linked recessive trait[69] and is characterized by a very high turnover rate of the uric acid pool with high serum levels.[109] Recently the neuropathologic findings of perivascular demyelination and cerebellar granule cell degeneration were reported.[121]

Symptoms of the disorder begin early in life with developmental retardation, choreoathetosis and hyperuricemia. Patients show a peculiar tendency to mutilate themselves by biting their lips and fingertips. Gross uric acid crystalluria and hematuria are found. So far only boys have been reported with the disease.

Reduction of the hyperuricemia with allopurinol has been reported[106] in this rare degenerative disease and appears to be the only rational therapy at present, although its effect upon the clinical deficit is uncertain.[99] If the X-linked mode of inheritance is proved by a larger number of case reports, one can expect half the boys in a family to have the disease and half the girls to be carriers.

Hereditary Disease of Mineral Metabolism

Hepatolenticular Degeneration (Wilson's Disease)

PATHOGENESIS.—This relatively rare disease is inherited in an autosomal recessive fashion and causes cirrhosis of the liver and degenerative changes in the brain, especially in the caudate nucleus and putamen. Not yet completely understood,[112] the favored etiologic explanation holds that the disease, including the extrapyramidal signs, is due to a primary disturbance in copper metabolism and leads to chronic copper poisoning.[39] Supporting this concept are the following findings in patients with the disease: (1) absent or low quantities of ceruloplasmin (the protein to which 98% of circulating copper is attached), (2) high levels of "direct-reacting" copper (the copper which is measured in ordinary serum copper determinations and which is bound loosely to albumin) and (3) high levels of tissue copper (liver, brain and cornea).[24, 89, 146]

CLINICAL AND LABORATORY DIAGNOSIS.—Disease symptoms have their onset toward the end of the first or during the second decade of life. In the advanced case, cirrhosis of the liver, signs of basal ganglion disease and Kayser-Fleischer (K-F) corneal rings make diagnosis obvious. However, as laboratory diagnostic methods have been refined and clinical awareness has increased, it is recognized that the early clinical picture may vary greatly and present itself in unexpected ways. Episodes of "viral hepatitis" with jaundice may usher in the disease, followed later by the development of cirrhosis and hepatosplenomegaly. Less often and in younger patients acute hemolytic anemia with leukopenia and thrombocytopenia may be the first signs.[92,96] Such patients may have an acute, downhill and rapidly fatal course. Other patients in whom neurologic symptoms develop first may exhibit mild intellectual or emotional disturbances and frank schizophrenic states. In the classic neurologic syndrome the patient has bulbar signs (dysarthria, change in voice quality, dysphagia and chewing difficulty), parkinsonian signs (immobile facies, drooling, tendency to hold the mouth open, cog-wheel rigidity) and a coarse, rhythmic, "wing-flapping" tremor which is present at rest but is accentuated by volitional movement and emotional stress. In the advanced stages the typical greenish brown pericorneal K-F ring can be seen grossly, but in the early stages this zone of pigmentation can be seen only by slit-lamp examination. In the terminal stages the patient becomes almost helpless, with rigidity and dysphagia. Tube feeding then becomes necessary to prevent aspiration.

The diagnosis of Wilson's disease should be considered in any young patient with hepatitis, cirrhosis, acute hemolytic anemia of obscure etiology, schizophrenia, intellectual deterioration, early parkinsonism, obscure movement or tone disorder, or in patients with unexplained bulbar symptoms and signs. Also, of course, the diagnosis must be considered strongly in any relative of a patient with an established or suspected diagnosis of Wilson's disease.

Hypocupremia, hypoceruloplasminemia, hypercupruria and generalized aminoaciduria[8] confirm the diagnosis. One or more of the laboratory examinations should be performed, despite their technical difficulty, if the diagnosis is in doubt.

MANAGEMENT AND PROGNOSIS.—As soon as diagnosis has been made a regimen should be instituted to minimize the absorption of dietary copper and to promote the excretion of copper already deposited in the tissues. This treatment should be continued indefinitely. Administration of a low-copper diet which is high in protein is advised, together with oral administration of potassium sulfide.[123] Copper-chelating agents such as oral penicillamine[60,68] (this drug of choice is given in divided doses with a total daily dose of 0.3–2 gm./day), BAL (2,3, dimercaptopropanol) or Versenate effect the mobilization of tissue copper stores and increased urinary copper excretion. With intensive therapy clearing of some symptoms can be expected in some patients. Disappearance of mental symptoms occurs commonly but neurologic signs improve with less consistency. The K-F rings will fade on therapy, but the hepatic defect remains unchanged. Several authors have stressed the desirability of not only instituting early treatment of symptomatic cases, but early diagnosis and prophylactic treatment of high-risk, suspect cases in whom biochemical laboratory evidence is diagnostic. Isolated cases of penicillamine-induced optic neuritis have been reported. Presumably penicillamine causes a pyridoxine deficiency, because vitamin B_6 therapy reverses the complication promptly.[142]

This progressive disease is invariably fatal if it goes untreated, but longevity varies from a few months to 10 years. The absence of symptoms or signs in eight treated asymptomatic patients who have been followed up to 6 years[135] speaks strongly in favor of early diagnosis and treatment.

Degenerative Diseases of Unknown Etiology

Spinocerebellar Ataxia (Friedreich)

PATHOGENESIS.—This familial and hereditary disorder is inherited usually but not always as an autosomal recessive trait and, although it is a rare disease, it represents the commonest type of hereditary cerebellar ataxia. The disease is associated with degenerative changes of selected long tracts in the spinal cord and sometimes the cerebellum and brain stem. The posterior columns, the dorsal roots, dorsal and ventral spinocerebellar tracts and the corticospinal tracts show degeneration and extensive gliosis. In many cases interstitial myocarditis is found. Necrosis and degeneration of cardiac muscle fibers are seen, together with focal cellular infiltrates. The underlying metabolic defect is totally obscure.

CLINICAL AND LABORATORY DIAGNOSIS.—Ataxia is usually the first sign of the disease and makes its appearance in middle or late childhood. Occasionally there is a history of delayed walking and clumsy gait since infancy. Later, frank incoordination appears in the upper extremities. The incoordination results from real cerebellar ataxia and loss of proprioception from posterior column degeneration. Loss of deep tendon reflexes occurs uniformly and Babinski signs reflect pyramidal tract involvement. Pes cavus (Fig. 21.22) or clubfoot deformities and scoliosis appear in a high percentage of cases. Dysarthria, optic atrophy, nystagmus, pseudoathetosis (from loss of position sense) and muscle atrophy appear as the disease progresses. In the terminal stages the patient may be helpless because of ataxia, muscle atrophy and deforming scoliosis. Dementia occurs rarely and then only in advanced cases. Many authors have called attention to both the clinical and the ECG signs of myocarditis. Tachycardia, arrhythmias and cardiomegaly result from the myocarditis and in part from the restricted lung capacity in patients with severe kyphoscoliosis.

Fig. 21.22.—Typical high-arched foot deformity (pes cavus) in a patient with Friedreich's ataxia.

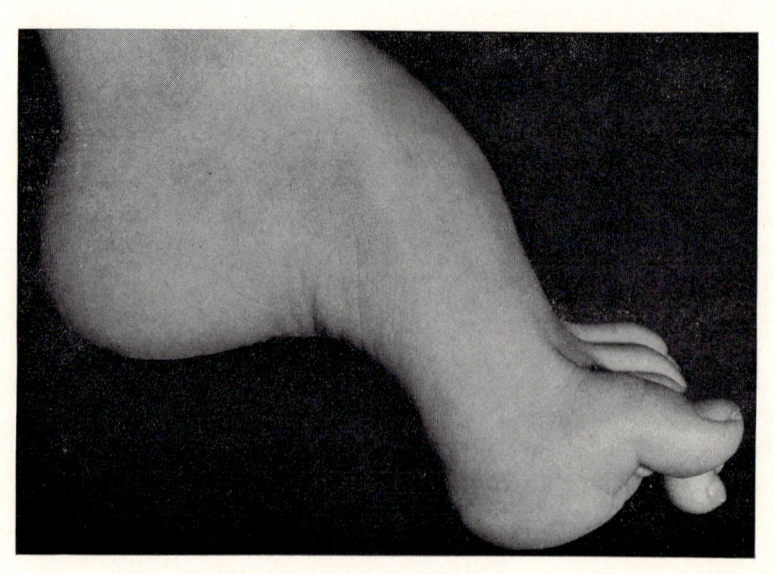

No laboratory studies contribute to a diagnosis except for ECG evidence of myocarditis and arrhythmias and x-ray demonstration of the scoliosis.

Differential diagnosis is easy if one can elicit a history of the disease in the family. In sporadic cases one must differentiate spinal cord tumors, multiple sclerosis, other chronic types of ataxia (Table 9.1, p. 95), other causes of scoliosis (Table 10.1, p. 97) and other disorders which can cause the type of focal deficit mentioned in Chapter 9.

MANAGEMENT AND PROGNOSIS.—Effective treatment is limited to physical therapy, tendon lengthening and tendon transplants to relieve foot deformities.

The recurrence risk in subsequent siblings or children of affected individuals is significant and depends upon the mode of inheritance operating within the given kindred (see Pathogenesis). Serious disability usually develops between 20 and 30 years of age and death often results from myocardial disease or pulmonary infections.

Chronic Progressive Hereditary Chorea (Huntington)

PATHOGENESIS.—This strongly dominant hereditary disorder is characterized by progressive chorea and dementia. Widespread degenerative changes in the brain are seen, with marked shrinkage of the caudate nucleus and atrophy of the cerebral cortex. There are degenerative changes in nearly all of the basal nuclei and profound glial reaction is seen microscopically. No systemic pathologic changes occur and clues to the basic etiology are entirely lacking.

CLINICAL AND LABORATORY DIAGNOSIS.—The disease has its usual onset in early or middle adult life but occasionally begins in childhood. The symptomatic state may be ushered in by either the movement disorder or mental changes. Involuntary choreiform movements, bizarre grimacing, irregular respiratory rhythm and articulatory speech difficulty appear, and irregular, abrupt, jerky movements of the extremities impart a "prancing" quality to the gait. Attention and stress increase the severity of the movements, whereas the movements disappear during sleep. In the early stages the patient may appear just restless or "fidgety" but gradually the grimacing and amplitude of the movements increase. Eventually the patient becomes completely incapacitated and is bed-ridden. The earliest mental changes may also be subtle, with forgetfulness, irritability and personality changes. Gradually progressive memory loss, intellectual deterioration and carelessness with personal appearance and hygiene supervene. Jervis[72a] and Byers and Dodge[20b] have pointed out that in the juvenile form seizures, mental retardation and rigidity rather than chorea occur more commonly than in adults.

Pneumoencephalography reveals rather typical enlargement of the lateral ventricles as a result of caudate nucleus atrophy. The electroencephalogram may show loss of alpha pattern and diffuse, nonspecific, low voltage slowing. No other laboratory studies contribute to the diagnosis.

The differential diagnosis presents no difficulty if one encounters a history of the disease in a family member. Sydenham's chorea is distinguished by evidence of acute rheumatic fever and by its nonprogressive course. Hepatolenticular degeneration is recognized by liver disease, K-F rings, low or absent serum ceruloplasmin and increased copper excretion. Hemiballismus behaves as do most strokes in that it appears abruptly, is unilateral and tends to improve with time. Sporadic cases of chorea in later life may present considerable diagnostic difficulty.

MANAGEMENT AND PROGNOSIS.—Although no therapy alters the natural course of the disease the severity of the choreiform movements can often be reduced by giving chlorpromazine (10–25 mg. three times daily) or reserpine. In terminal stages of the illness the patient must often be fed, and restraints become necessary to prevent self-inflicted injury from the uncontrollable movements.

The members of affected families quickly become aware of the strong likelihood of passing this affliction on to their offspring, and they are usually urged not to have children. Death from this distressing disease results usually from intercurrent infection, but suicide and chronic alcoholism are seen commonly because of the severe associated depression.

Progressive Myoclonus Epilepsy (Unverricht)

PATHOGENESIS.—This rare autosomal recessive disorder can be suspected clinically by the occurrence of seizures, myoclonus and dementia and is characterized pathologically by a special type of widespread neuronal degeneration. The involved neurons contain round inclusion bodies (Lafora) in the cytoplasm, which stain like amyloid and are most conspicuous in the substantia nigra, the thalamus and the dentate nucleus.[71a] Histochemical studies of Lafora bodies suggest that they are composed, in part at least, of an acid mucopolysaccharide. In addition to the inclusion bodies, cortical nerve cell loss and reactive gliosis are seen.

CLINICAL AND LABORATORY DIAGNOSIS.—Onset is in late childhood, with convulsive seizures, true myoclonus and eventually dementia. One must make a clear distinction between the isolated convulsive myoclonic jerks which are an extremely common seizure type in childhood and the myoclonus in this condition. The myoclonus is frequent, repetitive and often violent. The movements interfere with the normal use of the hands and with speech, and they may serve to fling the erect patient to the ground if the muscles of the hips or lower extremities are involved. The movements may occur spontaneously but are also provoked by various light and sound stimuli. In late stages of the disease cerebellar ataxia and rigidity may appear along with severe dementia.

Routine laboratory studies are normal except that the electroencephalogram may exhibit diffuse slowing in the delta and theta ranges mixed with diffuse single and multiple spike discharges. Usually photic stimulation easily evokes both the epileptiform EEG discharges and the myoclonic movements.

The differential diagnosis includes all of the conditions which are characterized by myoclonic activity. Schilder's disease, subacute sclerosing leukoencephalitis (Chapter 18) and juvenile amaurotic idiocy may be indistinguishable without pathologic examination of nerve tissue. Early Huntington's chorea, Sydenham's chorea and hepatolenticular degeneration must be distinguished by their distinctive laboratory features, which have been described.

MANAGEMENT AND PROGNOSIS.—Treatment with anticonvulsant drugs (Chapter 2) may control the generalized seizures, but the myoclonic activity and dementia are not benefited. Patients with this degenerative disease survive for 10–20 years.

The pattern of inheritance is said to be recessive, but the number of documented case reports is so limited that accurate genetic counseling is difficult.

Hallervorden-Spatz Disease

PATHOGENESIS.—This unusual familial disorder, characterized by rigidity, choreoathetosis, torsion spasm and dementia, can be identified pathologically by the deposition of brown or greenish blue pigment in the globus pallidus and substantia nigra. The areas of increased pigmentation take a heavy iron stain but nobody has proved that this is a reflection of disordered iron metabolism. In fact, nothing is known about any basic biochemical defect. The findings of neuronal loss, gliosis and demyelination have been inconsistent in different reports.

CLINICAL AND LABORATORY DIAGNOSIS.—Retrospective clinical review of autopsy-proved cases indicates that this familial disease has its usual onset in middle childhood with cog-wheel rigidity, dysarthria, pes cavus deformities and dementia. Later in the illness a parkinsonian tremor, athetosis, dystonic postures and Babinski signs may be present. Moderate optic atrophy often develops and dementia becomes severe.

This diagnosis can be considered in any progressive familial extrapyramidal disorder (hepatolenticular degeneration, chronic progressive chorea, dystonia musculorum deformans, juvenile paralysis agitans), but it can be proved only by autopsy. The progressive course suffices to differentiate this disease from static extrapyramidal disorders seen in early childhood (kernicterus, anoxic encephalopathy and congenital athetosis, rigidity or chorea). No diagnostic laboratory tests are helpful.

MANAGEMENT AND PROGNOSIS.—No specific therapy is available for this condition, which runs a fatal course in 5 to 20 years. Patients are usually confined to a wheelchair in later stages and they require nasogastric tube feeding because of pseudobulbar dysphagia.

In families in which affected children run a typical clinical course or in which diagnostic autopsy evidence is available, parents should be warned about the high recurrence risk.

Dystonia Musculorum Deformans (Torsion Spasm)

PATHOGENESIS.—This specific disease entity of unknown etiology occurs more commonly in Russian Jews and may be familial or sporadic. The pattern of inheritance is not clear but some regard it as dominant. Pathologic findings have been inconsistent, partly because in some reported cases dystonia has been due to other causes. In the disease itself degenerative changes are seen primarily in the putamen and caudate nuclei. Although the findings are rather nonspecific they serve to rule out other causes of dystonia (Chapter 3). The fundamental metabolic defect is totally obscure.

CLINICAL AND LABORATORY DIAGNOSIS.—The disease has its onset in middle childhood, usually with abnormalities of gait which are often attributed to psychogenic factors. The bizarre movements may increase the normal lumbar lordosis and cause twisting of the pelvis. Later the slow, sustained twisting, turning and writhing movements of all skeletal muscles appear. Muscles of the trunk, pelvis and shoulder girdles are most involved although the facial and extremity muscles are also affected. The involuntary movements cause facial grimacing, dysarthria and torticollis. The powerful spasms which occur as the disease progresses may cause pain and may be strong enough to fracture long bones. Psychologic stress and voluntary movement exaggerate the spasms but the movement disorder subsides in sleep. No other neurologic signs are seen except for moderate dementia in the terminal stages. Joint contractures and muscle wasting often develop late in the course.

MANAGEMENT AND PROGNOSIS.—The most striking benefit for some of these pathetic patients has resulted from placing surgical lesions in the globus pallidus (pallidotomy) or thalamus (thalamotomy). Unfortunately the striking initial improvement is often only transient, and the patient may revert to his helpless state. Medical therapy with agents such as chlorpromazine and reserpine is usually tried, but the effects are limited. Paralyzing agents such as curare and myanesin are strictly and temporarily palliative.

The disease is usually progressive although it may remain stationary for years. Death usually occurs in 5 to 10 years. The possibility of recurrence in subsequent siblings should be called to the parents' attention.

Weakness, Atrophy, Areflexia and Sensory Deficit

Degenerative Diseases of Unknown Etiology

Hereditary Sensory Radicular Neuropathy

PATHOGENESIS.—This rare familial disorder behaves as a progressive degenerative disease in some cases[38] with a dominant mode of inheritance. Degeneration of the posterior spinal nerve roots, ganglia and posterior columns has been described. Also, degeneration of the cochlear and vestibular nuclei is found. The etiology is completely obscure.

CLINICAL AND LABORATORY DIAGNOSIS.—The condition may appear in childhood or early adult life with perforating ulcers of the feet, followed by bone atrophy and severe foot deformities. Pain, thermal sensation and tendon reflexes are lost below the knees, but muscle atrophy is not described. Lightning pains may occur, and later the hands may be involved. Mild ataxia and deafness has been noted in some cases.

The disorder must be differentiated from tabes dorsalis, congenital insensitivity to pain[137] and a similar but nonprogressive sensory neuropathy described more recently.[111]

MANAGEMENT AND PROGNOSIS.—Treatment of this rare disorder is symptomatic, attention being directed to the prevention of trauma. The physician must be aware that this clinical syndrome can run either a progressive or a nonprogressive course and that it has been described repeatedly as a dominant hereditary trait.

Progressive Bulbar Palsy (Fazio-Londe)

PATHOGENESIS.—This rare disorder may occur sporadically or as a familial disorder. Few autopsy studies have been reported, but it can result from the absence of anterior horn cells in the cranial nerve nuclei. Gomez et al.[60a] reported a well-documented example of this disorder which they regard simply as a variant of motor neuron disease or progressive spinal muscular atrophy (Chapter 19).

CLINICAL AND LABORATORY DIAGNOSIS.—Slowly progressive, symmetrical weakness and atrophy of any or all of the bulbar muscles characterizes the disease. Patients usually have paralysis of extraocular movements, ptosis of the lids, dysphagia, dysarthria and facial weakness. Atrophy of the tongue is also seen. Electromyography helps to distinguish a neural from a myopathic etiology. Careful muscle biopsy may also be necessary and useful. When evidence of pyramidal tract or motor neuron disease is superimposed upon the signs of bulbar weakness, the more common clinical diagnosis of amyotrophic lateral sclerosis or progressive muscular atrophy must be considered.

The differential diagnosis should include myasthenia gravis, brain stem glioma, myotonic dystrophy, late-onset ocular myopathy, inflammatory mass lesions of the brain stem and polyneuritis.

MANAGEMENT AND PROGNOSIS.—The disease runs a very slowly progressive course and lifespan is limited because of pulmonary disorders such as atelectasis and pneumonia which complicate pharyngeal paralysis. Accurate diagnosis and good symptomatic therapy provide the patient with the best long-term comfort.

Loss of Vision

Hereditary Optic Atrophy (Leber)

PATHOGENESIS.—This disorder which causes optic atrophy and loss of vision is inherited in different ways. Although the considerably higher incidence in males has suggested a sex-linked recessive trait, additional evidence indicates that the same clinical syndrome can appear in a dominant (Fig. 21.23, *A*) or autosomal recessive pattern. The limited number of pathologic studies which have been done show atrophy and degeneration of the ganglion cells in the retina, together with degeneration of the optic nerves, chiasm and geniculate bodies. The clinical resemblance in some reported families to the general group of heredofamilial ataxias suggests that the pathologic changes would be more widespread if autopsy data were available.

CLINICAL AND LABORATORY DIAGNOSIS.—Onset of visual loss usually begins in late childhood but may appear early (Fig. 21.23,*B*). Vision at first deteriorates rapidly and then reaches a plateau in a few months, after which there is usually little progression. Both eyes are involved eventually, with large central scotomata and relative preservation of the temporal fields. Examination in the early stages may show congestion and edema, but this is soon replaced by obvious optic atrophy. Additional clinical findings in some patients, such as clubfeet, ataxia, spasticity,

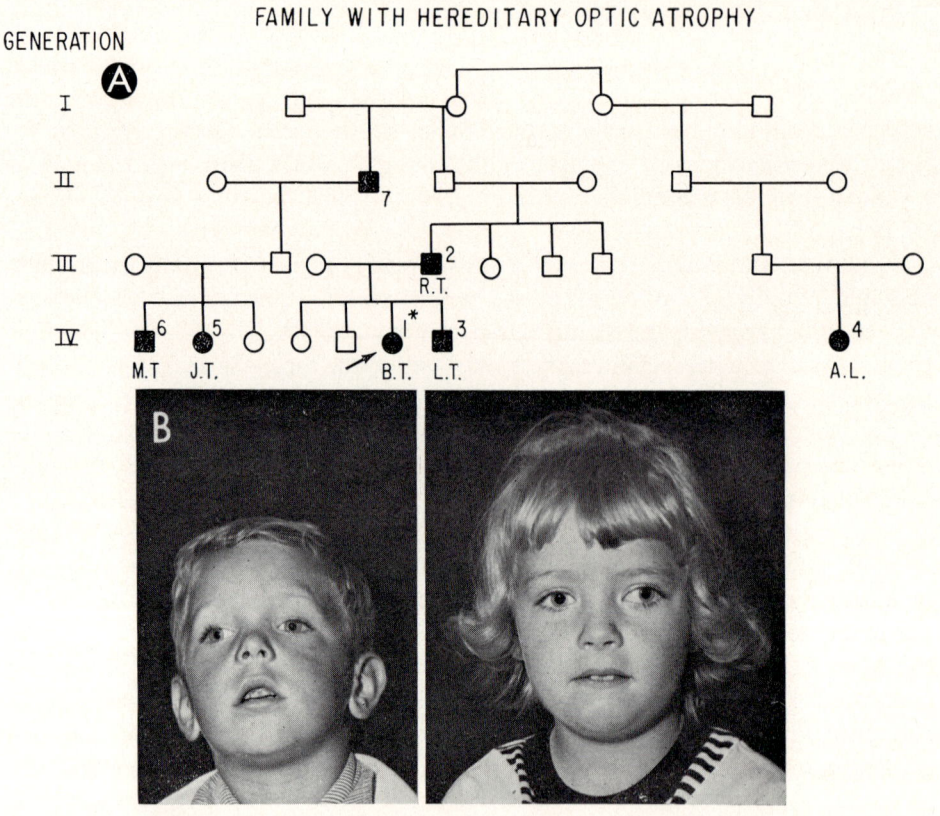

444 HEREDITARY METABOLIC AND DEGENERATIVE DISEASES

Fig. 21.23.—Hereditary optic atrophy (Leber). **A**, kindred diagram of family shows: **1**, girl, 5½, with visual defect, optic atrophy and nystagmus. After three years she alone shows signs of spastic diplegia. **2**, man, 28, with visual defect and optic atrophy. **3**, boy, 2 years 9 months, with visual defect, optic atrophy and squint. **4**, girl, 3½, with ocular squint, visual defect and nystagmus but no apparent optic atrophy. **5**, girl, 16, and **6**, man, 21, with visual defect and optic atrophy. **7**, man with noncorrectible visual defect for years. Siblings B.T. and L.T. are shown in **B**.

This family with hereditary optic atrophy demonstrates several important clinical features: (1) The disorder in this family behaves as an autosomal dominant trait. (2) Age of onset and severity of symptoms vary among different relatives. (3) Some, but not all, affected individuals have ocular squint. (4) Some, but not all, have nystagmus. (5) One patient (A.L.) has visual defect, a squint and nystagmus but no optic nerve pallor.

hyperreflexia and mental defect, suggest a fundamental relationship to the hereditary cerebellar ataxias.[48c]

Hereditary optic atrophy may be difficult to distinguish from optic neuritis and retrobulbar neuritis unless one can ascertain that a close relative has the same disease.

MANAGEMENT AND PROGNOSIS.—No therapy for the failing vision is available. Special education using the Braille system may be essential in many cases.

If a consistent pattern of inheritance emerges in a family, this information can be employed in genetic counseling. Although in most patients deterioration of vision becomes stationary in a few months, visual loss progresses to almost total blindness in a minority of patients.

Pigmentary Degeneration of the Retina

Retinitis Pigmentosa

PATHOGENESIS.—This strongly hereditary disorder usually affects only the eye and is transmitted in a variable manner. The genetic evidence suggests that for apparently the same clinical disease different inheritance patterns are involved in different kindreds—autosomal or X-linked, dominant or recessive.[134] Degeneration of the layer of rods and cones of the retina is followed by atrophy of the optic nerve fibers. Later the melanin-containing cells of the pigment layer are displaced to a more superficial position in the retina.

CLINICAL AND LABORATORY DIAGNOSIS.—Symptoms may have their onset at almost any age, the first symptom usually being night blindness in childhood. The visual fields are reduced concentrically from the periphery to the center, with concomitant loss of visual acuity. Funduscopic appearance may be normal at first, but soon large deposits of dark brown or black pigment are seen in the midportion of the retina between the central region and the extreme periphery. Eventually pallor of the optic nerves develops and central blindness occurs last. Although loss of vision is usually the only symptom, some patients give evidence of congenital neurologic defect in the form of deafness, mental retardation and seizures.

In the differential diagnosis one must consider (1) the Laurence-Moon-Biedl syndrome (obesity, mental retardation, sexual infantilism, diabetes insipidus and sometimes polydactlyly), (2) Hallervorden-Spatz disease (see under Ataxia), (3) juvenile amaurotic familial idiocy (see Cerebral Lipidoses) (4) Refsum's syndrome (chronic symmetrical polyneuritis, retinitis pigmentosa with concentric constriction of the visual fields, cerebellar signs with nystagmus, and increased CSF protein) and (5) progressive neural muscular atrophy (Charcot-Marie-Tooth). Recent studies report that patients with Refsum's disease have high levels of phytanic acid in serum and tissues, suggesting that it is a disorder of lipid metabolism.[1,115]

MANAGEMENT AND PROGNOSIS.—The visual loss usually progresses steadily but the rate of loss varies. As indicated, this disorder can affect several members of a sibship and can occur in successive generations.

No therapy alters the course of the disease and patients may be forced to learn the Braille reading system.

Familial Dysautonomia

PATHOGENESIS.—This disorder of autonomic function[117a] is inherited as a recessive trait and occurs in Jews most frequently but not exclusively. Disseminated lesions of the brain stem reticular formation have been described[30] but the limited number of studies cannot be considered significant. Recent physiologic studies of patients using histamine and methacholine are interesting but they do not answer the fundamental question as to whether this disorder is a single specific inborn metabolic degenerative disorder or a broader functional disturbance of the autonomic nervous system.

CLINICAL AND LABORATORY DIAGNOSIS.—During infancy there are symptoms of dysphagia, drooling and recurrent lower respiratory infections. Later, a lack of tearing, blotchy skin with excessive sweating, feeding problems and poor temperature regulation are noted. These infants show rather marked irritability and have episodic hypertension and postural hypotension. Their impaired pain perception leads at times to corneal ulcerations and they manifest mental and physical retardation with hypotonia, hyporeflexia and poor coordination. Riley and Moore[117] have recently reviewed carefully the criteria for diagnosis.

Recurrent respiratory infections are accompanied by x-ray evidence of pulmonary infiltrates and atelectasis. Recently it has been suggested that most or all patients with the disease have no taste buds on their tongues and this may be the simplest, most reliable diagnostic sign.[36] The failure of pain and erythema to develop around an intradermal histamine wheal is typical in patients with this disorder and may have diagnostic value. The development of pupillary miosis with instillation of 2.5% methacholine into the conjunctival sac is a less reliable diagnostic procedure because it does not occur in all patients who have the disease.

The differential diagnosis should include other types of neuropathy, myopathy and the many causes of mental retardation, including Hartnup disease, congenital insensitivity to pain and acrodynia. In the differential diagnosis of recurrent pneumonia one must consider food sensitivities, cystic fibrosis, foreign body aspiration, congenital pulmonary and vascular anomalies, and agammaglobulinemia.

MANAGEMENT AND PROGNOSIS.—Treatment is limited to the prevention and eradication of pulmonary infections, the prevention of corneal ulcerations, the management of hypertension and vomiting and the judicious use of sedatives and tranquilizing agents.

If these children survive the complications seen in early childhood, a satisfactory adjustment in adult life can be expected. The fact that more than one child in a family can be affected must be considered in family counseling.

BIBLIOGRAPHY

1. Alexander, W. S.: Phytanic acid in Refsum's syndrome, J. Neurol. Neurosurg. & Psychiat. 29:412, 1966.
2. Allen, R. J.: Personal communication.
2a. Armstrong, M. D., and Robinow, M.: A case of hyperlysinemia: biochemical and clinical observations, Pediatrics 39:546, 1967.
3. Auerbach, V. H., et al.: Histidinemia, J. Pediat. 60:487, 1962.
4. Austin, J., et al.: Metachromatic form of diffuse cerebral sclerosis, Arch. Neurol. 14:259, 1966.
5. Austin, J. H.: Metachromatic form of diffuse cerebral sclerosis: I. Diagnosis during life by urine sediment examination; II. Diagnosis during life by isolation of metachromatic lipids from urine, Neurology 7:415, 716, 1957.
5a. Avery, M. E., et al.: Transient tyrosinemia of the newborn: Dietary and clinical aspects, Pediatrics 39:378, 1967.
6. Baron, D. N., et al.: Hereditary pellagra-like skin rash with temporary cerebellar ataxia, constant renal amino-aciduria and other bizarre biochemical features, Lancet 2:421, 1956.
7. Bartler, F. C.: Hypophosphatasia, in Stanbury, J. B., Wyngaarden, J. B., and Fredrickson, D. S. (eds.): *The Metabolic Basis of Inherited Disease* (2d ed.; New York City: McGraw-Hill Book Company, Inc., 1966), ch. 43.
8. Bearn, A. G.: Wilson's Disease, in Stanbury, J. B., Wyngaarden, J. B., and Fredrickson, D. S. (eds.): *The Metabolic Basis of Inherited Disease* (2d ed.; New York City: McGraw-Hill Book Company, Inc., 1966), ch. 34.
9. Bellanti, J. A., et al.: Ataxia-telangiectasia: immunologic and virologic studies of serum and respiratory secretions, Pediatrics 37:924, 1966.

10. Berlow, S., and Efron, M. L.: Studies in cystathioninemia. (Abstract) J. Pediat. 67:714, 1965.
11. Berry, H. K., and Spinanger, J.: A paper spot test useful in study of Hurler's syndrome, J. Lab. & Clin. Med. 55:136, 1960.
12. Berry, H. K., et al.: Detection of phenylketonuria in newborn infants, J.A.M.A. 198: 1114, 1966.
13. Berry, H. K., et al.: Phenylketonuria, *Disease-a-Month* (Chicago: Year Book Medical Publishers, Inc.), December, 1966.
14. Berry, H. K., et al.: Treatment of phenylketonuria, Am. J. Dis. Child. 113:2, 1967.
15. Bessman, S. P., and Baldwin, R.: Imidazole aminoaciduria in cerebromacular degeneration, Science 135:789, 1962.
15a. Blaw, M. E., et al.: Sudanophilic leukodystrophy and adrenal cortical atrophy, Arch. Neurol. 11:626, 1964.
16. Boder, E., and Sedgwick, R. P.: Ataxia-telangiectasia: Familial syndrome of progressive cerebellar ataxia, oculocutaneous telangiectasia and frequent pulmonary infection, Pediatrics 21:526, 1958.
17. Bracken, M. M., and Bragdon, F. H.: Von Recklinghausen's disease of the central nervous system, Am. J. Clin. Path. 26:1456, 1956.
18. Brady, R. O.: The sphingolipidoses, New England J. Med. 275:312, 1966.
19. Brand, E., et al.: Cystinuria: The excretion of a cystine complex which decomposes in the urine with the liberation of free cystine, J. Biol. Chem. 86:315, 1930.
20. Bray, P. F.: Sex-linked neurodegenerative disease associated with monilethrix, Pediatrics 36:417, 1965.
20a. Budd, M. A., et al.: Isovaleric acidemia, New England J. Med. 277:321, 1967.
20b. Byers, R. K., and Dodge, J. A.: Huntington's chorea in children, Neurology 17:587, 1967.
21. Carr, E. A., et al.: The various types of thyroid malfunction in cretinism and their relative frequency, Pediatrics 28:1, 1961.
22. Carson, N. A. J., and Neill, D. W.: Metabolic abnormalities detected in a survey of mentally backward individuals in Northern Ireland, Arch. Dis. Childhood 37:505, 1962.
23. Carson, N. A. J., et al.: Homocystinuria: New inborn error of metabolism associated with mental deficiency, Arch. Dis. Childhood 38:425, 1963.
24. Cartwright, G. E.: Hepatolenticular Degeneration, in Harrison, T. R., et al. (eds.): *Principles of Internal Medicine* (5th ed.; New York City: McGraw-Hill Book Company, Inc., 1966), ch. 103.
25. Centerwall, W. R., and Miller, M. M.: Ataxia, telangiectasia, and sinopulmonary infections—a syndrome of slowly progressive deterioration in childhood, A.M.A. Am. J. Dis. Child. 95:385, 1958.
26. Childs, B., et al.: Idiopathic hyperglycinemia and hyperglycinuria: New disorder of amino acid metabolism. I, Pediatrics 27:522, 1961.
27. Chutorian, A., and Rowland, L. P.: Lowe's syndrome, Neurology 16:115, 1966.
27a. Cobb, W., et al.: Cerebral lipidosis: An electroencephalographic study, Brain 75:343, 1952.
28. Cochrane, W. A.: Idiopathic infantile hypoglycemia and leucine sensitivity, Metabolism 9:386, 1960.
29. Cochrane, W. A., et al.: Familial hypoglycemia precipitated by amino acids, J. Clin. Invest. 35:411, 1956.
30. Cohen, P., and Solomon, N. H.: Familial dysautonomia, J. Pediat. 46:663, 1955.
31. Colombo, J. P., et al.: Congenital lysine intolerance with periodic ammonia intoxication, Lancet 1:1014, 1964.
32. Colombo, J. P., et al.: Lysine intolerance with periodic ammonia intoxication, Am. J. Dis. Child. 113:138, 1967.
33. Cornblath, M., et al.: Hereditary fructose intolerance, New England J. Med. 269:1271, 1963.
34. Crowe, F. W., et al.: *Multiple Neurofibromatosis* (Springfield, Ill.: Charles C Thomas, Publisher, 1956).
35. Cusworth, D. C., et al.: Amino-aciduria in galactosemia, Arch. Dis. Childhood 30:150, 1955.
36. Dancis, J., and Smith, A. A.: Familial dysautonomia, New England J. Med. 274:207, 1966.
37. Dancis, J., et al.: Intermittent branched-chain ketonuria: Variant of maple-syrup-urine disease, New England J. Med. 276:84, 1967.
38. Denny-Brown, D.: Hereditary sensory radicular neuropathy, J. Neurol. Neurosurg. & Psychiat. 14:237, 1951.
39. Denny-Brown, D.: Hepatolenticular degeneration (Wilson's disease), New England J. Med. 270:1149, 1964.

40. Denny-Brown, D., *et al.*: Difficulty in walking and petit mal attacks in a child, New England J. Med. 267:1198, 1962.
41. DiGeorge, A. M., *et al.*: Elevated serum insulin associated with leucine induced hypoglycemia, Soc. Ped. Res. (abstract), 1960.
42. Donnell, G. N., *et al.*: Hypoglycemia in maple syrup urine disease, Am. J. Dis. Child. 113:60, 1967.
43. Dunn, H. G., *et al.*: Homocystinuria, Neurology 16:407, 1966.
44. Efron, M. L.: Aminoaciduria, New England J. Med. 272:1058, 1107, 1965.
45. Efron, M. L.: Disorders of Proline and Hydroxyproline Metabolism, in Stanbury, J. B., Wyngaarden, J. B., and Fredrickson, D. S. (eds.): *The Metabolic Basis of Inherited Disease* (2d ed.; New York City: McGraw-Hill Book Company, Inc., 1966), ch. 18.
46. Efron, M. L.: Treatment of hydroxyprolinemia and hyperprolinemia, Am. J. Dis. Child. 113:116, 1967.
47. Eisen, A. H., *et al.*: Immunologic deficiency in ataxia telangiectasia, New England J. Med. 272:18, 1965.
48. Engel, W. K., *et al.*: Protein abnormalities in neuromuscular diseases: I, J.A.M.A. 195:754, 1966.
48a. Feigin, I., and Wolf, A.: A disease in infants resembling Wernicke's encephalopathy, J. Pediat. 45:243, 1954.
48b. Feigin, I., *et al.*: The infantile spongy degenerations, Neurology 18:153, 1968.
48c. Ferguson, F. R., and Critchley, M.: Leber's optic atrophy and its relationship with heredo-familial ataxias, J. Neurol. Psychopath. 9:120, 1928.
48d. Fisch, R. O., *et al.*: Prenatal and postnatal developmental consequences of maternal phenylketonuria, Pediatrics 37:979, 1966.
49. Ford, F. R.: *Diseases of the Nervous System in Infancy, Childhood and Adolescence* (5th ed.; Springfield, Ill.: Charles C Thomas, Publisher, 1966).
50. Freeman, J. M., *et al.*: Ammonia intoxication due to a congenital defect in urea synthesis (abstract) J. Pediat. 65:1039, 1964.
51. Frimpter, G. W., *et al.*: Cystathioninuria, New England J. Med. 268:333, 1963.
52. Frimpter, G. W., *et al.*: Reversible "Fanconi syndrome" caused by degraded tetracycline, J.A.M.A. 184:111, 1963.
53. Frimpter, G. W., *et al.*: Cystathioninuria: Management, Am. J. Dis. Child. 113:115, 1967.
54. Gentz, J., *et al.*: Dietary treatment in tyrosinemia (tyrosinosis), Am. J. Dis. Child. 113:31, 1967.
55. Gerritsen, T., and Waisman, H. A.: Homocystinuria: Absence of cystathionine in the brain, Science 145:588, 1964.
56. Gerritsen, T., and Waisman, H. A.: Hypersarcosinemia, an inborn error of metabolism, New England J. Med. 275:66, 1966.
57. Gerritsen, T., *et al.*: A new type of idiopathic hyperglycinemia with hypo-oxaluria, Pediatrics 36:882, 1965.
58. Ghadimi, H., and Partington, M. W.: Salient features of histidinemia, Am. J. Dis. Child. 113:83, 1967.
59. Ghadimi, H., *et al.*: Hyperlysinemia associated with retardation, New England J. Med. 273:723, 1965.
60. Goldstein, N. P., *et al.*: Copper balance studies in Wilson's disease, Arch. Neurol. 12:456, 1965.
60a. Gomez, M. R., *et al.*: Progressive bulbar paralysis in childhood (Fazio-Londe's disease), Arch. Neurol. 6:317, 1962.
61. Greenfield, J. G., *et al.*: *Neuropathology* (2d ed.; Baltimore: Williams & Wilkins Company, 1963).
62. Grosfeld, J. C. M., *et al.*: Argininosuccinic aciduria in monilethrix, Lancet 2:789, 1964.
63. Grumbach, M. M., and Kaplan, S. L.: Amino acid and alpha-keto acid-induced hyperinsulinism in leucine-sensitive type of infantile and childhood hypoglycemia, J. Pediat. 57:346, 1960.
64. Haddad, H. M., *et al.*: Leucine-induced hypoglycemia, New England J. Med. 267:1057, 1962.
65. Hagberg, B., *et al.*: Clinical and laboratory diagnosis of metachromatic leucodystrophy, Cerebral Palsy Bull. 3:438, 1961.
66. Halvorsen, S.: Dietary treatment of tyrosinosis, Am. J. Dis. Child. 113:38, 1967.
67. Harris, H., *et al.*: Cystathioninuria, Ann. Human Genet. 23:442, 1959.
68. Herring, V. G., *et al.*: Hepatolenticular degeneration: Observations on a case treated with D-penicillamine, J. Pediat. 63:550, 1963.
69. Hoefnagel, D., *et al.*: Hereditary choreoathetosis, self-mutilation and hyperuricemia in young males, New England J. Med. 273:130, 1965.

69a. Hoefnagel, D., et al.: Addison's disease and diffuse cerebral sclerosis, J. Neurol. Neurosurg. & Psychiat. 30:56, 1967.
69b. Hogan, G. R., and Richardson, E. P.: Spongy degeneration of the nervous system (Canavan's disease), Pediatrics 35:284, 1965.
70. Hooft, C., et al.: Methionine malabsorption in a mentally defective child, Lancet 2:20, 1964.
71. Horner, F. A., et al.: Termination of dietary treatment of phenylketonuria, New England J. Med. 266:79, 1962.
71a. Janeway, R., et al.: Progressive myoclonus epilepsy with Lafora inclusion bodies, Arch. Neurol. 16:565, 1967.
72. Jepson, J. P.: Hartnup Disease, in Stanbury, J. B., Wyngaarden, J. B., and Fredrickson, D. S. (eds.): *The Metabolic Basis of Inherited Disease* (2d ed.; New York City: McGraw-Hill Book Company, Inc., 1966), ch. 57.
72a. Jervis, G. A.: Huntington's chorea in childhood, Arch. Neurol. 9:244, 1963.
73. Joseph, R., et al.: Maladie familiale associant, des convulsions à début très précoce, une hyperalbuminorachie et une hyperaminoacidurie, Arch. franc. pédiat. 15:374, 1958.
74. Kalckar, H. M., et al.: Galactosemia, a congenital defect in a nucleotide transferase, Biochim. et biophys. acta 20:262, 1956.
75. Kampine, J. P., et al.: Diagnosis of Gaucher's disease and Niemann-Pick disease with small samples of venous blood, Science 155:86, 1967.
75a. Kapp, J. P., et al.: Brain tumors with tuberous sclerosis, J. Neurosurg. 26:191, 1967.
76. Karpati, G., et al.: Ataxia-telangiectasia, Am. J. Dis. Child. 110:51, 1965.
77. Kennedy, C., et al.: Homocystinuria: A report in two siblings, Pediatrics 36:736, 1965.
78. Kiloh, L. G., and Osselton, J. U.: *Clinical Electroencephalography* (2d ed.; London: Butterworth & Co., Ltd., 1966).
79. Kogut, M. D., et al.: Tyrosinosis, Am. J. Dis. Child. 113:47, 1967.
80. Komrower, G. M.: Dietary treatment of homocystinuria, Arch. Dis. Childhood 41:666, 1966.
80a. Komrower, G. M., and Westall, R.: Hydroxykyneninuria, Am. J. Dis. Child. 113:77, 1967.
81. LaDu, B. N.: Histidinemia, Am. J. Dis. Child. 113:88, 1967.
82. Lahey, M. E., et al.: Hypoparathyroidism, Clin. pediat. 2:43, 1963.
83. Lake, B. D.: A reliable rapid screening test for sulphatide lipidosis, Arch. Dis. Childhood 40:284, 1965.
84. Landing, B. H., et al.: Familial neurovisceral lipidosis, Am. J. Dis. Child. 108:503, 1964.
85. Lesch, M., and Nyhan, W. L.: A familial disorder of uric acid metabolism and central nervous system function, Am. J. Med. 36:561, 1964.
86. Levin, B.: Argininosuccinic aciduria, Am. J. Dis. Child. 113:162, 1967.
87. Levin, B., and Russell, A.: Treatment of hyperammonemia, Am. J. Dis. Child. 113:142, 1967.
88. Levin, B., et al.: Argininosuccinic aciduria, an inborn error of amino acid metabolism, Arch. Dis. Childhood 36:622, 1961.
89. Lygren, T.: Hepatolenticular degeneration (Wilson's disease) and juvenile cirrhosis in the same family, Lancet 1:275, 1959.
90. Mabry, C. C., et al.: Mental retardation in children of phenylketonuric mothers, New England J. Med. 275:1331, 1966.
90a. Malamud, N.: Neuropathology of phenylketonuria, J. Neuropath. & Exper. Neurol. 25:254, 1966.
90b. Martin, L. W., et al.: Rectal biopsy as an aid in the diagnosis of diseases of infants and children, J. Pediat. 62:197, 1963.
91. McFarlin, D. E., et al.: Immunoglobulin: A production in ataxia telangiectasia, Science 150:1175, 1965.
92. McIntyre, N., et al.: Hemolytic anemia in Wilson's disease, New England J. Med. 276:439, 1967.
93. McKusick, V. A., et al.: The genetic mucopolysaccharidoses, Medicine 44:445, 1965.
94. McMurray, W. C., et al.: Citrullinuria, Pediatrics 32:347, 1963.
95. Mellman, W. J., et al.: Indolylacroyl glycine excretion in a family with mental retardation, Clin. chim. acta 8:843, 1963.
96. Menkes, J. H.: Metabolic Diseases of the Nervous System, in Brennemann-Kelley: *Practice of Pediatrics* (Hagerstown, Md.: W. F. Prior Company, Inc., 1966), ch. 6N.
97. Menkes, J. H., et al.: A new syndrome: Progressive familial infantile cerebral dysfunction associated with an unusual urinary substance, Pediatrics 14:462, 1954.
98. Menkes, J. H., et al.: A sex-linked recessive disorder with retardation of growth, peculiar hair, and focal cerebral and cerebellar degeneration, Pediatrics 29:764, 1962.
99. Michener, W. M.: Hyperuricemia and mental retardation, Am. J. Dis. Child. 113:195, 1967.

100. Milne, M. D.: Disorders of amino-acid transport, Brit. M. J. 1:327, 1964.
101. Mohyuddin, F., et al.: Studies on amino acid metabolism in citrullinuria, Am. J. Dis. Child. 113:152, 1967.
102. Morris, M. D., et al.: Late-onset branched-chain ketoaciduria (maple syrup urine disease), Journal-Lancet 86:149, 1966.
103. Morrow, G.: Citrullinemia, Am. J. Dis. Child. 113:157, 1967.
104. Moser, H. W., et al.: Argininosuccinic aciduria, Am. J. Med. 42:9, 1967.
105. Mudd, S. H., et al.: Homocystinuria: An enzymatic defect, Science 143:1443, 1964.
106. Newcome, D. S., et al.: Treatment of X-linked primary hyperuricemia with allopurinol, J.A.M.A. 198:315, 1966.
107. Norman, R. M., et al.: Pelizaeus-Merzbacher disease: A form of sudanophil leucodystrophy, J. Neurol. Neurosurg. & Psychiat. 29:521, 1966.
108. Nyhan, W. L.: Treatment of hyperglycinemia, Am. J. Dis. Child. 113:129, 1967.
109. Nyhan, W. L., et al.: A familial disorder of uric acid metabolism and central nervous system function: II, J. Pediat. 67:257, 1965.
110. O'Flynn, M. E., et al.: Hyperphenylalaninemia without phenylketonuria, Am. J. Dis. Child. 113:22, 1967.
111. Ogden, T. E., et al.: Some sensory syndromes in children: Indifference to pain and sensory neuropathy, J. Neurol. Neurosurg. & Psychiat. 22:267, 1959.
112. O'Reilly, S.: Problems in Wilson's disease, Neurology 17:137, 1967.
112a. Perry, T. L., et al.: Carnosinemia, New England J. Med. 277:1219, 1967.
112b. Perry, T. L., et al.: Cystathioninuria in two healthy siblings, New England J. Med. 278:590, 1968.
113. Peterson, R. D. A., et al.: Ataxia-telangiectasia: A possible clinical counterpart of the animals rendered immunologically incompetent by thymectomy, J. Pediat. 63:701, 1963.
114. Peterson, R. D. A., et al.: Ataxia-telangiectasia: Its association with a defective thymus, immunological-deficiency disease, and malignancy, Lancet 1:1189, 1964.
115. Rake, M., and Saunders, M.: Refsum's disease: A disorder of lipid metabolism, J. Neurol. Neurosurg. & Psychiat. 29:417, 1966.
116. Reed, W. B., et al.: Cutaneous manifestations of ataxia-telangiectasia, J.A.M.A. 195:746, 1966.
117. Riley, C. M., and Moore, R. H.: Familial dysautonomia differentiated from related disorders, Pediatrics 37:435, 1966.
117a. Riley, C. M., et al.: Central autonomic dysfunction with defective lacrimation: I. Report of five cases, Pediatrics 3:468, 1949.
118. Robins, M. M.: Pyridoxine dependency convulsions in a newborn, J.A.M.A. 195:491, 1966.
119. Robins, M. M., et al.: Morquio's disease: An abnormality of mucopolysaccharide metabolism, J. Pediat. 62:881, 1963.
119a. Robinson, F., et al.: Necrotizing encephalopathy of childhood, Neurology 17:472, 1967.
119b. Rosenberg, R. N., et al.: The interrelationship of neurofibromatosis and fibrous dysplasia, Arch. Neurol. 17:174, 1967.
120. Russell, A., et al.: Hyperammonemia: A new instance of an inborn enzymatic defect of the biosynthesis of urea, Lancet 2:699, 1962.
121. Sass, J. K., et al.: Juvenile gout with brain involvement, Arch. Neurol. 13:639, 1965.
122. Schafer, I. A., et al.: Familial hyperprolinemia, cerebral dysfunction and renal anomalies occurring in a family with hereditary nephropathy and deafness, New England J. Med. 267:51, 1962.
123. Scheinberg, I. H., and Sternlieb, I.: Environmental treatment of a hereditary illness: Wilson's disease, Ann. Int. Med. 53:1151, 1960.
124. Schimke, R. N., et al.: Homocystinuria, J.A.M.A. 193:711, 1965.
125. Schwartz, J. F., et al.: Bassen-Kornzweig syndrome: Deficiency of serum beta-lipoprotein, Arch. Neurol. 8:438, 1963.
126. Scriver, C. R.: Vitamin B_6-dependency and infantile convulsions, Pediatrics 26:62, 1960.
127. Scriver, C. R.: Hartnup disease, New England J. Med. 273:530, 1965.
128. Scriver, C. R.: Membrane transport in disorders of amino-acid metabolism, Am. J. Dis. Child. 113:170, 1967.
129. Scriver, C. R., et al.: Hereditary tyrosinemia and tyrosyluria in a French Canadian geographic isolate, Am. J. Dis. Child. 113:41, 1967.
130. Smith, D. W., et al.: The mental prognosis in hypothyroidism of infancy and childhood, Pediatrics 19:1011, 1957.
131. Snyderman, S. E., et al.: Maple syrup urine disease, with particular reference to dietotherapy, Pediatrics 34:454, 1964.
132. Southren, A. L., et al.: An unusual neurologic syndrome associated with hyperserotoninemia, New England J. Med. 260:1265, 1959.

133. Stanbury, J. B.: Familial Goiter, in Stanbury, J. B., Wyngaarden, J. B., and Fredrickson, D. S. (eds.): *The Metabolic Basis of Inherited Disease* (2d ed.; New York City: McGraw-Hill Book Company, Inc., 1966), ch. 10.
134. Stern, C.: *Principles of Human Genetics* (San Francisco: W. H. Freeman and Co., 1960).
135. Sternlieb, I., and Scheinberg, I. H.: The diagnosis of Wilson's disease in asymptomatic patients, J.A.M.A. 183:747, 1963.
136. Strich, S. J.: Pathological findings in three cases of ataxia-telangiectasia, J. Neurol. Neurosurg. & Psychiat. 29:489, 1966.
137. Swanson, A. G.: Congenital insensitivity to pain with anhydrosis, Arch. Neurol. 8:299, 1963.
138. Tada, K., *et al.*: Congenital tryptophanuria with dwarfism, Tohoku J. Exper. Med. 80:118, 1963.
139. Tada, K., *et al.*: Hypervalinemia, Am. J. Dis. Child. 113:64, 1967.
140. Tanaka, K., *et al.*: Isovaleric acidemia: A new genetic defect of leucine metabolism, Proc. Natl. Acad. Sc. 56:236, 1966.
140a. Terry, K., and Linker, A.: Distinction among four forms of Hurler's syndrome, Proc. Soc. Exper. Biol. & Med. 115:394, 1964.
141. Thomas, R. P., *et al.*: Homocystinuria and ectopia lentis in Negro family, J.A.M.A. 198:560, 1966.
142. Tu, J., *et al.*: DL-penicillamine as a cause of optic axial neuritis, J.A.M.A. 185:83, 1963.
143. Waisman, H. A.: Variations in clinical and laboratory findings in histidinemia, Am. J. Dis. Child. 113:93, 1967.
144. Waldinger, C.: Pyridoxine deficiency and pyridoxine dependency in infants and children, Postgrad. M. J. 35:415, 1964.
145. Wallace, B. J., *et al.*: Mucopolysaccharidosis type III, Arch. Path. 82:462, 1966.
146. Walshe, J. M.: Wilson's disease: The presenting symptoms, Arch. Dis. Childhood 37:253, 1962.
147. Westall, R. G.: Treatment of argininosuccinic aciduria, Am. J. Dis. Child. 113:160, 1967.
147a. Westall, R. G.: Dietary treatment of maple syrup urine disease, Am. J. Dis. Child. 113:58, 1967.
148. White, H. H., *et al.*: Homocystinuria, Arch. Neurol. 13:455, 1965.
148a. Williams, T. F., *et al.*: Familial (Hereditary) Vitamin D-Resistant Rickets with Hypophosphatemia, in Stanbury, J. B., Wyngaarden, J. B., and Fredrickson, D. S. (eds.): *The Metabolic Basis of Inherited Disease* (2d ed.; New York City: McGraw-Hill Book Company, Inc., 1966), ch. 51.
149. Woody, N. C.: Hyperlysinemia, Am. J. Dis. Child. 108:543, 1964.
150. Yudell, A., *et al.*: The neuropathy of sulfatide lipidosis (metachromatic leukodystrophy), Neurology 17:103, 1967.
151. Ziter, F. A., *et al.*: The clinical findings in a patient with nonketotic hyperglycinemia, Pediatric Research 2:250, 1968.

22

Demyelinating Disease

Primary Demyelinating Diseases
    Encephalomyelitis
        Acute disseminated encephalomyelitis   Retrobulbar neuritis
        Optic neuritis   Neuromyelitis optica
        Transverse myelitis   Acute hemorrhagic
    Multiple Sclerosis   encephalomyelitis
    Leukodystrophies (Chapter 21)
Secondary Demyelinating Diseases
    Postinfectious or Postvaccinal Encephalomyelitis (Chapter 18)
Miscellaneous*
    Hereditary Metabolic Defects (Phenylketonuria[6,17])
    Malignancy (Progressive Multifocal Leukoencephalopathy—Hodgkin's Disease[2])
    Ischemic Vascular Disease
    Intoxications (e.g., Central Pontine Myelinolysis—Leukemia[19] and Alcohol[1])
    Nutritional Deficiencies (Subacute Combined Degeneration of the Cord—Vitamin B_{12}[11])
    Infections (Subacute Inclusion-Body Encephalitis[7])

CLASSIFICATION.—On the basis of available information it remains appropriate to segregate a group of conditions known as *demyelinating diseases* because demyelinating represents the primary pathologic process in these disorders of unknown etiology. In fitting these disorders into an outline it must be conceded that demyelination is also seen secondarily as part of other disease processes. In the latter conditions not only is there a discrete cause for the demyelination but other pathologic tissue changes are also seen. At present the conditions are divided into nonfamilial and familial disorders. It then seems best to segregate the primary demyelinating disorders along a continuous spectrum, with the classic nonrecurrent condition at one end (acute disseminated encephalomyelitis) and the classic recurrent disorder at the other end (multiple or disseminated sclerosis). All the other conditions tend to fall into either the recurrent or the nonrecurrent diseases,

---

*These disorders are included in the outline for orientation purposes. They are discussed in a limited way in other chapters and appropriate references are provided here.

though many exceptions to this generalization can be expected. Optic neuritis generally does not recur, whereas retrobulbar neuritis can be expected to. In the middle of this schema are patients with transverse myelitis and neuromyelitis optica, which may or may not recur. Admittedly, the size and shape of this outline will change as new information accrues.

Primary Demyelinating Diseases
ENCEPHALOMYELITIS

PATHOGENESIS.—The pathologic changes in this condition are essentially the same for postexanthematous, postvaccinal (Chapter 18) and postinfectious encephalomyelitis. Perivenous demyelination, perivascular round-cell infiltration and microglial reaction characterize the histologic changes. The lesions may be distributed diffusely or in a focal fashion, thereby producing varying constellations of clinical signs. Whereas the cause-and-effect relationship with postexanthematous and postvaccinal disease is fairly clearcut, so-called postinfectious encephalomyelitis usually follows a nonspecific upper respiratory or influenza-like infection. The reader should realize that the acute course and isolated temporal character of these syndromes represent the only justification for separating them. However, if the long-term course is punctuated by remissions and exacerbations, the diagnosis of multiple or disseminated sclerosis is made.

A whole new approach to the pathogenesis of multiple sclerosis and other degenerative diseases of obscure etiology has recently been undertaken,[4] based upon the observations that "slow virus infections" in animals (scrapie, Aleutian disease in mink, and Visna) and a single human virus infection (parkinsonism resulting from von Economo encephalitis) can cause demyelinating disease of the nervous system. Efforts are being made to reproduce diseases such as multiple sclerosis and amyotrophic lateral sclerosis in a wide variety of laboratory animals. Gajdusek[9] has already successfully reproduced Kuru-like disease (a diffuse cerebellar degeneration seen in selected populations in New Guinea) in chimpanzees.

CLINICAL AND LABORATORY DIAGNOSIS.—*Acute disseminated encephalomyelitis.*—In mild forms of the disease the patient has headache, fever, drowsiness and perhaps weakness restricted to one limb with one or two cranial nerve palsies. In severely affected patients there are deepening coma, hemiplegia or paraplegia and multiple brain stem signs (cranial nerve palsies, nystagmus and impairment of vital signs).

Optic neuritis.—The patient usually notes the rather sudden loss of vision, often in both eyes, and examination reveals swelling of the optic nerve heads, i.e., hyperemia, venous tortuosity, indistinct disc margins and sometimes even hemorrhages. One may elicit a history of pain behind the eyes, but children often localize the pain poorly and may complain of frontal headache. The average physician cannot usually differentiate papillitis (as a sign of demyelinating disease) from papilledema (as a result of increased intracranial pressure). However, in optic neuritis the pupils are often dilated and fail to respond to light. If visual loss is incomplete, one can plot scotomata in the central field of vision with relative sparing of the peripheral fields.

Optic neuritis may occur as a sole neurologic finding or it may be associated with a transverse myelitis or evidence of brain stem involvement. Evidence of multiple sclerosis was eventually turned up by Kennedy and Carroll[13] in eight of 41 children with a diagnosis of optic neuritis, indicating the close relationship between the two conditions and the difficulties with classification and prognosis. Kennedy and Carter[14] stated that simultaneous bilateral optic neuritis with papillitis more often led to the eventual diagnosis of multiple sclerosis in children than in adults. The clinical syndrome of optic neuritis can appear as a complication of measles,[20] mumps[21] and varicella,[12] and it can result from malnutrition,[5] including vitamin B_{12} deficiency.[3]

Transverse myelitis.—At first the patient exhibits a flaccid paraplegia and may be areflexic, with bilateral Babinski signs. Variable sensory loss is found below the level of the lesion, and there is urinary retention. Later a spastic paraplegia supervenes with hyperreflexia. Gradual improvement usually occurs but there may be residual weakness and atrophy. Recovery of sensation is usually complete. Occasionally the acute transverse myelitis is succeeded by an ascending paralysis which leads to death. Because this disorder is often ushered in by pain in the mid-back, it must always be differentiated from spinal epidural abscess.

Neuromyelitis optica (Devic's disease).—Seen more often than isolated cases of either optic neuritis or transverse myelitis is a combination of signs involving both optic nerves and a spinal cord lesion. We have seen several cases in which the child had complained of frontal headache and choked discs had been noted without an appreciation of any visual loss. The subsequent development of pyramidal tract signs and sensory deficit misled the physician into studying the patients in detail for an intracranial tumor, only to have the patients gradually lose their vision and eventually recover during observation.

Acute hemorrhagic leukoencephalitis.—Although some have placed this disorder in a separate category, it seems most likely that it represents a severe, fulminating form of acute disseminated encephalomyelitis. The disorder has received recognition as an entity in its own right because, in addition to perivenous demyelination, histologic study reveals multiple small hemorrhages around necrotic blood vessels. The clinical findings do not differ significantly from those of other severe forms of acute disseminated encephalomyelitis. In a review of the literature Lander[15] emphasized that the clinical features are characterized by the sudden onset of speech disturbances, motor paralyses and urinary incontinence.

The cerebrospinal fluid in all forms of encephalomyelitis generally shows a slight lymphocytic pleocytosis (25–250 cells) and a slight elevation in protein content—nonspecific findings.

MANAGEMENT AND PROGNOSIS.—The course and prognosis of all types of encephalomyelitis vary considerably. With severe forms of the *acute disseminated* disease, one can expect a high mortality. In milder cases, residual neurologic deficit (paraplegia, hemiplegia) is common. Recent uncontrolled therapy of acute disseminated encephalomyelitis with corticotropin or adrenal steroids by Ziegler[23] suggests a beneficial effect which parallels institution of therapy and a worsening which parallels discontinuation. *Transverse myelitis* has a lower mortality rate but a high incidence of neurologic deficit. In patients with *optic neuritis* significant visual loss may develop with the attack, and good function may be recovered either rapidly or over a period of time. Most patients wtih the syndrome of *neuromyelitis optica* are left with residual visual loss and a paraplegia of varying severity. Dispute continues about the incidence of recurrent symptoms, but we agree with those who state that patients with neurologic exacerbations should rationally be labeled with the diagnosis of multiple sclerosis, not neuromyelitis optica. Almost by definition the condition of *acute hemorrhagic leukoencephalitis* is uniformly fatal since the diagnosis cannot be established with certainty unless the characteristic histologic abnormalities are found.

Multiple Sclerosis (Disseminated Sclerosis)

PATHOGENESIS.—This common degenerative neurologic disorder disables adults frequently, most often between the ages of 20 and 40, and is seen only rarely in children (Low et al.[16]). A disease of unknown etiology, it occurs more frequently in temperate than in tropical climates and in Caucasians more often than in Negroes. It is not inherited and, despite studies and reports by many workers, no one has proved that the original disease or its relapses are precipitated by external factors such as trauma, infections, pregnancy, lumbar punctures or psychic stress. A recent surge of research interest in the possible role of "slow viruses" in the etiology of multiple sclerosis and other chronic neurodegenerative diseases has developed.[4] The recovery of filterable agents from animals with chronic diseases, such as scrapie, Visna and Aleutian disease of mink, which are characterized by pathologic changes suggesting demyelinating or degenerative diseases, has aroused interest in the possible role of pathogenic "slow viruses" in the central nervous system of man.

The pathologic changes in the syndrome have been described in great detail. The lesions or *plaques* have notoriously disseminated locations, they vary in size and they affect white matter and cranial nerve roots and periventricular areas in the cerebrum primarily. Cerebral white matter, optic nerves, long tracts in the spinal cord and nuclei in the brain are affected most frequently, although essentially no areas are spared. Histologically, new lesions may resemble those in acute encephalomyelitis in that they have a perivenous location, but older lesions show mainly sizeable, sharply outlined areas of demyelination with little cellular infiltrate except for gliosis.

CLINICAL AND LABORATORY DIAGNOSIS.—A proper understanding of the distribution of "M.S." plaques will make it easier for the reader to understand the variable character of the clinical picture. It has been said that "the disease must be disseminated both in time and in space" in order for the diagnosis to be entertained. We agree that one must document with certainty both remissions and exacerbations and more than one lesion in the nervous system on the basis of careful regional diagnosis. Having laid down these criteria, one adds little by dividing cases into "acute" multiple sclerosis (realizing that such cases may be indistinguishable from acute disseminated encephalomyelitis) and "chronic relapsing" multiple sclerosis. For the sake of clinical convenience it may be helpful to divide cases into the commonly occurring clinical syndromes:

1. Retrobulbar neuritis (with recurrences of lesions elsewhere, by definition)
2. Paraplegia or hemiplegia (less common)
3. Focal brain stem or cerebellar deficit

In *retrobulbar neuritis* "the patient sees nothing and the doctor sees nothing."

Young adults are affected more often than children and the disease is unilateral much more often than is optic neuritis, which as a rule is bilateral. The patient first complains of blurred vision with or without retroorbital pain. The pupil on the affected side is large and reacts poorly to light. Usually there is a central scotoma on tangent screen visual field examination. Later the disc may show signs of papillitis and at a remote later date optic nerve pallor ensues. Recurrent attacks of retrobulbar neuritis are common. It is assumed by most workers that in many of these patients clinical signs of multiple sclerosis eventually develop, sometimes only after a symptom-free interval of many years.

Patients may have pyramidal tract signs in both legs or one arm and one leg and have gait disability, ataxia, posterior column deficit (impaired vibratory, position, stereognostic and two-point sensation) and bladder-bowel dysfunction ("automatic" emptying of the bladder and constipation). If hemiplegia occurs, it may develop rapidly in an apoplectiform fashion and the physician may think first of a neoplasm or a vascular accident.[8,18]

Patients with *brain stem-cerebellar* deficit may have the Charcot triad of scanning speech, nystagmus and intention tremor. Vertigo disables many patients acutely as a result of lesions in the vestibulocerebellar pathways, and diplopia and internuclear ophthalmoplegia (horizontal nystagmus in the abducting eye and paralysis of adduction) often occur.

Less commonly, patients with multiple sclerosis may have mental disturbances, symptoms of tic douloureux or seizures as a result of the disseminated lesions.

The differential diagnosis of necessity must include an extremely wide range of neurologic disorders, but the physician especially must not overlook a neoplasm (especially slow-growing intraspinal tumors in the cervical canal or foramen magnum or benign intracranial masses) or chronic meningitis (such as lues). The hereditary degenerative disorders (Chapter 21), including hereditary optic atrophy (Leber), may be mistaken for multiple sclerosis. Gall and associates[10] have pointed out that multiple sclerosis in children differs very little from the disease in adults in mode of onset, symptoms, signs and CSF findings.

The CSF examination reveals a mild lymphocytic pleocytosis (20 cells) and a slight protein elevation in one-fourth of the patients. More recent studies[22] have shown that the gamma globulin content of the cerebrospinal fluid is elevated, in the absolute sense or relative to the total protein content, in two-thirds of the patients (usually those with the acute fulminating form or chronic advanced cases). For the same reason a first-zone rise is seen in the colloidal gold curve of the cerebrospinal fluid.

MANAGEMENT AND PROGNOSIS.—The variable course makes long-term prediction difficult in the individual case. Remissions which occur early in the course may last so long that the physician may doubt the original diagnosis, but follow-up examinations by experienced neurologists usually show eventual signs of relapse. Most patients succumb to intercurrent respiratory infections.

A vast array of drugs, diets, hormones and physical modalities has been used in therapy of multiple sclerosis. Most recently the adrenal corticosteroids have been employed extensively, but, despite the fact that some workers have been impressed with their value in optic and retrobulbar neuritis, controlled proof of their usefulness is lacking. Physical therapy should be given, when indicated, together with good general care. When relapse occurs the patient should be encouraged sincerely to believe that he can expect a remission. Anyone who deals with many of these patients realizes quickly that little is gained by confronting the patient with all the distressing complications that may ensue. Instead, one can feel justified in assuming that any given patient may be among the fortunate ones who enjoy a significant and prolonged remission.

BIBLIOGRAPHY

1. Adams, R. D., et al.: Central pontine myelinolysis: A hitherto undescribed disease occurring in alcoholics and malnourished patients, A.M.A. Arch. Neurol. & Psychiat. 81: 154, 1959.
2. Aström, K. E., et al.: Progressive multifocal leukoencephalopathy: A hitherto unrecognized complication of chronic lymphatic leukaemia and Hodgkin's disease, Brain 81:93, 1958.
3. Björkenheim, B.: Optic neuropathy caused by vitamin-B_{12} deficiency in carriers of the fish tapeworm, Diphyllobothrium latum, Lancet 1:688, 1966.
4. Brody, J. A., et al.: Soviet search for viruses that cause chronic neurologic diseases in the U.S.S.R., Science 147:1114, 1965.
5. Carroll, F. D.: Nutritional retrobulbar neuritis, Am. J. Ophth. 30:172, 1947.
6. Crome, L., and Pare, C. M. B.: Phenylketonuria: Review and report of the pathological findings in four cases, J. Ment. Sc. 106:862, 1960.
7. Dawson, J. R.: Cellular inclusions in cerebral lesions of epidemic encephalitis, Arch. Neurol. & Psychiat. 31:685, 1934.
8. Ford, F. R.: *Diseases of the Nervous System in Infancy, Childhood and Adolescence* (5th ed.; Springfield, Ill.: Charles C Thomas, Publisher, 1966).
9. Gajdusek, C. D.: Slow-virus infections of the nervous system, New England J. Med. 276: 392, 1967.
10. Gall, J. C., et al.: Multiple sclerosis in children, Pediatrics 21:703, 1958.
11. Greenfield, J. G. (ed.): *Neuropathology* (2d ed.; Baltimore: Williams & Wilkins Company, 1963).
12. Hatch, H. A.: Bilateral optic neuritis following chickenpox, J. Pediat. 34:758, 1949.
13. Kennedy, C., and Carroll, F. D.: Optic neuritis in children, A.M.A. Arch. Ophth. 63:747, 1960.
14. Kennedy, C., and Carter, S.: Relation of optic neuritis to multiple sclerosis in children, Pediatrics 28:377, 1961.
15. Lander, H.: Acute hemorrhagic leuco-encephalitis, Australasian Ann. Med. 7:55, 1958.
16. Low, N. L.: and Carter, S.: Multiple sclerosis in children, Pediatrics 18:24, 1956.
17. Malamud, N.: Neuropathology of phenylketonuria, J. Neuropath. & Exper. Neurol. 25: 254, 1966.
18. Prockop, L. D., and Heinz, E. R.: Demyelinating disease presenting as an intracranial mass lesion, Arch. Neurol. 13:559, 1965.
19. Rosman, N. P., et al.: Central pontine myelinolysis in a child with leukemia, Arch. Neurol. 14:273, 1966.
20. Ström, T.: Acute blindness as post-measles complication, Acta paediat. 42:60, 1953.
21. Woodward, J. H.: The ocular complications of mumps, Ann. Ophth. 16:7, 1907.
22. Yahr, M. D., et al.: Further studies on the gamma globulin content of cerebrospinal fluid in multiple sclerosis and other neurological diseases, Ann. New York Acad. Sc. 58:613, 1954.
23. Ziegler, D. K.: Acute disseminated encephalitis, Arch. Neurol. 14:476, 1966.

23

Neurologic Complications of Systemic Disease

Diseases of the Blood and Blood Vessels
    Hemorrhage
        Acute leukemia
        Aplastic anemia
        Hemorrhagic disease of the newborn
        Idiopathic thrombocytopenic purpura
        Hemophilia
        Anaphylactoid purpura
        (see below)
        Hypoprothrombinemia
        Scurvy
        Hypertension
    Embolization
        Congenital heart disease with right-to-left shunt
        Rheumatic heart disease with mitral stenosis and atrial fibrillation
        Ventriculocardiovascular shunts for obstructive hydrocephalus
        Subacute bacterial endocarditis with mycotic embolus and abscess formation
        Myocarditis
        Fat embolus
        Air embolus
    Vasculitis (Collagen Vascular Disease)
        Rheumatic chorea (Sydenham)
        Polyarteritis nodosa
        Systemic lupus erythematosus
        Anaphylactoid purpura
        Dermatomyositis (Chapter 19)
    Thrombosis (Occlusive Vascular Disease)
        Cyanotic congenital heart disease
        Perinatal complications
        Infections: meningitis, mastoiditis, otitis media, sinusitis
        Diseases of blood and blood vessels
            Sickle cell disease
            Thrombotic thrombocytopenic purpura
            Systemic lupus erythematosus
            Hemolytic-uremic syndrome
        Miscellaneous
            Trauma
            Metastatic tumor
            Hypertension
            Homocystinuria
            Spontaneous (idiopathic) arterial occlusion

Hyperbilirubinemia with Kernicterus

Renal Disease

    Thrombosis, Hemorrhage and Hypertension with Cerebral Edema

    Metabolic Complications (Hypocalcemia, Hyponatremia, Metabolic Acidosis)

    "Reverse Urea" Effect from Dialysis Therapy

Chronic Respiratory Disease

    Hypercapnea with Papilledema

    Neurologic Deficit from Correction of Hypercapnea

Liver and Gastrointestinal Disease

    Hepatic Coma

    Malabsorption with Hypoglycemia

    Bacillary Dysentery

Deficiency Disease

    Vitamin C   Vitamin B_1

    Vitamin D   Malnutrition (Kwashiorkor)

    Vitamin B_6

Diseases of the Blood and Blood Vessels

PATHOGENESIS

IN THE ABSENCE OF large autopsy series one can only guess at the frequency with which ischemic occlusive cerebrovascular disease causes "strokes" in children. Cerebrovascular accidents undoubtedly are less common in children now than a generation ago because of fewer venous thromboses and less rheumatic heart disease. The severity of brain damage due to occlusive blood vessel disease depends upon (1) the rapidity with which obstruction occurs (more rapid and severe with embolic infarcts because the vascular bed has no chance to develop a collateral circulation), (2) the size of the occluded vessel (usually greater damage with a larger vessel—also more common with emboli) and (3) the vulnerability of different cells (greater in the case of neurons and less with most of the supporting glial structures). In highly vascular sections of ischemic brain, such as cortex, *hemorrhagic infarcts* develop, whereas *necrosis* often develops in the white matter. These lesions may at times be differentiated clinically by the presence of blood in the cerebrospinal fluid. Large areas of infarction can cause swelling of the cerebral hemisphere and lead to the complication of uncal herniation (Chapter 8).

Occlusive arterial disease, such as that seen in atherosclerosis, and frank hemorrhagic disease present no problems in classification, but in patients with vasculitis, embolization or hypertension ischemic infarction is often associated with or complicated by hemorrhage.

Hemorrhage

Most of the blood disorders (see preceding outline) produce neurologic deficit by causing intracranial hemorrhage, which in turn may cause marked brain swelling and uncal herniation (Chapter 8).

Embolization

Diseases which cause embolization probably account for the majority of clinically recognizable cerebrovascular accidents in childhood at present. The striking advances in the field of cardiovascular surgery have dramatically lowered the mortality rate among children with congenital heart disease, but a significant number of strokes result from aseptic embolic infarcts and mycotic abscesses.[7,9,21,50] Although the incidence of subacute bacterial endocarditis has dropped along with that of rheumatic fever, many large medical centers are grappling with an increasing number of cases of septic emboli from bacterial endocarditis, a complication of the "universal shunt" therapy of hydrocephalus. The problem of cerebral embolization as a consequence of mural thrombi, secondary to atrial fibrillation and mitral stenosis, primarily affects adults with long-standing rheumatic heart disease. Myocarditis, a disorder of diverse infectious and unknown etiologies, causes a small number of strokes in young children.

Vasculitis (Collagen Vascular Disease)

Although rheumatic fever secondary to group A, beta-hemolytic streptococcal infections may represent the commonest form of cerebral vasculitis in children, this disorder does no significant permanent damage to the brain. Most of the collagen vascular diseases listed in the outline cause cerebral vasculitis occasionally, but they occur uncommonly in children. (Some examples are given under Clinical and Laboratory Diagnosis.) No attempt will be made here to describe the different pathologic characteristics of the cerebral blood vessels in these rare manifestations in children.

Arterial Thrombosis

Occasionally "idiopathic" (obscure cause[4,16]) arterial thrombosis, especially that involving the carotid vessels in the neck, is seen in the adolescent, but this occurrence is rare.[1] Thrombosis can result spontaneously or from trauma.[18] Most often trauma to the internal carotid artery in children results when an object held in the mouth penetrates the paratonsillar area. A thrombus may then propagate distally and cause massive cerebral infarction and death. Equally uncommonly one sees arteriolar thrombosis in children and young adults with rare conditions such as essential hypertension and homocystinuria. Arterial degenerative disease (not atherosclerosis) has been incriminated in isolated cases of arterial thrombosis by some workers, as has dissecting aneurysm of the cerebral arteries.[53] Occasionally in centers with large neurologic services carotid thrombosis complicating diagnostic arteriography has been reported.

Rare disorders of the blood characterized by "hypercoagulability" can cause intracranial arterial or venous thromboses.

Venous or Sinus Thrombosis

In most countries of the world where the population is well nourished, enjoys good hygiene and has access to modern medical care, nervous system damage from venous or sinus thrombosis is not commonly diagnosed. This vascular problem is a complication of dehydration, diarrhea, marasmus, sepsis, meningitis and chronic purulent infections of the mastoid, middle ear and sinuses, especially in very young children. It is seen commonly in autopsies on children who have had cyanotic congenital heart disease.[1] Lateral sinus thrombosis occasionally complicates mastoiditis, otitis media and eosinophilic granuloma, giving rise to cerebral edema, increased intracranial pressure and so-called otitic hydrocephalus (Chapter 8). Cavernous sinus thrombosis may result from adjacent infections of the face and soft tissue, and any of the major venous sinuses can become thrombosed as a complication of head trauma or tumor metastasis (especially neuroblastoma).

Congenital or Neonatal Cerebrovascular Accidents

Arterial thrombosis or embolism can occur in early life, either prenatally[1,6] or in the early neonatal period.[24] The etiology of these vascular accidents is often obscure and the causes are probably multiple. Banker has stated that, "Although there are a number of clinical reports of thrombosis of the internal carotid artery in children, pathologically confirmed cases of the idiopathic type are distinctly rare."[1] Multiple emboli may originate from an infarcted placenta. Thrombotic lesions may be secondary to trauma, infection, embolism from cardiac vegetations or hypercoagulation states, such as polycythemia.

CLINICAL AND LABORATORY DIAGNOSIS (TABLE 23.1)
Hemorrhage

In patients with bleeding disorders the diagnosis is usually made without much difficulty by (1) careful examination of the blood and bone marrow and (2) a study of coagulation. Apoplexy associated with blood in the cerebrospinal fluid is common in the terminal stages of *acute leukemia,* in *aplastic anemia, hemophilia*[47] and *congenital malformations*. The diagnosis of acute leukemia is made by finding "blast" forms of leukocytes in the blood or bone marrow. In the early stages of the disease these patients often have pancytopenia without circulating "blasts." Children with aplastic anemia have pancytopenia but no "blasts," and one commonly finds that the patient has been receiving a marrow-suppressing drug. The diagnosis of a bleeding vascular malformation is made with an angiographic study (Chapter 13).

Large intracranial hemorrhages can also result from *hypoprothrombinemia* (newborn infants with hemorrhagic disease and older patients receiving anticoagulant drugs such as Dicumarol[12]). This diagnosis is made by finding a prolonged prothrombin time in an oxalated sample of the patient's whole blood. Small hem-

TABLE 23.1.—DIFFERENTIAL DIAGNOSIS OF CEREBROVASCULAR DISEASES IN CHILDHOOD

Manifestation	Probable Cerebrovascular Disease	Other Diseases
1. Abrupt onset of focal neurologic deficit	Embolization (see text and outline) Hemorrhage Arterial occlusion Vascular malformation with hemorrhage (venous or sinus thrombosis)	Tumors Abscess Postictal paresis (without history of seizure) Demyelinating disease (acute M.S. or Schilder's disease) Trauma—subdural or epidural hematoma
2. Neurologic deficit with signs of cardiovascular disease	Embolization (see text and outline) Hypertension Venous or sinus thrombosis	Abscess
3. Neurologic or psychiatric symptoms in patients with evidence of systemic disease	Vasculitis (see outline) Hemorrhagic bleeding disorders (see outline) Small-vessel thrombosis in patients with polycythemic heart disease	Homocystinuria
4. Increased intracranial pressure	Sinus thrombosis with otitic hydrocephalus Brain abscess secondary to congenital heart disease Large infarcts or hemorrhages with cerebral swelling	Subdural or epidural hematoma Tumor Congenital hydrocephalus Chronic granulomatous meningitis (tuberculosis) Demyelinating disease (including optic neuritis) Other causes of pseudotumor cerebri (intoxication with water, lead, cortisone, vitamin A)
5. Blood in the CSF	Hemorrhagic bleeding disorders Hemorrhage from vascular malformations Hemorrhagic infarct	Trauma with subarachnoid hemorrhage (head trauma, birth trauma to cord) Bleeding associated with a malignant tumor (e.g., medulloblastoma) Acute hemorrhagic leukoencephalitis

orrhages may occur with less severe bleeding disorders, such as idiopathic thrombocytopenic purpura (Fig. 23.1), or in patients with steroid-induced hypertensive encephalopathy or hemorrhage.

Ischemic or hemorrhagic cerebrovascular disease should be suspected:

1. If there is an *abrupt* or *apoplectiform onset of focal neurologic deficit*—hemiparesis, cranial nerve palsy, aphasia or a demonstrable hemianopia (embolization, hemorrhage, venous or sinus thrombosis, arterial occlusion, vascular malformation). Occasionally patients with tumors, demyelinating disease (acute multiple sclerosis or Schilder's disease), brain abscess or postictal paresis will report the strokelike onset of symptoms.

2. If *focal neurologic deficit*, regardless of the rapidity of its onset, occurs in any patient with cardiovascular disease (embolization associated with congenital heart disease, rheumatic heart disease, subacute bacterial endocarditis, myocarditis), or in patients with hypertension.

3. If *focal neurologic deficit, increased intracranial pressure or psychiatric symptoms* are seen in patients with evidence of diffuse vascular disease, such as vas-

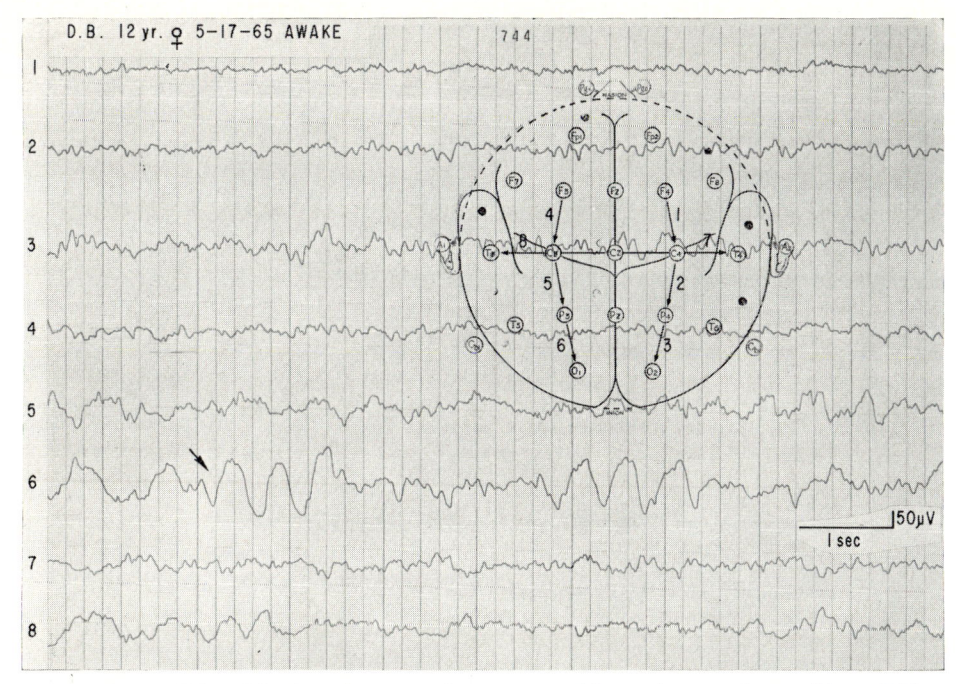

Fig. 23.1.—Idiopathic thrombocytopenic purpura with cerebrovascular accident. Diffuse skin petechiae, lethargy and headache developed over one week in girl, 12. She then had a right focal seizure and was found to have a mild right hemiparesis, a right hemianopia, mental obtundation with a diffuse, left-sided slow wave EEG focus (illustrated). Blood smear revealed a scanty number of platelets with a count of 50,000 (lower normal, 150,000) and the cerebrospinal fluid contained 31 RBC/mm.³ The patient recovered completely with prednisone therapy and a blood transfusion. Three months later she had no clinical neurologic deficit. Presumably a small intracerebral hemorrhage caused the seizure, the focal neurologic deficit and the EEG focus.

culitis (collagen vascular disease) or a bleeding disorder. In such patients one must also rule out rare systemic disorders which promote hypercoagulability, such as the hemolytic-uremic syndrome,[20] thrombotic thrombocytopenic purpura[34] or homocystinuria.

Embolization

When a cerebral embolus complicates *congenital heart disease* with a right-to-left shunt, the presence of the basic heart defect is usually well known and the stroke mechanism is easily recognized (Fig. 23.2). However, embolization occasionally occurs in a patient who has previously been considered well, who has not been handicapped by his defects and who may not have an impressive murmur or heart enlargement. Hence, any child who suffers a stroke should have a careful heart examination (including blood pressure and pulse in all extremities), a search for minimal cyanosis and clubbing, an electrocardiogram and chest x-rays. These procedures will uncover the evidence of congenital heart disease in nearly all cases. However, differentiation of a brain abscess from a large aseptic infarct may be difficult. The septic course, percussion skull tenderness and a well-defined delta wave

464 NEUROLOGIC COMPLICATIONS OF SYSTEMIC DISEASE

EEG focus typify an abscess. Increased pressure can prevail with both lesions but is commoner with abscess.

In the older patient with well-established *rheumatic heart disease, mitral stenosis and atrial fibrillation,* aseptic cerebral emboli are common. The history, the typical murmurs, fluoroscopic and x-ray evidence of left atrial enlargement and the absence of another etiology identify the rheumatic basis of the heart trouble.

Patients with *subacute bacterial endocarditis* (associated with congenital or rheumatic heart disease or secondary to a ventriculoatrial shunt for obstructive hydrocephalus) often have strokes as well as embolic phenomena in other parts of the

Fig. 23.2.—Cerebral embolus secondary to tetralogy of Fallot. Boy, 9, was born with congenital heart defect but was neurologically intact. One month before planned operative correction of the heart defect he suddenly became confused, "hysterical," didn't recognize familiar persons and lost consciousness for six hours. Upon awakening he had a left hemiparesis which became permanent. Later he had left-sided focal motor seizures and hyperactive behavior, with destructiveness, temper tantrums and short attention span. Examination showed microcephaly, obvious left hemiparesis and right-sided epileptiform EEG abnormalities. Full Scale IQ score was 83.

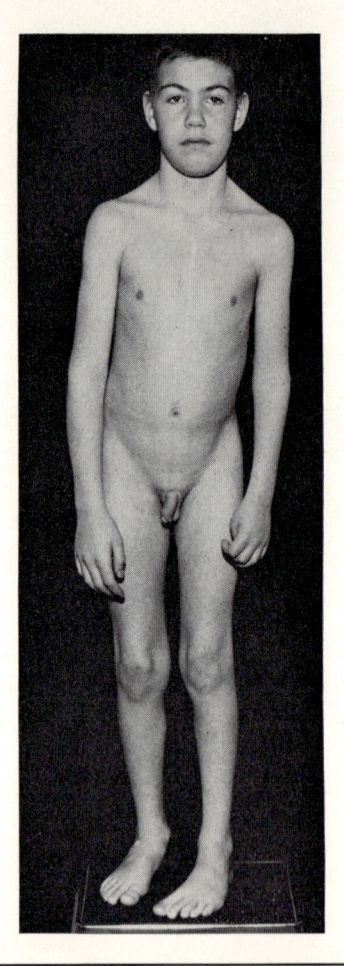

Fig. 23.3.—Myocarditis with secondary cerebral embolus. In this 18-month-old boy a flulike illness was followed in 10 days by lethargy, fever and vomiting. He then had a "cyanotic" spell with sweating and limpness but no loss of consciousness. In the hospital, cardiomegaly was noted (**A**) and an electrocardiogram showed a big Q wave, inverted T waves and elevated S-T segments in leads V_5 and V_6 (**B**). The latter findings suggested an infarct and the total clinical picture was compatible with the diagnosis of myocarditis. He had signs of congestive failure and was treated accordingly. One week later he was found with a flaccid right hemiplegia (paretic side is on reader's left in **C**). Subsequently the pulses in two extremities were lost. Diagnosis was multiple arterial emboli secondary to myocarditis. Recovery has been slow and incomplete. **D** documents the area of cerebral infarction. Note the marked amplitude suppression over the left frontoparietal area (arrows).

DISEASES OF THE BLOOD AND BLOOD VESSELS 465

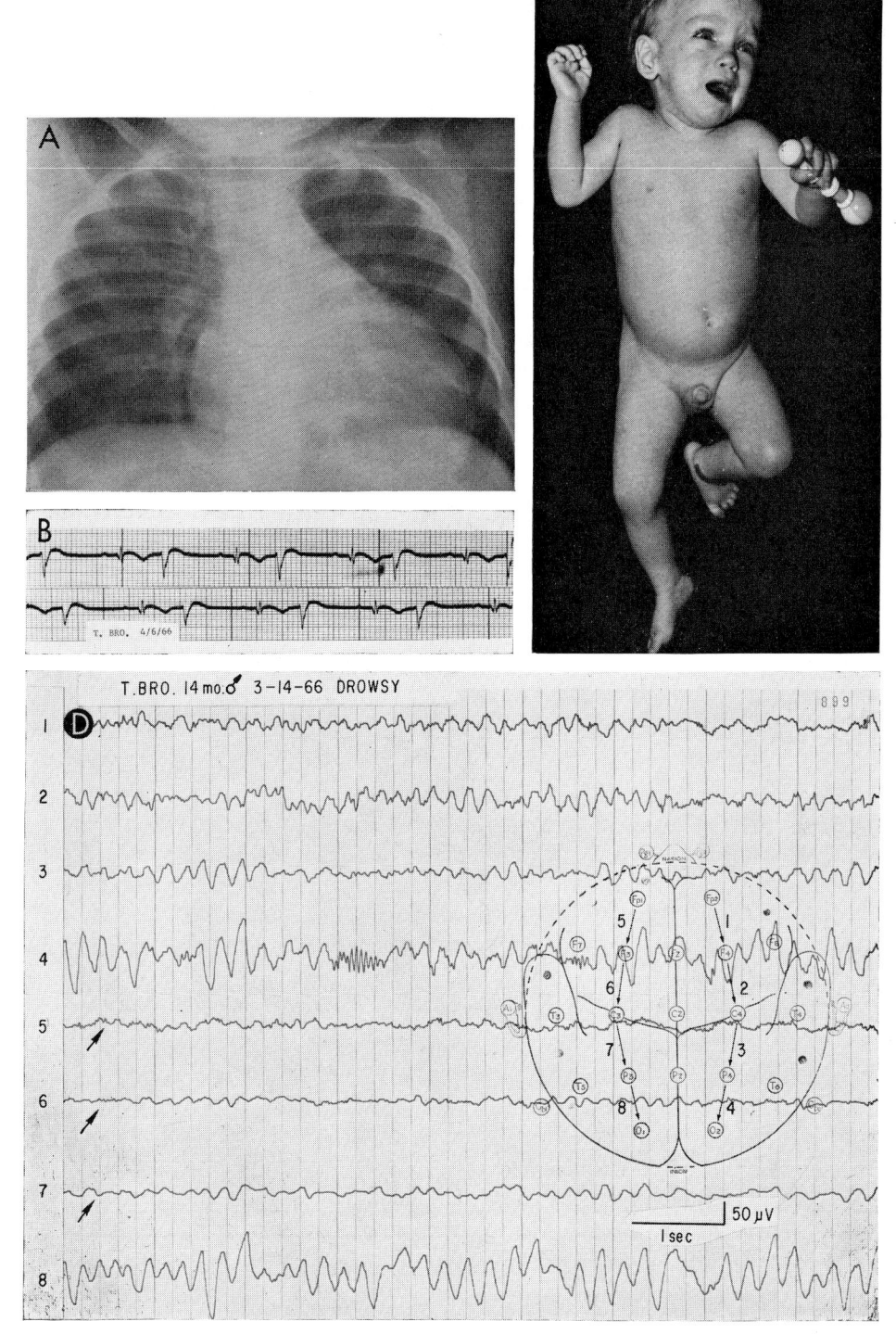

Fig. 23.3.—For legend see opposite page.

body. The diagnosis is established by positive blood culture results and by finding anemia, leukocytosis and splinter hemorrhages or petechiae.

Less commonly *myocarditis* (of multifactorial etiology) causes an embolic cerebrovascular accident (Fig. 23.3), the basic cause of which can be recognized by the associated cardiomegaly, tachycardias, arrhythmias, evidence of congestive failure and abnormalities in the electrocardiogram (S–T segment elevation and T wave inversion). Focal slow waves and flattening of the amplitude appear on the electroencephalogram.[32]

Clinically serious *fat* and *air emboli* occur infrequently but inflict a high fatality rate. Fat emboli complicate extensive long bone fractures by allowing fat from the marrow to enter the circulation where it then causes diffuse petechial hemorrhages in the white matter of the brain, with clinical signs of coma, seizures, focal deficit and often death.[43] Air emboli enter the bloodstream as a result of trauma or at the time of operation and cause cardiac ventricular arrhythmias. Large air emboli may cause blindness, bilateral or focal paralysis and dementia.

Vasculitis

Sydenham's chorea (St. Vitus' dance).—This common condition is an important, late manifestation of rheumatic fever. It should be emphasized that the rheumatic chorea can be one-sided and that it is nearly always aggravated by attention, stress or excitement. The latter phenomenon, which characterizes all involuntary movement disorders, often leads erroneously to a psychiatric explanation for the problem. Concomitant neurologic signs include hypotonia with slight generalized weakness, "hung-up" tendon reflexes and variable changes in the mental state, progressing at times to an organic delirium state with confusion and hallucinations. Although chorea is almost self-limiting and usually benign, it should always be considered a manifestation of rheumatic activity and not psychogenic.

This movement disorder is commoner in girls than in boys and varies greatly in its severity. It can range from a mild, ticlike jerkiness or twitching of small muscle groups which resembles simple restlessness or a neurotic habit spasm to gross and violent involuntary muscle contractions. Patients may be unable to walk, feed themselves or speak distinctly, and at times they require physical restraints in bed for self-protection. Distinctive postural abnormalities include (1) pronation of the forearms when the arms are held outstretched above the head and (2) flexion of the wrists with hyperextension of the fingers when the hands are stretched forward horizontally. Choreic movements produce an audible "click" of the tongue during speech and an audible "gasp" when the diaphragm is involved.

Generalized EEG slowing occurs inconstantly in many of these patients, the severity of changes usually being proportional to the severity of the chorea.[2] Inasmuch as it represents a late major manifestation of rheumatic fever, many of the usual clinical and laboratory evidences of rheumatic activity are not found. However, complete studies including heart examination, electrocardiography, chest x-ray, determination of antistreptolysin O titer, C-reactive protein, mucoprotein and erythrocyte sedimentation rate should be carried out.

Polyarteritis nodosa.—This disease produces peripheral neuropathies more often than any other neurologic sign. Seizures, which are sometimes associated with hypertension, and focal deficit, such as hemiparesis, aphasia and hemianopia, may occur late in the disease and not always abruptly since they result from occlusion of medium-sized or small blood vessels.[31] The diagnosis of polyarteritis is based most firmly upon positive results of skin and muscle biopsy, although fever, eosinophilia, hypertension, renal disease and an asthma-like syndrome should suggest the diagnosis.

Systemic lupus erythematosus.—This uncommon disorder occurs much more frequently in girls than in boys. In the series of Gold and Yahr,[22] 90% of the children had neurologic manifestations. Convulsions are common and organic psychosis, hemiparesis and cortical sensory deficit have also been noted frequently.[19,35] Diffuse EEG abnormalities, including slowing and epileptiform discharges, are often seen, as are the clinical syndromes of polyneuritis[42] and acute disseminated encephalomyelitis.[52] Physical evidence of diffuse systemic disease includes the typical "butterfly" facial rash, hypertension, renal disease, petechiae of the skin and mucous membranes, hepatosplenomegaly and signs of carditis. Common laboratory abnormalities include the L.E. cell phenomenon (the most definitive test), anemia, thrombocytopenia and leukopenia.

Anaphylactoid purpura (Schönlein-Henoch syndrome).—This disease is caused by vasculitis of the small blood vessels similar to that in systemic lupus erythematosus, but it carries a much better prognosis. The etiology for the vasculitis is un-

Fig. 23.4.—Anaphylactoid purpura with small subdural hematoma. A 20-month-old white boy had onset of purpura followed by progressive lethargy, irritability and nuchal rigidity. Lumbar puncture showed CSF pressure of 350 mm. H_2O with 10 RBC/mm.^{3}, and the fundi showed distention and tortuosity of retinal veins. An electroencephalogram showed diffuse theta and delta activity, more marked on the right, compatible with the other signs of increased intracranial pressure. A brain scan revealed an abnormal uptake of isotope in the right frontoparietal area, compatible with an area of hemorrhage. A right subdural tap disclosed 3–4 ml. of xanthochromic fluid. Impressive improvement occurred in two days without further aspirations, and recovery was complete within a month. In this patient with anaphylactoid purpura an intracranial hemorrhage (subdural hematoma) caused mildly increased intracranial pressure.

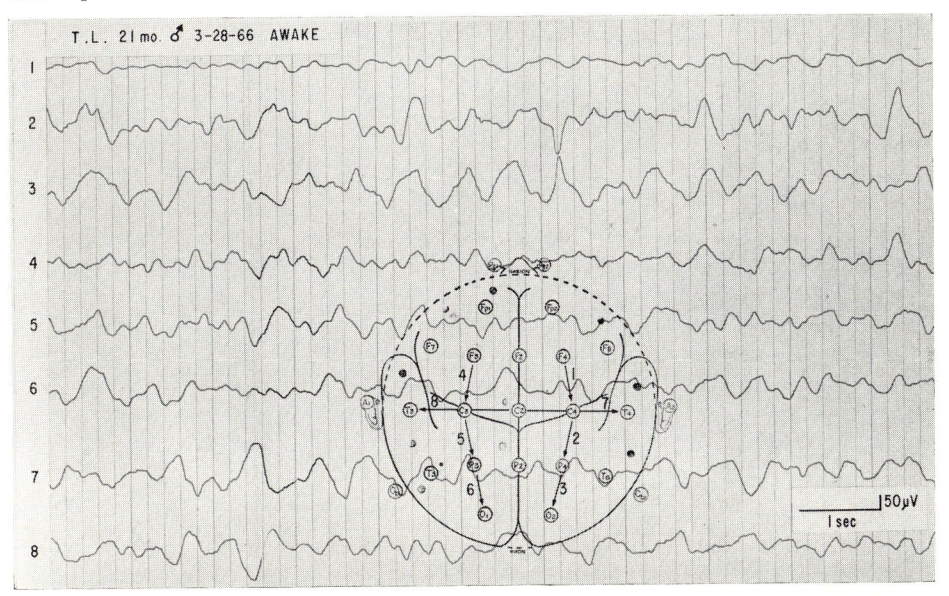

known. Purpura develops in the skin, the gastrointestinal tract and the kidneys. Neurologic symptoms such as convulsions and stupor may occur but are usually associated with severe renal disease and hypertension, suggesting the diagnosis of hypertensive encephalopathy.[30] Undoubtedly petechial hemorrhages from arterioles and capillaries in the brain can cause the neurologic manifestations.

No laboratory test is diagnostic of this disorder, and one should realize that these patients have no abnormalities in blood or bone marrow and have normal findings in coagulation studies, including the tourniquet test. One may find increased intracranial pressure on spinal puncture and diffuse slowing on EEG examination (Fig. 23.4). The cerebrospinal fluid will contain small numbers of red blood cells if the neurologic signs are the result of bleeding from small vessels in the brain, or it may contain no cells if the syndrome is caused by renal hypertension. The patient shown in Figure 23.4 had a small subdural hematoma which was demonstrated with a technetium brain scan.

Thrombosis (Occlusive Vascular Disease)

Most clinicians think that occlusion of cerebral blood vessels is rare in infants and children. However, if one looks at careful autopsy studies (Table 23.2), a surprisingly high incidence of thrombosis is noted. Obviously, series of cases may be heavily weighted or biased by the fact that large centers which publish their experiences act as referral points for special problems such as congenital heart disease, blood disorders and tumors. On reviewing the literature it is extremely difficult to draw reliable conclusions about the pathogenesis of strokes in children because few patients are followed to autopsy and angiography is carried out infrequently. No laboratory test other than an abnormal angiogram provides definitive diagnostic evidence to the clinician.

Certain pathophysiologic mechanisms seem to predispose children to vascular occlusions. These include states of *increased blood coagulability, sepsis* and *dehydration*. Clinical conditions which are associated with these states are (1) *cyanotic congenital heart disease* with polycythemia, (2) *complications* of the *perinatal period,* (3) *infections* such as meningitis, mastoiditis, otitis media and sinusitis in febrile, dehydrated or malnourished children and (4) *diseases of the blood*

TABLE 23.2.—OCCLUSIVE VASCULAR DISEASE IN CHILDHOOD*
(48 CASES (8.7%) OF 555 CONSECUTIVE COMPLETE AUTOPSIES)

	VENOUS	ARTERIAL	SMALL VESSEL
Incidence	28 (58%)	16 (33%)	4 (8%)
Etiology			
Congenital heart disease	9	4	—
Sepsis	9	8	—
Tumor	4	—	—
Perinatal complications	2	3	—
Systemic lupus	—	—	3
Miscellaneous (trauma, idiopathic, hypertension, homocystinuria)	4	1	1

*Modified from Banker.[1]

and blood vessels such as sickle-cell disease,[23] thrombotic thrombocytopenic purpura, systemic lupus erythematosus and the hemolytic-uremic syndrome.

Venous and small-vessel thrombosis.—Careful autopsy studies indicate that, in contrast to the situation in adults, occlusive venous disease is more common than arterial thrombosis in children.[1] Since venous thrombosis may develop insidiously, in contrast to the apoplectiform arterial occlusion, the clinician may overlook the disease entity and the pathologist may be impressed with its common occurrence. In addition to the diseases listed above, venous sinus thromboses also result uncommonly from metastatic tumor such as neuroblastoma (Chapter 17), but in such a situation one usually finds signs of increased pressure.

Arterial thrombosis.—In contrast to its common occurrence in adults, thrombosis occurs rarely in children. *Spontaneous (idiopathic) occlusion* of the large carotid vessels in the neck or of the middle cerebral artery or its branches can cause a typical stroke in children.[48] Assessing the frequency of this phenomenon is extremely difficult since the patients generally recover and since angiography has been carried out in few children with acute hemiplegia. *Injury* to the paratonsillar area from an object carried in child's mouth can cause internal carotid artery thrombosis. If the thrombus propagates distally, massive cerebral infarction and death may ensue.[37] Occasionally this clinical sequence of events is found in children who have evidence of essential *hypertension*. On reviewing the literature it is extremely difficult to draw reliable conclusions about the pathogenesis of the catastrophe because so few patients have come to autopsy and arteriograms have not been done in many cases. No laboratory tests other than an abnormal angiogram provide definitive diagnostic evidence.

Recently a new inborn error of metabolism called *homocystinuria* has been associated with spontaneous arterial thrombosis. Patients with this disease have dislocated lenses, tall stature, a positive urinary nitroprusside test, mental defect and a history of similar disease in siblings.

Management and Prognosis

Hemorrhage

A detailed plan for the therapy of acute leukemia and aplastic anemia cannot be given here, but the preferred therapeutic drugs and their doses are listed in Table 23.3 (also see Chapter 17). The drug prophylaxis and therapy of other bleeding disorders are also given in Table 23.3.

Idiopathic thrombocytopenic purpura is self-limiting in most cases, and initial therapy should be conservative. Although the effectiveness of corticosteroid therapy is questionable, prednisone is often used, and in some refractory cases splenectomy is carried out. The patient should be kept at bed rest, with sedation if necessary. Antihypertensives should be used if necessary, as well as hypertonic agents to reduce cerebral edema. Depending upon the patient's general systemic condition and prognosis, one may wish to evacuate intracerebral clots surgically.

The management of congenital vascular malformations which cause subarachnoid bleeding is covered in Chapter 13. Patients with massive intracerebral hemorrhage have a grave prognosis and a high early fatality rate. With smaller hemorrhages, however, prognosis is much better, although patients may be left with permanent deficits such as seizures or organic behavior disorders (Fig. 23.1).

Occlusive Vascular Disease (Embolization, Vasculitis, Thrombosis)

GENERAL THERAPY

Patients who have suffered acute strokes from aseptic emboli (including patients who have congenital heart disease, rheumatic heart disease or myocarditis and those with ventriculoatrial shunts for hydrocephalus) often need supplemental *oxygen* via nasal tube or tent. If they are stuporous or comatose, they should be placed on one side with the head lowered slightly to promote drainage of secretions and vomitus. Some will require tracheostomy to insure an adequate airway.

Careful attention should be directed to proper maintenance therapy of *fluids* and *electrolytes* (Appendix 3). *Antibiotics* should be given prophylactically if prolonged stupor or coma is present, and they should be given therapeutically for any well-defined infection, such as pneumonia (Appendix 5). Consideration of surgical intervention is discussed under Specific Therapy. *Anticonvulsants* should be used immediately to treat status epilepticus or as maintenance prophylactic therapy (Chapter 2). Patients with restlessness and anxiety, especially those with evidence of a large subarachnoid or intracerebral hemorrhage, should be kept in bed and given sedatives. If circulatory collapse results from hemorrhagic shock or cardiovascular hypotension, pressor agents should be used to maintain adequate blood pressure. When cerebral edema develops it should be treated promptly (Appendix 2). Patients who survive cerebrovascular accidents may be left with chronic residual neurologic deficits such as (1) mental retardation, (2) convulsive disorders, (3) cerebral palsy, (4) behavior problems, (5) sight or hearing deficit and (6) impaired vision. The management of these chronic symptoms and signs is covered in Part I.

SPECIFIC THERAPY

Embolization.—Although much controversy surrounds the general use of *anticoagulants,* most workers agree that these agents should be given to prevent further embolic cerebrovascular accidents, provided that a lumbar puncture reveals no evidence of intracranial bleeding.[13] An initial heparin dose of 50 units/kg. is given by intravenous drip, followed by 100 units/kg. every four hours.[45] Because of the ever-present danger of bleeding after heparin therapy, the patient's clotting time must be followed with great caution. A preheparin measurement is made, followed by another two hours after start of therapy; two determinations are then carried out daily. The aim is to keep the clotting time between 15 and 20 minutes or two to three times the preheparin rate. If the clotting time reaches an excessively high value or if any sign of bleeding develops, 1 mg. of protamine sulfate is given promptly by intravenous drip for every 1 mg. of heparin administered in the previous four hours. Anticoagulant therapy is usually discontinued arbitrarily after three days because of the impracticality of continuous heparinization and the risks of long-term oral use of anticoagulants in children.

Congestive heart failure commonly accompanies embolization in patients with myocarditis and sometimes occurs with other conditions (Table 23.3). For details of *digitalization* dosage at different ages the reader should consult other references.[28,45] In children over age 2 the dosage is 0.02–0.04 mg./kg. Digoxin intramuscularly or intravenously over a 16-hour period. A maintenance daily dose of Digoxin (one-fourth the digitalizing dose if given orally or one-fifth the digitalizing dose if given intramuscularly or intravenously) is started 12 hours later and given in two equally divided doses. Patients receiving any digitalis preparation should be watched carefully for signs of intoxication both clinically and with serial electrocardiograms. *Oxygen, low-salt diet* and 0.1 mg./kg. *morphine sulfate* for sedation should be used. A diuretic is given every other day.[40]

Circulatory collapse can occur and should be managed with vasopressor drugs as outlined in Appendix 4. Cardiac arrhythmias occur commonly with all types of heart disease that lead to cerebral embolism. In addition to digitalis, quinidine remains the preferred therapy.[45] Although its value in the treatment of myocarditis is questionable, *prednisone* is recommended by some; dosage is 0.25–0.5 mg./kg./day given in four equally divided doses.

Patients who have congenital heart lesions with a right-to-left shunt should be evaluated and operated upon as early as possible to prevent embolic catastrophes (Fig. 23.2). However, certain surgical procedures which relieve the cardiovascular disability (e.g., the creation of an atrial septal defect in patients with transposition of the great vessels) heighten the risk of embolization and abscess formation. The age-old problem of embolic cerebrovascular accidents which complicate rheumatic heart disease is being reduced by intensive prophylactic therapy in patients with acute rheumatic fever (see Vasculitis). Whenever embolization is noted in a hydrocephalic patient with a ventriculoatrial shunt tube in place, the shunt should be removed and revised as soon as possible. The management of brain abscess is covered in Chapter 18.

Prognosis for improvement in patients with embolic strokes is related to the size of the vessel which has been obstructed. Most patients who sustain such vascular accidents are left with significant neurologic defects (Figs. 23.2 and 23.3) because large vessels are usually involved and collateral circulation has not had time to develop.

Vasculitis.—Patients with *rheumatic chorea* are given penicillin therapeutically and prophylactically (Table 23.3) until at least age 21. The vigor of therapy for chorea should be proportional to the severity of the movement disorder. Phenobarbital, chlorpromazine and reserpine (Table 23.3) are used by graduating from smallest doses to those which prove effective. In many patients the sedative or other side effects of the drug preclude the use of full doses. Chorea, unlike the other manifestations of rheumatic fever, is not affected appreciably by salicylates or corticosteroids. In his therapeutic zeal the physician should remember the basically self-limiting nature of this problem (usual duration about four to 10 weeks). Despite this reassurance, one must realize that chorea as a sign of rheumatic fever continues to be associated with a high incidence of mitral stenosis in later life and hence calls for full penicillin prophylaxis.

No good medical therapy has been found for *polyarteritis*. The prognosis is poor and anticoagulation therapy is contraindicated. Prednisone 1 mg./lb./day has been used but is of dubious value.

TABLE 23.3.—Therapy of Systemic Disease in Patients with Cerebrovascular Disorders

Type of Cerebrovascular Disorder	Clinical Indication	Drug Schedule and Dosage

Embolization
Congenital heart disease with right-to-left shunt
Rheumatic heart disease with atrial fibrillation
Myocarditis
Ventriculoatrial shunts for hydrocephalus
Subacute bacterial endocarditis with mycotic embolus and abscess formation
	Embolic infarcts
	
	Congestive failure
	
	Arrhythmia
	
	Myocarditis
	Brain abscess
		Anticoagulants
		Heparin 50 units/kg. I.V. stat; 100 units/kg. I.V. every 4 hr.
		See text regarding careful follow-up
		Digitalization
		Digoxin
		  Digitalizing dose (age 2 and over) 0.02–0.04 mg./kg. I.M. or I.V.
		  Maintenance dose (in 2 divided doses)
		    Oral: ¼ digitalizing dose
		    I.M., I.V.: ⅕ digitalizing dose
		Morphine sulfate 0.1 mg./kg.
		Diuretics[28]
		Quinidine[39]
		Pressor drugs (Appendix 4)
		Prednisone 1 mg./lb./day (in 4 divided doses)
		See Chapter 18

Vasculitis
Rheumatic fever
Polyarteritis
Systemic lupus erythematosus
Anaphylactoid purpura
	Chorea	*Penicillin*[25]
		Therapy:
		  Oral: 250,000 units penicillin G or V every 6 hr. for 10 days
		  I.M.: (over 5 yr.) 1,200,000 units C-R bicillin every 4 days × 2
		    (under 5 yr.) 600,000 units C-R bicillin every 4 days × 2
		Prophylaxis (patient weighing 40–150 lb.):
		  Sulfadiazine (oral) 0.5 Gm. twice daily
		  Penicillin G (oral) 250,000 units twice daily
		  Benzathine penicillin (I.M.) 1,200,000 units a month
		Sedation
		Phenobarbital 16–32 mg. every 6–8 hr.
		Thorazine 10–50 mg. every 6–8 hr.
		Reserpine 0.02 mg./kg./day

Arterial thrombosis	Focal neurologic deficit Cerebral edema	Antibiotics (Appendix 5) Fluids and blood (Appendix 3) Anticonvulsants (Chapter 2) Hypertonic agents (Appendix 2)

Bleeding disorders
Acute leukemia
 	
Aplastic anemia
	
	Intracranial hemorrhage
	
	Intracranial hemorrhage
		Prednisone 1 mg./lb./day; give every 48 hr. for chronic administration
		Methotrexate 2.5–5 mg./day
		6 MP 2.5 mg./kg./day
		Cytoxan 5 mg./kg./day
		    2.5 mg./kg./day
		Vincristine 0.05–0.15 mg./kg./day
		Blood (Appendix 3)
		Fluids (Appendix 3)
		Antibiotics (Appendix 5)
		Prednisone 1 mg./lb./day
		Testosterone (oral) 1–2 mg./kg./day
		    (I.M.) 100–200 mg. every 3 wk.
		Blood (Appendix 3)
		Fresh platelets

TABLE 23.3.—THERAPY OF SYSTEMIC DISEASE IN PATIENTS WITH
CEREBROVASCULAR DISORDERS—CONTINUED

Type of Cerebrovascular Disorder	Clinical Indication	Drug Schedule and Dosage
Hemorrhagic disease of the newborn		Prophylaxis: Vitamin K_1 1 mg. I.M. in delivery room

Hypoprothrombinemia	Intracranial hemorrhage	Treatment: Vitamin K_1 repeat prophylactic dose
		Blood transfusion 20 ml./kg. stat
		Vitamin K_1 1 mg./day I.M. in infants
		    5 mg./day I.M. in older children
		    2–3 ml./kg./hr. for 6–10 hr., then 1 ml./kg./hr. for 3–4 days

Hemophilia		Fresh plasma
Idiopathic thrombocytopenic purpura		Prednisone 1 mg./kg./day
Scurvy		Vitamin C (ascorbic acid) 100–200 mg./day
Congenital vascular malformations	Intracranial hemorrhage	Pressor drugs (Appendix 4) Blood transfusion (Appendix 3) Anticonvulsants (Chapter 2) Water and electrolytes (Appendix 3)

Systemic lupus erythematosus should be treated with corticosteroids (Table 23.3) over an extended period of time if necessary. Physicians who manage this rare disorder should be familiar with the problems of long-term steroid therapy (edema, hypertension). Recently immunosuppressive therapy (azathioprine or Imuran) has been used successfully in a number of cases, but this drug is not yet generally available. Use of anticoagulants for systemic lupus erythematosus is contraindicated. In the past more than 50% of patients have died within two years, but intensive combined therapy with prednisone and azathioprine (Imuran) offers much greater hope for prolonged remissions.

Anaphylactoid purpura causes neurologic signs only occasionally (Fig. 23.4). When evidence of group A beta-hemolytic streptococcal infection is found, a full course of penicillin therapy should be given (Table 23.3.—chorea). Although most patients with the disorder require only symptomatic therapy because of the benign course, occasional cases are severe or fatal. In these cases prednisone therapy should be employed.

Arterial thrombosis.—The primary management is directed at good general supportive care. Anticoagulant therapy is contraindicated. Seizures, status epilepticus and cerebral edema occur commonly; management is outlined in Appendices 1 and 2. Currently a controversy is raging about the value of surgical endarterectomy in patients who have occlusive arterial disease in the extracranial neck vessels. In selected cases such a procedure may have value, but such instances rarely arise in children. In those rare cases in which essential hypertension accompanies the thrombosis, antihypertensive agents such as reserpine (Table 23.3) or other agents[45] should be used. Most patients survive these childhood strokes if they do not die in status epilepticus, but they are left with fixed neurologic deficits of varying severity.

Venous sinus thrombosis.—These patients should receive the best possible supportive care. Special attention should be given to fluid and electrolyte control, antibiotic and anticonvulsant therapy, blood transfusion and the treatment of cerebral edema. Patients with persistent intracranial hypertension sometimes require surgical decompression, especially if one is dealing with arterial sinus thrombosis and otitic hydrocephalus secondary to mastoiditis. The prognosis for both life and serious neurologic disability is always serious.

Hyperbilirubinemia with Kernicterus

PATHOGENESIS.—Neonatal hyperbilirubinemia causes selective damage to the immature nervous system for reasons not fully understood.[11] Most commonly this disorder results from hemolytic disease of the newborn due to blood group (Rh or A-B-O system) incompatibility. Less commonly hyperbilirubinemia of the premature causes kernicterus and the mechanism is potentiated by other factors, including drugs such as sulfisoxazole and vitamin K. Rarely the disorder results from the autosomal recessive inheritance of a deficiency in the liver enzyme, glucuronyl transferase. This disease is called congenital familial nonhemolytic jaundice (Crigler-Najjar syndrome). Although bilirubin preferentially stains certain portions of the nervous system, such as the basal ganglia, brain stem and cerebellum, extensive studies by Haymaker and co-workers[26] have shown that the neurologic damage is widespread and not always proportional to the degree of tissue jaundice. Clinical deafness has been attributed by some workers to degeneration of the cochlear nuclei.

CLINICAL AND LABORATORY DIAGNOSIS.—The clinical signs of kernicterus vary with the patient's age. During the first week of life the infant looks seriously but nonspecifically ill, with respiratory distress, an impaired Moro reflex, high-pitched cry, poor suckle and hypotonia. This gives way to generalized hypertonia or opisthotonos and eventually athetosis.[51] Seizures may occur at this early age but are rarely seen later. In infants who survive, the characteristic and permanent signs of kernicterus gradually develop between age 3 months and 2 years; these include muscular rigidity, bilateral choreoathetosis, facial grimacing and an explosive type of dysarthria. Paralysis of upward gaze and bilateral high-tone nerve deafness distinguish kernicterus from other types of chronic extrapyramidal syndromes. Nerve deafness has been detected in patients who were jaundiced as newborn infants but who did not develop athetoid cerebral palsy.[15] The rigidity in the arms varies greatly but may be severe enough to prevent all useful hand function. Pyramidal tract signs may or may not appear. Intelligence has been found within normal limits in at least half the reported patients[5] but one can expect much individual variation.

MANAGEMENT AND PROGNOSIS.—Treatment of choreoathetosis leaves much to be desired. No one has shown that restricting the purposeless and unsightly movements helps the patient to develop useful motor activity, although its psychotherapeutic value may be considerable. Tranquilizing agents such as chlorpromazine may quiet the patient slightly by virtue of their sedative action, but their effect is limited. Few of these patients ever become suitable candidates for basal ganglia surgery. Byers[5] reports that in some patients the deafness is benefited by mechanical hearing aids despite its alleged neural basis. These patients often adjust quite well to their motor limitations because of their relatively good intelligence.

Obviously, immediate exchange transfusion of subsequent erythroblastotic siblings should be carried out to prevent damage to the nervous system.

Renal Disease

PATHOGENESIS.—Pathologic changes in the brain occur commonly in both acute and chronic renal disease, usually in association with hypertension. The complex changes consist of focal edema, necrosis and hemorrhage, and they are due to severe hypertension, thrombosis or vessel spasm. The interpretation of the mechanism is complicated in isolated cases by prolonged, high-dose therapy of the basic disease with adrenal corticosteroids and by dialysis to correct uremia.

CLINICAL AND LABORATORY DIAGNOSIS.—Patients with renal failure often have nervous system manifestations such as irritability, muscular twitching, stupor and convulsions. There may be systemic hypertension, papilledema, retinal hemorrhages, signs of tetany and eventually focal neurologic deficit. Encephalopathy in some cases may result from states of extreme systemic acidosis. Posner and Plum[38] have shown that encephalopathy is related quite directly to the pH of the cerebrospinal fluid and is not seen in patients who have normal CSF pH even though systemic acidosis may be pronounced.

Uremic neuropathy occurs frequently in adults with chronic renal insufficiency,[14,26a,49] but its rarity in children places its discussion outside the scope of this text.

Common laboratory abnormalities include azotemia, hypocalcemia, hyponatremia, evidence of acidosis, elevated CSF pressure and blood in the subarachnoid space.

MANAGEMENT.—Special attention is called here to the many factors involved in treatment, especially in patients already on some therapy: (1) hypocalcemic tetany, (2) hyponatremic seizures, (3) stupor resulting from severe acidosis and dehydration, (4) intracranial hypertension and cerebral edema due to intensive corticosteriod therapy and (5) the "reverse urea effect" produced by dialysis.

"Reverse urea effect" from dialysis therapy.—Several groups (Scribner,[44] Peterson,[36] Kennedy et al.[29]) have called attention to the fact that headache, confusion, agitation, seizures and even death have occurred in patients undergoing dialysis for uremia and chronic renal disease. These neurologic complications presumably result from the development of cerebral edema when the BUN (blood urea nitrogen) is lowered too abruptly. It is assumed that the mechanism causing the edema is the reverse of that which occurs when cerebral edema is improved acutely by the administration of hypertonic urea. Kennedy and associates[29] state that a dialysis solution of high glucose concentration (1.52 Gm./100 ml.) is a simple and effective way to prevent neurologic signs and cerebral edema. The neuropathy associated with chronic uremia seems to improve with intermittent dialysis therapy.[26a]

The reader is referred to other general texts for the management of renal failure, hypertension and uremia.

Chronic Respiratory Disease

PATHOGENESIS.—Chronic respiratory disease with hypercapnia can cause a variety of central nervous system manifestations, including papilledema, often in association with heart failure (Chapter 8). Some workers have subdivided the etiologic disorders into (1) chronic pulmonary disease, e.g., chronic bronchitis, emphysema and pulmonary insufficiency (cystic fibrosis is the commonest example of this type in children) and (2) the pulmonary insufficiency resulting from alveolar hypoventilation (either from central causes such as motor neuron disease and poliomyelitis or from peripheral causes such as muscular dystrophy,[33] severe chest deformities or the pickwickian syndrome).

CLINICAL AND LABORATORY DIAGNOSIS.—*Hypercapnia with papilledema.*—Typical signs of papilledema have been reported in a variety of clinical conditions, the common denominator of which has been chronic pulmonary insufficiency with hypercapnia. Although CO_2 retention is known to be associated often with an elevated CSF pressure, a measurably elevated pressure is not always found in these patients.[33]

Neurologic deficit from correction of hypercapnia.—Somewhat paradoxically, it has been observed that neurologic signs (seizures, coma and chorea-like movement disorders) may appear *de novo* when chronic hypercapnia from obstructive pulmonary disease is corrected rapidly with mechanical methods.[41] These latter patients did *not* have papilledema or elevated CSF pressure. Few significant brain changes have been noted in autopsied patients, suggesting that clinical signs result from transient metabolic defects induced by alkalosis or too-rapid correction of hypercapnia.

MANAGEMENT AND PROGNOSIS.—In patients with papilledema from hypercapnia the CO_2 tensions should be lowered slowly, with careful monitoring of blood CO_2, pH and electrolytes. If any neurologic signs develop during the corrective therapy, 5% CO_2 in O_2 should be given. In the careful study of two patients with "pulmonary encephalopathy," Bulger *et al.*[3] emphasized the need to reduce CO_2 tension in treating patients with obscure acid-base disorders. They stress the value of studying cerebrospinal fluid, pH, bicarbonate ion and CO_2 tension rather than focusing attention solely upon blood pH.

Liver, Gastrointestinal and Other Systemic Diseases

Hepatic coma.—In patients with hepatic insufficiency from cirrhosis or severe hepatitis, coma and a "flapping" tremor of the arms may be associated with ammonia intoxication. This complication occurs more often in adults than in children.

Malabsorption with hypoglycemia.—Gastrointestinal malabsorption can lead to hypoglycemic seizures and in some cases permanent mental retardation (Chapter 2).

Severe bacillary dysentery is often ushered in with delirium, convulsions and coma (acute toxic encephalopathy—Chapter 2).

Primary hereditary endocrinopathies which affect the nervous system are discussed in Chapter 21. For a discussion of endocrinopathies which begin later in life and cause neuromuscular symptoms, such as hypothyroid myopathy, the reader is referred to general textbooks of internal medicine.

Deficiency Diseases

Neurologic symptoms and signs can and do result from specific dietary deficiencies, but their occurrence is rare. Scurvy (vitamin C deficiency) has been responsible for an occasional case of subdural hematoma (Chapter 16), vitamin D deficiency can cause tetany (Chapter 2) and vitamin B_6 deficiency causes essentially the same clinical picture as pyridoxine dependency (Chapter 21). The reader is referred to Ford[17] and other texts for the classic descriptions of neurologic syndromes caused by pellagra (nicotinic acid deficiency) and beriberi (thiamine deficiency). Infants with clinical signs of thiamine deficiency (beriberi) have typical pathologic signs of Wernicke's encephalopathy (superior hemorrhagic polioencephalitis).[8,1]

Feigin and Wolf[14a] described lesions in the brains of three children which resemble closely those seen in patients with Wernicke's encephalopathy, a neurologic manifestation of vitamin B_1 deficiency. The diet of these children did not appear deficient in retrospect. Whether the neuropathologic lesions resulted from an excessive thiamine need or from an unrelated cause remains conjectural.

Kahn and Falcke[27] have reported a transient neurologic syndrome in some South African Bantu children recovering from malnutrition (kwashiorkor). The syndrome is characterized by coarse tremors and posturing of the extremities, hyperreflexia, myoclonus and irritability, insomnia and excessive sweating in some cases. The neurologic signs were not seen while the babies were still severely ill with malnutrition, but instead had their onset one to four weeks after high protein diets were started. The signs persisted from several weeks to several months and then disappeared completely in most cases.

A large body of evidence suggests that chronic and severe malnutrition in infancy (kwashiorkor) can cause mental subnormality in later life. Obviously such observations, if true, have extremely important public health implications. The many and complex factors which enter into an evaluation of this problem have left the issue unsettled.

BIBLIOGRAPHY

1. Banker, B. Q.: Cerebral vascular disease in infancy and childhood: I. Occlusive vascular disease, J. Neuropath. & Exper. Neurol. 20:127, 1961.
2. Bray, P. F.: Unpublished observations.
3. Bulger, R. J., et al.: Spinal-fluid acidosis and the diagnosis of pulmonary encephalopathy, New England J. Med. 274:433, 1966.
4. Byers, R. K., and McLean, W. T.: Etiology and course of certain hemiplegias with aphasia in childhood, Pediatrics 29:376, 1962.
5. Byers, R. K., et al.: Extrapyramidal cerebral palsy with hearing loss following erythroblastosis, Pediatrics 15:248, 1955.
6. Clark, R. M., and Linell, E. A.: Case report: Prenatal occlusion of the internal carotid artery, J. Neurol. Neurosurg. & Psychiat. 17:295, 1954.
7. Clarkson, P. M., et al.: Central nervous system complications following Blalock-Taussig operation, Pediatrics 39:18, 1967.
8. Cochrane, W. A., et al.: Superior hemorrhagic polioencephalitis (Wernicke's disease) occurring in an infant—probably due to thiamine deficiency from use of a soya bean product, Pediatrics 28:771, 1961.
9. Cohen, M. M.: The central nervous system in congenital heart disease, Neurology 10:452, 1960.
10. Davis, R. A., and Wolf, A.: Infantile beriberi associated with Wernicke's encephalopathy, Pediatrics 21:409, 1958.
11. Diamond, I., et al.: Kernicterus: Revised concepts of pathogenesis and management, Pediatrics 38:539, 1966.
12. Dooley, D. M., and Perlmutter, I.: Spontaneous intracranial hematomas in patients receiving anticoagulation therapy, J.A.M.A. 187:396, 1964.
13. Editorial: Anticoagulants and cerebral infarction, Lancet 1:245, 1966.
14. Editorial: Uremic neuropathy, Lancet 1:749, 1966.

14a. Feigin, I., and Wolf, A.: A disease in infants resembling chronic Wernicke's encephalopathy, J. Pediat. 45:243, 1954.
15. Fisch, L., and Norman, A. P.: Hyperbilirubinaemia and perceptive deafness, Brit. M. J. 2:142, 1961.
16. Fisher, R. G., and Friedmann, K. R.: Carotid artery thrombosis in persons fifteen years of age or younger, J.A.M.A. 170:1918, 1959.
17. Ford, F. R.: *Diseases of the Nervous System in Infancy, Childhood and Adolescence* (5th ed.; Springfield, Ill.: Charles C Thomas, Publisher, 1966).
18. Frantzen, E., et al.: Cerebral artery occlusions in children due to trauma to the head and neck: A report of six cases verified by cerebral angiography, Neurology 11:695, 1961.
19. Fulton, W. H., and Dyken, P. R.: Neurological syndromes of systemic lupus erythematosus, Neurology 14:317, 1964.
20. Gianantonio, C., et al.: The hemolytic-uremic syndrome, J. Pediat. 64:478, 1964.
21. Gilman, S.: Cerebral disorders after open-heart operations, New England J. Med. 272:489, 1965.
22. Gold, A. P., and Yahr, M. D.: Childhood lupus erythematosus: A clinical and pathological study of the neurological manifestations, Tr. Am. Neurol. A., 1960, p. 96.
23. Greer, M., and Schotland, D.: Abnormal hemoglobin as a cause of neurologic disease, Neurology 12:114, 1962.
24. Gross, R. E.: Arterial embolism and thrombosis in infancy, Am. J. Dis. Child. 70:61, 1945.
25. Grossman, B. J., and Dorfman, A.: Rheumatic Fever, in Gellis, S. S., and Kagan, B. M. (eds.): *Current Pediatric Therapy* (Philadelphia: W. B. Saunders Company, 1964).
26. Haymaker, W., et al.: Kernicterus and Its Importance in Cerebral Palsy, in *American Academy for Cerebral Palsy,* Swinyard, C. A. (ed.) (Springfield, Ill.: Charles C Thomas, Publisher, 1961).
26a. Jebsen, R. H., et al.: Natural history of uremic polyneuropathy and effects of dialysis, New England J. Med. 277:327, 1967.
27. Kahn, E., and Falcke, H. C.: A syndrome simulating encephalitis affecting children recovering from malnutrition (kwashiorkor), J. Pediat. 49:37, 1956.
28. Kaplan, S.: Treatment of Cardiac Failure, in Nelson, W. E. (ed.): *Textbook of Pediatrics* (Philadelphia: W. B. Saunders Company, 1964).
29. Kennedy, A. C., et al.: The pathogenesis and prevention of cerebral dysfunction during dialysis, Lancet 1:790, 1964.
30. Lewis, I. C., and Philpott, M. G.: Neurological complications of Schönlein-Henoch syndrome, Arch. Dis. Childhood 31:369, 1956.
31. Malamud, N.: Case of periarteritis nodosa with decerebrate rigidity and extensive encephalomalacia in five-year-old child. J. Neuropath. & Exper. Neurol. 4:88, 1945.
32. Marquardsen, J., and Harvald, B.: The electroencephalogram in acute cerebrovascular lesions, Neurology 14:275, 1964.
33. McCormack, W. M., and Spalter, H. F.: Muscular dystrophy, alveolar hypoventilation and papilledema, J.A.M.A. 197:957, 1966.
34. O'Brien, J. L., and Sibley, W. A.: Neurologic manifestations of thrombotic thrombocytopenic purpura, Neurology 8:55, 1958.
35. O'Connor, J. F., and Musher, D. M.: Central nervous system involvement in systemic lupus erythematosus, Arch. Neurol. 14:157, 1966.
36. Peterson, H. D.: Acute encephalopathy associated with renal hemodialysis: The reverse urea effect, Neurology 13:358, 1963.
37. Pitner, S. E.: Carotid thrombosis due to intraoral trauma, New England J. Med. 274:764, 1966.
38. Posner, J. B., and Plum, F.: Spinal-fluid pH and neurologic symptoms in acidosis, New England J. Med. 277:605, 1967.
39. Rashkind, W. J.: Cardiac Arrhythmias (Treatment), in Gellis, S. S., and Kagan, B. M. (eds.): *Current Pediatric Therapy* (Philadelphia: W. B. Saunders Company, 1964).
40. Robinson, S. J.: Heart Failure, in Gellis, S. S., and Kagan, B. M. (eds.): *Current Pediatric Therapy* (Philadelphia: W. B. Saunders Company, 1964).
41. Rotheram, E. G., et al.: CNS disorder during mechanical ventilation in chronic pulmonary disease, J.A.M.A. 189:993, 1964.
42. Scheinberg, L.: Polyneuritis in systemic lupus erythematosus, New England J. Med. 255:461, 1956.
43. Schneider, R. C.: Fat embolism: A problem in the differential diagnosis of craniocerebral trauma, J. Neurosurg. 9:1, 1952.
44. Scribner, B. H.: Discussion, in Brown, H. W., and Schreiner, G. E.: Prolonged hemodialysis with bath refrigeration, Tr. Am. Soc. Artif. Organs 8:195, 1962.
45. Shirkey, H. C.: *Pediatric Therapy* (St. Louis: The C. V. Mosby Company, 1966).

45a. Shirkey, H. C., and Barba, W. P.: Drug Therapy, in Nelson, W. E. (ed.): *Textbook of Pediatrics* (8th ed.; Philadelphia: W. B. Saunders Company, 1964).
46. Siekert, R. G., and Clark, E. C.: Neurologic signs and symptoms as early manifestations of systemic lupus erythematosus, Neurology 5:84, 1955.
47. Silverstein, A.: Intracranial bleeding in hemophilia, A.M.A. Arch. Neurol. 3:141, 1960.
48. Stevens, H.: Carotid artery occlusion in childhood, Pediatrics 23:699, 1959.
49. Tenckhoff, H. A., *et al.*: Polyneuropathy in chronic renal insufficiency, J.A.M.A. 192:1121, 1965.
50. Tyler, H. R., and Clark, D. B.: Cerebrovascular accidents in patients with congenital heart disease, A.M.A. Arch. Neurol. & Psychiat. 77:483, 1957.
51. Van Praagh, R.: Diagnosis of kernicterus in the neonatal period, Pediatrics 27:870, 1961.
52. Vejjajiva, A.: Systemic lupus erythematosus presenting as acute disseminated encephalomyelitis, Lancet 1:352, 1965.
53. Wisoff, H. S., and Rothballer, A. B.: Cerebral arterial thrombosis in children, Arch. Neurol. 4:258, 1961.

APPENDIX 1

Treatment of Prolonged Acute Convulsions and Status Epilepticus*

Anticonvulsant Medication[1,2,3]

Prolonged or repeated intermittent convulsions

1. Sodium phenobarbital (I.M.)   2. Sodium Seconal (rectal)

Dose	Age	Dose
32 mg.	Under 1 year	65 mg.
50 mg.	1–2 years	100 mg.
65 mg.	2–5 years	150 mg.
100 mg.	Over 5 years	200 mg.

3. Paraldehyde (I.M.)
   Dose: 1 ml./year of age; not to exceed 5 ml.

Status Epilepticus

1. Sodium phenobarbital (I.V.)
   Initial dose: 5 mg./kg. *slowly*
   Additional dose: 3 mg./kg. *slowly*
2. Paraldehyde

Rectally	Intramuscularly	Intravenously
0.3 ml./kg. *or*	1 ml./year of age *or* (not to exceed 5 ml.)	4 ml. in 100 ml. normal saline

3. Diazepam (Valium)[4,5]
   Dose: 2.5–10 mg. *slowly, intravenously*
   This drug, introduced recently, has proved useful in terminating status in patients with chronic seizure disorders but, like other agents, it is less useful in patients with acute cerebral disorders.

General Supportive Care

1. Put the patient on his side in the Trendelenburg position.
2. Provide an adequate airway.
3. Give adequate oxygen by nasal catheter.
4. Place a padded tongue depressor between the teeth.

Treat Cerebral Edema in Prolonged Status Epilepticus

See Appendix 2.

---

*We acknowledge that intravenous administration of anticonvulsants will stop severe convulsions effectively if large enough doses are given. However, the significant risk of producing respiratory arrest with this route of administration is a *contraindication to its routine use*. Intravenous barbiturates and paraldehyde should be given (1) only to patients in true status epilepticus, (2) only in conservative doses and (3) *slowly*, while vital signs are monitored continuously.

REFERENCES

1. Farmer, T. W.: *Pediatric Neurology* (New York City: Paul B. Hoeber, Inc., 1964).
2. Gold, A. P., and Carter, S.: Pediatric Neurology in Shirkey, H. C. (ed.): *Pediatric Therapy* (2d ed.; St. Louis: C. V. Mosby Company, 1966).
3. Livingston, S.: Seizure Disorders in Gellis, S. S., and Kagan, B. M. (eds.): *Current Pediatric Therapy* (Philadelphia: W. B. Saunders Company, 1966–67).
4. Lombroso, C. T.: Treatment of status epilepticus with diazepam, Neurology 16:629, 1966.
5. Prensky, A. L., et al.: Intravenous diazepam in the treatment of prolonged seizure activity, New England J. Med. 276:779, 1967.

APPENDIX 2

Treatment of Cerebral Edema

1. Provide adequate airway and oxygen (tracheostomy if necessary).
2. Treat the *acute brain swelling*.
   a) "One-shot" therapy*
      (1) 30% urea: 1 Gm./kg. I.V. in 30 minutes
      (2) 20% mannitol: 1.5 Gm./kg. I.V. in 20 minutes
   b) Glucocorticoid therapy†

Drug and Manufacturer	Equivalent Doses (Mg.)	Frequency of Administration (I.M.)‡
Cortisone acetate (I.M. only) (many manufacturers)	125	6 to 72 hr.
Hydrocortisone (many manufacturers)	100	6 to 72 hr.
Prednisolone		
Hydeltrasol (Merck)	25	6 to 24 hr.
Sterane (Pfizer) (I.M. only)	25	6 to 24 hr.
Meticortelone (Schering)	25	6 to 24 hr.
Methylprednisolone		
Depo-Medrol (Upjohn) (I.M. only)	20	7 to 15 days
Solu-Medrol (Upjohn)	20	6 to 24 hr.
Triamcinolone (I.M. only)		
Aristocort Forte (Lederle)	20	up to 28 days
Kenalog (I.M.) (Squibb)	20	up to 28 days

*When the physician uses urea or mannitol to reduce cerebral edema, he must not give too much too fast because cases have been documented (and we have seen such a case) in which the acute brain shrinkage has led to the formation of a subdural hematoma.[1]

†It seems likely that most of the parenteral preparations of prednisolone, methylprednisolone, triamcinolone, dexamethasone and betamethasone have the same basic therapeutic effect in equivalent doses.

Many other hypertonic solutions for the relief of cerebral edema, including 50% glucose, 50% magnesium sulfate, 50% sucrose and concentrated human albumin, have been used. Although all of these agents have a prompt beneficial effect on the edema, most of them cannot be used repeatedly and a prompt rebound in the swelling often occurs. At present the glucocorticoids are enjoying the most favor, and they can be continued for seven to ten days without major side effects. Urea should not be used in patients with poor renal function, dehydration or intracranial hematomas. Some have stated that mannitol may cause less rebound than urea[2] but this has not been proved.

Drug and Manufacturer	Equivalent Doses (Mg.)	Frequency of Administration (I.M.)‡
Dexamethasone		
Decadron (Merck)	3.75	6 to 24 hr.
Hexadrol (Organon)	3.75	6 to 24 hr.
Betamethasone (I.M. only)		
Celestone Soluspan (Schering)	3	up to 7 days

Reprinted with permission from *The Medical Letter on Drugs and Therapeutics*: Glucocorticoids for parenteral administration, 7:111, 1965.

‡Except for preparations marked "I.M. only" these agents can be given intramuscularly or intravenously. All intravenous preparations should be given at intervals of 2 to 8 hours.

EXAMPLE: Dexamethasone (Decadron—I.V. or I.M.)

"Stat" dose: 4 mg. (equivalent to 100 mg. hydrocortisone)
Maintenance dose: 0.5–1.5 mg. every 4 hours
This dose can be continued for 4 to 5 days, then tapered completely by 7 to 10 days.

3. Treat the associated disease (Chapter 8).

REFERENCES

1. Marshall, S., and Hinman, F.: Sudural hematoma following administration of urea for diagnosis of hypertension, J.A.M.A. 182:813, 1962.
2. Matson, D. D.: Treatment of cerebral swelling, New England J. Med. 272:626, 1965.

APPENDIX 3

*Water, Electrolyte and Transfusion Therapy (Parenteral)**

1. *Initial rapid hydration to establish urine flow* (place catheter in bladder to measure urine flow)
   a) Amount: Give 30 ml./kg. of a solution in Table 1 in the first hour or two.
   b) Type solution

TABLE 1

Solution	Supplier	Na	K	Cl	HCO₃†	Ca	Mg
Hartmann's	Abbott; Cutter; McGaw	131	4	110	28	3	—
Ionosol D-CM	Abbott	138	12	108	50	5	3
Normosol R	Abbott	140	5	98	27	—	3
Plasmalyte	Baxter	140	10	103	55	5	3
Polysal	Cutter	140	10	103	55	5	3
Equivisol	McGaw	140	—	103	55	5	3
"1–2"		150	—	100	50	—	—

(Milliequivalents per Liter)

"1–2" is a nonproprietary mixture of one part M/6 lactate and two parts normal saline.
†Or HCO₃ precursors.

*The information on parenteral water and electrolyte solutions is based on material published in *The Medical Letter on Drugs and Therapeutics,* vol. 7, p. 65, 1965.

2. *Fluid therapy for 24–48 hours after urine flow is established*
   a) Amount of fluid from Table 2 solution per 24 hours:
       Infants   125 ml./kg.
       Older children   100 ml./kg.
       Adults   70 ml./kg.
   b) Type solution

TABLE 2

Solution	Supplier	Na	K	Cl	HCO$_3$	Ca	Mg	P
Darrow's	Abbott; Baxter; Cutter; McGaw	121	35	103	53	—	—	—
		Dilute with equal parts 10% dextrose						
Electrolyte 75	Cutter	40	35	40	20	—	—	15
Ionosol B	Abbott	57	25	49	25	—	5	13
Normosol	Abbott	40	13	40	16	—	3	—
Electrolye 2	Baxter	61	25	50	25	—	6	13
Polysal M	Cutter	40	16	40	24	5	3	—
Electrolyte 2	McGaw	58	25	51	25	—	6	13
"1–2–7"		46	†	30	16	—	—	—

"1–2–7" is a nonproprietary mixture consisting of one part M/6 lactate, two parts normal saline and 7 parts 10% dextrose-water.

†Add sufficient potassium (as acetate) to provide 25 mEq./L.

3. *Maintenance therapy*
   a) Amount: 1,600 ml./M.^{2} body surface per 24 hours (maintenance water based on surface area—see Table 4)
   b) Type solution
   All maintenance solutions should contain at least 5% dextrose. A liter of satisfactory maintenance solution can be made with the following ingredients:
   (1) 150 ml. M/6 sodium lactate *or* isotonic sodium bicarbonate (25 mEq. sodium and either lactate or bicarbonate)
   (2) 20 ml. of 1M KCl (20 mEq. potassium and chloride)
   (3) 830 ml. of 5% dextrose in water

TABLE 3.—Premixed Electrolyte Solutions for Maintenance

Solution	Supplier	Na	K	Cl	HCO$_3$	Mg	P
Ionosol MB	Abbott	25	20	22	23	3	3
Electrolyte 4	Baxter	35	15	22	20	—	3
Electrolyte 48	Cutter	25	20	22	23	3	3
Electrolyte 4	McGaw	30	15	22	20	—	3
Isolyte P	McGaw	25	20	22	23	3	3

TABLE 4.—Weight and Surface Area

Body Weight Kg.	Lb.	Surface Area M^2	Approximate Maintenance Water Ml./24 Hr.
3	6.6	0.21	300
6	13.2	0.30	500
10	22	0.45	700
20	44	0.80	1,300
30	66	1.05	1,700
40	88	1.30	2,100
50	110	1.50	2,400
60	132	1.65	2,600
70	154	1.75	2,800
80	176	1.85	3,000

4. *Blood transfusion* to correct severe anemia. (See Appendix 4 for treatment of shock.)
    a) Amount of blood
       Hemoglobin concentration
       Under 5 Gm./100 ml.:   Give the *same number* of cc. of blood/lb. as the hemoglobin concentration in Gm./100 ml.
       5–10 Gm./100 ml.:   Give 10 cc./lb.

APPENDIX 4

Treatment of Shock

The physician can treat shock effectively only if he assesses the cardiovascular disturbance accurately. One or a combination of the following three factors cause shock: (1) volume depletion, (2) cardiac failure and (3) peripheral vascular failure.

Hemorrhagic shock results primarily from volume deficit and should be treated with restoration of lost blood or plasma.

EMERGENCY RESTORATION OF BLOOD OR PLASMA LOSS

FLUID	INDICATIONS
Use in the following order:	
1. Lactated Ringer's solution	Immediate restoration of plasma volume
2. Plasma	Restoration of plasma volume when blood cell loss is not great
3. Blood	Restoration of blood volume especially when blood loss is extensive
4. Dextrans	Use when other materials are not available

Amount of fluid and rate of administration: 30 ml./kg. in 30–45 minutes

COMMERCIAL FLUIDS FOR USE IN SHOCK*

PRODUCT	MANUFACTURER
Normal human plasma USP	Courtland; Hyland; and others
Normal human serum albumin USP 5%	Hyland; Merck (Albumisol 5%)
Normal human serum albumin USP 25%	Cutter; Hyland; Merck (Albumisol 25%)
Plasma protein fraction USP	Cutter (Plasmanate); Hyland
Dextran 6% in saline	Abbott; Baxter (Gentran); Cutter
Dextran 6% in dextrose	Abbott
Dextran 6%, invert sugar 10%, in water	Baxter (salt-free Gentran)

*Reprinted from *The Medical Letter on Drugs and Therapeutics*, Vol. 8, p. 25, 1966.

Septic shock, on the other hand, often results from a combination of the factors: (1) volume depletion, (2) peripheral vascular failure and (3) cardiac failure. These can be evaluated by the *measurement of central venous pressure* (for details of recording see Weinstein and Klainer[1]).

If the central venous pressure is low (less than 5 cm. of water), one is dealing with *volume depletion* or *peripheral vascular failure.* These two situations can be distinguished from each other on the basis of the response to fluid administration. If administered fluid raises the central venous and blood pressures to normal (8–12 cm. of water), a fluid deficit has existed; however, a transient or unsustained rise in central venous pressure indicates peripheral vascular failure. Peripheral vascular failure can be treated with large doses of corticosteroids every four hours for 48 hours and intensive measures to correct acid-base imbalance.

If the central venous pressure is high (more than 10 cm. of water) and there are clinical signs of shock, one is dealing with *cardiac failure*. This is treated with:
Intravenous isoproterenol, 0.05–4 µg./minute. (1 vial to 200 cc. of 5% dextrose in water is equal to 1 µg./ml.) The blood and central venous pressures should be monitored continuously.

Vasopressor agents.—Despite their widespread use in the past, many authorities on the management of shock discourage the use of vasopressor agents. In fact, their use should probably be limited to emergencies in which the blood pressure is unrecordable. Use of metaraminol (Aramine) is recommended until the blood pressure is raised to 35 or 40 mm. of mercury. This establishes sufficient blood flow to permit the administration of the fluids, electrolytes and drugs discussed above.
Metaraminol administration (Aramine—Merck)[2]
    Single subcutaneous or intramuscular dose: 0.04–0.2 mg./kg. *or* 1–5 mg./M.[2]
    Intravenous infusion: 0.3–2.0 mg./kg. *or* 10–60 mg./M.[2] in 500 ml. Ringer's lactate. Titrate rate of infusion by frequent blood pressure recordings.
Continuous supervision is *not* necessary and one can expect a more prolonged duration of action (especially via intramuscular and subcutaneous routes). Extravasation into tissues does not cause sloughing.

REFERENCES

1. Weinstein, L., and Klainer, A. S.: Management of emergencies: IV. Septic shock—pathogenesis and treatment, New England J. Med. 274:950, 1966.
2. Nelson, W.: *Textbook of Pediatrics* (8th ed.; Philadelphia: W. B. Saunders Company, 1964), p. 213.

APPENDIX 5

*Antimicrobial Therapy**

Infecting Organism	Drug of 1st Choice	Alternative Drugs
Gram-positive cocci		
Streptococcus pyogenes, groups A, B, C and G	A penicillin	Erythromycin; a cephalosporin
Streptococcus viridans	A penicillin with or without streptomycin	A cephalosporin
Enterococcus	Ampicillin with or without streptomycin	Penicillin G with or without streptomycin; erythromycin with streptomycin
Streptococcus anaerobius	A tetracycline	A penicillin
Pneumococcus	A penicillin	Erythromycin; cephalothin
Staphylococcus aureus		
Nonpenicillinase-producing	A penicillin	Erythromycin; lincomycin; cephalothin
Penicillinase-producing	A penicillinase-resistant penicillin	Vancomycin; cephalothin

*The information on antimicrobial therapy is based on material published in *The Medical Letter on Drugs and Therapeutics,* Vol. 7, p. 81, 1965 (revised 1968).

Infecting Organism	Drug of 1st Choice	Alternative Drugs
Gram-negative cocci		
Meningococcus	A penicillin	A cephalosporin; erythromycin
Gonococcus	A penicillin	Erythromycin; a tetracycline
Gram-positive bacilli		
Listeria monocytogenes	A penicillin	Erythromycin; a tetracycline
Clostridium tetani	A penicillin	A tetracycline
Corynebacterium diphtheriae	A penicillin	Erythromycin
Gram-negative bacilli		
Salmonella typhosa	Chloramphenicol	Ampicillin
Other salmonella	Ampicillin	
Shigella	Ampicillin	Kanamycin (oral); a tetracycline
Escherichia coli		
Enteropathogenic	Kanamycin (oral) or neomycin (oral)	Ampicillin; a tetracycline
Sepsis	Kanamycin (parenteral)	Chloramphenicol; a tetracycline; polymyxin B or colistimethate
Urinary infections	Ampicillin	A tetracycline; a sulfonamide; nitrofurantoin; methenamine mandelate; methenamine hippurate
Aerobacter aerogenes	A tetracycline with or without streptomycin	Kanamycin
Klebsiella pneumoniae	A tetracycline with or without streptomycin	Cephalothin; chloramphenicol with or without streptomycin; kanamycin
Proteus mirabilis	A penicillin	Cephalothin; chloramphenicol
Other Proteus	A tetracycline with or without streptomycin	Kanamycin
Pseudomonas aeruginosa	Polymyxin B or colistimethate	Gentamicin
Brucella	A tetracycline with or without streptomycin	Chloramphenicol with or without streptomycin
Pasteurella tularensis	Streptomycin	A tetracycline
Pasteurella pestis (bubonic plague)	Streptomycin with or without a sulfonamide	A tetracycline
Hemophilus influenzae		
Respiratory infections	Ampicillin	A tetracycline
Meningitis	Ampicillin	A tetracycline with or without streptomycin; chloramphenicol with or without streptomycin
Acid-fast bacilli		
Mycobacterium	Isoniazid plus aminosalicylic acid or ethambutol, with or without streptomycin	Cycloserine; viomycin; pyrazinamide; ethionamide; kanamycin
Atypical mycobacteria	Ethionamide	Streptomycin
Schizomycetes		
Treponema pallidum	A penicillin	Erythromycin; a tetracycline
Leptospira	A penicillin	A tetracycline
Nocardia	A sulfonamide with cycloserine	A tetracycline with cycloserine; streptomycin
Rickettsia (Rocky Mountain spotted fever, endemic typhus, Q fever)	A tetracycline	Chloramphenicol
Viruses		
Mycoplasma pneumoniae (atypical pneumonia)	Erythromycin	A tetracycline
Herpetic keratitis	Idoxuridine (topical)	No alternative

Infecting Organism	Drug of 1st Choice	Alternative Drugs
Fungi		
Histoplasma capsulatum	Amphotericin B	No alternative
Candida albicans	Nystatin (topical or oral)	Amphotericin B
Aspergillus	Amphotericin B	No dependable alternative
Cryptococcus neoformans	Amphotericin B	No dependable alternative
Mucor	Amphotericin B	No dependable alternative
Coccidioides immitis	Amphotericin B	No dependable alternative

APPENDIX 6

Deep-Sedation Mixture for Diagnostic and Therapeutic Procedures in Young Children

This deep-sedation mixture is used in conjunction with local anesthesia for diagnostic procedures such as pneumoencephalography, subdural taps, myelography, etc. The mixture is given intramuscularly at least 45 minutes before the procedure is started. An appropriate dose of atropine sulfate should be given simultaneously.

1 cc. of the sedative mixture contains:
- meperidine (Demerol)   25 mg.
- chlorpromazine (Thorazine)   6.25 mg.
- promethazine (Phenergan)   6.25 mg.

Dosage Schedule*

Body Weight (Lb.)	Dose of Sedative Mixture (Cc.)	Dose of Atropine Sulfate (Mg.)
10	0.4	0.04
15	0.5	0.06
20	0.75	0.09
25	0.85	0.10
30	1.0	0.13
40	1.5	0.18
50	1.6	0.22
60	1.7	0.27
70	1.8	0.30
80	1.9	0.36
90 and over	2.0	0.40

*For the sake of safety and to avoid idiosyncratic reactions, we suggest that *the dose be estimated with extreme care on the low side,* especially in acutely or chronically ill children. Repeated, fractional doses can be given if necessary at the time of the procedure.

APPENDIX 7

Normal Head and Chest Circumferences*

HEAD CIRCUMFERENCE OF BOYS

AGE	MEAN In.	MEAN Cm.	NO. OF CASES	STANDARD DEVIATION In.	STANDARD DEVIATION Cm.
Birth	13.9	35.3	125	0.5	1.2
3 months	16.1	40.8	117	0.5	1.2
6 months	17.3	44.0	115	0.4	1.0
9 months	18.0	45.8	108	0.4	1.0
1 year	18.5	47.1	102	0.4	1.1
1½ years	19.2	48.8	97	0.4	1.1
2 years	19.5	49.6	93	0.5	1.2
2½ years	19.7	50.1	99	0.5	1.2
3 years	19.8	50.4	86	0.5	1.2
4 years	20.1	51.0	74	0.5	1.2
5 years	20.2	51.3	75	0.5	1.2
6 years	20.4	51.9	56	0.5	1.2
8 years	20.7	52.7	26	0.5	1.3
10 years	20.9	53.1	113	0.4	1.1

CHEST CIRCUMFERENCE OF BOYS

AGE	MEAN In.	MEAN Cm.	NO. OF CASES	STANDARD DEVIATION In.	STANDARD DEVIATION Cm.
Birth	13.1	33.2	98	0.7	1.8
3 months	16.0	40.6	115	0.7	1.7
6 months	17.3	44.0	113	0.7	1.8
9 months	18.3	46.5	114	0.9	2.2
1 year	18.9	47.9	109	0.8	2.1
1½ years	19.6	49.9	104	0.8	2.1
2 years	20.1	51.0	99	0.8	2.0
2½ years	20.4	51.9	94	0.8	2.0
3 years	20.7	52.7	99	0.9	2.2
4 years	21.3	54.0	87	0.9	2.3
5 years	21.8	55.4	88	0.9	2.4
6 years	22.2	56.5	75	1.0	2.5

HEAD CIRCUMFERENCE OF GIRLS

AGE	MEAN In.	MEAN Cm.	NO. OF CASES	STANDARD DEVIATION In.	STANDARD DEVIATION Cm.
Birth	13.7	34.7	110	0.4	1.0
3 months	15.7	40.0	121	0.5	1.2
6 months	16.9	42.9	131	0.5	1.2
9 months	17.6	44.7	121	0.5	1.2
1 year	18.1	45.9	121	0.5	1.3
1½ years	18.7	47.4	107	0.5	1.2
2 years	19.0	48.2	104	0.6	1.4
2½ years	19.3	49.0	96	0.6	1.4
3 years	19.4	49.3	96	0.5	1.3
4 years	19.6	49.9	85	0.5	1.3
5 years	19.8	50.3	70	0.5	1.3
6 years	20.0	50.8	69	0.6	1.4
8 years	20.4	51.8	46	0.6	1.4
10 years	20.9	53.0	23	0.6	1.4

*From Vickers, V. S., and Stuart, H. C.: Anthropometry in the pediatrician's office: Norms for selected body measurements based on studies of children of North European stock, J. Pediat. 22:155, 1943.

Chest Circumference of Girls

Age	Mean In.	Mean Cm.	No. of Cases	Standard Deviation In.	Standard Deviation Cm.
Birth	13.0	32.9	111	0.6	1.6
3 months	15.7	39.8	120	0.7	1.7
6 months	17.0	43.2	130	0.7	1.9
9 months	18.0	45.6	120	0.7	1.9
1 year	18.6	47.2	123	0.8	2.0
1½ years	19.2	48.9	105	0.8	2.0
2 years	19.8	50.3	106	0.9	2.2
2½ years	20.3	51.5	95	0.9	2.2
3 years	20.5	52.1	103	0.9	2.4
4 years	21.1	53.5	86	1.0	2.6
5 years	21.5	54.6	87	1.0	2.5
6 years	22.0	56.0	68	1.0	2.6

APPENDIX 8

*Method of Determining Ventricular Enlargement**

The measurement, *A,* is taken along a line perpendicular to the longest oblique diameter, *B,* 5 mm. from the ventricular edge in the *body* of the lateral ventricle (*not the frontal horn*). This measurement is obtained best from an anteroposterior (A-P) upright film.

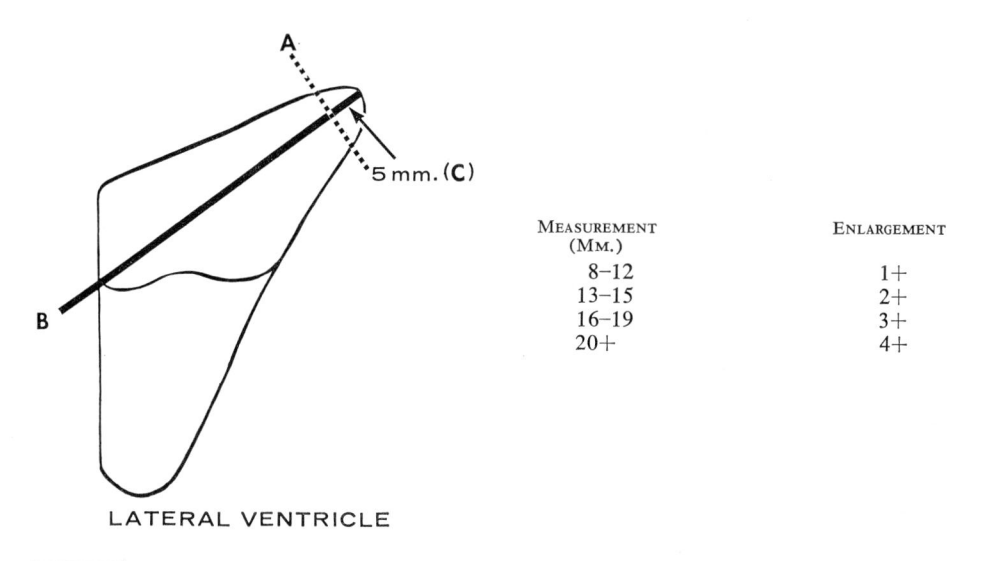

Measurement (Mm.)	Enlargement
8–12	1+
13–15	2+
16–19	3+
20+	4+

LATERAL VENTRICLE

*Modified from Taveras, J. M., and Wood, E. H.: *Diagnostic Neuroradiology* (Baltimore: Williams & Wilkins Company, 1964).

APPENDIX 9

Normal Ventricular Measurements of the Lateral Pneumogram

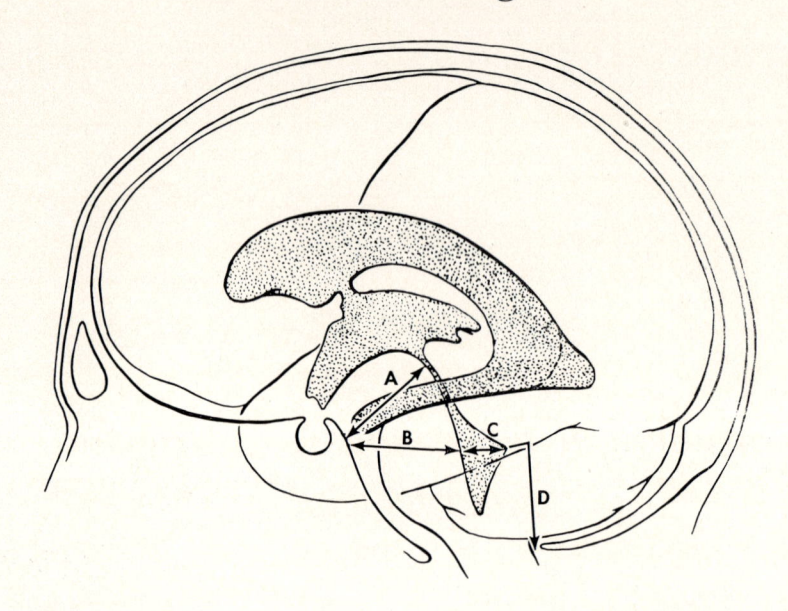

	Minimum (Cm.)	Maximum (Cm.)	Average
A: Aqueduct to dorsum sellae	3.0	3.9	3.4
B: Fourth ventricle to sella	3.3	4.0	3.6
C: Height of fourth ventricle†	1.0	2.0	1.5
D: Fourth ventricle to foramen magnum	3.0	4.0	3.3

*Modified from Taveras, J. M., and Wood, E. H.: *Diagnostic Neuroradiology* (Baltimore: Williams & Wilkins Company, 1964).
†In the frontal pneumogram the width of the floor of the fourth ventricle ranges from 1.5 to 2 cm., with an average width of 1.7 cm.

APPENDIX 10

Upper Limits of Normal Vertebral Interpediculate Distances[1,2]

	Usual Upper Limits (Cm.)	Extreme Upper Limits (Cm.)
Cervical		
2	3.0	3.1
3	3.0	3.2
4	3.2	3.4
5	3.2	3.3
6	3.2	3.4
7	3.1	3.3

	Usual Upper Limits (Cm.)	Extreme Upper Limits (Cm.)
Thoracic		
1	2.7	3.0
2	2.3	2.5
3	2.2	2.2
4	2.0	2.0
5	2.0	2.1
6	2.0	2.1
7	2.0	2.1
8	2.0	2.2
9	2.2	2.2
10	2.1	2.3
11	2.3	2.7
12	2.6	3.0
Lumbar		
1	2.8	3.0
2	2.9	3.2
3	3.0	3.5
4	3.1	3.5
5	3.3	3.9

REFERENCES

1. Elsberg, C. A., and Dyke, C. G.: The diagnosis and localization of tumors of the spinal cord by means of measurements made on the x-ray films of the vertebrae and the correlation of clinical and x-ray findings, Bull. Neurol. Inst. New York, 3:359, 1934.
2. Taveras, J. M., and Wood, E. H.: *Diagnostic Neuroradiology* (Baltimore: Williams & Wilkins Company, 1964).

APPENDIX 11

Estimation of Enlargement of the Pituitary Fossa

Taveras and Wood[1] recommend that enlargement of the pituitary fossa be estimated by measuring the greatest anteroposterior (A-P) diameter. They consider this distance the most reliable single measurement. Generally any A-P diameter greater than 17 mm. can be considered pathologic.

The A-P diameter is taken from the most anterior to the most posterior margins (arrows). In selecting the most posterior point of the dorsum sellae, one must measure carefully to the anterior margin of the midportion of the dorsum (heavy line) and not to the lateral edges (faint line).

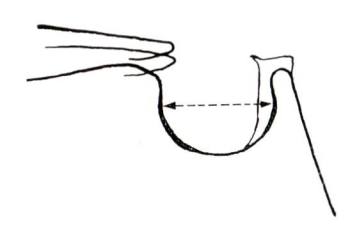

Silverman[2] has studied the normal variation in children with sex and age, using the area as the index of enlargement.

REFERENCES

1. Taveras, J. M., and Wood, E. H.: *Diagnostic Neuroradiology* (Baltimore: Williams & Wilkins Company, 1964).
2. Silverman, F. N.: Roentgen standards for size of the pituitary fossa from infancy through adolescence, Am. J. Roentgenol. 78:451, 1957.

APPENDIX 12

Normal Cerebrospinal Fluid Values

Determination	Normal Value
Amount in newborn	Up to 5 ml.
Increases with age to adult figure	100–150 ml.
Initial pressure	70–200 mm. of water
Cell count	
Under 1 year	Up to 10 cells/cu. mm.
1–4 years	Up to 8 cells/cu. mm.
Over 5 years	0–5 cells/cu. mm.
Chloride	
7 days to 3 months	108.8–122.5 mEq./L.
4–12 months	112.7–128.5 mEq./L.
13 months to 12 years	116.8–130.5 mEq./L.
Glucose*	
6 months to 10 years	71–90 mg./100 ml.
Over 10 years	50–80 mg./100 ml.
Protein	
Ventricular fluid	6–15 mg./100 ml.
Cisterna magna fluid	15–25 mg./100 ml.
Lumbar CSF	20–45 mg./100 ml.
Albumin	87% of total protein
Globulin	13% of total protein

*Normal cerebrospinal fluid glucose levels are about two-thirds the blood glucose levels.

APPENDIX 13

Normal Blood Values

Chemical Constituents of Blood

Determination	Material	Normal Value
Acid-Base Constituents		
Sodium*	Serum	136–143 mEq./L.
Potassium*	Serum	4.1–5.6 mEq./L.
Calcium*	Serum	10–12 mg./100 ml.
		5–6 mEq./L.

CHEMICAL CONSTITUENTS OF BLOOD *(Cont.)*

DETERMINATION	MATERIAL	NORMAL VALUE
Magnesium*	Serum	2–3 mg./100 ml.
In the newborn a value as low as 1.3 mEq./L. would be considered normal.		1.65–2.5 mEq./L.
Phosphorus, inorganic, as P	Serum	4–6.5 mg./100 ml.
Slightly higher in the newborn (in infants, up to 8 mg./100 ml. considered normal)		1.29–2.1 mM/L.
HPO_4—/H_2PO_4 (average valence 1.8 at pH 7.4)		2.3–3.8 mEq./L.
Standard bicarbonate (Astrup)	Serum	21–25 mEq./L.
Carbon dioxide content	Serum from venous blood	45–70 vol.% 20.3–31.5 mM/L.
Miscellaneous		
Copper	Serum	0.08–0.235 mg./100 ml.
Lead	Serum	0.001–0.003 mg./100 ml.
Iodine, protein-bound	Serum	0.003–0.008 mg./100 ml.
Thiamine	Blood	5.5–9.5 μg./100 ml.
Osmolarity	Plasma	270–285 milliosmols/L. plasma water

*In human red blood cells an average concentration of sodium would be about 21 mEq./L. of red blood cells; of potassium, about 86 mEq./L.

The level of calcium in serum is influenced by the concentration of serum protein because part of the calcium is associated with or bound to the protein. Practically all the calcium in blood is in the plasma.

APPENDIX 14

Normal Urinary Values

DETERMINATION	NORMAL VALUE	MINIMAL QUANTITY REQUIRED	NOTE
Calcium	Under 150 mg./day	24-hr. specimen	Collect in special bottle with 10 cc. of concentrated HCl.
Catecholamines	Epinephrine: under 10 μg./day Norepinephrine: under 100 μg./day	24-hr. specimen	Should be collected with 12 cc. of concentrated HCl (pH should be between 2 and 3).
Copper	0–100 μg./day	24-hr. specimen	
Coproporphyrin	50–250 μg./day Children under 80 lb: 0–75 μg./day	24-hr. specimen	Collect with 5 Gm. of sodium carbonate.
Creatine	Under 100 mg./day or less than 6% of creatinine. In pregnancy: up to 12%. In children under 1 year: may equal creatinine. In older children: up to 30% of creatinine	24-hr. specimen	Also order creatinine.
Creatinine	15–25 mg./kg./day	24-hr. specimen	
Creatinine clearance	150–180 L./day/1.73 sq. mm. of body-surface area	24-hr. specimen	
Lead	0.08 μg./ml. or 120 μg. or less/24 hr.	24-hr. specimen	

Determination	Normal Value	Minimal Quantity Required	Note
Phosphorus (inorganic)	Varies with intake; average 1 Gm./day	24-hr. specimen	Collect in special bottle with 10 cc. of concentrated HCl.
Porphobilinogen	0	10 cc.	Use freshly voided sample.

Index

A

Abdomen
  congenital absence of muscles, 345
  ruptured viscus, and head injury, 214
Abiotrophy, 388
Abortifacients, congenital anomalies due to, 175
Abscess, intracranial, 296 ff.
  with congenital heart disease, 462
  diagnosis, 297 f.
  management, 298
  in meningitis, 283
  with penetrating injury, 210
"Absence" attacks, 25, 185, 186
Acanthocytosis, 435 f.
Acetazolamide
  in hydrocephalus, 139
  in petit mal seizures, 31
  in pseudotumor cerebri, 84
Achalasia of esophagus, 151
Achondroplasia, see Chondrodystrophy
Acidosis, 9
  metabolic
    in methanol poisoning, 365
    in salicylate poisoning, 374
Acoustic nerve deficits, traumatic, 200
Acrocephalosyndactyly, 157
Acrodynia, 381
Actinomycin D, in Wilms' tumor, 265
Adamantinoma, see Craniopharyngioma
Adenoma
  pancreatic, 45, 46
  sebaceum, in tuberous sclerosis, 428, 429
Adie's syndrome, 92
Adiposogenital dystrophy, 103
Adversive attacks, 25, 26
Adynamia episodica hereditaria, 342 f.
Aerocele formation, 217
  complicating fracture, 211
Agammaglobulinemia, recurrent meningitis in, 283
Agenesis
  cerebellar, 146
  of corpus callosum, 141, 142 f.
Agraphia, developmental, 70
Akathizia, in chlorpromazine therapy, 95
Akinetic episodes, 25
Albright's syndrome, with fibrous dysplasia, 165
Alcohol poisoning, 355, 365 f.
Allergy to anticonvulsants, 30 ff., 33 ff.
Alpers' disease, 433
Amblyopia
  causes of, 77
  ex anopsia, 77 f., 88, 89
Amino acids
  metabolic defect, movement disorders in, 433 ff.
  transport, disorders of, 403 f.
Aminoacidurias
  patterned type, 403
  primary, 388 ff.

Aminophylline intoxication, 355, 379 f.
Aminopterin, congenital anomalies due to, 175
Ammonia
  defective renal production, 391, 404
  intoxication, 398 f.
  periodic, hyperlysinemia with, 399 f.
Ammons Picture Vocabulary Test, 6
Ammons' Quick Test, 6
Amnesia
  for night terrors, 49
  post-traumatic, 200
Amphetamine derivatives, toxic reactions to, 355, 373 f.
Amphotericin B, in meningitis, 296
Ampicillin, in purulent meningitis, 289, 290 f.
Amylopectinosis, 324
Amyoplasia congenita, 346, 348
Amyotonia congenita, 52, 53
Analgesia
  in management of poisonings, 358
  for painful diagnostic and therapeutic procedures, 111, 487
Anemia
  aplastic, 461, 469
    drug-induced, 34, 35, 39
    drug therapy in, 472
  severe, 231
    blood transfusion in, 484
Anencephaly, 128, 135
Aneurysms
  arterial, 155 f.
  of vein of Galen, 153
Angiography, 111
  in arterial aneurysm, 155, 156
  in brain tumors, 244, 253, 255
  carotid, in epidural and subdural hematoma, 202, 205, 206 f.
  indications for, 112
Angiomas of brain, 151 ff.
  arteriovenous, 153 f.
  capillary, 152
Angiomatosis, encephalotrigeminal, 152
Anisocoria, 92
Anomalies, see Malformations, congenital; specific names of anomalies
Anoxia; see Hypoxia
Anticancer drugs, neurotoxicity, 370, 378
Anticholinesterase agents, in myasthenia, 338, 340
Anticoagulants, in cerebral embolization, 470, 472
Anticonvulsants
  in breathholding spells, 41
  in centrencephalic epilepsy, 30 ff.
  for focal cerebral seizures, 32 ff.
  in grand mal seizures, 32 ff.
  guidelines for dosage, 27 f.
  in headaches, 48
  maintenance therapy in febrile convulsions, 36
  in minor motor epilepsy, 28

Anticonvulsants (*cont.*)
  in organic psychoses, 18
  for prolonged acute convulsions, 480
  in status epilepticus, 480
  structure-activity interrelationships, 40
  toxic reactions to, 30 ff., 33 ff.
    prevention and treatment, 39
Antidiuretic hormone, inappropriate secretion of, 101 f.
Antidotes
  recommended, for specific poisons, 359
  universal, 357
Antifreeze, poisoning due to, 355, 365
Antimicrobial agents
  of choice, in various infections, 485 ff.
  in purulent meningitis, 288 ff.
  toxic reactions to, 355, 370, 374 ff.
  See also specific agents
Anti-migraine drugs, 49
Antimongolism, 171 f.
Antitoxin
  botulism, 367
  horse serum sensitivity, 370, 382
Antivenin
  coral snake, 369
  pit viper, 369
  for spider bites, 368
Apert's syndrome, 157 f.
Aphasia
  acquired, 19, 72 f.
  apparent deafness in, 79
  causes of, 72 f., 239
  EEG abnormalities in, 117
  with left subfrontal astrocytoma, 259
  motor, developmental, 72
Apnea, causes of, 231, 233, 236
Arachnidism, 355, 368
Arachnoiditis, chronic adhesive, 83
Arboviruses, 287
  nervous system infections, 280 f., 292
Argininosuccinicaciduria, 8, 9, 389, 398, 399
Arhinencephaly, 136
  with trigonencephaly, 157, 158
Arnold-Chiari malformation, 129
Arsenic poisoning, 355, 360
  antidotes, 359, 360
Arteries
  carotid
    aneurysms of, 155 f.
    internal, injuries to, 198, 460
  cerebral, arteriovenous malformations involving, 153
  middle meningeal, injury to, 196, 208
  thrombosis of, 460 f.
Arteriovenous fistula, complicating head injury, 198, 208
Arthrogryposis, 346, 348
Asphyxia
  causing brain hemorrhage, 235
  severe, causes, 231
Astereognosis, 239
  in spastic hemiplegia, 56
Astrocytoma
  brain stem, 249
  cerebellar, 242
    clinical and laboratory diagnosis, 245 ff.
    management and prognosis, 247
  cerebral, 252
    left subfrontal, with diencephalic syndrome, 258, 259
    of temporal lobe, 254
  intramedullary, 268, 269
A.T. 10, in chronic hypoparathyroidism, 425

Ataxia
  acute, opsoclonus in, 91 f.
  cerebellar, acute, 95
  with cerebellar astrocytoma, 245
  diagnosis, 57
  differential diagnosis, 95
  diseases causing, 94 f.
  with posterior third ventricle tumors, 261
  spinocerebellar, 438 f.
Ataxia-telangiectasia, 152, 433 ff.
Atlantic City Eye Test, 78
Atonic diplegia, 52, 53, 54, 142, 146
Atrophy, 316
  cerebral, 141, 143
  muscular
    hereditary spastic paraplegia, 331 ff.
    infantile spinal, 53, 326 ff.
    juvenile proximal spinal, 330 f.
    progressive neural, 329 f.
  neurogenic, 316
  occipital lobe, in status epilepticus, 238
  optic
    hereditary, 443, f.
    with left subfrontal astrocytoma, 259
    with optic glioma, 260
Atropine, for muscarinic effects of poisoning, 359, 361, 367
Audiometric tests, 79 f.
Auditory imperception, congenital, 71 f.
Aura, in generalized seizures, 27
Autism, early infantile, 20
Automobile driving, by patients with epilepsy, 190
Autonomic nervous system
  disorder of, 445 f.
  structural malformations of, 150 ff.
Autosomes, 166
  abnormalities in number, 167 ff.
Azathioprine, in systemic lupus erythematosus, 473

B

BAL therapy
  in arsenic poisoning, 359, 360
  in Wilson's disease, 437
Barany's caloric test, 91
Barbiturate
  -amphetamine intoxication, 374
  for convulsions in strychnine poisoning, 362
  intoxication, 371 f.
  See also Phenobarbital
Barr body, 166
Basal ganglia
  congenital anomalies of, 145, 147
  état marbré in, 236
Basilar impression, 163
Bassen-Kornzweig disease, 435 f.
"Battered-child" syndrome, 203
  subdural hematoma in, 197, 203
Behavior
  antisocial, 21
  criminal, and XYY chromosome anomalies, 169 f.
  withdrawn, 20
Behavior disorders, 13 ff.
  autistic, 20
  diagnostic workup, 7
  drug therapy in, 17 f.
  EEG in, 116 f.
  hyperactive
    diagnosis, 14 ff.
    management, 16 f.
  hypoxia causing, 239

post-traumatic, 200 f.
psychogenic, 20 f.
psychotic, 18 f.
in spastic hemiplegia, 56
in status epilepticus, 237
Bell's palsy, 73
  drug therapy in, 301, 305
  etiology, 301, 304
Bender-Gestalt test, 6, 14 ff.
Benedict's test, in galactosemia, 406
Benzathine penicillin, in rheumatic chorea, 472
Beriberi, encephalopathy in, 477
Betamethasone, in cerebral edema, 482
Bielschowsky's disease, 412, 414
Biopsy
  in diagnosis, 118, 120 f.
  muscle, technique, 120 f.
Birth injuries
  to head, 221 ff.
  intracranial, 222 ff.
  spinal cord, 224 ff.
Bites
  snake, 368 ff.
    causing flaccid weakness, 94
  spider and tick, 355, 368
Blind spots, enlarged, 114
  with increased intracranial pressure, 82, 83
Blindness
  cortical, 76 f.
    caused by hypoxia, 239
  in degenerative diseases, 388 ff.
  impaired language development with, 68
Blood
  chemical constituents of, 492 f.
  determinations in poisonings, 356
  diagnostic tests, 118
    screening, 9
  diseases, 459 ff.
    treatment of, 472 f.
  normal values, 492 f.
Blood transfusions
  in blood disorders, 472 f.
  in severe anemia, 484
Blood vessel
  aneurysms, 153, 155 ff.
  angiomas, 151 ff.
  congenital malformations, intracranial hemorrhage in, 462, 473
  diseases, 459 ff.
    differential diagnosis, 462
    occlusive, 468 ff.
    treatment, 471 ff.
  radiographic studies, 111 f.
Bobble-head doll syndrome, 91
Body, abnormal size with neurologic deficit, 8
Bone
  brittleness, in osteopetrosis, 164
  formation
    disorders of, 164 f.
    osteoid, defect in, 402
Bone marrow suppression, due to anticonvulsants, 39
Bornholm disease, 336 f.
Botulism, 355, 367
Bourneville's disease, 427 ff.
Brachial plexus
  birth injuries of, 226
  neuritis, with antiserum therapy, 382
Brachycephaly, 157, 158
Brain
  abscess, see Abscess, intracranial
  anoxic damage, 231 ff.
    complicating febrile seizures, 35
  diagnosis, 238 f.
    differential diagnosis, 239
  atrophy, 141, 143, 144, 238
    changes in meningoencephalitis, 281 f.
  congenital vascular malformations of, 151, ff.
  damage
    hypoxic, 231 ff.
    ischemic postseizure, 36
    in occlusive vascular disease, 459
    in renal disease, 475
    reproductions in Bender-Gestalt test, 15
  degeneration
    of gray matter, 433
    spongy, of white matter, 432 f.
  developmental failure of, 135, 136
  edema, treatment, 245, 481 f.
  external decompression in encephalitis, 292
  growth, 59
    failure of, 60 f.
  hemorrhage
    in blood disorders, 460
    clinical signs, 238 f.
    due to hypoxia, 233, 235 f.
  herniation of temporal lobe uncus, 84 ff., 236 ff.
  hypoplasia, 141, 143, 144
  injuries
    birth, 222 ff.
    postnatal (direct), 195 ff.
  lipidoses, 411 ff.
  mass lesions, 48, 117
  occult anomalies of, 47, 141 ff.
  shrinkage causing subdural hematoma, 481
  size and macrocrania, 61 f.
  subdural and epidural empyema, 298
  tumors, see Tumors
  vasculitis in, 460
  ventricle
    enlargement, determining, 489
    normal measurements, 490
Brain scans, radioisotopic, 112
  in cerebral hemisphere tumors, 253
Brain stem
  congenital anomalies, 146 f.
  deficit in multiple sclerosis, 455, 456
  gliomas, 249 ff.
  vs. acute cerebellitis, 303
Breathholding spells, 39, 41
  EEG in, 116
Bromides, in seizures, 33, 35
Brown-Sequard syndrome, 227
Brudzinski sign, 282

C

Café-au-lait spots, 8
  in optic glioma, 259
Cafergot, for headaches, 49
Calciferol, in chronic hypoparathyroidism, 425
Calcification
  defective, in hypophosphatasia, 391
  intracranial
    evaluation of, 109
    in hypoparathyroidism, 424
    in neonatal infections, 174
    in pseudohypoparathyroidism, 425 f.
    in Sturge-Weber syndrome, 152
    in pineal gland region, 262
  subcutaneous, in polymyositis, 334
Calcium excretion, measurement, 425
Calvarium, evaluation of thickness, 108
Camptodactyly, 346, 348
Canavan's disease, 432 f.
Caput succedaneum, 223

INDEX

Carbohydrate metabolism, disturbances, 104
Carbon monoxide poisoning, 355, 362 f.
Cardiac seizures, 47
Carotid arteries
  aneursysm of, 155 f.
  internal, trauma to, 198, 460
  occlusion, causing stroke, 469
Carpopedal spasm, in tetany, 41
Cataplexy, 50
Cataracts
  congenital, after maternal rubella, 173
  in Lowe's oculocerebrorenal syndrome, 405
Catell Infant Intelligence Scale, 6
Cat-scratch fever, 311
Celiac disease, hypocalcemic tetany in, 42, 43
Celiac-like syndrome, with neuroblastoma, 273, 275
Cell division, nondisjunction in, 166, 167 f.
Cellulitis, chronic orbital, 309 f.
Central core disease, 314, 326
Cephalohematomas
  differentiated from encephaloceles, 133
  in newborn, 222, 223, 224
"Cerebellar fits," 247
Cerebellitis, acute, 95, 303 f.
Cerebellum
  astrocytoma of, 245
  congenital anomalies of, 145 f., 147
  herniation, 85 f.
  medulloblastoma of, 247 ff.
Cerebral artery, arteriovenous malformations involving, 153
Cerebral palsy, 52 ff., 68
  diagnostic workup, 7
Cerebritis, in bacterial meningitis, 281
Cerebrospinal fluid
  in anaphylactoid purpura, 467, 468
  in arterial aneurysm with hemorrhage, 156
  blood in, diseases causing, 461, 462
  in brain abscess, 298
  in chronic granulomatous meningitis, 288
  in CNS leukemia, 264 f.
  decreasing production of, in hydrocephalus, 139
  diagnostic tests on, 118 ff.
  in encephalomyelitis, 301
  findings in newborn, 222 f.
  in meningoencephalitis, 285, 286 ff.
  in multiple sclerosis, 456
  in neonatal cord injury, 226
  normal values, 492
  otorrhea, 211, 213, 217
  pH, and encephalopathy of renal disease, 475
  pressure, abnormal readings, 83
  protein, in leukodystrophies, 418
  rhinorrhea, tests for, 210 f., 213
  in sarcoidosis, 311
  sediment, India ink stains, 288
  shunting procedures, 139 f., 215
  in subacute inclusion encephalitis, 309
Cerebrovascular accidents, 459 ff.
  in bleeding disorders, 461 f.
  in cerebrovascular disease, 459, 462
  congenital and neonatal, 461
  in congenital heart disease, 460, 463 f.
  severity of brain damage in, 459
  therapy, 469 ff.
Cerebrovascular disease, 459 ff.
  differential diagnosis, 462 f.
  management and prognosis, 469 ff.
Cerebrum, see Brain
Charcoal, activated: as universal antidote, 357
Charcot triad, in multiple sclerosis, 456

Charcot-Marie-Tooth atrophy, 329 f.
Chest, normal circumferences at various ages, 488 f.
Chickenpox, see Varicella infection
Chloramphenicol, in purulent meningitis, 289 f.
Chlordane poisoning, 355, 362
Chloroquine neurotoxicity, 376
Chlorpromazine
  adverse reactions to, 359, 373
  in amphetamine intoxication, 359, 373
  in behavior disorders, 17
  for choreiform movements, 58, 440, 471, 472, 474
  in deep-sedation mixture, 487
  unusual movements caused by, 95
Chondrodystrophy, 164
Chordomas, spinal extradural, 276
Chorea, 95
  chronic progressive hereditary, 439 f.
  rheumatic, 466
    drug therapy in, 471, 472
    psychotic reactions in, 18
Choreoathetosis, 57 f.
  in kernicterus, 474
Chromatin study, buccal smear, 10, 166
Chromatography in diagnosis, 118, 119
Chromosomes
  abnormalities in number, 167 ff.
  abnormalities in structure, 166, 170 ff.
  deletions, 166, 171, 172
  ring configurations, 166, 170, 171
  translocations, 166, 170
Chvostek's sign, 41
Citrullinemia, 9, 390, 398, 399
Clubfoot, 346
  in Friedreich's ataxia, 438
Cold intolerance, with craniopharyngioma, 256, 257
Collagen vascular disease, 460, 462
  myositis in, 335
  neurologic complications of, 466 ff.
    therapy in, 470, 471 f.
  psychotic behavior in, 18
Colobomas, 136
Coma, 9
  causes of, 47
  hepatic, 476
Concussion, 196, 199, 201
  with fracture, 208
Conduction velocity studies, in diagnosis, 119
Consciousness, loss of, 25 ff.
Contractures of muscles, congenital, 346 ff.
Contusion, cerebral, 196
Conversion reaction, hysterical, 21 f.
  convulsion as, 47
  dysarthria as, 73
Convulsions
  as conversion reaction, 47
  febrile, 35 f, 37, 189, 234, 236
    EEG in, 116
    resulting in status epilepticus, 237
  management, in poisoning, 358
  prolonged acute, treatment of, 480 f.
Corpus callosum, agenesis of, 141, 142 f.
Corticosteroids, adrenal
  in bacterial meningitis, 290
  in cerebral edema, 481 f.
  neurotoxic reactions to, 370, 377
  in tuberculous meningitis, 296
  See also specific compounds
Cortisone
  replacement therapy after surgery for craniopharyngioma, 258

in therapy of cerebral edema, 481
Counseling
　genetic, in mongolism, 172
　of parents of retarded child, 10
Cover test, in examination for squint, 88
Coxsackie virus infections, 284
　causing paralysis, 285
Coyotillo, 367 f.
Cranial nerves
　anomalies of, 146 f.
　deficits
　　post-traumatic focal, 200, 208
　　in subdural effusions, 283
　See also names of specific nerves
Cranial sutures
　diastasis due to trauma, 209
　premature closure, see Craniosynostosis
Craniofacial dystosis, 158
Craniolacunia, 130
Craniopharyngiomas, 242, 256 ff.
　diagnosis, 256, 258
　management and prognosis, 258
　radiation therapy in, 245
Craniorhachischisis, 127 ff.
Craniosynostosis, 62, 83, 156 ff.
　associated anomalies, 157
　causing microcrania, 60
　management, 160 f.
　physical findings, 156 ff.
Cranium bifidum, with meningoencephalocele, 132-133
Creatine phosphokinase, in childhood dystrophy, 317, 319
Creatinuria, in classic muscular dystrophies, 317
Cretinism, 8, 421 ff.
　recurrence risk, 424
　thyroid therapy in, 423
Cri du chat syndrome, 170 f.
Crigler-Najjar syndrome, 474
Crouzon's disease, 158, 159
Cyanide-nitroprusside drop test, in diagnosis of homocystinuria, 401
Cystathioninuria, 9, 390, 400 f.
Cystinosis, 8, 9
Cysts
　colloid, of third ventricle, 262 f.
　dermoid, 65, 266
　　intraspinal, 271
　epidermoid, of skull, 134
　fluid, in craniopharyngioma, 258
　leptomeningeal, formation with fracture, 209, 210
　suprasellar, see Craniopharyngioma
Cytomegalovirus infection, 8
　and microcephaly, 61
Cytoxan, in intracranial hemorrhage, 472

D

Dandy-Walker anomaly, 63, 136, 137
Davidoff-Dyke-Masson syndrome, 55
Deafness
　apparent, 78, 79
　in brain stem glioma, 250, 251
　conduction, 79, 80
　congenital, after maternal rubella, 173
　conservation-of-hearing programs, 80
　EEG in diagnosis, 116
　nerve, 8
　　causes of, 79, 80
　　in kernicterus, 474
　speech impairment in, 68, 72
　true
　　causes of, 79, 80
　　distinguishing from apparent deafness, 78 f.
　word, developmental, 71 f.
Decerebrate rigidity, 99 f.
Deficiency diseases, nervous system manifestations in, 476 f.
Degenerative diseases of nervous system
　diagnostic tests, 118, 389 ff.
　hereditary, transmission, 388
　indications for complete metabolic studies, 118
　progressive, 13
　psychotic behavior in, 18
　seizures in, 236, 388 ff.
　of unknown etiology, 438 ff., 442 f.
Dehydration, dangers of correction, 290
Deletions, chromosome, 171
　in cell divisions, 166
　chomosome 18-deletion syndrome, 172
Delirium, acute: EEG in, 116
Dementia
　in anoxia, 239
　apparent deafness in, 79
　in degenerative diseases, 388 ff.
　differential diagnosis, 13
　Heller's infantile, 20, 416
　in metabolic disorders, 388 ff.
　myoclonus in, 57
　from postnatal ischemic brain damage, 37
　progressive, of unknown etiology, 432 f.
Demyelinating diseases, 452 ff.
Dermal sinuses, 128 f.
Dermatomyositis, 333 ff.
Development
　areas of, 4 f.
　milestone failures in, 5
　normal, signs of, 5
　progress of child, in retardation, 11
Devic's disease, 454 f.
Dexamethasone, in cerebral edema, 482
Dexedrine, in narcolepsy, 50
Diabetes
　insipidus, 101 f.
　　with craniopharyngioma, 256, 257
　　management, 104
　　in reticuloendothelioses, 307 ff.
　maternal, effects on fetus, 176
Dialysis
　peritoneal, for hypernatremia, 377
　reverse urea effect, 475
　in therapy of poisoning, 359
Diaphragm, congenital absence of hemidiaphragm, 345
Diastasis, traumatic, 209
Diastematomyelia, 161
Diazepam, in status epilepticus, 480
Diazoxide, in hypoglycemia, 46
Diencephalic syndromes, 101 ff., 258, 259
Diets
　adverse reactions to, 370, 378 f.
　free of milk and dairy products, 407
　in hyperglycinemia, 398
　low-calcium, 378 f.
　low-methionine, 401, 404
　low-phenylalanine, 394, f.
　low-protein, 398
　　in ammonia intoxication, 399, 400
　in maple syrup disease, 396
Digoxin, in cerebral embolization, 471, 472
Dihydrotachysterol, in chronic hypoparathyroidism, 425
Dimethadione
　in petit mal seizures, 31
　reactions to, 39

Diphenylhydantoin
  for generalized and focal seizures, 32 ff.
  for maintenance anticonvulsant therapy, 36
  toxic reactions to, 32 f., 34
Diphenylthiocarbazone, in thallotoxicosis, 355, 361
Diphtheria antitoxin, dosage, 300
Diplegia, 55
  spastic, 56
Diplopia
  with brain stem glioma, 250
  with brain tumor, 243, 245
  head tilt to avoid, 93
  and paralytic squint, 88, 90
Dithizon, see Diphenylthiocarbazone
Dizziness, episodic, 49
Dolichocephaly, 156, 157
Down's syndrome, 168
Draw-a-Man test, 6
Drug therapy
  adverse reactions to
    adrenal corticosteroids, 377
    anticonvulsants, 30 ff., 33 ff., 370 ff.
    antimicrobial agents, 355, 374 ff.
    insulin, 377
    prevention and treatment, 24, 39, 371 ff.
    sedatives, 371 f.
    stimulants, 373 f., 379
  allergic manifestations, 30 ff., 33 ff.
  congenital malformations due to, 175 f.
  postinjection neuropathies, 220 f.
  See also specific drugs and conditions
Duane's syndrome, 146 f.
Duchenne's dystrophy, 318 f.
Dwarfism, 8
  chondrodystrophic, 164
  with craniopharyngioma, 256, 257
  microcephalic, 171
Dysarthria
  acquired, causes of, 73, 93
  developmental, 71
Dysautonomia, familial, 149, 445 f.
Dysentery, bacillary: encephalopathy in, 476
Dyslexia, developmental, 69 f.
Dysphagia, 93
Dysphonia, 93
Dystonia
  in chlorpromazine therapy, 95
  musculorum deformans, 441 f.
Dystrophy, 316
  childhood (Duchenne), 318 f.
  classification, 315, 317
  facioscapulohumeral (Landouzy-Déjerine), 319 f.
  Limb-girdle, 322 f.
  myotonic (Steinert), 320 ff.
    differentiated from peroneal muscular atrophy, 330
  oculocerebrorenal, see Lowe's syndrome
  pathogenesis, 317
  Schilder's sudanophilic, 412, 418, 420 f.

E

ECHO virus infections, 284
  causing paralysis, 285
Echoencephalography, 112
  in intracranial hematoma, 202
  in localization of brain tumors, 243, 244, 253
Ectodermal dysplasia, hereditary, 149
Eczema, 8
Edema, cerebral
  in acute toxic encephalopathy, 35, 36 f., 237
  in dialysis, effects of, 475
  from direct injury, 196
  drug therapy in, 245, 481
  in lead poisoning, 363, 365
  treatment, 481 f.
EDTA therapy, in lead poisoning, 359, 365
Effusions, subdural: in meningitis, 283, 290
Electric current, injuring nervous system, 228
Electrocorticography, 115
Electrodes, EEG: positioning of, 114 f.
Electroencephalography
  arousal response, in detecting hearing loss, 79
  in brain abscess, 297, 298
  in brain tumors, 243, 244, 254, 255
  in cerebrovascular accident, 463, 465
  defining "life or death" in cerebral anoxia, 117
  in diagnosis, 114 ff.
  discharges, 117
  in epidural hematoma, 202
  in epilepsy
    age-distribution curve, 189
    focal, 187 ff.
    petit mal, 184 ff., 188
  in febrile convulsions, 35 f.
  interpretation, 115 f.
  in minor motor seizures, 28, 29
  in phenylketonuria, 389
  principles of recording, 114 f.
  prognostic value, 116
  provocative techniques, 115 f.
  in retardation, 9
  serial
    in encephalomyelitis, 301
    in "fugue" state, 19
    in meningoencephalitis, 292, 293
    in subacute inclusion encephalitis, 309
    in subdural hematoma, 205 f., 467
Electrolytes
  administration
    parenteral therapy, 482 f.
    in poisoning, 358
    premixed solutions for maintenance, 483
  determinations in diagnosis, 118
  metabolism, disturbances, 102
Electromyography, in diagnosis, 118 f.
Ellsworth-Howard test, in diagnosis of pseudohypoparathyroidism, 426
Emaciation syndrome of Russell, 103
Emboli
  air, 466
  fat, 466
Embolization, cerebral
  in bacterial endocarditis, 464, 466
  in congenital heart disease, 463 f.
  differential diagnosis, 462
  diseases causing, 460
  in myocarditis, 464 ff.
    congestive heart failure in, 470 f.
  therapy, 470 ff.
Emotional incontinence, 55
Empyema
  epidural, 298
  subdural, 210, 298
Encephalitis
  herpes simplex, therapy, 292
  in infectious mononucleosis, 306
  Marie-Strümpell, 36 f.
  pontine, 95, 251, 303 f.
  subacute inclusion, 282, 309
Encephalocele
  with anencephaly, 135
  with nervous system anomalies, 132 f., 134 f.
  orbital, proptosis due to, 65

Encephalomyelitis, 300 ff., 453 ff.
  acute disseminated, 453, 454
  equine, 282
  postinfectious, 300 ff.
  postvaccinal, 300, 301
Encephalomyelopathy, necrotizing, 433
Encephalopathy
  acute toxic, 35, 36 f., 83, 237, 370
  anoxic, 231
  hypertensive, 83
  postseizure, 36 f., 237
  in renal disease, 475
  Sabin's nontoxoplasmic vascular, 174
  Wernicke's, 477
Endocarditis, bacterial
  septic emboli from, 460
  subacute
    cerebral embolization in, 464, 466
    drug therapy in, 472
Endocrine disorders
  myopathies secondary to, 326
  and neurologic disease, 101 ff.
Enterovirus infections, 280 f., 284 ff.
  cerebrospinal fluid in, 287
Environmental factors
  in congenital malformations, 127, 165 f.
    drugs, 175 f.
    irradiation, 176
    maternal infections, 173 ff.
  and headaches, 49
  and hyperactive behavior, 16 f.
Enzyme deficiencies
  in aminoacidurias, 389 ff.
  in fructosuria, 407
  in glycogen storage diseases, 323, 324
  in hyperammonemia, 398
  in hyperbilirubinemia, 474
Enzymes
  serum, in childhood dystrophy, 317, 319
  therapy, in meningitis, 290
Ependymomas
  intramedullary, 268
  intraventricular, 263
Epilepsy, 13
  abdominal, 26
  acquired aphasia in, 73
  automobile driving by patients, 190
  centrencephalic (petit mal), 26, 28, 184
    drug therapy in, 30 ff.
    EEG recordings, 115, 116, 117, 184 ff., 188
    ketogenic diet in, 32
    light-sensitive, 186
    prognosis, 190 f.
    recurrence risk in sibling, 191 f.
  clinical categories, 184 ff.
  differential diagnosis, 189 f.
  EEG abnormalities, 117, 184 ff., 188
    age distribution curve of petit mal, 189
  familial incidence, 183 f., 185, 187 f.
  focal, 25, 26, 186 ff.
    drug therapy in, 32 ff.
    refractory, 35
  general management of patient, 190
  generalized (grand mal), 27, 189
    drug therapy in, 32 ff.
    refractory, 35
  genetic basis of, 183 f.
  minor motor, 25 f., 28, 29, 57
  pathologic findings in brain, 184
  post-traumatic, 199
  progressive myoclonus, 440 f.
  psychomotor, 25, 26, 116, 186, 234
    drug therapy in, 32 ff.

  reading, 38
  reflex, 38
  subcortical, 26
  temporal lobe, 234
  See also Seizures
Epinephrine, in hypoglycemia, 46
Erb's dystrophy, 322
Esophagus, achalasia of, 151
Etat marbré in basal ganglia, 236
Ethanol poisoning, 355, 365
Ethosuximide, in petit mal seizures, 30 f.
Ethylene glycol poisoning, 355, 365
von Eulenberg's disease, 344
Eupractone, *see* Dimethadione
Exanthem subitum, 300
  convulsions in, 302
Exophthalmos
  in children, 65 f.
  in optic nerve glioma, 258
Eyes
  clinical signs
    in congenital hydrocephalus, 138
    in neurological disorders, 8
  congenital anomalies of structures, 136
  cover test for squint, 88
  deviations, 88 ff.
  interorbital distance, in diagnosis, 63
  "lazy," 77 f., 88
  motor apraxia, 90 f.
  neurological signs of focal deficit, 87 ff.
    in cranial nerve injuries, 200

F

Face
  in Crouzon's disease, 158, 159
  deformities of, 63 f.
  in gargoylism, 409
  in infantile hypercalcemia syndrome, 145
  weakness or asymmetry, 92
Facial nerve
  birth injuries, 226
  effects of injury, 200
Facioscapulohumeral dystrophy, 319 f.
Fanconi's syndrome, 8, 9
Fat deposition, disturbances in, 103
Fazio-Londe palsy, 443
Fever
  glandular, 306 f.
  seizures due to, 35 f., 37, 116, 236, 237
Fibrous dysplasia, 165
  polyostotic, proptosis due to, 65
Filter paper "spot test," for gargoylism, 410
Fistula, arteriovenous: complicating head injury, 198, 208
Flashing lights, provoking seizures, 38
Floppy babies, 53
  differential diagnosis, 328
  hyperlysinemia in, 400
Fluid therapy
  maintenance, by weight and surface area, 483
  parenteral, 482 f.
  in poisoning, 358
Fontanel, anterior: time of closure, 62
Food poisoning, 367 f.
Foreign bodies, intracranial: and recurrent meningitis, 283
Formula
  cow's milk
    adverse reactions to, 370, 378 f.
    and hypocalcemic tetany, 41
  lactose-free, 407
  for leucine-sensitive infants, 46

502 INDEX

Formula (*cont.*)
 low-calcium, 379
 low-phenylalanine, 395
 See also Diets
Fracture-dislocation, of spine, 218
Fractures
 skull, 198, 208 ff.
  basal, 198, 208 f.
  comminuted, 209 f.
  complications, 210 f., 213, 216 f.
  compound, 198, 210
  depressed, 198, 209, 222, 224
  diastatic, 209
  "ping-pong ball," 222, 224
 spinal, 218 ff.
  compression, 218
  with subdural hematoma ("battered-child" syndrome), 203, 204
Friedreich's ataxia, 73, 438 f.
Froehlich's syndrome, 103, 256, 257
Fructose tolerance test, 407
Fructosuria, with hypoglucosemia, 407
Fugue state, 18, 19
Fungus infections
 drug therapy of, 487
 meningoencephalitis, 281

G

Galactosemia, 391, 406 f.
 metabolic pathway block in, 406
 transferase assay test in, 406
Gamma globulin
 deficiency, in ataxia-telangiectasia, 433
 in measles encephalitis, 302
Gantrisin, neurotoxicity, 370, 376
Gargoylism, 409 f.
 classic, 408
 head enlargement in, 61
Gas gangrene infection, 336
Gaucher's disease, 9, 412 ff.
Gemonil, *see* Metharbital
Gesell
 adaptive performance test, 240
 areas of development, 4 f.
 copying test, 16
 Developmental Schedules, 4, 5, 6
Gifted children
 antisocial behavior in, 21
 poor school adjustment in, 22
Gigantism, cerebral, 103
Glaucoma, in Lowe's oculocerebrorenal syndrome, 405
Gliomas
 anterior third ventricle, 258, 259
 brain stem, 249 ff.
  vs. acute cerebellitis, 303
  diagnosis, 250 f.
  incidence, 242
  management and prognosis, 251 f.
  radiation therapy in, 245
  seeding, 250
 cerebral hemisphere, 242, 252, 253 f., 256
 intramedullary, 266, 268 f.
 optic nerve, 65, 76, 258 ff.
  neurofibromatosis in, 259
  radiation therapy in, 245
 slow-growing, 244
Glucose
 in dialysis, 475
 in isovaleric acidemia, 402
 tolerance test, intravenous, 45
Glue sniffing, 366

Glycine, defective metabolism of, 397
Glycogen storage diseases, 323 f.
Glycogenoses, muscle, 323 ff.
Gonads
 agenesis, 103
 dysgenesis, with sex chromosome abnormality, 167
Gower's maneuver, 318
Granulomas
 eosinophilic, 307
 in reticuloendothelioses, 307
Grasp reflex, 5
Growth
 defect, in hypophosphatasia, 402
 intrauterine retardation, 176, 177 f.
 somatic, disturbances in, 103
 See also Development
Growth hormone, human: in hypoglycemia, 46
Guillain-Barré syndrome, 305 f.
Guthrie test for phenylketonuria, 393 f.

H

Hair, in neurological disorders, 8, 389 ff.
Hallervorden-Spatz disease, 441
Hallucinations, in psychomotor seizures, 25
Hand dominance
 age of, 5
 in dyslexia, 70
 in stuttering, 71
Hand-Schüller-Christian syndrome, 307
Hartnup disease, 8, 9, 391, 403
 treatment, 404
Head injuries
 acute focal deficits with, 200
 birth, 221 ff.
 closed and open, 195
 coma in, 47
 irradiation, 227
 management
  depressed and compound fractures, 213, 216 f.
  with increased intracranial pressure, 212, 215
  with loss of consciousness, 212, 213 f.
  with no loss of consciousness, 212 f.
 postnatal (direct), 195 ff.
  to brain substance, 195 f.
  diagnosis, 198 ff.
  vascular, 196 ff.
 prognostic value of EEG in, 116
 seizures following, 199
 transient central blindness following, 77
Head shape
 abnormal, 62 ff.
 with premature closure of sutures, 156 ff.
Head size
 abnormal, 59 ff., 108
 in diagnosis of hydrocephalus, 138
 evaluation of, 108
 large, 61 f.
  in cerebellar astrocytoma, 245
  in hydranencephaly, 135
 measurement of, 59 f.
 normal circumferences at various ages, 488
 small, 59
  causes of, 60 f.
  in hypophosphatasia, 403
  in hypotensive hydrocephalus, 109
Head tilt, 93
Headaches, 47 ff.
 with cerebral hemisphere tumors, 252
 in hysteria, 21
 migraine, 48 f.

INDEX

organic, 47 f.
psychogenic, 48
Head-bobbing episodes, 25
Hearing deficit
  diagnosis, 7, 78 ff.
  management, 80
  prevention, 80
  screening tests for, 79 f.
  See also Deafness
Heart
  failure
    congestive, with cerebral artery aneurysm, 153
    isoproterenol in therapy, 485
  seizures, 47
  septal defects, brain abscesses in, 296 ff.
Heart disease
  congenital
    brain abscess in, 296 ff., 462
    cerebrovascular accidents in, 460
    cyanotic, thromboses in, 461
    embolization in, 463 f., 471, 472
    after maternal rubella, 173
  rheumatic, cerebral embolization in, 464
Heller's infantile dementia, 20, 416
Hemangioma, proptosis due to, 65
Hematoma
  epidural (extradural), 196, 201 f.
  intracerebral, 198, 206 ff.
  management, 212 f., 215 f.
  subdural, 196 f., 202 ff.
    in anaphylactoid purpura, 467
    of anterior, middle or posterior fossa, 196, 206, 207
    calcified, 215
    chronic relapsing juvenile, 206, 207
    convexity, 196 f., 206
    following treatment of cerebral edema, 481
    head enlargement in, 61
    infection in, 210
    prognosis, 215 f.
    subdural tap in diagnosis, 202, 203 ff.
    symptoms and signs, 203
  uncal herniation due to, 237
Hemianopia
  bitemporal, 114
  causes of, 76, 239
Hemiparesis
  following seizure, 36, 37
  following status epilepticus, 237
  in uncal herniation, 85
Hemiplegia
  acute infantile, following seizure, 36 f.
  management, 55 f.
  spastic, 55
Hemispherectomy
  indications, 144
  in spastic hemiplegia, 55, 56
Hemolytic disease of newborn, hyperbilirubinemia in, 474
Hemorrhage
  into brain stem, in uncal herniation, 85
  intracranial, 83
    asphyxia causing, 235
    in blood disorders, 263, 460 f.
    clinical signs, 238 f.
    differential diagnosis, 206 f.
    diseases causing, 263, 461 ff.
    drug therapy in, 472 f.
    hypoxic, 222, 233, 235 f.
    from injury, 196 ff., 222
    neonatal, 222 ff.
    in vascular disease, therapy, 469 f.
  with ischemic brain infarction, 459
  management, in head-injured patient, 214
  retinal, 88
  subarachnoid, 197, 235
    with spinal cord birth injury, 225
Hemorrhagic disease of newborn, therapy in, 473
Heparin
  bleeding following administration of, 470
  in cerebral embolization, 470, 472
Hepatitis, toxic: anticonvulsant-induced, 39
Hepatolenticular degeneration, 391, 436 f.
Hepatomegaly in neurologic disorders, 9
Herbicide poisoning, 355, 360 ff.
Heredity
  of achondroplasia, 164
  in classic muscular dystrophies, 317, 319
  in degenerative diseases of nervous system, 388, 389 ff.
  in idiopathic or centrencephalic epilepsy, 183 f.
  in neurologic anomalies, 127
Herniation
  of cerebellar tonsils, 85 f.
  of temporal lobe uncus, 84 ff., 236 ff.
Herpes simplex encephalitis, 282
  therapy, 292
Herpes zoster
  infection, with Bell's palsy, 304
  radiculitis, 284, 285, 292
Heteroptopias, 142, 143
Hippocampal-uncal-amygdaloid sclerosis, 233 f., 236
Hirschsprung's disease, 150 f.
Histidinemia, 389, 397
Histiocytosis X, 307 ff.
Homocystinuria, 8, 9, 390, 401
  metabolic pathway blocks in, 400
  in scoliosis patient, 98
  with spontaneous arterial thrombosis, 469
Horner's syndrome, ptosis in, 92
Horse antiserum, complications of therapy, 370, 382
Hunter's disease, 408, 410
Huntington's chorea, 439 f.
Hurler's disease, 408, 409 f.
Hydranencephaly, 135
Hydrocarbons, chlorinated: poisoning due to, 355, 362
Hydrocephalus, 60, 61
  Arnold-Chiari malformation with, 129
  congenital, 136 ff.
    communicating, 136 f., 139
    management, 139 ff.
    noncommunicating, 136, 139
    obstructive, 83
    pathogenesis, 136 f.
  head enlargement in, 61
  hypertensive, 109
  hypotensive, 109, 234
  after meningocele repair, 131 f.
  obstructive
    Dandy-Walker anomaly, 63
    with intracranial tumors, 242, 261, 262, 263
    in meningitis, 282, 283
    shunt procedures for, 262
  otitic, 83
  with platybasia, 163
  shunt procedures for, 139 f., 262
    complications of, 460, 471, 472
Hydrocortisone, in cerebral edema, 481
Hydromyelia, 147
Hydrops, meningeal, 83
Hydroxyprolinemia, 9

504 INDEX

Hygroma, subdural, 198, 208
Hyperactivity, with drug intoxication, 95
Hyperammonemia, 9, 390, 398 f.
Hyperbilirubinemia, neonatal, 474 f.
Hypercalcemia
    from excess dietary ingestion of calcium, 378 f.
    infantile, 145
Hypercapnia, 475 f.
    neurologic deficit from correction, 476
    with papilledema, 476
Hyperglycinemia, 9, 389, 397 f.
Hyperkalemia, in periodic paralysis, 342 f., 344
Hyperlysinemia, with periodic ammonia intoxication, 390, 399 f.
Hypernatremia, 370, 377
Hyperopia, convergent squint with, 89
Hyperprolinemia, 9
Hypertelorism, orbital, 63 f.
Hypertension, intracranial, 83
Hyperthermia, 104
Hyperuricemia, X-linked primary, 436
Hyperventilation
    in EEG recording, 115
    in evoking petit mal seizure, 186
Hypocalcemia
    correction, 42
    tetany due to, 41 f.
Hypoglycemia, 104
    classification of, 42, 44
    diagnosis, 42, 44 ff.
        sequence of tests in, 45
    idiopathic, 404 ff.
    in malabsorption, 476
    neonatal, 44, 405
        management, 46
    organic, 44, 45
    treatment, 46
Hypokalemia, in periodic paralysis, 342, 343 f.
Hyponatremia
    in Landry-Guillain-Barré syndrome, 305 f.
    and water intoxication, 370, 376 f.
Hypoparathyroidism, idiopathic, 43, 424 f.
Hypophosphatasia, 8, 160, 391, 402 f.
Hypoplasia, cerebral, 141, 143, 144
Hypoprothrombinemia
    intracranial hemorrhage with, 461
    treatment, 473
Hypotelorism, orbital, 63
Hypothalamus
    anterior lesions, and sexual infantilism, 103
    damage to
        in craniopharyngioma, 256, 257
        from head trauma, 198, 201
    neuroendocrinologic syndromes involving, 101 ff.
    posterior lesions, and sexual precocity, 103
Hypothermia
    in hypothalamic syndromes, 104
    in neonatal meningitis, 283
    therapeutic, in head injuries, 214
Hypothyroidism
    congenital, 421 ff.
    secondary to craniopharyngioma, 257
Hypotonia, 52
    acute, 94
    benign congenital, 53
    cerebral, 52, 53, 54
    management, 53 f.
Hypoxia
    anemic, 231
    anoxic, 231
    cerebral, defining "life or death" in, 117
    clinical signs, 238 f.
    etiologies, 230 ff., 236
    ischemic, 231
    management and prognosis, 239 f.
    maternal, and congenital anomalies, 176
    neonatal, 231 ff., 238 ff.
        intracranial hemorrhage due to, 222
    neuropathologic states caused by, 230 ff., 235 f., 239
    in occult anomalies of brain, 142
    postnatal, 231, 236 ff.
        chronic deficits resulting from, 239
    prenatal, 231, 238 ff.
        cerebral, 232
    primary cortical neuron, 236
    stagnant, 231
    tissue, due to uncal herniation, 236
Hypsarrhythmia, 28, 29
Hysteria, 21 f.
    dysarthria in, 73
    seizures in, 24, 47

I

Idiocy, amaurotic familial, 412
    types of, 414 ff.
Idoxuridine, in herpes simplex encephalitis, 292
Illiterate E test, 75, 78
Immunizations, neurotoxic reactions to, 378
Imuran, in systemic lupus erythematosus, 473
Inclusion disease
    cytomegalic in newborn, 174, 175
    subacute inclusion encephalitis, 309
Incontinentia pigmenti, 144 f.
Infantilism, sexual, 103
Infants
    chloramphenicol therapy in, 289
    evaluation of vision in, 74
    febrile convulsions in, 35
    low birth weight, 176 f.
    meningitis in, 282 f.
Infants, newborn
    cerebral seizures in, 38
    chloramphenicol therapy in, 289
    coma in, 47
    hemorrhagic disease, treatment, 473
    hyperbilirubinemia and kernicterus in, 474 f.
    hypoglycemia in, 44
    hypoxia in, 231 ff.
        clinical signs, 238 f.
        management and prognosis, 239 f.
    injuries
        to head, 221 ff.
        of peripheral nerves, 226 f.
        to spine and spinal cord, 224 ff.
    muscle tone in, 98
    neuroblastoma in, 273, 274 f.
    opisthotonus in, 98 f.
    phenylketonuric, 392
        Guthrie test in, 393 f.
Infants, premature, *see* Prematurity
Infarction, hemorrhagic cerebral, 459
Infections
    antimicrobial agents of choice in, 485 ff.
    complicating skull fracture, 210, 213, 217
    cytomegalovirus, and microcephaly, 61
    intrauterine, 239
    maternal, malformations due to, 173 ff.
    nerve deafness due to, 79
    of nervous system, 83, 279 ff.
        causing head pain, 48
        with neurotoxic organisms, 298 ff.
        prognostic value of EEG in, 116
        virus, 284 ff., 287, 292, 300 ff.

INDEX 505

orbital, 65
organic psychosis due to, 18
pyogenic, of skeletal muscle, 336
respiratory, in familial dysautonomia, 446
systemic, causing headaches, 47 f.
Injuries
  birth, 221 ff.
    causing intracranial hemorrhage, 222, 235
    to head, 221 ff.
  postnatal (direct), 195 ff.
    to brain substance, 195 f.
    causing psychotic behavior, 18
    classification, 194
    diagnosis, 198 ff.
    electric current causing, 228
    management, 211 ff.
    paratonsillar, causing carotid artery thrombosis, 469
  to peripheral nerves, 220 f.
    skull fractures, 198, 208 ff.
    to spine and spinal cord, 217 ff.
    vascular accidents, 196 ff.
  radiation, 227
  skeletal, with subdural hematoma, 203, 204
Insecticide poisoning, 355, 361 f.
Insulin
  therapy causing hypoglycemia, 370, 377 f.
  tolerance tests, hazards of, 45
Insuloma, 45, 46
Intelligence
  and learning disabilities, 22
  in patients with idiopathic epilepsy, 191
Intelligence quotient
  distribution curve, 4
  function
    in child with systemic disease, 6
    over- and underestimation, 4, 6
  in hemiplegic children, 55
  in hypocalcemic syndromes, 43
  in mentally retarded, 3 f.
  psychometric tests, 6
Intervertebral disk, calcified, 113
Intoxication
  ammonia, 398 f.
    periodic, hyperlysinemia in, 399 f.
  causing cerebral edema, 83
  causing psychotic behavior, 18
  chloramphenicol, 289
  drug
    hyperactivity due to, 95
    nystagmus due to, 91
  water, 290
  See also Poisoning
Intracranial pressure, increased, 82 ff.
  cerebellar herniation in, 85 f.
  cerebrovascular diseases causing, 462 f.
  with craniopharyngioma, 256
  diagnosis, 82 f.
  differential diagnosis, 83, 243 f.
  injuries with, management, 212, 215
  management, 84
  meningismus with, 98
  with platybasia, 163
  uncal herniation in, 84 ff.
  in vascular accidents, 201, 202
  visual deficit due to, 75 f.
Isochromosomes, 166
Isoniazid
  neurotoxicity, 296, 370, 375
  in tuberculous meningitis, 295 f.
Isopropanol poisoning, 355, 366
Isoproterenol, in cardiac failure, 485

Isotopes, radioactive: for brain scans, 112
Isovaleric acidemia, 8, 9, 390, 402

J

Jaundice
  familial nonhemolytic, 474
  neonatal, 8
Jaw-jerking, in reading epilepsy, 38
Joint, contractures, in arthrogryposis, 348
Jolly reaction, in myasthenia gravis, 339

K

Kanamycin
  neurotoxicity, 376
  in purulent meningitis, 289 f.
Karyotype, 166
Kernicterus, clinical signs, 474
Kernig sign, 282
Kerosene, toxicity due to, 355, 366
Keto acids, branched-chain: in maple syrup disease, 396
Ketogenic diet, for drug-refractory seizures, 32
Ketonil, 394
Ketonuria, branched-chain, 8, 9
Kidney
  disease
    brain pathology in, 475
    in neurological disorders, 9
  insufficiency, hypocalcemic tetany in, 42
Klinefelter's syndrome, 8, 167, 169
Klippel-Feil deformity, 58, 161 f.
Krabbe's disease, 412, 416 f., 418
Kufs' disease, 412, 414
Kugelberg-Welander atrophy, 330 f.
Kwashiorkor, effect on nervous system, 477
Kyphoscoliosis, etiologies, 97 f.

L

Laboratory studies
  of anoxic brain damage, 239
  diagnostic, 106 ff.
  in metabolic and degenerative disorders, 118
  in poisonings, 356
Labyrinth, Barany's caloric test, 91
Labyrinthitis, acute, 304
Lacerations
  cerebral, 196, 212
  of peripheral nerves, 220
  of scalp, 211, 217
Lafora's disease, 57
Landouzy-Déjerine dystrophy, 319 f.
Landry-Guillain-Barré syndrome, 305 f.
Language development, 5
Language disorders, 67 ff.
  acquired, 72 f.
  congenital, 68
  developmental, 69 ff.
  diagnostic workup, 7
  psychogenic, 73
Laurence-Moon-Biedl syndrome, 103
Lavage, gastric: in poisoning, 357
Lead poisoning, 355, 363 ff.
  antidote, 359, 365
  head enlargement in, 61
Learning disabilities, 22
Leber's optic atrophy, 443 f.
Leigh's disease, 433
Letterer-Siwe disease, 307
Leucine
  metabolism, defect in, 402

506 INDEX

Leucine (*cont.*)
  sensitivity
    milk formula in, 46
    test, 46
Leukemia
  acute
    diagnosis, 461
    nervous system involvement in, 263 ff.
    treatment of intracranial hemorrhage in, 472
  central nervous system, 266
    clinical syndromes, 264 f.
    radiation therapy, 245
  spinal epidural, 271 ff.
Leukodystrophies, 416 ff.
  differential diagnosis, 412
  globoid cell, 412, 416 f., 418
  metachromatic, 418 ff.
  Pelizaeus-Merzbacher, 418
  sudanophilic, 418, 420 f.
Leukoencephalitis
  acute hemorrhagic, 454, 455
  subacute sclerosing, 309
Leukomalacia, periventricular: due to hypoxia, 233 f.
Levallorphan, in narcotic poisoning, 359, 372
Leyden-Möbius dystrophy, 322
Light stimulation, in petit mal seizure, 186
Lightwood syndrome, 379
Lindane poisoning, 355, 362
Lipid storage disorders, 411 ff.
Lipidoses
  cerebral, head enlargement in, 61
  foam cells in, 413
  neural, 8, 411
    differential diagnosis, 412
  sulfatide, 418 ff.
Lipomas, intraspinal, 271
Locasol formula, 379
Lockjaw, 299
Lofenalac formula, 394 f.
Louis-Bar disease, 152, 433 ff.
Lowe's snydrome, 8, 9, 136, 391, 404 f.
Lückenschädel, 130
Lumbar puncture
  in chronic granulomatous meningitis, 286
  diagnostic tests, 119 f.
  importance of, 286
  in infants with possible meninigtis, 282 f.
  in pseudotumor cerebri, 84
  in spinal epidural leukemia, 272
Luminal, in petit mal seizures, 30
Lupus erythematosus, systemic, 467
  drug therapy in, 472, 473
Lysine intolerance, congenital, 9, 390
  with periodic ammonia intoxication, 399 f.

M

McArdle's syndrome, 323
Macrocrania, 59, 61 f., 108
Macula, degeneration, 8
Malabsorption
  with hypocalcemia, 42
  with hypoglycemia, 476
  methionine, 391, 404
  tryptophan, 403
Malathion poisoning, 359, 361
Malformations, congenital, 8, 125 ff.
  of autonomic nervous system, 150 f.
  of basal ganglia, cerebellum and brain stem, 145 ff.
  of brain, 47, 53, 141 ff.
  chromosome abnormalities, 166 ff.
  defects in development of ventricular system, 136 ff.
  drugs causing, 175 f.
  excess irradiation causing, 176
  of head, 62 ff.
  from incompelte closure of neural tube, 127 ff.
  infantile hypercalcemia syndrome, 145
  in infants of diabetic mothers, 176
  and learning impairment, 22
  maternal infections causing, 173 ff.
  of muscles, 345 ff.
  in myositis ossificans, 335
  and neonatal seizures, 38
  of skull and spine, 156 ff.
  of speech organs, 68
  of spinal cord and peripheral nerves, 147 ff.
  vascular, 151 ff.
  See also specific anomalies
Malingering, 21
Malnutrition
  effect on nervous system, 477
  maternal, and congenital anomalies, 176
Mannitol, in cerebral edema, 481
Maple syrup disease, 389, 396
Marcus Gunn phenomenon, 146
Marfan's syndrome
  in scoliosis patient, 98
Marie-Strümpell encephalitis, 36 f.
Measles
  encephalomyelitis, 300, 301 ff.
  German, *see* Rubella
Median nerve injuries, 220, 221
Medulla, congenital anomalies of, 147 ff.
Medulloblastoma, cerebellar, 242, 245, 247 ff.
Megacolon, aganglionic, 150 f.
Megalencephaly, 61 f., 142
Megaloureters, 151
Meiosis, nondisjunction in, 166, 167 f.
Memory for Designs test, 6
Meninges, laceration and avulsion of, 211, 217
Meningioma, 269
Meningismus, 93, 98, 99
Meningitis, 47
  acute bacterial, 280 ff.
    brain changes in, 281 f.
    etiologic agents, 280 f.
    diagnosis, 282 f., 286 f.
    meningismus with, 98
    prevention, 291
    prognosis, 291
    specific therapy, 289, 291
    unknown etiology, therapy, 288 ff.
  age distribution, 284
  aseptic, 99, 306
  chronic, head enlargement in, 61
  chronic granulomatous, 83, 282, 283, 286, 288
    specific therapy, 295 f.
  coccidioidal, 286, 288
    therapy, 296
  with compound skull fracture, 210, 213
  cryptococcal, 286, 288
    therapy, 296
  leptospiral, 286
  neonatal, 283
  purulent, 283, 286 f.
    microorganisms causing, 289, 291
    therapy, 288 ff.
  recurrent, 283
  tuberculous, 282, 286
    therapy, 295 f.
Meningocele
  lacunar skull with, 150

INDEX

orbital, 133
spinal, 128
Meningococcemia, petechiae in, 282
Meningoencephalitis, 279
  cerebrospinal fluid profiles, 286 f.
  congenital, 280
  EEG in, 117, 292, 293
  epidemiology, 280 f.
  pathogenesis, 280 f.
  viral
    diagnosis, 283 f., 287 f.
    pathology in, 282
    prevention, 292
    prognosis, 292
    therapy, 291 f.
  See also Meningitis, acute bacterial
Meningoencephalocele
  cranium bifidum with, 132 ff.
  management, 130 ff.
  spina bifida with, 128 ff.
Mental retardation, 3 ff.
  apparent deafness in, 79
  with chromosomal abnormalities, 167, 168, 169 f., 171
  counseling of parents, 10
  developmental progress, 5, 11
  diagnosis, 4 ff., 7
  differential diagnosis, 6 ff.
  educable children, 3
  etiologic factors, 7 ff.
  impaired language development in, 68
  medical therapy, 10
  pathologic, 3 f.
  physiologic, 3 f.
  prognosis, 10 f.
  recommendation for institutionalization, 12
  recurrence risks, 12 f.
  sociopathic tendencies in, 13
  special educational help, 11 f.
  trainable children, 4
Meperidine, in deep-sedation mixture, 487
Mephenesin, in strychnine poisoning, 362
Mephenytoin
  reactions to, 39
  in seizure control, 33, 34
Mephobarbital, for generalized and focal seizures, 33, 34
6-Mercaptopurine, neurotoxicity, 370
Mercury poisoning, 355, 359, 370, 381
Merrill-Palmer test, 6
Mestinon, for myasthenia gravis, 340
Metabolic disorders, 47
  with anomalies of brain, 142
  causing cerebral seizures, 38, 236, 388 ff.
  diagnosis, 118, 239
  hereditary, 99, 388 ff., 436 f.
  muscle glycogenoses, 323 ff.
  neuropathology, 101 ff.
Metal intoxication, 13
Metaraminol, in shock, 485
Methanol poisoning, 355, 365
Metharbital, in generalized and focal seizures, 33, 34
Methicillin
  in purulent meningitis, 288 ff.
Methionine
  malabsorption, 8, 391, 404
  metabolism, disorders of, 400
Methotrexate
  in CNS leukemia, 265
  in intracranial hemorrhage, 472
Methsuximide, in petit mal seizures, 31
Methylphenidate, in narcolepsy, 50

Methylprednisolone, in cerebral edema, 481
Methysergide maleate
  for headaches, 49
  toxic reactions to, 381
Microcephaly, 59, 60, 61
Microcrania, 59, 60 f., 108, 142
Microphthalmia, 136
Micropolygyria, 142, 143
Migraine
  abdominal, 26
  classic, 48, 49
Mineral metabolism, hereditary disease of, 436 f.
Mirror movements, 58, 162
Mirror writing, 69, 70
Mitosis, nondisjunction in, 166
Möbius' syndrome, 146
Mongolism, 168
  chromosomal abnormalities in, 167, 168, 170, 171
  recurrence risk in, 172
Mononucleosis, infectious, 306 f.
Monosomy, 166, 169
  partial 18, 172
  partial 21, 171
Moro reflex, 5
Morphine sulfate sedation, with digitalization, 471, 472
Morquio's disease, 408, 410 f.
Motor deficit, see Motor disorders; Perceptual-motor disabilities
Motor disorders
  acute involuntary, 95
  acute motor neuron weakness, 93 f.
  chronic, 52 ff.
  speech difficulties in, 68
  focal neurological signs, 87 ff.
  in hysteria, 21 f.
  See also specific disorders
Mucopolysaccharide disorders, 408 ff.
Mull-soy formula, 407
Mumps meningoencephalitis, 286, 287, 300, 302
Muscles
  biopsy, 120 f.
  congenital absence of, 345 f.
  congenital contractures, 346 ff.
  disorders of, 314 ff.
  extraocular, imbalance, 88 ff.
  glycogenoses, 323 ff.
  tone, see also Hypotonia
    in neonate, 98
    sudden loss of, 50
  weakness, see also Paralysis
    acute, 93
    biopsy in evaluation, 120
    periodic, 94
Mushroom poisoning, 355, 359, 367
Myasthenia gravis, 337 ff.
  juvenile, 338 f., 340
  neonatal, 339 f.
  Tensilon test for, 239
  ptosis in, 92
Myelitis, transverse, 454
Myelography, 113 f.
Myelomalacia, from irradiation, 227
Myocarditis
  cerebral embolization in, 464 ff.
    congestive failure following, 470 f.
  drug therapy in, 471, 472
Myoclonus, 25, 57
Myoglobinuria, familial, 325
Myopathies, 314, 316 ff.
  biopsy in diagnosis, 120
  distal, 322

Myopathies (*cont.*)
 hereditary, 316 ff.
  with distinctive structural defects, 325 f.
 nonhereditary, 326
 ocular, 322
Myophosphorylase deficiency, 323, 324
Myopia, divergent squint with, 89
Myositis, 316, 333 ff.
 microbial and parasitic, 336 f.
 in orbital cellulitis, 309 f.
 ossificans, 335 f.
 of unknown etiology, 333 ff.
Myotonia congenita, 344
Myotonia dystrophica, 320 ff.

N

Nalorphine, in narcotic poisoning, 359, 372
Narcolepsy, treatment, 50
Narcotic poisoning, 355, 372
 antidotes, 359
Nemaline myopathy, 326
Nephroblastoma, *see* Wilms' tumor
Nephrosis, drug-induced, 31, 39
Neural tube, incomplete closure, 127 ff.
Neurilemmomma, extramedullary intradural, 269
Neurinoma
 acoustic, 91, 108
 extramedullary intradural, 269
Neuritis
 of facial nerve, *see* Bell's palsy
 optic, 453 f.
 retrobulbar, 455 f.
Neuroblastoma, 65, 273, 275 f.
Neuroblastomas, irradiation in, 245
Neurofibroma, 65
 of cranial and spinal nerves, 269, 430 f.
Neurofibromatosis, 8, 430 ff.
 with extramedullary intradural tumors, 269 f.
Neurofibrosarcoma, 270
Neuromuscular transmission, disorders of, 315, 316, 337 ff., 341 ff.
Neuromyelitis optica, 48, 454 f.
Neurons, cortical: loss due to anoxia, 233 f., 236
Nevus, port-wine facial, 152
Nicotinamide, in Hartnup disease, 404
Niemann-Pick disease, 9, 411 f., 413
Nightmares, 49
Nitrofurantoin, neurotoxicity, 375
Nondisjunction, in cell division, 166, 167 f.
Numbness, 96
Nutramigen formula, 407
Nystagmus, 91 f.
 optickinetic, 74
 pendular, 75

O

"Oasthouse urine" disease, 404
Obstetric injuries
 of head, 222 f.
 of spinal cord, 53, 224 ff.
Oculocerebrorenal syndrome, 8, 9, 136, 391, 404 f.
Oculomotor apraxia, 70, 90 f.
Odors, in diagnosis of neurological disorders, 8, 389 ff.
Olfactory nerve, injury to, 200
Opisthotonus, 98
 etiology, 99
 in meningitis, 282
 in tetanus, 299
Opsoclonus, 91 f.

Optic chiasm
 gliomas in, 258 ff.
 lesions and visual deficit, 75 f.
Optic foramen, x-ray evaluation, 108
Optic nerve
 atrophy, 76, 87 f., 259, 443 f.
 avulsion of, 200
 congenital aplasia, 136
 gliomas, 65, 76, 108, 258 ff.
 head, papilledema, 84
 inflammation, 453 f.
 lesions of, 75 f.
 leukemic infiltration, 264
Optic tract, lesions of, 76
Orbit
 chronic cellulitis of, 309 f.
 fibrous dysplasia of, 165
 infections, 65
 tumors causing proptosis, 65 f.
Osteomas, skull, 277
Osteopetrosis, 164 f.
Otorrhea
 cerebrospinal fluid, management, 213, 217
 with compound fracture, 211, 213
Oxycephaly, 157, 158
Oxygen therapy
 adverse reactions, 370, 382
 in management of poisonings, 358, 363

P

Pachygyria, 142, 143
Pain
 abdominal
  in hysteria, 21
  in visceral seizures, 26
 congenital insensitivity to, 149 f.
 of neural origin, 96
Pallidotomy, 58, 442
Palsy, *see* Bell's palsy; Cerebral palsy; Paralysis
PAM therapy, in organic phosphate poisoning, 359, 362
Papilledema, 84, 114
 in acute meningitis, 283
 in brain stem glioma, 251
 differential diagnosis, 84
 with hypercapnia, 476
 in Landry-Guillain-Barré syndrome, 305
Papilloma, choroid plexus, 249, 262
Para-aminosalicylic acid
 side effects, 296
 in tuberculous meningitis, 295 f.
Paraldehyde, in status epilepticus, 480
Paralysis
 congenital facial, 146
 extraocular muscle, 88
 familial periodic, 341 ff.
 Landry's ascending, 305
 oculomotor, 92
 progressive bulbar, 443
 pseudobulbar, 54 f., 56
 sixth nerve, 82, 90, 146
 third nerve, 85, 90, 92, 146
 tick, 355, 368
 in virus infections, 284, 285
Paramethadione
 in petit mal seizures, 31
 reactions to, 39
Paramyoclonus multiplex, 57
Paramyotonia congenita, 344
Paraplegia, 55, 56 f.
 hereditary spastic, 331 ff.
 in multiple sclerosis, 455, 456

INDEX 509

Parathion poisoning, 359, 361 f.
Parathormone deficiency, 424 f.
Parinaud syndrome, 261
Parkinsonism, postencephalitic, 292
Pelizaeus-Merzbacher disease, 412, 418
Penicillamine, in Wilson's disease, 437
Penicillin
  in congenital syphilis, 175
  neurotoxicity, 370, 375
  in purulent meningitis, 288 ff.
  in rheumatic chorea, 471, 472
Perceptual-motor disabilities
  psychometric evaluation, 6, 14 ff.
  special education in, 16
  tests for, 6
Peripheral nerves
  disorders, differentiation, 330
  hereditary sensory radicular neuropathy, 149
  injuries to, 220 f.
    birth, 226
    radiation, 227
  neurofibromatosis, 430
Personality
  changes
    with brain tumors, 242 f.
    due to postseizure encephalopathy, 37
    post-traumatic, 201
  disorders, EEG in, 116
Pertussis encephalomyelitis, 300, 302
Pes cavus, in Friedreich's ataxia, 438
Pesticide poisoning, 355, 360 ff.
PGSR test, 79 f.
Phenacemide
  causing toxic hepatitis, 39
  in seizures, 33, 34 f.
Phenistix test, 393
Phenobarbital
  in behavior disorders, 17
  in cerebral seizures, 30, 33, 240
  maintenance anticonvulsant therapy, 36
  in rheumatic chorea, 471, 472
  sodium
    in prolonged convulsions, 480
    in status epilepticus, 480
Phenothiazines
  antidote for, 359, 373
  toxic reactions, 372 f.
Phenoxyacetic acids, chlorinated: poisoning due to, 355, 360 f.
Phensuximide, in petit mal, 31
Phenylalanine level
  dietary control of, 394 f.
  in phenylketonuria, 392
Phenylketonuria, 8, 9, 389
  low-phenylalanine diet in, 394 f.
  maternal, 396
  metabolic pathway block in, 392
  screening tests for, 393 f.
  status epilepticus in, 238
Phosphates, organic: poisoning due to, 355, 359, 361
Phosphofructokinase deficiency, muscle, 324, 325
Photic stimulation
  in EEG recording, 115
  of petit mal seizure, 186
Physical examination
  in children with proptosis, 65
  in mentally retarded, to determine etiology, 7 f.
Physical therapy in spastic hemiplegia, 55 f.
Pineal gland
  calcified, on skull x-ray, 108
  tumor, 261, 262
Pitressin, in diabetes insipidus, 104

Pituitary
  damage
    in basal fracture, 198
    with craniopharyngioma, 256, 257
  fossa, estimation of enlargement, 491 f.
Placenta
  abnormalities, 231
  insufficiency, 232
  vascular accidents causing anoxic brain damage, 231
Plagiocephaly, 157
Platybasia, 162 ff.
Pleurodynia, epidemic, 336 f.
Pneumoencephalography, 107, 109, 110 f.
  in brain stem glioma, 250, 251
  in cerebellar astrocytoma, 247
  in congenital hydrocephalus, 137, 138
  in localization of brain tumors, 244
  in occult anomalies of brain, 142 f.
  in optic glioma, 260
  in pseudotumor cerebri, 83
  in retardation, 9 f.
  in subdural hematoma, 205
Pneumography, 107, 109
  cerebral, discovery of diagnostic value, 211
  complications, 111
  in diagnosis of cranial anomalies, 133 f.
  pneumoencephalography vs. ventriculography, 110 f.
Pneumonia
  chemical, kerosene causing, 366
  in poisonings with volatile hydrocarbons, 356, 358
Poison control centers, 354
Poisoning, 352 ff.
  causing stupor in children, 47
  clinical manifestations, 354 ff.
  laboratory diagnosis, 356
  list of toxic agents, 352, 355
  management, 356 ff.
  poison prevention kit, 357
  See also Intoxications; specific agents
Poliomyelitis
  bulbar, 285, 292
  immunization, 292, 294 f.
  nervous system changes in, 282
  paralytic, 284
Polyarteritis nodosa, 466 f.
  prednisone in, 471
Polymyositis, 333 ff.
Polymyxin B, in meningitis, 289 f.
Polyneuritis
  diphtheritic, 300
  infectious, 305 f., 328
Polysaccharidoses, 407 ff.
Pompe's disease, 323
Porencephaly, 141, 142, 143
Potassium, serum: in familial periodic paralysis, 341, 343
Prednisolone, in cerebral edema, 481
Prednisone
  in Bell's palsy, 301, 305
  in CNS leukemia, 265
  in encephalomyelitis, 302
  in herpes zoster radiculitis, 292
  in hypoglycemia, 46
  in idiopathic thrombocytopenic purpura, 463, 473
  in intracranial hemorrhage, 472, 473
  in minor motor epilepsy, 28
  in myocarditis, 471, 472
  in polyarteritis, 471

Prednisone (cont.)
　in sarcoidosis, 311
　in systemic lupus erythematosus, 472, 473
Pregnancy
　complications causing fetal brain damage, 8
　infections causing malformations, 173 ff.
Prematurity
　brain hemorrhage in, 233, 235 f.
　head asymmetry in, 62
　in infants of diabetic mothers, 176
　neonatal hypoxia in, 231 ff.
　neurologic complications of, 176 f.
　placental abnormalities in, 231
Primidone, in seizures, 33, 34
Promethazine, in deep-sedation mixture, 487
Proptosis, 65 f., 133
Prostigmin test, in myasthenia gravis, 339
Protamine sulfate, in heparin therapy, 470
Protein, cerebrospinal fluid
　in diagnosis, 119 f.
　in leukodystrophies, 418
Protozoa, causing meningoencephalitis, 281
Pseudobulbar palsy, 54 f., 56
Pesudo-Hurler's disease, 411
Pseudohypoparathyroidism, 425 f.
Pseudoprematurity, 177 f.
Pseudotumor
　cerebri, 76, 83 f.
　orbital, 309 f.
Psychogalvanometric skin-resistance test, 79 f.
Psychometric tests of intellectual functioning, 6
Psychosis
　functional, in childhood, 18
　organic
　　drug therapy in, 18
　　EEG in, 116
Ptosis, 92, 345
Pupils
　in hysteria, 21
　inequality of, 92
　in posterior third ventricle tumors, 261
Purpura
　anaphylactoid, 467 f.
　　drug therapy in, 472, 473
　idioapthic thrombocytopenic
　　with cerebrovascular accident, 463
　　treatment, 463, 469, 473
Pyloric stenosis, 151
Pyridoxine deficiency and dependency, 426 f.
Pyrimethamine, in toxoplasmosis, 175

Q

Quadriplegia, 55, 56
Quinine, effect on fetus, 175

R

Rabies, 286
　postexposure treatment, 294, 295
Radial nerve injuries, 220, 221
Radiation
　effect on fetus, 176
　injury to nervous system, 227
Radiation therapy
　in brain stem glioma, 251 f.
　in brain tumors, 245
　in cerebellar medulloblastoma, 248 f.
　in cerebral hemisphere tumors, 256
　in CNS leukemia, 265
　in ependymoma, 249
　in neuroblastoma, 275
　in optic glioma, 261
　in Wilms' tumor, 265
Radiculitis, herpes zoster, 285
Radioisotopic scans
　in cerebellar astrocytoma, 246
　in localization of brain tumors, 243, 244
Ramsay-Hunt syndrome, 57, 304
Rathke's pouch cyst, see Craniopharyngioma
Reading disabilities, in oculomotor apraxia, 90 f.
Reading epilepsy, 38
Reading retardation, 69 f., 73
von Recklinghausen's disease, 65, 430 ff.
Reflexes
　grasp, 5
　Moro, 5
　primitive, 5
　in spinal bifida with meningomyelocele, 128
Refractive errors, estimating, 75
Reserpine, in rheumatic chorea, 471, 472
Respiratory disease, chronic: nervous system manifestations, 475 f.
Respiratory distress
　with cord injury at birth, 225, 226
　management, in head-injured patient, 214
　relief, in poisonings, 358
Resuscitation, in neonatal hypoxia, 239 f.
Reticuloendothelioses, 411 ff.
　diagnosis, 307, 412
　treatment, 307 ff.
Retina
　hemorrhages, 88
　lesions, 8
　pigmentary degeneration of, 445
Retinitis pigmentosa, 445
Retrolental fibroplasia, oxygen therapy and, 382
Rhabdomyosarcoma, 65
Rhachischisis, complete, 128
Rheumatic disease
　chorea in, 18, 466
　　drug therapy, 471, 472
　of heart, cerebral emboli in, 464
Rhinorrhea
　cerebrospinal fluid
　　management, 213, 217
　　tests for, 210 f., 213
　in head injuries, 210
Rickets, vitamin-D-resistant, 8, 9, 41
Riley-Day snydrome, 149
Ring chromosomes, 166, 170, 171
Rinne test, 80
Ritalin, in narcolepsy, 50
Rodenticide poisoning, 355, 360 ff.
Rorschach test, 6
Rubella
　encephalitis, 300, 302
　maternal, malformations due to, 173
　prophylaxis, 173, 295
　syndrome, 136

S

St. Vitus' dance, see Chorea
Salaam attacks, 25
Salicylate intoxication, 355, 374
Salivary gland virus, prenatal infection with, 174, 175
Salt, overload, 370, 377
Sanfillipo's disease, 408, 410
Sarcoidosis
　diagnosis, 311
　nervous system involvement in, 310 f.
Sarcoma
　giant cell, of cerebral hemisphere, 255

intraspinal, 266, 270, 276
  skull, 277
Scalp, avulsion of, 211, 217
Scaphocephaly, 156, 157, 160
Scapula, congenital malposition of, 347 f.
Scheie's disease, 408, 411
Schilder's disease, 77, 83, 412, 420 f.
Schönlein-Henoch syndrome, 467 f.
Schwannoma, extramedullary intradural, 269
Sciatic nerve injuries, from intramuscular injections, 220 f.
Sclerosis
  diffuse cerebral, 412, 416 ff.
  hippocampal-uncal-amygdaloid, 233 f., 236
  juvenile amyotrophic lateral, 331 ff.
  multiple, 455 ff.
    clinical syndromes in, 455 f.
    and optic neuritis, 454
  tuberous, 8, 427 ff.
Scoliosis
  etiology, 97 f.
  with syringomyelia, 131
Scotomata, 114
Screening test of intellectual functioning, 6
Seconal sodium, in prolonged convulsions, 480
Sedatives
  in behavior disorders, 17 f.
  in cerebral seizures, 27, 30, 33, 240
  with digitalization, 471, 472
  mixture for diagnostic and therapeutic procedures, 487
Seizures
  absence, 25, 185, 186
  in asphyxiated neonates, 240
  cardiac, 47
  clinical types, 25 ff.
  in degenerative diseases, 388 ff.
  in drug intoxications, 370
  drug therapy, 27 ff.
    of prolonged acute, 480 f.
  in exanthem subitum, 302
  febrile, 35 f., 37, 189, 234, 236 f.
  focal cortical origin of, 26
  fugue state and aphasia with, 18, 19
  in hereditary metabolic disorders, 388 ff.
  in hypoxia, 236, 239
  hysterical, 24, 47
  in intracranial tumors, 243, 252 f., 254
  Jacksonian, 25
  in meningitis, 282, 290
  neonatal, 38
  in poisoning, 358, 364
  post-traumatic, 199
  psychomotor, 25, 26, 32, 116, 186, 254
  surgery for, 38
  as systemic sign in neurological deficit, 9
  with vascular malformations, 152
  in water intoxication, 290
  See also Epilepsy
Sella turcica
  deformity, in optic glioma, 259, 260
  in skull x-rays, 108
Sense of smell: loss, with head injury, 200
Sense of taste: loss, with head injury, 200
Sensory neuroapthy, hereditary radicular, 442
Sensory stimuli, provoking seizures, 38
Sensory symptoms, hysterical, 21
Septicemia, 47
Serum
  chromatography, in maple syrup disease, 396
  rabies, hyperimmune, 294, 295
  sickness, 382
Sex chromosomes, 166

abnormalities
  and criminal behavior, 169 f.
  in number, 167, 169 f.
  triplo-X complement, 169
Sexual development
  delayed, 103
  precocious, 102 f.
  with pineal tumors, 261
Shagreen patches, 8
Shock
  cause of, 484
  treatment, 484 f.
    commercial fluids in, 484
    in head-injured patient, 214
    in poisoning, 358
Shoulder, congenital elevation of, 346, 347
Shoulder-girdle weakness, 94
Shunt procedures
  in craniopharyngioma, 257
  for hematoma, 215
  for hydrocephalus, 139 f.
Sinuses
  air, fractures into, 208, 211
  dermal, 128 f., 283
Skeletal deformities
  in hypophosphatasia, 402 f.
  in neurological disorders, 8
Skin
  clinical signs in neurological disorders, 8
  lesions
    in dermatomyositis, 333 f.
    in neurofibromatosis, 430, 431
    in tuberous sclerosis, 428, 429
  vascular nevi with angiomas, 152
Skull
  abnormalities, 8
    in diagnosis, 62 f.
    head enlargement in, 61
  defects, with meningocele, 132 ff.
  epidermoid cyst, 134
  fibrous dysplasia of, 165
  lacunar, 130
  sutures
    premature closure of, 156 ff.
    x-ray interpretation, 108
  thickening of, evaluation, 108
  traction, for spinal injuries, 218 f.
  tumors of, 276 f., 307, 308
  x-rays
    in cerebellar astrocytoma, 246, 247
    in craniostenosis, 159 f.
    in diagnosis, 107, 108 f.
    in diagnosis of increased pressure, 82
    in hemiparesis, 55
    in localization of brain tumors, 244
    in optic glioma, 259
    in tuberous sclerosis, 428
Skull fractures, 198
  basal, complications, 198, 210 f., 283
  comminuted, 209 f.
  complications, 210 f., 213, 216 f.
  compound, 198, 208, 210
    treatment, 213, 217
  depressed, 198, 209, 222, 224
    treatment, 213, 216 f.
  diastatic, 209
  linear, 198, 208 f.
  neonatal, 222, 224
  "ping-pong ball," 222, 224
Sleep
  deprivation, EEG recordings after, 116
  EEG recordings, 115
Sleepiness, excessive, 50

Smallpox encephalomyelitis, 300, 302
Snake bites, 368 ff.
Snellen charts, 75, 78
Sodium glutamate, in hypoglycemia, 46
Solvents
    poisoning due to, 365, 366
    sniffing of, 366 f.
Spasm, torsion, 441 f.
Spasmus nutans, 90
Spasticity, 54 ff.
    in degenerative diseases, 388 ff.
Speech
    development, 5, 68
        slow, 68, 239
    disorders, 68, 70 f., 73, 78
    therapy, 68
Spelling problems, in dyslexia, 69
Spider bites, 355, 368
Spielmeyer-Vogt disease, 412, 414
Spina bifida
    with meningomyelocele, 128 ff.
    prognosis, 131
    occulta, 128 f., 132
Spinal canal
    incomplete closure of, 128
    width, measurements of, 113
Spinal cord
    compression
        with extramedullary tumor, 271
        treatment of, 219
    congenital anomalies of, 147 ff., 161
    injuries
        obstetric, 224 ff.
        postnatal, 217 ff.
    tumors, 266 ff.
Spine
    anomalies, head enlargement in, 61
    cervical, failure of vertebral segmentation, 161 f.
    deformities, 97 f.
        mirror movements in, 58
    sprain, subluxation and fracture, 217 ff.
    upper limits of normal vertebral interpediculate distances, 490 f.
    x-rays, interpretation, 112 f.
Splenomegaly, 9
Sprain, of neck and lower back, 217 f.
Sprengel's deformity, 162, 346, 347
Squint
    in brain stem glioma, 250
    in cerebellar astrocytoma, 245
    convergent, 89
    divergent, 89
    long-standing, effect on vision, 77 f., 88
    nonparalytic, 88 f.
    paralytic, 90
    therapy and prognosis, 77 f., 89
Stammering, see Stuttering
Stanford-Binet test, 6, 240
Status epilepticus, 36, 37, 83
    hypoxic brain damage following, 237, 238
    treatment, 480 f.
Steinert's disease, 320 ff.
Stick test, in phenylketonuria, 393
Stimulants, in behavior disorders, 17 f.
Stomach
    aspiration, in poisonings, 357
    lavage, in poisoning, 357
Strabismus, see Squint
Streptomycin
    in meningitis, 289, 295 f.
    neurotoxicity, 296, 370, 375
Strokes, see Cerebrovascular accidents

Strychnine poisoning, 355, 362
Stupor, 9
Sturge-Weber syndrome, 152
Stuttering, 70 f.
Subdural space
    cerebrospinal fluid in, 198, 205
    empyema, 210
    See also Hematoma, subdural
Subdural tap, 202
    technique, 203 ff.
    in treatment of hematoma, 215
Subluxation of spine, 218, 219
Sulfadiazine
    in neonatal toxoplasmosis, 175
    in purulent meningitis, 289, 291
    in rheumatic chorea, 472
Sulkowitch test, 425
Sutures, see Cranial sutures
Sweat, inability to, 149
Sydenham's chorea, 466
Syncope, 41
Syndactyly, with craniostenosis, 157, 159
Syphilis, congenital, 65, 174 f.
Syringobulbia, 129, 147, 148 f.
Syringomyelia, 58, 129, 147 f., 161 f.

T

Tachycardia, paroxysmal auricular, 47
Talipes, congenital, 346
Tay-Sachs disease, 412, 414, 415
Temperature, body: disturbances in regulation, 104
Tensilon test, in myasthenia gravis, 239, 339, 340
Teratomas, 65, 266, 276
    intraspinal, 271
Testosterone, oral: in aplastic anemia, 472
Tetanus, 298, ff.
    antitoxin, dosage, 299
    toxoid, dosage, 300
Tetany, 41 f.
    hypocalcemic, differential diagnosis, 41, 43
Tetracyclines, neurotoxicity, 370, 374
Tetralogy of Fallot, cerebral embolization in, 464
Thalidomide, congenital anomalies due to, 147, 175 f.
Thallium poisoning, 355, 359, 361
Thematic Apperception Tests, 6
Thomsen's disease, 344
Thrombocytopenic purpura, with cerebrovascular accident, 463
Thrombosis
    arterial, 460 f., 469
        therapy, 472, 473
    incidence in childhood, 468
    mechanisms predisposing to, 468 f.
    septic, 296 f.
        treatment, 474
    venous, 461, 462, 469
        in meningitis, 281, 283
Thymectomy, in myasthenia, 341
"Thymic syndrome," in ataxia-telangiectasia, 433
Thyroid, dessicated: in cretinism, 423
Tick paralysis, 355, 368
Tingling, 96
Todd's palsy, 36, 93
Tolbutamide tolerance test, 45
Torticollis, 346, 347
Toxoplasmosis, 8, 174, 175
Tracheostomy, for head-injured patient, 214
Transferase assay test, for galactosemia, 406
Tranquilizers
    in behavior disorders, 17 f.

toxic reactions, 355, 359, 372 f.
   See also Chlorpromazine
Transillumination
   in brain anomalies, 135, 143, 144, 238
   in diagnosis of cranial defects, 133, 134
   in subdural bleeding, 203
Translocation of chromosomes, 166, 170
Trauma, see Injuries
Trephination, in treatment of hematoma, 212 f., 215
Triamcinolone, in cerebral edema, 481
Trichinosis, 337
Trigeminal nerve, injury to, 200
Trigonencephaly, 157, 158 f.
Trimethadione
   in petit mal seizures, 31
   reactions to, 39
Triplo-X syndrome, 167, 169
Trismus, in tetanus, 299
Trisomy, 166, 167, 168 f., 170
   in D group, 136, 167, 169
   in E group, 167, 168 f.
   in G group, 167, 168
Tromethamine therapy, in extreme acidosis, 374
Trousseau's sign, 41, 42
Tuberculomas, intracranial, 286
Tumors
   cerebellar, 245 ff.
   congenital, 256, 266, 276 f.
      location, 269, 271
   intracranial, 61, 83, 241 ff.
      brain stem, 249 ff., 303
      calcification in, 109
      clinical diagnosis, 242 f.
      diagnostic procedures in localization, 108 f., 243 f., 254, 255
      diencephalic, 103
      differential diagnosis, 243 f.
      head enlargement in, 61
      incidence, 242
      intraventricular, 247 ff., 261, 262
      management and prognosis, 244 f.
      metastatic, 263 ff.
      optic nerve, 65, 76, 108, 258 ff.
      parasellar, 256 ff.
      posterior fossa, 245 ff., 252
      subtentorial, 245 ff.
      supratentorial, 252 ff.
   intraspinal
      differential diagnosis, 266 ff.
      extradural, 266, 271 ff.
      extramedullary intradural, 267, 269 ff.
      intramedullary, 267, 268 f.
   myelography in, 113 f.
Tunnel vision, 114
Turner's syndrome, 8, 169, 170
Turricephaly, 157, 158
2,4-D poisoning, 355, 360 f.
Tyrosinemia, neonatal, 401 f.
Tyrosinosis, 8, 9, 390, 401 f.

U

Ulegyria, occipital, 238
Ulnar nerve injuries, 220, 221
Umbilical cord torsion, causing anoxic brain damage, 231
Uncal herniation, 84 ff., 236 ff.
Unverricht's disease, 57, 440 f.
Urea
   in cerebral edema, 481
   subdural bleeding complicating, 197
   cycle, hereditary metabolic defects in, 398 f.

Uric acid metabolism, inherited defect in, 436
Urine
   chromatography
      in maple syrup disease, 396
      for o-OH phenylacetic acid, 395
   diagnostic tests, 9, 118, 119
      in lead and arsenic poisoning, 356
      for maple syrup disease, 396
   drop test, false-positive results, 393
   normal values, 493 f.

V

Vaccination, encephalomyelitis after, 300, 302
Vaccine
   duck embryo, in rabies, 294, 295
   poliomyelitis, 292, 294 f.
   for rubella, 295
   triple, toxic reactions to, 378
Vagal stimulation, in cardiac seizures, 47
Valium
   in minor motor epilepsy, 28
   in status epilepticus, 480
Varicella infection, 284, 292
   with Bell's palsy, 301, 304
Vasculitis, see Collagen vascular disease
Vasopressor agents, in shock, 485
Velban, in reticuloendothelioses, 307 f.
Ventricles
   colloid cyst of, 262 f.
   defects in development, 136 ff.
   enlargement
      determining, 489
      in differentiation of hydrocephalus, 109
   normal measurements of lateral pneumogram, 490
   tumors of, 247 ff., 261 f.
Ventriculography
   air, in localization of brain tumors, 244, 249
   choice over pneumoencephalography, 110 f.
   combined with pneumoencephalography, in glioma, 251
   Pantopaque, 111
   in localization of brain tumors, 244, 246
Versenate therapy, in Wilson's disease, 437
Vertebrae
   anomalies, 113
   atlantoaxial dislocation, 218
   cervical, failure of segmentation, 161 f.
   fractures of, 218
   upper limits of interpediculate distances, 490 f.
Vertigo, 26
   periodic, 49
Vinblastine
   neurotoxicity, 370, 378
   in reticuloendothelioses, 307 f.
Vincristine
   in intracranial hemorrhage, 472
   neurotoxicity, 370, 378
Vineland Social Maturity Scale, 6
Virus infections
   acute cerebellitis as, 303
   encephalomyelitis as complication, 300 ff.
   maternal, effects in newborn, 175
   rubella, 173
   salivary gland, 174, 175
   of muscle, 336 f.
   of nervous system, 280 f.
      cerebrospinal fluid findings, 287
      diagnosis, 283 ff.
      pathology, 282
   See also specific viruses and diseases
Visceral seizures, 26

Vision
  acuity, evaluation of, 74 f.
  conservation-of-sight programs, 78
  field of
    evaluation in diagnosis, 114
    in supratentorial tumors, 253, 255
    hereditary degenerative diseases, 443 ff.
    with increased intracranial pressure, 82
    in methanol poisoning, 365
    neurologic causes, 75 ff.
    ocular causes, 77 f.
    screening tests for, 75, 78
  impairment of, 74
    with brain tumors, 243
    central, 75
    in cerebellar astrocytoma, 245
    diagnostic workup, 7
  See also Blindness
Visual-Motor Gestalt test, 6
Visual perception, impaired, 6
Visual seizures, 26
Vitamin
  A intoxication, 379, 380
  B_6
    administration, 427
    deficiency and dependency, 426 f.
    therapeutic trial, 118
  D
    deficiency, and tetany, 41 f.
    hypersensitivity, 370, 378
  D_2, in chronic hypoparathyroidism, 425
  deficiencies, effects on nervous system, 476 f.
  K
    adverse reactions to, 370, 379
    prophylaxis of hemorrhage in newborn, 223 f.
  K_1, in intracranial hemorrhage, 473
Vitiligo, 8
Vomiting, induction in poisoning, 356 f.

W

Walking, age of, 5

Water
  intoxication, and hyponatremia, 370, 376 f.
  therapy, parenteral, 482 f.
Waterhouse-Friedrichsen syndrome, 282, 291
Weakness
  acute, 93 f.
  flaccid, 94
  muscle biopsy in diagnosis, 120
  neurogenic, 93 f.
Weber test, 80
Wechsler Adult Intelligence Scale, 6
Wechsler Intelligence Scale for Children, 6
Wechsler Preschool and Primary Scale of Intelligence, 6
Werdnig-Hoffmann atrophy, 326 ff.
Wernicke's encephalopathy, 477
Wilms' tumor
  neurologic picture, 265
  radiation therapy in, 245
Wilson's disease, 391, 436 f.
Word blindness, developmental, 69 f.
Word deafness, developmental, 71 f., 79
Wound infections, 210, 213, 217
Wryneck, 346, 347

X

Xanthines, toxic reactions to, 373
Xanthochromia, cerebrospinal fluid, 113, 119
X-rays
  skull
    in brain tumors, 244, 246, 247, 259
    in congenital hydrocephalus, 137, 138
    determining ventricular enlargement, 489
    in diagnosis of increased pressure, 82
    in diagnosis of poisonings, 356
    in epidural and subdural hematoma, 201, 202, 206, 207
    in hemiparesis, 55
    in retardation, 9
    in tuberous sclerosis, 428 f.
    value in diagnosis, 107, 108 f.
  spine, interpretation, 112 f.